Kyoto Symposia

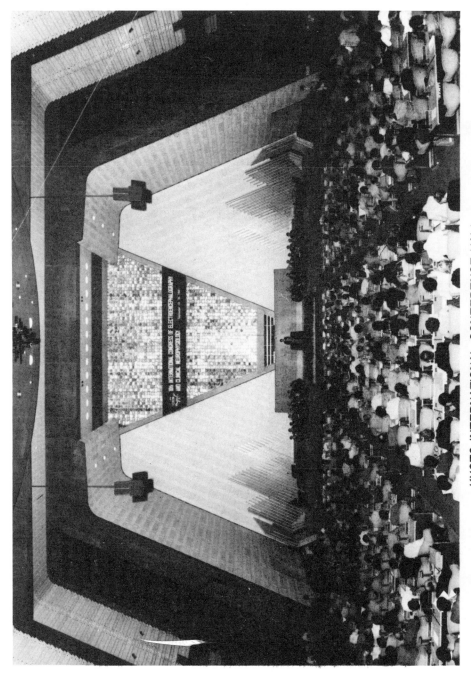

KYOTO INTERNATIONAL CONFERENCE HALL, SEPTEMBER 13-18, 1981

Kyoto Symposia

Being the invited contributions to Symposia and Workshops of the 10th International Congress of Electroencephalography and Clinical Neurophysiology held in Kyoto, Japan, September 13–18, 1981

EDITED BY

P.A. BUSER

Université Pierre et Marie Curie, Paris 75005 (France)

W.A. COBB

The National Hospital, Queen Square, London WC1N 3BG (England)

and

T. OKUMA

Tohoku University School of Medicine, Sendai 980 (Japan)

ELECTROENCEPHALOGRAPHY AND CLINICAL NEUROPHYSIOLOGY
SUPPLEMENT NO. 36
1982

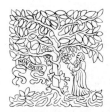

ELSEVIER BIOMEDICAL PRESS
AMSTERDAM · NEW YORK · OXFORD

Electroenceph. clin. Neurophysiol., 1982, Suppl. 36

ELSEVIER BIOMEDICAL PRESS
P.O. BOX 211, 1000 AE AMSTERDAM, THE NETHERLANDS

ELSEVIER/NORTH-HOLLAND, INC.
52 VANDERBILT AVENUE
NEW YORK, NEW YORK 10017
U.S.A

Library of Congress Cataloging in Publication Data

International Congress of Electroencephalography and
    Clinical Neurophysiology (10th : 1981 : Kyoto,
    Japan)
    Kyoto symposia.

    (Electroencephalography and clinical neurophysiology.
Supplement ; no. 36)

    1. Electroencephalography--Congresses. 2. Neuro-
physiology--Congresses. 3. Neuropharmacology--
Congresses. I. Buser, Pierre A., 1921-   .
II. Cobb, W. A. (William Albert) III. Okuma, Teruo,
1926-   . IV. Title. V. Series.
RC386.6.E43I55 1981   616.8   82-24237
ISBN 0-444-80436-6

Printed in The Netherlands.

PRESIDENTIAL ADDRESS

The President of an International Federation has duties to perform whose importance varies but, in every case, the responsibility is his own.

Among these duties, and not the least of them, is to organize, with the help of the governing bodies of the Federation which he presides over, the Congress which closes the fiscal period for which he has been responsible.

To organize a Congress is not easy, even if one has only the scientific responsibility and the choice of the country where it is to be held.

This time was of particular importance, because it concerned the Tenth Congress. To go from single to double figures, from one to ten, is in itself an event to which many of us attach a special importance. And, what is more, the means of investigation of the nervous system have considerably developed in the last few years and it was necessary to take stock concerning the durability of the importance of EEG and Clinical Neurophysiology in the diagnosis and treatment of illnesses which affect this system. Moreover, we must be aware that, in order to remain competitive, it is our duty not to ignore these new techniques but, on the contrary, to try to take advantage of them so as to increase our understanding of the many problems which remain unsolved.

Two notions must guide both the experimenter and the clinician:

(1) Any model is only a relative model, there is never identity between the model and reality; caution must prevail when faced with extrapolation from one model to another and, equally, from one species to another.

(2) Any new technique, no matter how sophisticated it may be, brings with it enthusiasm and disillusion; in spite of all the recent discoveries, electrophysiology is not dead and, if we know how to defend it, its best days are far from being behind us.

This Tenth Congress is thus of importance from the scientific point of view and it should bear a stamp which makes it a landmark in the constellation of stages which, every four years, reunite the younger generation with the older, those who never lose their youthful enthusiasm. Here today, I salute all of you.

The choice of these stages has almost always been made possible thanks to the influence of the Men and Societies who have built our Federation, and to whom we pay tribute. Until now, those who have left their mark on the history of our Federation came only from the western world and, with only one exception, were to be found in the countries bordering the North Atlantic and the Mediterranean. And the choice of city always adds a special something to which the participants are never indifferent. The aura of a town or region, through the Art of past civilisations which it offers to us, participants, is part of the necessary enrichment of our culture without which Science would have no value.

If few of you discovered London and Paris thanks to the Federation (it was in its infancy), many of us have discovered the New World thanks to the Congresses in Boston and San Diego, as others have been conquered by the splendours of the monuments and museums, and the richness and diversity of Europe's contribution to culture, thanks to the Congresses of Brussels, Rome, Amsterdam and Marseilles.

However, it should not be thought that all EEG and Clinical Neurophysiology could be found only in those countries where our Congresses were held! That would be proof of ignorance.

During this time, for example, in the Far East, in Japan, a Society of Electroencephalography and Electromyography was created and has developed into one of the most thriving in the world. This Society has known, much better than others, how to attract to each of its annual meetings, the most eminent specialists in a certain field of the Neurosciences, and each time the occasion has been transformed into an event. I had the good fortune to participate in one of these national meetings, at Kanazawa, and was very impressed by it.

Electroencephalography is not a recent Science in this country. In the nineteen thirties some studies were carried out on animals, in Japan itself, by Hasama (1934, 1935), Ito and Kaketa (1937) and Ito and Kitamura (1939); and in England, a Japanese, Yamagiwa, carried out a fundamental study with Adrian on "The origin of the Berger rhythm" (Adrian and Yamagiwa 1935).

In the 1940's, Motokawa, who in 1935, in Boston, was the first Japanese to participate in an international Congress, carried out with his colleagues a detailed investigation of a normal electroencephalogram in order to make clear its value. A mathematical and statistical analysis of the EEG was undertaken as well as a detailed survey of electroencephalographic distribution over the entire scalp (Motokawa 1942, 1943a, b, c, 1944a, b ; Motokawa and Mita 1942a, b ; Motokawa and Tuziguti 1943, 1944). The analysis of the EEG was, incidentally, continued through the 1950's by several researchers of whom some have played important roles in the initiation and organization of this Congress ... Imabori and Suhara (1947, 1949), Shimazono (1947), Sato and Nakane (1948), Sato (1950), Fujimori et al. (1958) and others.

Although, as early as 1942, one of the activities of the Japan Society for the Promotion of Science was the establishment of a research committee on electroencephalography headed by Katsunuma and Motokawa, data recording was usually done until 1951 by electromagnetic oscillograph. It is to Sakamoto and Takagi, from the Faculty of Engineering of the University of Tokyo, that the Japanese owe the knowledge necessary for the manufacturer of good multichannel inkwriters. This development allowed rapid and widespread dissemination of the clinical application of the EEG, and within a few years EEG apparatuses were established in a large majority of university hospitals, large general hospitals and hospitals dealing with psychiatric and neurological diseases.

The cooperative system of research by medical doctors, electroengineering researchers and manufacturers that was established then provided the opportunity for the development of medical electronics and resulted in the establishment of the Japan Society of Medical Electronics and Biological Engineering in 1962.

It was in 1952 that the first meeting of the Japan EEG Society was held in Tokyo, under President Shimizu. Following this first meeting, gatherings took place once a year in various parts of Japan. The Japan EEG Society consisted of researchers in basic medicine such as neurophysiology, in clinical medicine such as psychiatry, neurology, neurosurgery, pediatrics, etc..., and scientists who specialized in psychology and medical electronics. It was characteristic that those who specialized in the various fields had a common interest in electroencephalograms, electromyograms and functions of the nervous system and they had frequent scientific exchanges. A total of 217 papers were presented at the 20th meeting of this Society in 1971.

In 1959 Yoshii, with whom I had the good fortune to work in Marseilles, undertook to publish a monthly journal, "Clinical Electroencephalography", and this contributed to the exchange of knowledge of the EEG for researchers and doctors.

At the same time, in 1951, about 200 researchers participated in the first meeting on electromyography; this was organized primarily by the sorely missed Tokizane and by Tsuyama. Meetings were held twice a year for a time, but since 1955 it has been called "The Japan Society of EMG" and meetings are held annually. Scientists engaged in basic medical studies such as neurophysiology, and in clinical medicine, such as orthopaedics, neurology, neurosurgery, otorhinolaryngology, ophthalmology, etc... have participated in these meetings. The fundamental thrust of this Society has been the evolution of a neurophysiological basic theory and the development of the applied field following the line of its basic evolution. Japanese research on electromyograms has tended to focus particularly on the activity of spinal motoneurones and the functions of higher centres through the activities of the neuromuscular unit and other related subjects. Seventy papers were presented at the 24th meeting of this Society in 1971.

Annual meetings of the Japan EEG Society and the Japan EMG Society had been held jointly since 1958 and in 1971 the two societies were combined and the Japan Society of Electroencephalography and Electromyography was established. At the first meeting of the new joint group held that same year under President Tokizane, 270 papers were presented and about 1200 persons participated. Meetings have been held annually since then, with the number of papers and participants increasing each year.

A new constitution was drawn up in 1971 and Tokizane was nominated as the Society's first chairman, followed by Yoshii, the current chairman. Editorial, Analysis of EEG and EMG and Technicians committees are currently included. The "Japanese Journal of Electroencephalography and Electromyography" has been issued quarterly since 1972.

I hope to have shown you that the Japan Society of Electroencephalography and Electromyography well and truly exists, and is thriving. I think that you will realize this for yourselves in participating in the work of this Congress and that, like myself, you will consider that the Federation owed it to itself to come here to appreciate on the spot the quality of the work carried out in our field of research in this country.

To welcome our Federation, our Japanese colleagues have offered us Kyoto, which was one of their most prestigious capitals and remains one of their jewels, a city about which I will be careful not to say too much, others being more competent than I.

We can but thank them for having chosen such a town for this Tenth Congress. What a landmark for future years!

Before finishing this speech, which is also one of my duties as President, I would like, in the name of all of you, to thank the various personalities who have helped us in the realization of the scientific programme, all those who have agreed to participate and special thanks to our Japanese colleagues and, in particular, to Professors Shimazono, Ebe and Shimazu for all the practical organization necessary for this Congress.

I would like also personally to thank Dr. Yasuo Shimazono who was so very kind to instruct me regarding the history of Electroencephalography and Electromyography in Japan.

Robert Naquet

REFERENCES

Adrian, E.D. and Yamagiwa, K. The origin of the Berger rhythm. Brain, 1935, 58: 323–351.

Fujimori, B., Yokota, T., Ishibashi, Y. and Takei, T. Analysis of the electroencephalogram of children by histogram method. Electroenceph. clin. Neurophysiol., 1958, 10: 241–252.

Hasama, B. Über die elektrischen Begleiterscheinungen an der Riechsphäre bei der Geruchsempfindung. Pflügers Arch. ges. Physiol., 1934, 234: 748–755.

Hasama, B. Hirnrindenerregung durch Reizung des peripheren Geschmacksorgans im Aktionsstrombild. Pflügers Arch. ges. Physiol., 1935, 236: 36–43.

Imabori, K. and Suhara, K. On the statistical method of the brain wave study. Kagaku (Science), 1947, 17: 38–40 (in Japanese).

Imabori, K. and Suhara, K. On the statistical method in the brain wave study. Folia psychiat. neurol. jap., 1949, 3: 137–155.

Ito, G. und Kaketa, K. Zur Frage der Lokalisation des Grosshirnaktionsstromes. Tohoku J. exp. Med., 1937, 30: 546–560.

Ito, G. und Kitamura, K. Vergleichende Untersuchung über den Grosshirnaktionsstrom einiger Säugetiere (Untersuchung über den Grosshirnaktionsstrom II). Tohoku J. exp. Med., 1939, 37: 106–112.

Motokawa, K. Die Analyse der Perioden im normalen Elektrenkephalogramm des Menschen. Tohoku J. exp. Med., 1942, 42: 9–20.

Motokawa, K. Ein statistisches Gesetz über die Zellorientierung in der Grosshirnrinde des Menschen und seine physiologische Bedeutung. Tohoku J. exp. Med., 1943a, 45: 96–107.

Motokawa, K. Praktische Methoden der quantitativen Beschreibung des Elektrenkephalogramms. Tohoku J. exp. Med., 1943b, 45: 309–322.

Motokawa, K. Eine statistisch-mechanische Theorie über das Elektrenkephalogramm (Dipoltheorie der Nervenzellen in der Grosshirnrinde). Tohoku J. exp. Med., 1943c, 45: 278–296.

Motokawa, K. Die Verteilung der elektrischen Aktivität auf der Kopfschwarte und ihre Beziehung zur Cytoarchitektonik der Grosshirnrinde des Menschen. Jap. J. med. Sci., III, Biophysics, 1944a, 10: 99–111.

Motokawa, K. Die Verteilung der elektrischen Aktivität auf der Grosshirnrinde des normalen Menschen. Tohoku J. exp. Med., 1944b, 46: 382–395.

Motokawa, K. und Mita, T. Das Wahrscheinlichkeitsprinzip über die gehirnelektrischen Erscheinungen des Menschen. Jap. J. med. Sci., III, Biophysics, 1942a, 8: 63–77.

Motokawa, K. und Mita, T. Die statistische Analyse des Elektrenkephalogramms des Menschen. Jap. J. med. Sci., III, Biophysics, 1942b, 8: 79–91.

Motokawa, K. und Tuziguti, K. Über die Verteilung der α-Wellen auf der Grosshirnrinde des Menschen im optisch erregten Zustand. Jap. J. med. Sci., III, Biophysics, 1943, 9: 135–144.

Motokawa, K. und Tuziguti, K. Die Phasendifferenzen der α-Wellen und Lokalunterschiede der elektrischen Aktivität der Grosshirnrinde des Menschen. Jap. J. med. Sci., III, Biophysics, 1944, 10: 23–38.

Sato, K. On general probability function of square amplitude in electroencephalogram. Folia psychiat. neurol. jap., 1950, 3: 227–233.

Sato, K. and Nakane, K. Note on the general probability function of the alpha wave in electroencephalogram. Folia psychiat. neurol. jap., 1948, 2: 44–57.

Shimazono, Y. On the result of a method of analysis of the brain wave. Rep. Res. Comm. EEG (1947), 1947: 11–24 (in Japanese).

List of Contributors

Alvarado, R., 257
Arasaki, K., 336
Arimura, K., 682
Arissian, K., 415
Arrigo, A., 688
Asanuma, H., 415
Barker, J.L., 19
Barragán, L.A., 257
Binnie, C.D., 504
Bittencourt, P.R.M., 467
Bossi, L., 482
Brinkman, C., 375
Burke, D., 172
Caldecott-Hazard, S., 30
Calvo, J.M., 257
Cannon, J.T., 30
Coleman, R., 709
Condés-Lara, M., 257
Congdon, W.C., 487
Coons, S., 641
Cracco, J.B., 358
Cracco, R.Q., 358
Curzi-Dascalova, L., 631
Czeisler, C., 709
Delwaide, P.J., 179
Deniker, P., 516
Desmedt, J.E., 106
Dickins, S., 328
Ding, R., 129
DuCharme, L.L., 487
Dyck, P.J., 39, 81
Eisen, A., 349
Endo, M., 216
Etevenon, P., 516
Evarts, E.V., 147, 385
Fernández-Guardiola, A., 257
Fink, M., 447
Flores-Guevara, R., 631
Gauthier, G.M., 730
Ghez, C., 409
Gloor, P., 579

Goddard, G.V., 288
Guidasci, S., 631
Guiheneuc, P., 91
Guilleminault, C., 641, 709
Hashimoto, I., 305
Hassan, N.H., 169
Hiraga, H., 603
Hoirch, M., 349
Honda, Y., 524
Hugelin, A., 625
Hugon, M., 730
Humphrey, D.R., 393
Ichijo, S., 603
Iida, M., 671
Irwin, P., 447
Ito, M., 139
Ito, T., 566
Ives, J.R., 612
Jansen, J.K.S., 129
Jonec, V., 264
Jones, E.G., 367
Kadefors, R., 750
Kagono, Y., 524
Kakegawa, N., 437
Karnes, J., 39
Kelly, J.J., 81
Kimura, J., 328
Kita, S., 524
Knutsson, E., 161
Kogi, K., 738
Kubota, M., 566
Kudo, N., 336
Kugler, J., 549
Kuorinka, I., 733
Kurata, K., 378
Kuroiwa, Y., 111
Lee, R.G., 422
Le Gal La Salle, G., 239
Leung, L.S., 274
Levy, R.H., 487
Lewis, J.W., 30

Contents

Part 1. Multiple Receptor Functions in the Nervous System

Part 2. Molecular, Physiological and Morphologic Basis of Impaired Nerve Conduction

Part 3. Neuroplasticity and Functional Compensation

Part 4. Electrophysiological Evaluation of Muscle Relaxants

Part 5. Kindling – Pharmacology and Physiology

Part 6. Brain Stem Evoked Potentials: Clinical Uses

Part 7. Functional Organization of Motor Areas in Primates and Patients with Movement Disorders

Part 8. Blood Levels of Drugs and the EEG

Part 9. Effects of Psychotropic Drugs on EEG

Part 10. Data Reduction in Intensive Care and Long-term Surveillance of Patients

Part 11. EEG Polygraphy in Respiratory Disorders and other Risk Conditions in Infancy

Part 12. Human Factors and Hazards in Industrial Work: EEG and EMG Contributions

1. Multiple Receptor Functions in the Nervous System

Kyoto Symposia (EEG Suppl. No. 36)
Editors: P.A. Buser, W.A. Cobb and T. Okuma
© 1982, Elsevier Biomedical Press, Amsterdam

Amino Acid Effects on Vertebrate Spinal Neurones in Vitro and in Vivo

A. NISTRI

Department of Pharmacology, St. Bartholomew's Hospital Medical College, University of London, Charterhouse Square, London EC 1M 6BQ (England)

In the late 50s and early 60s it was shown that a number of amino acids (physiologically present in the nervous tissue) potently changed the excitability of cat spinal motoneurones and interneurones (Curtis et al. 1959, 1960). The amino acid effects could broadly be divided into two major groups: (a) excitation due to membrane depolarization leading to repetitive neuronal firing (this was typically produced by dicarboxylic amino acids and in particular by the endogenous compound L-glutamate); (b) inhibition mainly due to membrane hyperpolarization and usually associated with a significant loss of resting resistance so that neuronal excitability (and hence the spike generating mechanisms) was depressed. Such an inhibitory action was evoked by many neutral amino acids which included γ-aminobutyric acid (GABA) and glycine, both found in the spinal cord tissue. Although the early studies on amino acids cast some doubts on their possible role as physiological transmitter of excitation and inhibition, in the last decade a more positive assessment of their neurotransmitter function has been made (cf. reviews by Curtis and Johnston 1974; Krnjević 1974; Nistri and Constanti 1979). In the present report I shall focus my attention on data concerning the cellular mechanism of action of glutamate and GABA on spinal neurones, with particular emphasis on some new effects which have only recently become apparent. It will emerge that both glutamate and GABA can induce multiple actions, each one contributing to the overall neuronal response (excitation or inhibition).

ACTIONS OF GLUTAMATE ON SPINAL NEURONES

The simplest method to investigate the action of this amino acid is to apply it to a central neurone via a current pulse through an extracellular microelectrode filled with a strong water solution of glutamate. This technique is termed iontophoresis and the most frequently studied neuronal response to such an application is the change in firing rate of interneurones. Fig. 1 shows representative excitatory responses (i.e. increased firing rates) of cat interneurones elicited by iontophoretic applications of glutamate and several chemically related analogues. A distinctive feature of these records is the variability in the onset and offset rates of the responses: for example, the slow onset of ibotenate or N-methyl-D-aspartate

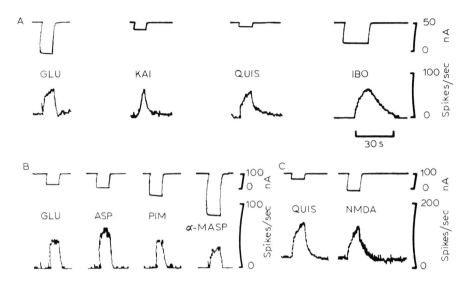

Fig. 1. Excitation of spinal interneurones by iontophoretically applied amino acids. A: top trace, iontophoretic currents (nA) used to eject amino acids; bottom trace, chart recordings of firing frequency (spikes/sec). Abbreviations: GLU, glutamate; QUIS, quisqualate; KAI, kainate; IBO, ibotenate. Same neurone for the 4 responses. B: as in A; abbreviations: ASP, aspartate; PIM, α-aminopimelate; α-MASP, α-methyl-aspartate. Different neurone from A. C: as A and B; abbreviation: NMDA, N-methyl-D-aspartate, different neurone from A and B. The time calibration (horizontal bar) applies to all responses. (Reproduced with permission from MacDonald and Nistri 1978.)

responses contrasts with the rapid onset of those to glutamate and aspartate. Several factors are probably involved in these phenomena: effective release of the compound from the iontophoretic pipette, distribution of the compound in the extracellular compartment, location of neuronal receptors and active removal of the substance by carrier-mediated transport.

The iontophoretic method coupled to extracellular recording is useful in order to obtain some quantitative data on amino acid actions. For instance, one can determine the apparent excitatory potency of a number of glutamate analogues synthesized through subtle changes in the chemical structure of the parent compound. Through a systematic analysis of many such drugs, this type of study represents a valuable approach to our understanding of the active groups of the glutamate molecule that can bind to the neuronal membrane receptor. Fig. 2 depicts some log-dose/response plots for glutamate and some related analogues: it is quite clear how, for example, quisqualate (a neuroexcitatory drug extracted from the seeds of *Quisqualis indica*) is a much more active compound than glutamate itself. Nevertheless, the usefulness of this technique stops here since one cannot directly examine any change in neuronal membrane potential or resistance: this drawback means that it is not possible to establish the cellular mode of action of a given compound at the level of the postsynaptic membrane. Furthermore, a very accurate analysis of amino acid-receptor interactions is prevented by the use of firing rates as the measure of receptor activation since, in a number of cases, there is a non-linear

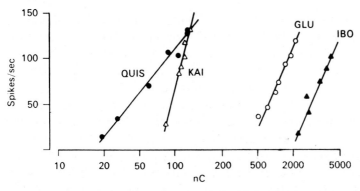

Fig. 2. 'Dose'-response relationships for the excitatory effects of glutamate (GLU), quisqualate (QUIS), kainate (KAI) and ibotenate (IBO) on a spinal interneurone. Abscissa: total applied charge (nC; log scale); ordinate: firing frequency (spikes/sec; linear scale). All the responses were obtained from the same neurone. Note that when all the results from different experiments were pooled and analysed statistically (Mann-Whitney U test), the slope values for kainate were found to be significantly different ($P < 0.008$) from those for glutamate. Quisqualate or ibotenate slope values did not differ from those for glutamate ($P < 0.12$ and < 0.15, respectively). (Reproduced with permission from MacDonald and Nistri 1978.)

relation between receptor occupancy and firing rates (see discussion in Nistri and Constanti 1979). In an attempt to overcome, at least in part, these problems, we have been using an in vitro slice preparation of the frog spinal cord (Constanti and Nistri 1976) initially described by Curtis et al. (1961). The advantages of this experimental preparation are many: no interference by anaesthetic agents with drug effects, controlled ionic composition of the incubating media, blockade of the amino acid active transport by low temperature or pharmacological agents. Furthermore, one can record from ventral roots and thus monitor the electrical activity of motoneurones. If such recordings are D.C. coupled, it is possible to evaluate the drug-evoked changes in membrane potential of the motoneuronal population. Similar recording from dorsal roots yields information on the synaptic and receptor mechanisms associated with presynaptic inhibition. Therefore, it has been possible to quantitate the potency of glutamate on frog motoneurones with an apparent dissociation constant of 300 μM (Nistri 1981a). The effect of glutamate consists of a neuronal depolarization dependent on the concentration of extracellular Na$^+$ but only intracellular recording with glass microelectrodes has revealed in a more direct fashion that such a depolarization is seemingly due to an increased membrane permeability to Na$^+$ and K$^+$ (Sonnhof and Bührle 1980). A more recent improvement of the technique for intracellular recording from frog motoneurones has been based on a very fast superfusion of the spinal slice preparation kept at low temperatures to minimize glutamate uptake (Arenson and Nistri 1981). Work currently in progress in our laboratory and based on this method indicates that glutamate (0.7–1 mM) and its more powerful synthetic analogue D,L-homocysteate (0.1–1 mM) can evoke complex responses from motoneurones. Quite often the earliest manifestation of the amino acid action (seen within 3–9 sec from the beginning of superfusion) is an enhancement of the so-called spike afterdepolarization, which is a late component of the antidromic spike (Arenson and Nistri 1982a). Although the precise mechanism generating the afterdepolarization has not yet been established, there is reason to believe it a dendritic invasion by the spike originated at the axon hillock (Schwindt 1976). Since in our experiments glutamate selectively affected this afterpotential, one is tempted to suggest that the primary site of action of this amino acid is at the level of dendrites. This early change in the afterdepolarization was not accompanied by significant changes in membrane potential or resistance. Shortly afterward, the more conventional action of glutamate (i.e. depolarization of the neuronal membrane) develops, although the associated resistance drop is unexpectedly rather small (about -20% on average) as also noted by Shapovalov et al. (1978). Several explanations may be offered for this small change in resistance. (a) The depolarization is caused by an electrogenic carrier-mediated Co-transport of glutamate and Na^+ (with more Na ions than glutamate molecules concentrated inside the cell) so that there is a net transfer of positive charges to the cell interior without the drastic decrease in membrane resistance which would be caused by the opening of many ionic channels activated by specific glutamate receptors. This is a possible phenomenon in vivo (and in vitro at room temperature) although in our experimental conditions the active transport of the amino acid was largely blocked. (b) The depolarization is chiefly generated at remote dendritic sites and any substantial resistance fall is not detected by the intracellular electrode located in the somatic region of the motoneurone. Our data on the afterdepolarization are consistent with this view, although other authors have reported that motoneuronal cell bodies are rather sensitive to glutamate (cf. Sonnhof et al. 1978). (c) The depolarization is generated by two opposite mechanisms: increase in Na^+ permeability and decrease in K^+ permeability so that the overall change in membrane resistance is small. Recent experiments (A. Nistri and M.S. Arenson, unpublished) with K^+ channel blockers (such as Cs^+) lend support to a K^+ channel blockade by glutamate since the depolarizing action of the amino acid is depressed by such a treatment. It is worth noting that a similar explanation has been proposed for the action of glutamate on cat motoneurones in vivo (Engberg et al. 1979).

Two further components of the glutamate-evoked response of frog motoneurones may also be detected (A. Nistri and M.S. Arenson, unpublished).

(a) A membrane hyperpolarization with a large resistance decrease frequently preceding the more conventional depolarization. Such a hyperpolarization, strongly reminiscent of a similar phenomenon noted in mammalian olfactory cortex neurones (Constanti et al. 1980a), is apparently different from other recently reported glutamate hyperpolarizations of brain neurones in vitro. The latter responses are thought to be due to increased K^+ permeability (Nicoll and Alger 1981; Wojtowicz et al. 1981) and display a long latency following (rather than preceding) the depolarization. Also our preliminary experiments with K^+ channel blockers are not consistent with a mechanism mainly based on a K^+ permeability increase to account for the glutamate hyperpolarizations in the frog spinal cord.

(b) A membrane resistance increase during the recovery phase following glutamate washout. This effect persists for a few minutes after the depolarization

TABLE I

EFFECTS OF GLUTAMATE ON SPINAL MOTONEURONES

Membrane potential change	Resistance change	Ionic mechanisms	Mode of action
Depolarization	Small (or no) decrease	$\uparrow gNa^+$; $\downarrow gK^+$ (or $\uparrow gK^+$)	Activation of glutamate receptors
Depolarization	No change	Electrogenic Na-glutamate transport	Binding to uptake sites
Hyperpolarization	Noticeable decrease	$\uparrow g\,Cl^-$ (?)	Not fully established
No change but spike after-depolarization $\uparrow$	No change	Unknown	Action on dendrites
Slight hyper-polarization or no change	Increase	Unknown	Unclear; the effect may be seen on washout

g = conductance.

has declined (cf. also Constanti et al. 1980a). Although a clear explanation of this event is at present lacking, it obviously increases the long-term excitability of motoneurones. Table I summarizes the different effects following glutamate application to spinal motoneurones.

Other features of the glutamate action deserve some comments: it seems that spinal interneurones are more sensitive to glutamate than motoneurones (Arenson and Nistri 1982b). This especially holds true for membrane resistance changes rather than amplitude of depolarizations; moreover, the application of glutamate to interneurones often results in sustained repetitive firing whereas the same application seldom evokes multiple action potentials from motoneurones. These contrasts between the two cell populations might indicate that the ionic mechanisms triggered by glutamate at membrane level differ between interneurones and motoneurones and, more significantly, that this amino acid can produce two different types of excitation: a fast one with prolonged action potential discharges from interneurones and a slower one (complicated by other responses as well) typically seen in motoneurones where the cells are reset to a state of more persistent depolarization (with small changes in resistance) that could conceivably amplify any incoming excitatory synaptic signal.

ACTIONS OF GABA ON SPINAL NEURONES

The neurochemical (and other) evidence favouring a transmitter function of GABA in the spinal cord has recently been reviewed in detail (Nistri 1983). It is now generally accepted that GABA is responsible for the mechanism of presynaptic inhibition; it is not unlikely, however, that GABA also plays an inhibitory transmitter role on spinal interneurones, and even motoneurones, alongside glycine (not discussed in the present paper), which appears to be a major inhibitory substance in mammals.

Focussing our attention on the effects of GABA on the cell bodies of spinal neurones, one notes that the predominant action of this amino acid is to reduce neuronal excitability. This is most convincingly demonstrated with intracellular recording from mammalian motoneurones *in vivo* (Krnjević et al. 1977) which rapidly lose (or largely impair) their ability to generate action potentials. A very characteristic finding is, however, a progressive diminution of the GABA effect ("fading") in spite of maintained application of this amino acid. This phenomenon is, by the way, quite commonly seen also in many other neurones of the brain and spinal cord (cf. Nistri and Constanti 1979) and greatly limits the duration of any GABA-evoked inhibition and thus the effectiveness of any attempted "long-term" exposure of neuronal receptors to GABA (no comparable fading of glutamate-induced excitation has been noted in the central nervous system). Krnjević and his associates (1977) also described the large fall in membrane resistance accompanying the fairly small and variable changes in membrane potential produced by GABA. Needless to say the changes in membrane potential and resistance quickly faded (within a few seconds) following sustained application of the amino acid. Krnjević (1976) pointed out that the majority of GABA actions on central neurones seem to be due to an increased membrane permeability to Cl^-. Cat motoneurones appear to be accommodated within this theory since the amplitude and polarity of their responses to GABA will chiefly depend on the cell membrane potential value with respect to the Cl^- equilibrium potential. If Cl^- moves in following the interaction of GABA with specific membrane receptors and opening of ionic channels, membrane hyperpolarization ensues; on the contrary, if Cl^- leaves the cell, depolarization will be produced. This view seems also to hold for frog motoneurones in vitro (Nistri and Morelli 1978).

How can the fading phenomenon be explained? The two simplest possibilities are: (a) receptor desensitization (analogue to the phenomenon occurring at the skeletal neuromuscular junction after sustained or closely spaced applications of acetylcholine); (b) active removal of GABA via an electrogenic Na^+-dependent transport system (Krnjević et al. 1977). If the latter explanation is correct (and there is a strong a priori argument to support it, especially for in vivo neurones), one should find some evidence for intracellular accumulation of Na^+ (as indeed has been the case; cf. Krnjević et al. 1977) and, more importantly, one should be able to produce GABA and Na^+ *extrusion* if GABA is injected into the cytoplasm of motoneurones. The electrical equivalent of Na^+ leaving the cell is, of course, a membrane hyperpolarization. This point has been demonstrated experimentally (Constanti et al. 1980b) through intracellular injections of GABA in cat motoneurones in vivo. Hence, in addition to the well known increase in Cl^- permeability, GABA appears to produce membrane depolarization or hyperpolarization, depending on whether it is taken up or pumped out by the motoneurone.

In summary then, there is convincing evidence to link the fading of GABA response to GABA uptake. Nevertheless, one still wonders how important receptor desensitization might be for the observed phenomenon. It is quite possible that the fading is concomitantly produced by GABA uptake and desensitization: this view is certainly supported by our recent experiments (A. Nistri and M.S. Arenson, unpublished) on frog motoneurones in vitro. When GABA uptake was minimized by a low incubating temperature (7°C), rapidly superfused GABA (1–3 mM) still produced fading responses. Moreover, muscimol (0.1 mM), a GABA analogue with little affinity for the GABA transport system, also elicited responses which faded away. If, as seems to be the case, GABA receptor desensitization really exists, one is still left with the unfinished task of explaining the molecular mechanisms of desensitization: much experimental work on this matter is eagerly needed.

The last topic I wish to examine here is the action of GABA on axons and their terminals. While no specific effect of GABA on the somatic spike configuration of spinal neurones can be detected, there is evidence that the amino acid can modulate some voltage-sensitive conductances in cultured ganglion neurones (Dunlap and Fischbach 1981). This action manifests itself as a decrease in the spike duration (i.e. enhanced repolarization) which has been suggested as due to blockade (by GABA) of an inward Ca^{2+} conductance. Shortening of the spike in the presence of GABA has also been noted with intracellular recording from motor axons (A. Nistri and M.S. Arenson, unpublished) although there is little support for a distinct Ca^{2+} conductance contributing significantly to the normal axon spike. Whatever the explanation for the GABA-evoked spike shortening may be, it is clear that such an event, if also present at (or near) the nerve terminals, may significantly reduce Ca^{2+}-dependent release of excitatory endogenous transmitters and lead to presynaptic inhibition. An alternative account of presynaptic inhibition and its relation to GABA is based on the GABA-induced depolarization of the nerve terminal membrane. Such a depolarization would reduce the amplitude of the incoming spike which would then liberate smaller amounts of transmitter. Although not devoid of uncertainties (cf. Krnjević 1979; Nistri 1983), this hypothesis is currently considered as the most plausible mechanism linking the action of GABA on nerve terminals with presynaptic inhibition.

What is the basis for this GABA-induced depolarization? The conventional answer (though only indirectly provided by recording from dorsal root ganglia) is efflux of Cl^- elicited by GABA receptor activation (Nishi et al. 1974). Nevertheless, it was first noted that Na^+ was also necessary to observe such a depolarization (Barker and Nicoll 1973): in spite of some resistance to accepting this finding, its validity has repeatedly been confirmed (Nistri and Corradetti 1978; Nicoll and Alger 1979). The early interpretation of the Na^+ dependence data postulated that GABA opened up Na^+ channels, thereby causing membrane depolarization. However, an alternative explanation suggests a GABA receptor modulation by Na^+ so that, in the absence of this ionic species, the amino acid affinity for its receptor is strongly reduced (although never abolished) (Nistri 1981b). This last interpretation is based only on indirect evidence collected from experiments on crustacean muscle where

TABLE II

EFFECTS OF GABA ON SPINAL NEURONES

On motoneurones		
(1)	Hyperpolarization or	$(Cl^-$ influx when $E_{Cl} > E_m)$
	depolarization	$(Cl^-$ efflux when $E_{Cl} < E_m)$
(2)	Depolarization or	$(Na^+$ uptake)
	hyperpolarization	$(Na^+$ extrusion)
On primary afferent fibres		
(1)	Depolarization	$(Cl^-$ efflux; $E_{Cl} < E_m)$; receptor might be modulated by Na^+
(2)	No change in membrane potential but shortening of spike duration	$(\downarrow g\ Ca^{2+})$

E_{Cl} = equilibrium potential for Cl^- (at this level no transfer of Cl^- occurs); E_m = membrane potential.

GABA clearly activates a Cl^- permeability increase. Here the action of GABA (and, in particular, that of some of its analogues) is reduced in Na^+-free media (Constanti and Nistri 1981). Also data on GABA receptor binding have recently lent further support to this view since Na^+ could powerfully modulate the binding of radiolabelled GABA to a rat brain membrane preparation (Kurioka et al. 1981).

To sum up then, it is by now evident that GABA possesses multiple actions (listed in Table II) on vertebrate spinal neurones. Some of these actions can produce postsynaptic inhibitory responses, such as decreased excitability, through stimulation of Cl^- permeability. The latter effect is, however, limited by the "fading" phenomenon and may be complicated by electrogenic uptake of GABA. Other GABA actions seem to be important to understand presynaptic inhibitory processes: in this context, GABA seems to regulate the configuration of the axonal action potential and to depolarize nerve terminals through Na^+-modulated receptors which open up Cl^- channels.

CONCLUSIONS

The large array of actions of amino acids on spinal neurones may appear bewildering but it certainly suggests a rather "economical" way of communicating many different signals with only a few transmitter substances acting via a considerable variety of neuronal mechanisms. Implicit in this idea is the concept that, in some circumstances, the main effect of a neurotransmitter may be self-limited by the concomitant activation of opposite responses; this process thus makes unnecessary or even implausible the simultaneous use of many different transmitters. In other words, specialization needed to transfer information might be efficiently achieved at the level of the postsynaptic membrane rather than through the presynaptic release of many substances.

REFERENCES

Arenson, M.S. and Nistri, A. Intracellular recordings from frog motoneurones superfused in vitro. J. Physiol. (Lond.), 1981, 319: 24P.

Arenson, M.S. and Nistri, A. The initial effect of glutamate on frog motoneurones consists in a selective change in the spike late afterdepolarization. J. Physiol. (Lond.), 1982a, 325: 26P–27P.

Arenson, M.S. and Nistri, A. Intracellular recordings reveal different sensitivity of frog spinal neurones to bath-applied glutamate and GABA. J. Physiol. (Lond.), 1982b, 326: 49P–50P.

Barker, J.L. and Nicoll, R.A. The pharmacology and ionic dependency of amino acid responses in the frog spinal cord. J. Physiol. (Lond.), 1973, 228: 259–277.

Constanti, A. and Nistri, A. A comparative study of the action of γ-aminobutyric acid and piperazine on the lobster muscle fibre and the frog spinal cord. Brit. J. Pharmacol., 1976, 57: 347–358.

Constanti, A. and Nistri, A. Differential effects of sodium-free media on γ-aminobutyrate and muscimol-evoked conductance increases recorded from lobster muscle fibres. Neuroscience, 1981, 6: 1443–1453.

Constanti, A., Connor, J.D., Galvan, M. and Nistri, A. Intracellularly-recorded effects of glutamate and aspartate on neurones in the guinea-pig olfactory cortex slice. Brain Res., 1980a, 195: 403–420.

Constanti, A., Krnjević, K. and Nistri, A. Intraneuronal effects of inhibitory amino acids. Canad. J. Physiol. Pharmacol., 1980b, 58: 193–204.

Curtis, D.R. and Johnston, G.A.R. Amino acid transmitters in the mammalian central nervous system. Ergebn. Physiol., 1974, 69: 97–188.

Curtis, D.R., Phillis, J.W. and Watkins, J.C. The depression of spinal neurones by γ-amino-n-butyric acid and β-alanine. J. Physiol. (Lond.), 1959, 146: 185–203.

Curtis, D.R., Phillis, J.W. and Watkins, J.C. The chemical excitation of spinal neurones by certain acidic amino acids. J. Physiol. (Lond.), 1960, 150: 656–682.

Curtis, D.R., Phillis, J.W. and Watkins, J.C. Actions of amino-acids on the isolated hemisected spinal cord of the toad. Brit. J. Pharmacol., 1961, 16: 262–283.

Dunlap, K. and Fischbach, G.D. Neurotransmitters decrease the calcium conductance activated by depolarization of embryonic chick sensory neurones. J. Physiol. (Lond.), 1981, 317: 519–535.

Engberg, I., Flatman, J.A. and Lambert, J.D.C. The actions of excitatory amino acids on motoneurones in the feline spinal cord. J. Physiol. (Lond.), 1979, 288: 227–261.

Krnjević, K. Chemical nature of synaptic transmission in vertebrates. Physiol. Rev., 1974, 54: 418–540.

Krnjević, K. Inhibitory action of GABA and GABA-mimetics on vertebrate neurons. In: E. Roberts, T.N. Chase and D.B. Tower (Eds.), GABA in Nervous System Function. Raven Press, New York, 1976: 269–281.

Krnjević, K. Pre- and post-synaptic inhibition. Adv. exp. med. Biol., 1979, 123: 272–286.

Krnjević, K., Puil, E. and Werman, R. GABA and glycine actions on spinal motoneurons. Canad. J. Physiol. Pharmacol., 1977, 55: 658–669.

Kurioka, S., Kimura, Y. and Matsuda, M. Effects of sodium and bicarbonate ions on γ-aminobutyric acid receptor binding in synaptic membranes of rat brain. J. Neurochem., 1981, 37: 418–421.

MacDonald, J.F. and Nistri, A. A comparison of the action of glutamate, ibotenate and other related amino acids on feline spinal interneurones. J. Physiol. (Lond.), 1978, 275: 449–465.

Nicoll, R.A. and Alger, B.E. Presynaptic inhibition: transmitter and ionic mechanisms. Int. Rev. Neurobiol. 1979, 21: 217–258.

Nicoll, R.A. and Alger, B.E. Synaptic excitation may activate a calcium-dependent potassium conductance in hippocampal pyramidal cells. Science, 1981, 212: 957–959.

Nishi, S., Minota, S. and Karczmar, A.G. Primary afferent neurones: the ionic mechanism of GABA-mediated depolarization. Neuropharmacology, 1974, 13: 215–219.

Nistri, A. Excitatory and inhibitory actions of ibotenic acid on frog spinal motoneurones in vitro. Brain Res., 1981a, 208: 397–408.

Nistri, A. New insights into the mechanism of action of inhibitory amino acids on frog spinal neurones. Adv. Biochem. Psychopharmacol., 1981b, 29: 263–269.

Nistri, A. Spinal cord pharmacology of GABA and chemically related amino acids. In: R.A. Davidoff (Ed.), Spinal Cord Pharmacology. Dekker, New York, 1983, 3: 45–104.

Nistri, A. and Constanti, A. Pharmacological characterization of different types of GABA and glutamate receptors in vertebrates and invertebrates. Progr. Neurobiol., 1979, 13: 117–235.

Nistri, A. and Corradetti, R. A comparison of the effects of GABA, 3-aminopropanesulphonic acid and imidazoleacetic acid on the frog spinal cord. Neuropharmacology, 1978, 17: 13–19.

Nistri, A. and Morelli, P. Effects of proline and other neutral amino acids on ventral root potentials of the frog spinal cord in vitro. Neuropharmacology, 1978, 17: 21–27.

Schwindt, P.C. Electrophysiological properties of spinal motoneurons. In: R. Llinás and W. Precht (Eds.), Neurobiology of the Frog. Springer, Berlin, 1976: 728–749.

Shapovalov, A.I., Shiriaev, B.I. and Velumian, A.A. Mechanisms of post-synaptic excitation in amphibian motoneurones. J. Physiol. (Lond.), 1978, 279: 437–455.

Sonnhof, V. and Bührle, Ch.Ph. On the postsynaptic action of glutamate in frog spinal motoneurons. Pflügers Arch. ges. Physiol., 1980, 388: 101–109.

Sonnhof, V., Grafe, P., Richter, D.W., Parekh, N., Krummikl, G. and Linder, M. Investigations of the effects of glutamate on motoneurons of the isolated frog spinal cord. In: R.W. Ryall and J.S. Kelly (Eds.), Iontophoresis and Transmitter Mechanisms in the Mammalian Central Nervous System. Elsevier, Amsterdam, 1978: 194–196.

Wojtowicz, J.M., Gysen, M. and MacDonald, J.F. Multiple reversal potentials for responses to L-glutamic acid. Brain Res., 1981, 213: 195–200.

Kyoto Symposia (EEG Suppl. No. 36)
Editors: P.A. Buser, W.A. Cobb and T. Okuma
© 1982, Elsevier Biomedical Press, Amsterdam

Multiple Receptor Functions in the Mammalian Brain as Studied in Vitro with Thin Brain Slices

C. YAMAMOTO

Department of Physiology, Faculty of Medicine, Kanazawa University, Kanazawa 920 (Japan)

Our understanding of the receptor functions in the nervous system has mostly been derived from the neuromuscular junction and sympathetic ganglia. This is partly because these tissues maintain their activities even if isolated in artificial media and can be used to study their receptor functions in vitro under more controlled conditions than in intact animals. In view of the usefulness of isolated preparations, I thought that if small pieces of the mammalian brain could maintain their functional activities in vitro, these preparations might be used to elucidate receptor functions in the brain and provide information which cannot be obtained in vivo. I have attempted, therefore, to develop techniques to prepare and maintain slices of the mammalian brain in which neuronal activities are preserved. In my presentation, I shall show that brain slices kept in artificial media exhibit electrical activities essentially identical with those observed in vivo, and then show some of our recent findings on receptor functions of central neurones revealed by our techniques.

ELECTRICAL ACTIVITIES RECORDED FROM BRAIN SLICES

When the guinea pig hippocampus is cut vertical to its long axis and transverse sections of about 0.4 mm thickness are prepared, the pyramidal cell layers in field CA1 to CA3 are clearly identified under a dissection microscope. In addition, the granular layer in the dentate gyrus is also well visualized. In our previous experiments (Yamamoto 1972) a stimulating electrode was inserted into the granular layer and potentials were recorded from region CA3. With recording electrodes of large tip diameter, mainly negative field potentials were recorded in response to granular layer stimulation. These negative waves reflected EPSPs and spikes generated in CA3 neurones. Since the field potentials disappeared after interruption between the site of stimulation and site of recording, the possibility may be ruled out that stimulating current spread to the recording site and directly activated neurones therein.

With electrodes of smaller tip diameter, intracellular potentials were easily recorded. A single shock to the granular layer in the dentate gyrus elicited EPSPs in CA3 neurones. When the EPSPs were large enough, action potentials of more than 60 mV were triggered. The EPSP was followed by a long IPSP. A second shock given to the granular layer elicited a markedly potentiated EPSP (Yamamoto et al. 1980).

Generation of these synaptic potentials is understood as follows. Axons of granule cells make synaptic contact with proximal dendrites of pyramidal cells. Activation of these axons, therefore, induces EPSPs monosynaptically in CA3 neurones. Action potentials triggered by the EPSPs conduct through axon collaterals of pyramidal cells and activate basket cells which in turn induce IPSPs in the impaled pyramidal cells. Thus, the synaptic machinery known in vivo works in thin hippocampal slices as well (Eccles 1964).

Electrical activities have also been recorded from slices prepared from other parts of the brain. For example, cell bodies of Purkinje cells are visualized with the aid of a microscope in thin slices of the cerebellum (Yamamoto 1975). With microelectrodes brought close to the cell bodies we can easily show that Purkinje cells regularly generate spontaneous discharges as in vivo, and white matter stimulation induces climbing fibre responses which are composed of bursts of action potentials.

ACTIONS OF NEUROTENSIN AND OPIOID PEPTIDE ON THE BED NUCLEUS OF THE STRIA TERMINALIS

One advantage of in vitro experiments is that one can administer chemicals reproducibly at known concentrations. This is especially important to examine actions of agents such as peptides which are effective at very low concentrations.

Nerve fibres from the amygdala pass through the stria terminalis and terminate in the bed nucleus of the stria terminalis. The latter sends fibres to the hypothalamus. Thus, the bed nucleus of the stria terminalis is the relay station between the amygdala and hypothalamus (Krettek and Price 1978). This nucleus has been found to receive nerve fibres containing neurotensin and enkephalin from the amygdala through the stria terminalis (Uhl et al. 1978; Uhl and Snyder 1979). If these peptides are transmitters, they are expected to have potent excitatory or inhibitory actions on neurones in the bed nucleus. To examine the actions of these peptides in vitro we prepared thin sections of the bed nucleus with incoming stria terminalis and incubated them in an artificial medium. A stimulating electrode was applied to the stria terminalis and potential activities were recorded from the bed nucleus. Single shocks to the stria terminalis elicited mainly negative field potentials in the bed nucleus with a latency of about 10 msec. Single cell discharges were often superimposed on the field potentials. Many cells also discharged spontaneously. The addition of neurotensin to the medium at as low a concentration as 10 μM caused marked increase in the number of evoked spikes and in spontaneous discharge frequency within 2 min of addition. The action of neurotensin was reversible (Sawada and Yamamoto 1980).

In our experiments, we can see clearly whether the action of neurotensin is due to increased release of excitatory transmitter from presynaptic terminals or due to direct excitatory effect on the postsynaptic neurones. This is another advantage of in vitro experiments. Namely, the action of neurotensin was not blocked in the medium containing Ca ions at low concentration and Mg ions at high concentration, whereas synaptic transmission was completely blocked. Therefore, we can conclude that neurotensin directly excites postsynaptic neurones in the bed nucleus.

An analogue of enkephalin, [D-Ala^2]-Met-enkephalinamide (EKA) was also effective at relatively low concentrations (Sawada and Yamamoto 1981). At 0.1 μM, EKA slightly suppressed the field potential elicited in the bed nucleus by stria terminalis stimulation. At 1 μM, the potential was suppressed to about half the control. Since the action of EKA was blocked by naloxone, the opioid peptide seems to affect specific receptors. EKA seems to affect directly the postsynaptic sites because firing induced by perfusion with a glutamate-containing medium was suppressed under the action of EKA.

In view of this postsynaptic action of the opioid peptide, a question naturally arises whether enkephalin actually mediates synaptic inhibition or not. As mentioned before, neurones in the bed nucleus fire with a latency of about 10 msec after stria terminalis stimulation. This excitation is followed by an inhibition lasting for about 100 msec. When naloxone, a specific blocker of opiate, was added to the medium at 1 μM, the inhibition decreased in magnitude and duration in 4 of the 11 neurones examined. This suggests that enkephalin is a transmitter mediating inhibition from the amygdala to the bed nucleus.

Summarizing our studies on the actions of peptides in the bed nucleus, we think that enkephalin-containing fibres mediate inhibitory outflow from the amygdala to the bed nucleus and neurotensin-containing fibres mediate excitatory influence.

GLUTAMATE RECEPTORS ON DENDRITES

A third advantage of the in vitro experiments is that the chemicals to be examined can be administered to the intended sites through micropipettes under direct visual control. We examined the sensitivity of dendrites of Purkinje cells to glutamic acid (Chujo et al. 1975). For this purpose, thin slices of the cerebellum were prepared and action potentials were recorded from cell bodies of Purkinje cells as mentioned previously. Then glutamate was administered electrophoretically to cell bodies or to the molecular layer. Administration of glutamate to cell bodies caused a moderate increase in spontaneous firing rate. Glutamate administered to some points in the molecular layer, however, induced much higher excitation in Purkinje cells. The sites sensitive to glutamate in the molecular layer extended over about 250 μm in the transverse direction and over about 300 μm from the inner portion of the molecular layer towards the pial surface. This extension of glutamate-sensitive sites almost coincided with the spread of Purkinje cell dendrites. These results indicate that glutamate sensitivity extends all over the surface of Purkinje cell dendrites, and lend support to the hypothesis that glutamate is the transmitter released from parallel fibres in the cerebellum (Young et al. 1974).

Recently, we have made more precise studies on dendritic glutamate sensitivity in

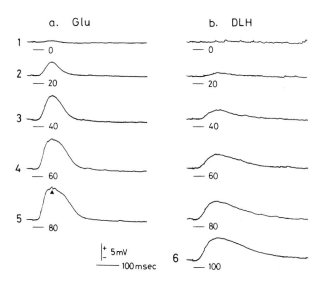

Fig. 1. Depolarizations induced by brief electrophoretic current pulses for L-glutamate (Glu) and DL-homocysteate (DLH). While intracellular potentials were recorded from a CA3 neurone, amino acids were ejected from a double-barreled electrode to a sensitive spot in the dendritic region. The periods of electrophoretic administration are indicated by the solid lines beneath the records. Intensities of currents are expressed in nanoamperes. Triangle in a5: generation of an action potential.

the hippocampus of the guinea pig. In these experiments we prepared slices of the hippocampus and a microelectrode filled with K acetate was inserted into the cell body of a CA3 neurone. While recording intracellular potentials from the impaled neurone, another electrode filled with 1 M glutamate was gently inserted into the area where dendrites of the impaled neurone were supposed to spread, and glutamate was ejected electrophoretically after every 5 μm advance of the pipette.

By this procedure we could show the presence of small spots very sensitive to glutamate (Fig. 1a). These spots were so sensitive that a pulse of ejection current lasting only 50 msec sometimes caused depolarization of more than 20 mV. The spots seemed to be highly localized in the tissue because a 5 μm movement of the glutamate pipette resulted in a marked increase or decrease in the amplitude of the depolarization. A feature of this depolarization was its fast decay. The slope of the falling phase of the potential was almost as steep as that of the rising phase. The fast decay may be explained by the presence of a high-affinity uptake for glutamate.

In the experiment shown in Fig. 1, a double-barreled electrode was used to administer excitatory amino acids. One barrel was filled with L-glutamate and another with DL-homocysteate. The tip of the electrode was brought to a glutamate-sensitive spot and the depolarizations induced by glutamate or DL-homocysteate were compared at various intensities of ejection current. In this illustration, the following two points are to be noted. First, the falling phase of homocysteate depolarization is much slower than that of glutamate depolarization. Secondly, while homocysteate has been reported by previous authors to be much more potent than glutamate (Crawford and Curtis 1964), homocysteate is less potent in this illustration, especially at low current intensities. How can we explain the discrepancy between high potency of homocysteate reported by previous authors and its low potency in our experiments?

Even in our experiments we can confirm the high potency of homocysteate if we administer the amino acid for more than several seconds, as other authors did. With such long ejecting currents, homocysteate induced very large depolarizations, particularly at sites a little remote from the glutamate-sensitive spots. These data can be explained by the assumption that, because of the absence of high-affinity uptake for homocysteate, homocysteate ejected in a large amount remains in the extracellular space for a considerable time and diffuses to remote unspecific or homocysteate-specific receptors to activate them.

Like homocysteate, N-methyl-D-aspartate has been reported to be one of the most potent excitants of central neurones. Tested with short pulses of ejecting current, however, N-methyl-D-aspartate was almost without effect at the glutamate-sensitive spots, while it induced very large and prolonged depolarization when ejected with a current of long duration.

Another discrepancy between previous data and ours concerns the potency of D-glutamate. Although D-glutamate was reported to be about 0.5 times as active as the L-isomer (Crawford and Curtis 1964), D-glutamate caused no marked depolarization in most of our cells. Again, however, the D-isomer induced considerable depolarization when ejected by current lasting for seconds.

In summarizing our experiments on glutamate receptors, I would like to say that we have succeeded in detecting the glutamate receptor function which is stereo-specific and apparently more sensitive to glutamate than to other excitatory amino acid analogues. I am not certain, however, whether the glutamate receptors exist at postsynaptic sites or at the extra-junctional membrane.

CONCLUSIONS

As a general conclusion of my presentation, I should like to emphasize the usefulness of the in vitro slice technique for research on receptor functions in the brain. Especially, in thin sections of the cerebellum, the surface of dendrites and the cell bodies of Purkinje cells are clearly visualized with the aid of a Nomarski microscope (Yamamoto and Chujo 1978). These cerebellar sections seem to be appropriate preparations for newly devised microtechniques to study transmitter-sensitive ion channels.

ACKNOWLEDGEMENTS

I thank Dr. J.C. Watkins for the gift of N-methyl-D-aspartate.
This study was supported by a grant from the Ministry of Education of Japan.

REFERENCES

Chujo, T., Yamada, Y. and Yamamoto, C. Sensitivity of Purkinje cell dendrites to glutamic acid. Exp. Brain Res., 1975, 23: 293–300.

Crawford, J.M. and Curtis, D.R. The excitation and depression of mammalian cortical neurones by amino acids. Brit. J. Pharmacol., 1964, 23: 313–329.

Eccles, J.C. The Physiology of Synapses. Academic Press, New York, 1964.

Krettek, J.E. and Price, J.L. Amygdaloid projections to subcortical structures within the basal forebrain and brainstem in the rat and cat. J. comp. Neurol., 1978, 178: 225–254.

Sawada, S. and Yamamoto, C. Electrical activity recorded from thin sections of the bed nucleus of the stria terminalis, and the effects of neurotensin. Brain Res., 1980, 188: 578–581.

Sawada, S. and Yamamoto, C. Postsynaptic inhibitory actions of catecholamines and opioid peptides in the bed nucleus of the stria terminalis. Exp. Brain Res., 1981, 41: 264–270.

Uhl, G.R. and Snyder, S.H. A neuronal pathway projecting from amygdala through stria terminalis. Brain Res., 1979, 161: 522–526.

Uhl, G.R., Kuhar, M.J. and Snyder, S.H. Enkephalin-containing pathway: amygdaloid efferents in the stria terminalis. Brain Res., 1978, 149: 223–228.

Yamamoto, C. Activation of hippocampal neurons by mossy fiber stimulation in thin brain sections in vitro. Exp. Brain Res., 1972, 14: 423–435.

Yamamoto, C. Recording of electrical activity from microscopically identified neurons of the mammalian brain. Experientia (Basel), 1975, 31: 309–311.

Yamamoto, C. and Chujo, T. Visualization of central neurons and recording of action potentials. Exp. Brain Res., 1978, 31: 299–301.

Yamamoto, C., Matsumoto, K. and Takagi, M. Potentiation of excitatory postsynaptic potentials during and after repetitive stimulation in thin hippocampal sections. Exp. Brain Res., 1980, 38: 469–477.

Young, A.B., Oster-Granite, M.L., Herndon, R.M. and Snyder, S.H. Glutamic acid: Selective depletion by viral induced granule cell loss in hamster cerebellum. Brain Res., 1974, 73: 1–13.

Kyoto Symposia (EEG Suppl. No. 36)
Editors: P.A. Buser, W.A. Cobb and T. Okuma
© 1982, Elsevier Biomedical Press, Amsterdam

Multiple Excitability Functions in Cultured Mouse Spinal Neurones

JEFFERY L. BARKER

Laboratory of Neurophysiology, National Institute of Neurological and Communicative Disorders and Stroke, National Institutes of Health, Bethesda, Md. 20205 (U.S.A.)

The excitability of the central nervous system (CNS) and the communication of excitability changes among CNS neurones are thought to determine activity levels in autonomic, endocrine, motor, sensory and cognitive systems. Much of the intercellular communication appears to be mediated by substances synthesized by, and secreted from, excitable elements. These "transmitters" diffuse to specific target cells where they react with receptor sites to induce changes in cellular excitability which in turn generate the complex and varied outputs characteristic of the CNS. Cellular excitability and the chemical substances which mediate changes in excitability between cells are thus fundamental to the physiology of the CNS and to all the behaviours elaborated by it.

Excitability is a membrane property expressed in most, if not all, evolutionary forms studied. In the vertebrate, excitable membrane mechanisms exist in a variety of neuronal and non-neuronal cell types (see Kuffler and Nicholls 1976). These mechanisms allow transmembrane movement of ionic charge, triggered either by changes in the electrical field across the membrane or by the presence of transmitter substance. Some details regarding chemical and electrical excitability in CNS neurones are now emerging with the advent of new strategies to study the physiology of central neurones. In this paper I shall briefly consider results from some recent experiments focussed on chemically excitable events in CNS neurones. Most of the data to be discussed are derived from experiments conducted in cultured spinal neurones, a preparation that allows ready accessibility to electrophysiological assays with high resolving power (Fig. 1). Although spinal neurones grow in culture as a virtual monolayer, they possess many of the properties characteristic of neurones recorded in vivo, including chemical and electrical forms of excitability (see recent text by Lieberman and Nelson 1981). These characteristics of the preparation make it suitable for resolving details of excitable events in CNS membranes.

GABA INHIBITS SPINAL NEURONES BY INCREASING CHLORIDE ION CONDUCTANCE

γ-Aminobutyric acid (GABA) is an amino acid endogenous to many, if not all

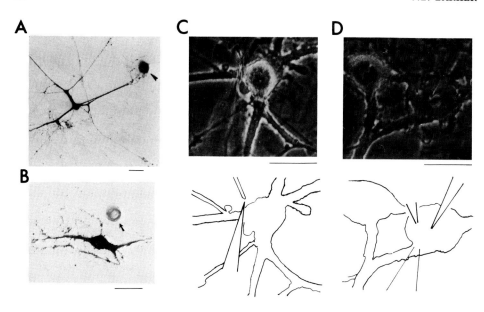

Fig. 1. Light micrographs of mammalian neurones growing in monolayer culture. Panels A and B show cells stained with immunohistochemical techniques for revealing the presence of the neuronal marker enzyme, nerve-specific enolase. The arrow heads point to sensory neurones which invariably stain less than spinal cord cells. The micrographs were made by Dr. Donald Schmechel. Panels C and D are phase contrast micrographs showing representative examples of spinal cord neurones used in studying chemical excitability functions. The tips of 2 microelectrodes are evident outside the cell shown in C and inside the right-hand cell in D. Schematic diagrams of the microelectrode placements are shown below the micrographs. Bars: 50 μm.

nervous systems (for review, see Nistri and Constanti 1979). It has been demonstrated in a variety of systems that GABA mediates synaptic signals which are inhibitory to electrical activity. Most mouse spinal neurones grown in tissue culture respond to pharmacological applications of GABA (Ransom et al. 1977; Barker and Ransom 1978a), and discrete applications of GABA to different parts of the same cell reveal that cultured neurones are not uniformly sensitive. For example, hyperpolarizing responses can usually be elicited when GABA is applied to the cell body or to nearby membrane on neuronal processes, while depolarizing responses or responses consisting of hyper- and depolarizing phases can be evoked from process membranes relatively distant from the cell body (Fig. 2). Many of the cultured neurones are invested with bouton-like structures that stain positively for the presence of glutamic acid decarboxylase, the enzyme converting glutamic acid to GABA (Barker et al. 1980d). In fact the topographic distribution of positively stained terminals often coincides with the distribution of membrane sites showing increased sensitivity to GABA (Study and Barker, unpublished observations), suggesting that the distributions may have physiological correlates. In this regard spontaneous inhibitory synaptic potentials can be recorded in many cultured spinal neurones and these can be affected by drugs which alter pharmacologically evoked responses to GABA, suggesting that some inhibitory synaptic events in cultured

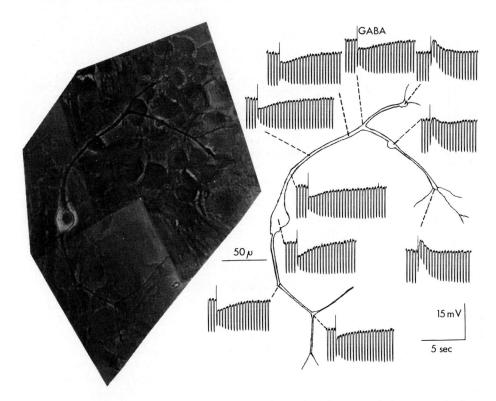

Fig. 2. Topographic distribution of GABA responses in a cultured mouse spinal neurone. A phase contrast micrograph of a neurone is on the left and a schematic outline of the cell is shown on the right. GABA has been applied to different sites on the cell surface with brief iontophoretic pulses. Membrane potential traces recorded with an intrasomatic microelectrode are shown during the GABA responses. Constant-current hyperpolarizing pulses have been injected, using a bridge circuit. Hyperpolarizing responses associated with an increase in membrane conductance can be evoked at sites near the cell body, while depolarizing or multiphasic responses can be elicited at sites on process membranes. Resting membrane potential: −51 mV. (Barker and Ransom, unpublished observation.)

spinal neurones may be mediated by GABA (Barker and McBurney 1979b; Choi et al. 1981).

The membrane potential responses to GABA and the pharmacologically sensitive synaptic events are always associated with an increase in membrane conductance. The ionic mechanism(s) underlying these events has been studied by changing the species and/or concentration of ions across the membranes. The results show that the inhibitory responses to GABA and the inhibitory synaptic potentials are largely, if not entirely, dependent on Cl⁻ ions; and further, that the polarity of the response is determined by the size and direction of the Cl⁻ ion gradient (Fig. 3). Similar results and conclusions have been drawn from results with pharmacological applications of two other naturally occurring neutral amino acids, glycine and β-alanine, each of which also inhibits excitability by increasing membrane conductance to Cl⁻ ions (Barker and Ransom 1978a).

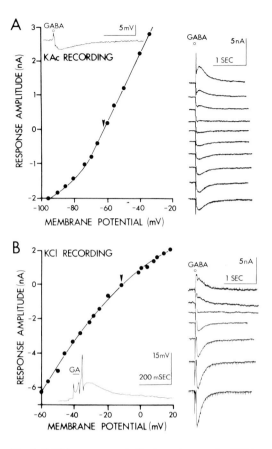

Fig. 3. GABA response polarity depends upon the Cl⁻ ion gradient. Intracellular records were made with 2 microelectrodes filled either with KAc (cell A) or KCl (cell B). GABA, applied by iontophoresis, hyperpolarizes cell A and depolarizes cell B, triggering an action potential. When the membrane potential is controlled by the voltage clamp technique and then varied over an 80 mV range, GABA evokes a family of membrane current responses (shown on right). Plots of membrane current amplitude as a function of membrane potential show that the current responses invert at −63 mV in cell A and −10 mV in cell B. (Barker and Smith, unpublished observations.)

INHIBITORY RESPONSES TO NEUTRAL AMINO ACIDS INVOLVE TWO STATE ION CHANNELS

The membrane mechanisms underlying Cl⁻-dependent responses to GABA, glycine and β-alanine in cultured spinal neurones have been investigated by the technique of "fluctuation analysis", introduced by Katz and Miledi (1972), who observed minute fluctuations occurring during membrane responses evoked by acetylcholine in muscle membranes. They analysed the fluctuations on the assumption that they represented fluctuations in the number of unitary events contributing to the membrane response. They reasoned that the unitary events were of uniform size but varying duration and that they occurred randomly and

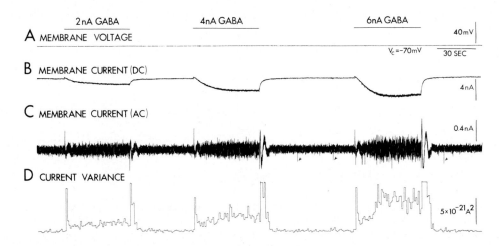

Fig. 4. Membrane current responses evoked by GABA in cultured mouse spinal neurones are associated with increased levels of "noise" in the current trace. An intracellular record was made with two KCl microelectrodes and GABA was applied by iontophoresis (marked in nA at top). A: the membrane voltage was clamped at −70 mV by the voltage clamp technique. B: iontophoresis of increasing amounts of GABA evokes membrane current responses of increasing amplitude. C: when the membrane current is amplified 10 × and filtered between 0.5 and 500 Hz, an increase in current "noise" proportional to the current response amplitude is evident. D: membrane current variance, integrated every second and displayed as a voltage, also increases in a dose-dependent manner. The arrowheads in panel C point to quantal synaptic events. (Barker and McBurney, unpublished observations.)

independently. Using this reasoning Katz and Miledi were able to estimate the electrical properties of the unitary events. More recent results, first by Anderson and Stevens (1973), then by Neher and Sakmann (1976) have confirmed and extended the original predictions of Katz and Miledi. It is now clear that two state (open-closed) unitary events underlie the action of agonist responses on many excitable membranes (for review, see Mathers and Barker 1982).

Membrane responses to GABA and the other amino acids are routinely associated with a marked thickening or "noise" in the membrane current trace (McBurney and Barker 1978) (Fig. 4). Fluctuation analysis of the current "noise" occurring during membrane responses shows that membrane responses evoked by different amino acids are comprised of two state Cl^- ion channel events with different properties (Barker et al. 1982) (Fig. 5). Experiments with the micropatch method, which allows study of the activities of individual channels in isolated patches of membrane, have confirmed that GABA does indeed activate two state channels (Mathers et al. 1981). The results thus indicate that each amino acid causes a membrane reaction resulting in a different amount of charge transfer across cultured neuronal membranes, the ratio of charge transfer being 1.00:0.74:0.32 for GABA, glycine, β-alanine.

The different electrical properties activated by each amino acid may lead to unique amplitudes and time courses of physiologically evoked conductance changes at synapses mediated by the neutral amino acids. The time course of the physiologically elaborated synaptic event corresponds closely to the average open

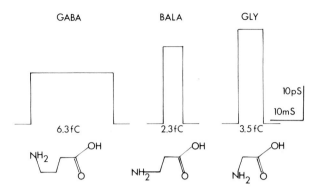

Fig. 5. Naturally occurring neutral amino acids activate Cl⁻ ion channels with unique properties in cultured mouse spinal neurones. The average properties of ion channels activated by GABA, β-alanine and glycine, estimated by fluctuation analysis of membrane current responses, are depicted as rectangular pulses of membrane conductance. The charge transferred during each averaged event has been calculated by integrating the elementary current over time and the values corresponding to the different events are given above the amino acid structures in femtocoulombs (fC). (Barker, McBurney and MacDonald, unpublished observations.)

time of the unitary channel event evoked pharmacologically by the putative transmitter substance (Katz and Miledi 1972; Dionne and Stevens 1975; Crawford and McBurney 1976; Ascher et al. 1979; Dudel et al. 1980; Faber and Korn 1980; Gardner and Stevens 1980; Miledi and Uchitel 1981). This suggests that the exponential decay in the synaptic conductance reflects the exponential distribution in lifetimes of the unitary events which comprise the synaptic conductance, rather than some other aspect of chemical transmission at synapses (e.g., diffusion, uptake, enzymatic inactivation). Thus, if the kinetics of Cl⁻ ion channels activated by the neutral amino acids also determine the kinetics of the conductance change generated under physiological circumstances, then each neutral amino acid should mediate an inhibitory signal of unique amplitude and time course. Whether this is true, and whether other substances which activate inhibitory, Cl⁻-dependent, responses, including peptides (Barker et al. 1980c), purines and pyrimidines (J.F. MacDonald et al. 1979; Barker et al. 1980a), also utilize similar two state ion channel mechanisms remain to be established. Furthermore, the physical arrangement of amino acid receptors and Cl⁻ ion permeation mechanisms also needs to be elucidated. In fact, there is preliminary evidence that several neutral amino acids may share the same Cl⁻ ion channel mechanism (Barker and McBurney 1979a).

PENTOBARBITAL AND DIAZEPAM MIMIC GABA'S INHIBITORY EFFECTS

Pentobarbital and diazepam are two clinically important drugs with somewhat overlapping therapeutic effects. Both drugs are used to depress the excitability of the CNS. When applied to cultured mouse spinal neurones, pentobarbital hyperpolarizes a majority of cells studied through an increase in Cl⁻ ion conductance (Barker and Ransom 1978b). Similar effects have recently been observed with diazepam, although in a minority of the cells recorded (Barker and Study 1981). These actions of the drugs are both associated with an increase in fluctuations of the membrane current trace and fluctuation analysis shows that both drugs activate channels whose conductance is similar to that of GABA (Mathers and Barker 1980; Barker and Study 1981). The average duration of the channel activated by the (−)-isomer of pentobarbital is about 4–5 times that activated by GABA. [The (−)-isomer has been used in the study because of its greater potency in activating Cl⁻ ion conductance (Huang and Barker 1980)]. Channels activated by diazepam are similar to that activated by GABA or slightly longer. Micropatch recordings of the effects of (−)-pentobarbital on cultured spinal neurones have confirmed that the drug activates two state ion channels (Mathers et al. 1981). The inhibitory effects of both the barbiturate and the benzodiazepine are blocked by agents which antagonize GABA (Barker and Ransom 1978b; Nicoll and Wojtowicz 1980; Study and Barker, unpublished observations). It is thus possible that the two state ion channels activated by the drugs involve either GABA receptors or the channel mechanisms coupled to GABA receptors. However, various invertebrate membranes with GABA receptors coupled to inhibitory, Cl⁻-dependent, mechanisms do not respond to either barbiturates or benzodiazepines (Adams and Banks 1980), and many cultured spinal neurones with functional GABA receptors are insensitive to the drugs (Study and Barker 1981). Thus, the "GABA-mimetic" properties of the drugs do not necessarily indicate that they are engaging GABA receptors or using Cl⁻ ion channels coupled to GABA receptors. The exact relationship between the drug responses and GABA receptor-coupled Cl⁻ ion channels has not been resolved yet.

PENTOBARBITAL AND DIAZEPAM MODULATE THE KINETICS OF GABA-ACTIVATED ION CHANNELS

Another type of excitability function has been observed in cultured mouse spinal neurones. This involves modulation of membrane responses to amino acids by peptides (Barker et al. 1980c) and by CNS-active drugs (Barker and McBurney 1979b; Barker et al. 1980b; Choi et al. 1981; R.L. MacDonald and Barker 1981; Study and Barker 1981). The results show that GABA responses are uniformly depressed by drugs which cause convulsant activity in vivo and consistently potentiated by drugs which depress CNS excitability (Fig. 6). Fluctuation analysis has recently been applied to GABA responses modulated by drugs. The convulsant drugs picrotoxin and bicuculline do not change the electrical properties of GABA-activated channels. Thus, those channels contributing to the (depressed) response have properties indistinguishable from normally activated channels. Diazepam increases the frequency of channel openings and does not change, or slightly prolongs, the average duration of an event while (−)-pentobarbital decreases the

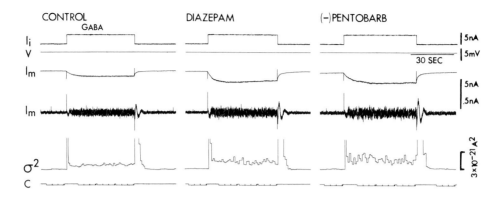

Fig. 6. Diazepam and (–)-pentobarbital potentiate membrane current responses evoked by GABA in a cultured mouse spinal neurone. The intracellular record was made with two KCl microelectrodes and the membrane potential was clamped at – 60 mV. The same amount of iontophoretic current (I) was used to apply GABA in the absence and presence of either 17 μM (–)-pentobarbital diffused passively from pipettes placed within 20 μM of the site on the cell body where GABA was applied. The current response to GABA is displayed as a DC signal in the upper I_m trace and then amplified 10 × and filtered 0.25–250 Hz in the lower I_m trace. The variance (σ^2) of the membrane current updated every second is shown below. The bottom trace (C) shows periods of data acquisition by the computer (downward deflections). Both drugs increase the amplitude of the GABA response and the variance associated with the response. (Study and Barker, unpublished observations.)

frequency of channel openings, but greatly increases the average duration of an event. These drug effects on channel kinetics can account, in a quantitative manner, for the potentiation observed. These results indicate that pharmacological potentiation of GABA-mediated inhibition can occur through different mechanisms. These mechanisms of drug-induced modulation at the level of the post-synaptic membrane may serve as useful references when studying examples of modulation mediated by naturally occurring substances.

MODULATION OF ACTION POTENTIAL ACTIVITY BY TRANSMITTERS AND DRUGS

Pharmacological applications of several endogenous substances, including the opioid peptides (Barker et al. 1980c) and GABA (Barker et al. 1980d), alter threshold and rheobase (current required to reach threshold) in a minority of cultured spinal neurones studied thus far. These effects occur in the absence of, or independent of, any other actions on membrane excitability, but multiple actions of the opioid peptides (including an increase in Cl^- conductance, modulation of glutamate responses, and an elevation in action potential threshold) have all been recorded in the same cultured neurones, with the different effects having different concentration requirements.

Clinically important drugs can also modulate the electrical excitability of cultured neurones independent of, or in the absence of, any other action on membrane

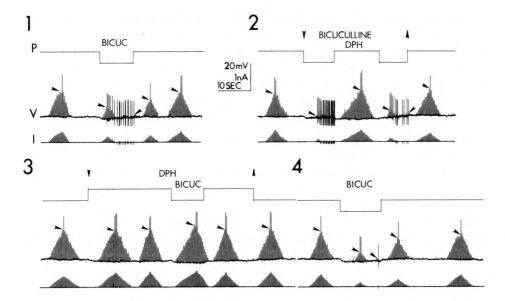

Fig. 7. Opposing actions of bicuculline (BICUC) and phenytoin (DPH) on the threshold for action potential generation in a cultured mouse spinal neurone. 10 mM MgCl₂ was added to the normal recording medium to suppress synaptic activity and noise threshold for triggering action potentials. The intracellular record was made with a KAc microelectrode. Bicuculline (50 μM) and DPH (10 μM) were applied by pressure (P) during the indicated periods. Depolarizing current pulses of varying amplitude (I) were used to assess the threshold for triggering an action potential (marked by tilted arrowhead). BICUC lowers threshold and induces spontaneous action potential activity (panel 1). DPH reverses this effect (panel 2) or prevents it (panel 3). The threshold lowering effects of BICUC recover (panel 4). Action potentials are not full-sized owing to the limited frequency response of the pen recorder. Resting membrane potential: -50 mV. (Barker and MacDonald, unpublished observations.)

properties (Barker et al. 1980d; Barker and MacDonald 1980). Three types of effect have been observed: (1) a change in threshold for evoking a single action potential without change in repetitive action potential activity; (2) no change in threshold for a single action potential with suppression of repetitive activity; and (3) reversal of drug-induced changes in threshold without evidence of other effects (Fig. 7). Drugs with convulsant properties in vivo lower threshold and/or enhance repetitive activity, while anticonvulsants elevate threshold and/or suppress repetitive activity. These actions may be cellular correlates of the pharmacological actions observed in vivo. Whether the effects of the drugs are related to the modulatory actions of endogenous ligands remains to be studied.

CONCLUSION

Mouse spinal neurones growing in cell culture have been used to study some details regarding chemically induced changes in excitability. Three functionally distinct types of excitable membrane process have been observed. They include (1) activation of two state Cl$^-$ ion channels, (2) modulation of amino acid responses and (3) modulation of electrical excitability. Each type of chemically excitable membrane event can be activated by both transmitter substances and clinically important drugs. All of the data obtained thus far have been derived from pharmacological experiments. For the endogenous ligands it will be important to demonstrate that similar excitability functions can be elaborated physiologically. For the exogenous ligands it will be important to resolve the relationship, if any, between the drug actions and the excitable membrane processes normally activated by transmitter substances. The excitability functions recorded in cultured mammalian neurones are some, but not all, of the types of chemical excitability reported thus far. The results suggest that chemically mediated forms of intercellular communication in the CNS are multiple and complex. Presumably, different chemical signals have evolved and been preserved through evolution because they comprise the cellular basis underlying the diverse array of functions characteristic of the CNS.

REFERENCES

Adams, P.R. and Banks, F.W. Actions of anesthetics and anticonvulsants on synaptic channels. In: B.R. Fink (Ed.), Molecular Mechanisms of Anesthesia. Raven Press, New York, 1980: 95–109.

Anderson, C.R. and Stevens, C.F. Voltage clamp analysis of acetylcholine produced end plate current fluctuations at frog neuromuscular junction. J. Physiol. (Lond.), 1973, 235: 655–691.

Ascher, P., Large, W.A. and Rang, H.P. Studies on the mechanisms of action of acetylcholine antagonists on rat parasympathetic ganglion cell. J. Physiol. (Lond.), 1979, 295: 139–170.

Barker, J.L. and MacDonald, J.F. Picrotoxin convulsions involve synaptic and non-synaptic mechanisms on cultured mouse spinal neurons. Science, 1980, 208: 1054–1056.

Barker, J.L. and McBurney, R.N. GABA and glycine may share the same conductance channel on cultured mammalian neurones. Nature (Lond.), 1979a, 277: 234–236.

Barker, J.L. and McBurney, R.N. Phenobarbitone modulation of post-synaptic GABA receptor function on cultured mammalian neurons. Proc. roy. Soc. B, 1979b, 206: 318–326.

Barker, J.L. and Ransom, B.R. Amino acid pharmacology of mammalian central neurons grown in tissue culture. J. Physiol. (Lond.), 1978a, 280: 331–354.

Barker, J.L. and Ransom, B.R. Pentobarbital pharmacology of mammalian central neurons grown in tissue culture. J. Physiol. (Lond.), 1978b, 280: 355–372.

Barker, J.L. and Study, R.E. Fluctuation analysis of direct inhibitory effects of diazepam and (−)-pentobarbital on the excitability of cultured mouse spinal neurons. Soc. Neurosci. Abstr., 1981, 10: 270.

Barker, J.L., Huang, L.M., MacDonald, J.F. and McBurney, R.N. Barbiturate pharmacology of cultured mammalian neurons. In: B.R. Fink (Ed.), Molecular Mechanisms of Anesthesia. Raven Press, New York, 1980a: 79–93.

Barker, J.L., Mathers, D.A., McBurney, R.N. and Vaughn, W. Convulsant actions on amino acid-activated channels. J. Physiol. (Lond.), 1980b, 308: 18P.

Barker, J.L., Gruol, D.L., Huang, L.M., MacDonald, J.F. and Smith, T.G. Peptides: three forms of chemical excitability on cultured mouse spinal neurons. Neuropeptides, 1980c, 1: 63–82.

Barker, J.L., MacDonald, J.F., Mathers, D.A., McBurney, R.N. and Oertel, W. GABA receptor functions in cultured mouse spinal neurons. In: F.V. DeFeudis and P. Mandel (Eds.). Amino Acid Neurotransmitters. Raven Press, New York, 1980d. 281–293.

Barker, J.L., McBurney, R.N. and MacDonald, J.F. Fluctuation analysis of neutral amino acid responses in cultured mouse spinal neurons. J. Physiol. (Lond.), 1982, 322: 365–387.

Choi, D.W., Farb, D.H. and Fischbach, G.D. Chlordiazepoxide selectively potentiates GABA conductance of spinal cord and sensory neurons in cell culture. J. Neurophysiol., 1981, 45: 621–631.

Crawford, A.C. and McBurney, R.N. On the elementary conductance event produced by L-glutamate and quanta of the natural transmitter at the neuromuscular junctions of *Maia squinado*. J. Physiol. (Lond.), 1976, 258: 215–225.

Dionne, V.E. and Stevens, C.F. Voltage dependence of agonist effectiveness of the frog neuromuscular junction: resolution of a paradox. J. Physiol. (Lond.), 1975, 251: 245–270.

Dudel, J., Finger, W. and Stettmeier, H. Inhibitory synaptic channels activated by γ-aminobutyric acid (GABA) in crayfish muscle. Pflügers Arch. ges. Physiol., 1980, 387: 143–151.

Faber, D.S. and Korn, H. Single shot channel activation accounts for duration of inhibitory post-synaptic potentials in central neurons. Science, 1980, 208: 612–615.

Gardner, D. and Stevens, C.F. Rate-limiting step of inhibitory post-synaptic current decay in *Aplysia* buccal ganglia. J. Physiol. (Lond.), 1980, 304: 145–164.

Huang, L.M. and Barker, J.L. Pentobarbital: stereospecific actions of (+) and (−) isomers revealed on cultured mammalian neurons. Science, 1980, 207: 795–797.

Katz, B. and Miledi, R. The statistical nature of the acetylcholine potential and its molecular components. J. Physiol. (Lond.), 1972, 224: 665–699.

Kuffler, S.W. and Nicholls, J. From Neuron to Brain. Sinauer Associates, Sunderland, Mass., 1976.

Lieberman, M. and Nelson, P.G. Excitable Cells in Tissue Culture. Plenum, New York, 1981.

MacDonald, J.F., Barker, J.L., Marangos, P., Paul, S.M. and Skolnick, P. Inosine may be an endogenous ligand for benzodiazepine receptors in cultured mouse spinal neurons. Science, 1979, 205: 715–717.

MacDonald, R.L. and Barker, J.L. Neuropharmacology of cultured mouse spinal neurons. In: M. Lieberman and P.G. Nelson (Eds.), Excitable Cells in Tissue Culture. Plenum Press, New York, 1981: 80–110.

Mathers, D.A. and Barker, J.L. (−)Pentobarbital opens ion channels of long duration in cultured mouse spinal neurons. Science, 1980, 209: 507–509.

Mathers, D.A. and Barker, J.L. Chemically-induced ion channels in nerve cell membranes. Int. Rev. Neurobiol., 1982, 23: 1–34.

Mathers, D.A., Jackson, M.G., Lecar, H. and Barker, J.L. Single channel currents activated by GABA, muscimol and (−)pentobarbital in cultured mouse spinal neurons. Biophys. J., 1981, 33: 14a.

McBurney, R.N. and Barker, J.L. GABA-induced conductance fluctuations in cultured spinal neurones. Nature (Lond.), 1978, 262: 596–597.

Miledi, R. and Uchitel, O.D. Properties of post-synaptic channels induced by acetylcholine in different frog muscle fibers. Nature (Lond.), 1981, 291: 162–165.

Neher, R. and Sakmann, B. Single-channel currents recorded from membrane of denervated frog muscle fibers. Nature (Lond.), 1976, 260: 799–802.

Nicoll, R.A. and Wojtowicz, J.M. The effects of pentobarbital and related compounds on frog motoneurons. Brain Res., 1980, 191: 225–237.

Nistri, A. and Constanti, A. Pharmacological characterization of different types of GABA and glutamate receptors in vertebrates and invertebrates. Prog. Neurobiol., 1979, 13: 117–235.

Ransom, B.R., Neale, E., Henkart, M., Bullock, P.M. and Nelson, P.G. Mouse spinal cord in cell culture. I. Morphology and intrinsic neuronal electrophysiologic properties. J. Neurophysiol., 1977, 40: 1132–1150.

Study, R.E. and Barker, J.L. Diazepam and (−)pentobarbital:fluctuation analysis reveals different mechanisms for potentiation of GABA responses in cultured central neurons. Proc. nat. Acad. Sci. (Wash.), 1981, 78: 7180–7184.

Kyoto Symposia (EEG Suppl. No. 36)
Editors: P.A. Buser, W.A. Cobb and T. Okuma
© 1982, Elsevier Biomedical Press, Amsterdam

The Epileptic and Anticonvulsant Properties of Opioid Peptides

J. TIMOTHY CANNON, SALLY CALDECOTT-HAZARD, YEHUDA SHAVIT,
JAMES W. LEWIS and JOHN C. LIEBESKIND

Department of Psychology, University of Scranton, Scranton, Pa. 18510 and
Department of Psychology, University of California, Los Angeles, Calif. 90024 (U.S.A.)

The identification of opiate receptors and their endogenous ligands has excited the neuroscience community as few discoveries have. Inevitably, attention focussed on the presumed involvement of endogenous opioid peptides in pain modulation, and significant progress has been made in this area (Cannon and Liebeskind 1979). It was clear early on, however, that whatever role opioids might play in pain mechanisms, this role was not apt to be an exclusive one (Goldstein 1976). In this paper, we shall review recent work on the relation of opioids to certain seizure phenomena. We shall first consider evidence that opioids provoke some epileptiform electrographic manifestations; next, more recent findings that opioids also possess an important anticonvulsant property will be discussed.

THE EPILEPTIC PROPERTIES OF OPIOID PEPTIDES

Urca et al. (1977) first reported that intracerebroventricular (ICV) injections of met-enkephalin caused epileptiform EEG activity in the rat. Typically, within the first minute after an injection, a 20–30 sec period of high frequency spike bursts could be seen in the cortical EEG. These bursts evolved into a period of lower frequency, large amplitude sharp waves (2–3/sec). A pattern of very small amplitude desynchronized EEG appeared next, lasting for approximately 30 sec, and was followed by a second build up of spike and wave complexes (1–2/sec). Finally, recurrent spike and polyspike and wave complexes appeared and continued at a frequency of 1 per 3–7 sec for a minimum of 3 min. These EEG events were virtually never associated with convulsions, although wet-dog shakes were often observed during the first minute of the seizure and occasionally thereafter. Myoclonic twitches of the trunk, head or limbs sometimes accompanied the recurrent spike and polyspike and wave complexes. Otherwise, the animals remained quiet and immobile. Subsequently it was shown in our laboratory that ICV leu-enkephalin or morphine elicited virtually identical epileptiform EEGs without convulsions (Frenk et al. 1978b), and other workers have made similar observations with these agents and other opioids (Henriksen et al. 1978; Tortella et al. 1978; Snead and Bearden 1980).

To establish that a phenomenon has as its basis a pharmacological interaction with opioid receptors, the fulfillment of 3 criteria is typically required. The epileptiform EEG activity induced by opiates or opioids has met these criteria as follows.

1. All EEG and behavioural manifestations provoked by ICV opioid and opiate injections in the rat are blocked by systemic administration of the opiate antagonist naloxone (Urca et al. 1977; Frenk et al. 1978b; Henriksen et al. 1978; Snead and Bearden 1980). That this antagonism typically requires the use of moderate to high doses of naloxone (3 mg/kg or greater) will be discussed below in relation to speculations concerning the type of opioid receptors involved in these EEG events.

2. Tolerance develops to these EEG effects with repeated enkephalin injections, as does cross-tolerance with morphine (Elazar et al. 1979; Tortella et al. 1979).

3. Stereospecificity has been established for the epileptogenic actions of levorphanol and dextrorphan administered ICV (Cannon et al. 1979; Lewis et al. 1981). Only levorphanol possesses an epileptogenic potential. As the following paragraph points out, however, this potential is only demonstrated under restricted conditions.

In our original work with ICV injections of levorphanol and dextrorphan tartrate, we were unable to produce epileptiform cortical discharges using either drug across a dose range that at its high end proved lethal to the majority of animals. The discovery by LaBella et al. (1979) that calcium chelators administered ICV have opiate-like effects led us to speculate that our ICV injections of morphine sulphate had been exerting at least part of their electrographic influences by means of the calcium chelating action of sulphate ions. Such an action would have been absent with injections of either levorphanol or dextrorphan tartrate. Subsequently we found that this was not the case in that ICV injections of morphine HCl were as potent as morphine sulphate in disrupting the cortical EEG of rats (Cannon et al. 1979). However, the addition of an equimolar concentration of sulphate ions to the levorphanol injection vehicle did result in electrographic phenomena identical to those produced by either morphine or the opioids. These manifestations were completely blocked by systemic naloxone administration. Importantly, the addition of sulphate ions at the same or higher concentrations did not result in dextrorphan having similar cortical EEG influences.

A potentially important additional finding of the above investigation was that, as the addition of sulphate ions was unmasking the epileptogenic action of levorphanol, it was reducing its efficacy as an analgesic. This apparent dissociation between the effects of sulphate ions on the analgesic and epileptogenic actions of levorphanol may not only speak to the importance of calcium chelation in the EEG influences of opiates and opioids but also support the arguments outlined below pointing to the analgesic and epileptogenic actions of opiates and opioids being mediated by qualitatively different opioid receptor populations.

Several lines of evidence indicate that the EEG changes and the analgesic effects of opioids and opiates are due to interactions with different opioid receptor types. We and others have found that approximately 3–5 mg/kg of systemic naloxone is necessary to block the EEG influences of opioids or morphine (Urca et al. 1977; Frenk et al. 1978b; Henriksen et al. 1978; Snead and Bearden 1980). Analgesia, in contrast, is typically sensitive to doses of naloxone in the 0.1–1 mg/kg range. In our work, an epileptiform EEG could be reliably produced by ICV injections of the enkephalins at doses as low as 25 μg and even at 10 μg in some animals (Frenk et al. 1978). Analgesia in these animals was only occasionally observed at 100 μg and never at the lower doses. In marked contrast to this pattern, morphine at 100 μg reliably produced profound analgesia but less consistently seizures. At 30 μg, morphine never produced seizures yet still elicited profound analgesia. Finally, in our experience the EEG effects of leucine-enkephalin last longer than those of methionine-enkephalin, suggesting that leucine-enkephalin has somewhat greater epileptogenic potency. Based upon such findings, Frenk et al. (1978a) suggested that enkephalin analgesia is mediated by μ receptors and enkephalin seizures by δ receptors. This suggestion is consistent with the work of Lord et al. (1977) using smooth muscle assays to characterize the relative affinities of various ligands for different opioid receptor types. They concluded that morphine had greater affinity for one kind of opioid receptor (μ), and that the enkephalins, especially leucine-enkephalin, had greater affinity for a different opioid receptor (δ).

There is also evidence that the EEG and analgesic effects of opioids rely on anatomically distinct receptor populations (Frenk et al. 1978a). Methionine-enkephalin (100 μg), injected directly into the ventral periaqueductal gray of the midbrain, caused analgesia without any alterations of cortical EEG. The same type of injections directed into the dorso-medial thalamus caused cortical EEG seizures without any evidence of analgesia. Overall, then, Frenk et al. (1978a) proposed that enkephalin seizures derive from interactions with the δ type of opioid receptor in the forebrain and analgesia from μ receptor interactions in the periaqueductal gray.

Subsequent work has indicated that the $\varkappa$ and σ opioid receptor types of Martin et al. (1976) are not involved in the production of seizure activity. ICV injections of agonists for these receptors, ketocyclazocine, cyclazocine or WIN-35, 197-2, failed to induce epileptiform EEG disturbances across a dose range in which high voltage spindle activity, analgesia and death could all be obtained (Cannon et al. 1979).

That enkephalin seizures in the rat are non-convulsive was the first clue that they may model petit mal epilepsy. Two recent findings by Snead and his colleagues (Snead et al. 1979; Snead and Bearden 1980) provide evidence supporting this idea. These investigators find that naloxone-sensitive leu-enkephalin seizures in the rat, having the same electrographic character as those described by our laboratory (Urca et al. 1977; Frenk et al. 1978b), are specifically blocked by drugs effective against human petit mal epilepsy. Drugs used to control human grand mal epilepsy were without effect in their study (Snead and Bearden 1980). Similarly, these authors report that seizures proposed to model petit mal epilepsy, provoked in rats by systemic administration of γ-hydroxybutyrate, are blocked by the opiate antagonists naloxone and naltrexone in moderately high doses (Snead et al. 1979). By contrast, we and others have been totally unsuccessful in blocking with opiate antagonists seizures that model grand mal epilepsy (see refs. in Lewis et al. 1981). To conclude this section, it seems that the epileptic activity of opioid peptides pharmacologically models petit mal epilepsy. It remains to be determined whether opioids are involved in the aetiology of this disease.

THE ANTICONVULSANT PROPERTIES OF OPIOID PEPTIDES

Frenk et al. (1979) reported that systemically administered morphine greatly prolonged, and naloxone greatly curtailed, the behavioural depression following convulsive seizures produced by amygdaloid stimulation in kindled rats (Holaday et al. 1978). At the same time, these drugs had no effect on the ictal phase of the seizure. It was suggested that opioids are released by ictus and are at least partly responsible for the postictal depression (Frenk et al. 1979). It was further postulated that opioids released by seizures may serve to forestall the onset or diminish the intensity of subsequent seizures (Frenk et al. 1979; Hardy et al. 1980). Some very recent evidence seems to confirm this anticonvulsant role of opioid peptides in two convulsive phenomena in rats: the first involves the amygdaloid kindling paradigm, considered to be a model of human temporal lobe epilepsy; the second deals with the clonic hind limb movements that occur in rats immediately after decapitation. We have found that these post-decapitation convulsions are diminished by acute administration of the clinically effective anti-grand mal drugs, diazepam (10 mg/kg) and phenobarbital (40 mg/kg), but not by phenytoin (40 or 100 mg/kg). In contrast, ethosuximide (300 mg/kg), an effective anti-petit mal agent, enhanced these convulsions after acute systemic administration (Cannon et al. unpublished observations).

Our principal findings in this area are the following:

Morphine, but only at high doses (>20 mg/kg), reduces the severity and/or duration of both decapitation convulsions (Cannon et al. unpublished observations) and repetitively stimulated seizures in amygdaloid kindled rats (Caldecott-Hazard et al. 1980). Naloxone blocks these opiate effects (Caldecott-Hazard et al. 1980; Cannon et al. unpublished observations). A systemically administered enkephalin analog (Eli Lilly) mimics morphine's action but is effective at a much lower dose (6 mg/kg), suggesting mediation by a receptor different from that for morphine (Caldecott-Hazard et al. 1980).

The severity of behavioural seizures in amygdaloid kindled rats is reduced by a naloxone-sensitive (opioid-mediated) form of stress analgesia, but not by a naloxone-insensitive (non-opioid) form (Shavit et al. 1982). Similarly, prior electroconvulsive shocks (ECS) reduce the severity of both the repetitive seizures (Shavit et al. 1981) and decapitation convulsions (Cannon et al. unpublished observations). That these ECS effects are also mediated by opioids is evidenced by the fact that they are partially blocked by naloxone (Cannon et al. unpublished observations; Shavit et al. 1981). These anticonvulsant effects of ECS appear to be more potent than those caused by morphine.

Naloxone given alone exacerbates decapitation convulsions (Cannon et al.

unpublished observations). This finding suggests that opioids exert a tonic suppressive action on the neural substrate mediating such convulsions. By contrast, naloxone facilitates repetitive seizures only after a series of stimulations, presumably once opioids have begun to be released in quantity by prior ictal events (Caldecott-Hazard et al. in preparation). Thus, tonic anticonvulsant effects of opioids are not obvious in this seizure model as they are after decapitation. Perhaps the spinal circuits mediating decapitation convulsions are more readily reached by circulating opioids than are the pathways mediating repetitive seizures. Consistent with this idea is the fact that adrenalectomy and adrenal demedullation enhance decapitation convulsions (Cannon et al. unpublished observations). These surgical procedures specifically block an opioid-mediated form of analgesia (Lewis et al. 1982), and appear to do so by eliminating adrenal medullary enkephalins. The suggestion that a peripheral store of opioids tonically modulates excitability in neurones mediating spinal convulsions offers intriguing possibilities for research on other convulsive phenomena and might have implications for our understanding of certain clinical epileptic states as well.

ACKNOWLEDGEMENT

Our research is supported by NIH Grant NS07628.

REFERENCES

Caldecott-Hazard, S., Ackermann, R.F., Shavit, Y., Liebeskind, J.C. and Engel, Jr., J. Anticonvulsant effects of opiates and opioids on kindled seizures in rats. Soc. Neurosci. Abstr., 1980, 6: 616.

Cannon, J.T. and Liebeskind, J.C. Descending control systems. In: R.F. Beers, Jr. and E.G. Bassett (Eds.), Mechanisms of Pain and Analgesic Compounds. Raven Press, New York, 1979: 171–184.

Cannon, J.T., Nahin, R.L., Ryan, S.M., Moskowitz, A.S. and Liebeskind, J.C. Relative analgesic and epileptic potencies of various opiate drugs. Soc. Neurosci. Abstr., 1979, 5: 190.

Elazar, Z., Motles, E., Ely, Y. and Simantov, R. Acute tolerance to the excitatory effect of enkephalin microinjections into hippocampus. Life Sci., 1979, 24: 241–248.

Frenk, H., McCarty, B.C. and Liebeskind, J.C. Different brain areas mediate analgesic and epileptic properties of enkephalin. Science, 1978a, 200: 335–337.

Frenk, H., Urca, G. and Liebeskind, J.C. Epileptic properties of leucine- and methionine-enkephalin: comparison with morphine and reversibility by naloxone. Brain Res., 1978b, 147: 327–337.

Frenk, H., Engel, Jr., J., Ackermann, R.F., Shavit, Y. and Liebeskind, J.C. Endogenous opioids may mediate post-ictal behavioral depression in amygdaloid-kindled rats. Brain Res., 1979, 167: 435–440.

Goldstein, A. Opioid peptides (endorphins) in pituitary and brain. Science, 1976, 193: 1081–1086.

Hardy, C., Panksepp, J., Rossi, III, J. and Zolovick, A.J. Naloxone facilitates amygdaloid kindled seizures in rats. Brain Res., 1980, 194: 293–297.

Henriksen, S.J., Bloom, F.E., McCoy, F., Ling, N. and Guillemin, R. Beta-endorphin induces nonconvulsive limbic seizures. Proc. nat. Acad. Sci. (Wash.), 1978, 75: 5221–5225.

Holaday, J.W., Belenky, G.L., Loh, H.H. and Meyerhoff, J.L. Evidence for endorphin release during electroconvulsive shock. Soc. Neurosci. Abstr., 1978, 4: 409.

LaBella, F.S., Havlicek, V. and Pinsky, C. Opiate-like excitatory effects of steroid sulfates and calcium-complexing agents given cerebroventricularly. Brain Res., 1979, 160: 295–305.

Lewis, J.W., Caldecott-Hazard, S., Cannon, J.T. and Liebeskind, J.C. Possible role of opioid peptides in pain inhibition and seizures. In: J.B. Martin, S. Reichlin and K.L. Bick (Eds.), Neurosecretion and Brain Peptides. Raven Press, New York, 1981: 213–224.

Lewis, J.W., Tordoff, M.G., Sherman, J.E. and Liebeskind, J.C. Adrenal medullary enkephalin-like peptides may mediate opioid stress analgesia. Science, 1982, 217: 557–559.

Lord, J.A.H., Waterfield, A.A., Hughes, J. and Kosterlitz, H.W. Endogenous opioid peptides: multiple agonists and rceeptors. Nature (Lond.), 1977, 267: 495–499.

Martin, W.R., Eades, C.G., Thompson, J.A., Huppler, R.E. and Gilbert, P.E. The effects of morphine and nalorphine-like drugs in the nondependent and morphine dependent chronic spinal dog. J. Pharmacol. exp. Ther., 1976, 197: 517–532.

Shavit, Y., Caldecott-Hazard, S. and Liebeskind, J.C. Anticonvulsant effects of electroconvulsive shock (ECS) on subsequent kindled seizures in rats. Soc. Neurosci. Abstr., 1981, 7: 579.

Shavit, Y., Caldecott-Hazard, S. and Liebeskind, J.C. The anticonvulsant effect of opioid peptides. Epilepsia, 1982, in press.

Snead, III, O.C. and Bearden, L.J. Anticonvulsants specific for petit mal antagonize epileptogenic effect of leucine enkephalin. Science, 1980, 210: 1031–1033.

Snead, III, O.C., Bearden, L.J. and Pegram, V. Response of the γ-hydroxybutyrate model of petit mal epilepsy to naloxone. Neurology (Minneap.), 1979, 29: 559.

Tortella, F.C., Moreton, J.E. and Khazan, N. Electroencephalographic and behavioral effects of D-ala[2]-methionine enkephalinamide and morphine in the rat. J. Pharmacol. exp. Ther., 1978, 206: 636–643.

Tortella, F.C., Moreton, J.E. and Khazan, N. Electroencephalographic and behavioral tolerance to and cross-tolerance between D-ala[2]-methionine-enkephalinamide and morphine in the rat. J. Pharmacol. exp. Ther., 1979, 210: 174–179.

Urca, G., Frenk, H., Liebeskind, J.C. and Taylor, A.N. Morphine and enkephalin: analgesic and epileptic properties. Science, 1977, 197: 83–86.

2. Molecular, Physiological and Morphologic Basis of Impaired Nerve Conduction

Kyoto Symposia (EEG Suppl. No. 36)
Editors: P.A. Buser, W.A. Cobb and T. Okuma
© 1982, Elsevier Biomedical Press, Amsterdam

The Morphometric Composition of Myelinated Fibres by Nerve, Level and Species Related to Nerve Microenvironment and Ischaemia*

PETER JAMES DYCK, JEANNINE KARNES, MARGARET SPARKS and PHILLIP A. LOW

Peripheral Nerve Laboratory, Mayo Clinic and Mayo Foundation, Rochester, Minn. 55905 (U.S.A.)

To understand the function, structure and pathological alterations of the peripheral nervous system one must evaluate not only the neural constituents (axons and supporting cells) but also their microenvironment. In nerve microenvironment we include the interstitial (endoneurial) fluid, the endoneurial barriers (perineurial, blood-nerve and other) and the blood supply. Early anatomists and neuropathologists emphasized anatomical differences at several peripheral neurone levels. Krücke (1955), reviewing this subject, lists a central (spinal cord) level, a root level, a root-nerve level (from exit of root through the dura to beginning of spinal ganglion), a ganglionic level and a peripheral nerve level. Some functional and morphological differences in microenvironment are characteristic for these levels. At the central level the amount of extracellular space is meagre – much less than at the other levels considered. At the root level the amount of interstitial fluid is increased. Here the fibres are separated from the cerebrospinal fluid (CSF) only by pia. The exact implications of this are not yet known, but possibly cerebrospinal fluid might act as a sink and prevent accumulation of metabolites in interstitial fluid. The root-nerve level has not yet been extensively studied. Such tracers as anionic dyes, bovine albumin and horseradish peroxidase (HRP) appear to pass freely between capillary endothelial cells in the spinal ganglion and possibly also at the root level (Waksman 1961; Malmgren and Olsson 1980). The fibres in nerve trunks, on the other hand, are protected by several dynamic barriers, notably the perineurial and capillary endothelial barriers (Olsson 1975).

Peripheral nerve fibres and their supporting cells receive their metabolic requirements and presumably rid themselves of waste products through 2 channels. The first is the axonal transport system (Malmgren and Olsson 1980). Macromolecules and enzymes synthesized in the perikaryon are transported to distal sites of utilization. Other materials from the periphery are transported back to the cell body. Axonal integrity and size are in part maintained by this axonal transport system (Ochs 1975). The second channel is through endoneurial capillaries and endoneurial fluid. This route must be especially important for cation and energy metabolism and remains largely unexplored.

---

* This investigation was supported in part by a Peripheral Neuropathy Clinical Center Grant from NINCDS (NS14304), a Center Grant from MDA (12), and Mayo, Borchard, Upton, and Gallagher Funds.

For the endoneurial space, perineurium offers a virtually complete barrier to bovine albumin and to HRP (Olsson 1975). Capillary endothelial cells of the endoneurium, because of their tight junctions, appear to inhibit albumin and HRP permeability, at least for adult nerves of most species (Malmgren and Olsson 1980). A small amount of HRP is probably transported through the endothelial cytoplasm by pinocytosis and is quickly taken up by macrophages (Lasek and Hoffman 1976; Dyck et al. 1980).

The nerve microenvironment is altered in various pathological states and may be involved in the mechanisms of fibre degeneration. A good example of such a relationship is the role of ischaemia in fibre degeneration in necrotizing angiopathic neuropathy. In this disorder a patchy central fascicular fibre degeneration, beginning at levels of poor perfusion, has been related to widespread focal occluded epineurial arterioles.

The role of the microenvironment for normal function and structure of nerve was further underscored by the observation that segmental demyelination developed after making an endoneurial window (Spencer et al. 1975). Subsequently it was shown that endoneurial fluid (EF) in healthy nerve is under a low pressure (Low et al. 1977). The segmental demyelination from the perineurial window may therefore relate to damage to fibres from shear forces near the window. An alteration of nerve microenvironment has also been apparent in neuropathies with oedema (Nichols et al. 1968; Sharma et al. 1976; Ohnishi et al. 1977; Powell and Lampert 1979), seen in man in Dejerine-Sottas disease (Dyck 1975), in inflammatory-demyelinating polyradiculoneuropathy (Dyck et al. 1968), in some patients with diabetic neuropathy (Thomas and Eliasson 1975), in acromegaly (Low et al. 1974), myxoedema (Nickel and Frame 1958), xanthomatosis (Thomas 1973, personal communication) and in other neuropathies. It is also a prominent feature in experimental neuropathies due to lead (Ohnishi et al. 1977), hexachlorophene (Powell and Lampert 1979) and galactose (Sharma et al. 1976). When measured, neuropathic disorders with oedema can also be shown to have raised endoneurial fluid pressure (EFP) (Low and Dyck 1977). Increased EFP has now been documented for several experimental neuropathies with oedema (Low and Dyck 1977; Powell et al. 1979a,b) but the pressure itself probably does not account for the fibre pathology. The degree of pressure depends not only on the rate of entry of fluid but also on the properties of the perineurium itself (Low et al. 1980). Equivalent degrees of pressure and oedema in lead and galactose neuropathy result in different types and amounts of fibre pathology indicating different underlying mechanisms.

The approach used here is to characterize morphometrically the number and diameter distribution of MFs and the myelinated fibre percentage of transverse endoneurial area (MF percentage area) considering species, nerve, level of nerve and age of animal. In particular we were interested in knowing whether, in transverse sections of nerve, the non-MF percentage of endoneurial area (an index of the amount of endoneurial fluid) was greater in peripheral nerve than root, was progressively greater toward the periphery, was greater with increasing age for a given level of nerve, and was greater in peripheral neuropathy. The results of this survey have shown that there are striking differences in fibre composition between different nerves (a fact extensively documented previously) with different levels of nerve, with age, and with species. These data may be found useful in considering the role of the microenvironment in health and disease.

THE MORPHOMETRIC COMPOSITION OF MYELINATED FIBRES BY NERVE, LEVEL AND SPECIES RELATED TO NERVE MICROENVIRONMENT

(A) Morphometric approaches

The number and size of myelinated fibres (MFs) of peripheral nerve trunks and fibre tracts have been measured almost since the advent of the light microscope, but earlier results varied so widely that their correctness could reasonably be questioned. With the use of good methodology (Dyck and Karnes 1981) it was possible to relate the peaks of diameter histograms to peaks of the compound action potentials (Erlander and Gasser 1933), to relate a selective sensory loss to degeneration or loss of a size category of an axon population (Dyck et al. 1971b; Lambert and Dyck 1975), to recognize nerve enlargement (Dyck et al. 1965), and oedema (Ohnishi et al. 1977) and to identify axon atrophy (Dyck et al. 1971a; Jakobsen 1976) or shrinkage (Dyck et al. 1981).

We have recently listed the reasons for the improved accuracy and reproducibility of morphometric measurements now possible (Dyck and Karnes 1981). These include improved fixation, selective staining of tissue components (e.g. myelin), use of improved embedding media and knives to make thin sections both for light and electron microscopic (EM) measurement, use of the electron microscope, especially for measurement of unmyelinated fibres and for ultrastructural relationships and for evaluation of cellular organelles, use of systematic sampling, use of larger numbers of nerves so that results could be statistically evaluated and use of specialized hardware and software in a computerized imaging system to tally, size and assess the shape of myelinated fibres.

The imaging system we have developed employs algorithms which automatically identify most MFs, border their inner myelin edge, and evaluate average myelin thickness (Zimmerman et al. 1980). The system is operator interactive so that an experienced observer can check results for accuracy of identification and bordering and can override the instrument in case of error. The system allows complete flexibility of analysis of results as all measurements for each fibre are individually stored.

(B) Material and methods

The nerves used were obtained for various other studies. Generally, the fixation and histological processing were comparable and consisted of fixation in slightly hyperosmolar glutaraldehyde in cacodylate buffer at pH 7.4, followed after washing in isosmolar buffer, by further fixation in isosmolar osmium tetroxide and embedding in epoxy. For animal nerves fixation was by whole body perfusion using a peristaltic pump or by in situ fixation. Human sural nerves were obtained in the operating room and immersed immediately in fixatives. For human nerve roots and large nerves, post-mortem specimens, usually obtained within 8 h of death, were obtained from patients who died of causes not known to be associated with peripheral neuropathy. For large nerves the specimen was split longitudinally and embedded in multiple epoxy blocks. Transverse sections were cut at 3/4 μm, and stained with phenylenediamine.

All of the analyses were performed by computer imaging. Initially the transverse fascicular area of nerve was obtained by tracing the outer edge of the endoneurial tissue. For small nerves every fascicle was used for analysis. For large nerves such as the segmental, sciatic and peroneal nerves, systematic sampling of fascicles and of microscopic frames within fascicles was employed. The first fascicle or frame within a fascicle to be analysed was chosen by chance. Thereafter, the fascicle or frame for analysis was taken at regular intervals in an x and y traverse of the section. Each MF profile in a frame was tallied, the inner edge of myelin bordered and myelin thickness determined by algorithms previously described. The diameter of an MF was calculated by taking the diameter of a circle whose area was equal to the measured area of the axon plus the measured area of myelin. The number of MFs per mm^2 of nerve was then derived and diameter histograms, using an exponential plot, were drawn.

(C) Results

To conserve space, only one representative MF diameter histogram will be drawn for the transverse section of a nerve. The single lines projecting downward from the baseline of the histogram show from left to right, the first percentile of the range of diameter, the position of the first peak, the position of the second peak, the position of the third peak (if a third peak is shown), and the 99th percentile of the range of diameters. The median diameter is shown by the short double lines. For some nerves the position of the peaks is not shown because of uncertainty regarding the number and location of peaks. For each of the nerves the MF percentage of endoneurial area is given in a column in the right hand column. The convention of showing only the baseline for other nerves conserves space and permits visual comparison of all the histograms. Mean values are shown in a mean distribution baseline at the bottom of the figure indicated by an asterisk.

Cat nerves

The MFs of ventral spinal root (VSR, n = 6, Fig. 1), of S1 segmental nerve (n = 23, Fig. 2), of peroneal nerve just above the knee (n = 12, Fig. 3), of proximal (midthigh) sural nerve (n = 6, Fig. 4), and of distal sural nerve (n = 6, Fig. 5) have been assessed.

The MFs of L5 VSR of the cat range in diameter from 2.3 to 18.3 μm with a median diameter of 12.1 μm. The non-MF percentage of area averages 53.2%. The 3 peaks occur at 3.9, 4.6 and 14.8 μm. These might be identified as axons small (A_s), axons intermediate (A_i) and axons large (A_l). The morphometric values of S1 segmental nerves of cat are shown in Fig. 2. As compared to VSR, the range is similar but because of a higher proportion of small to large fibres the median diameter is smaller (8 μm as compared to 12.1 μm). The non-MF percentage of area averaged 39.2%.

The morphometric values of peroneal nerve of the cat are not unlike those of the segmental nerve.

The MF diameter histograms of sural nerve of the cat are different from those shown above in that the range of diameters is less (2–14.2 μm) and median diameters are smaller.

In comparing the proximal (midthigh) and distal sural nerve several important differences are seen. The large axon (A_l) peak and the value of the P99 diameter

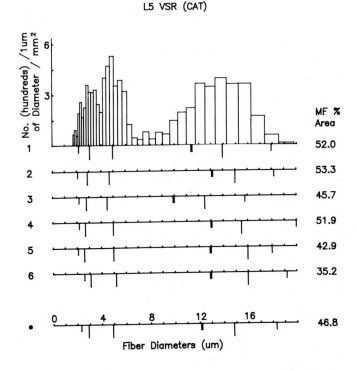

Fig. 1. See text for description.

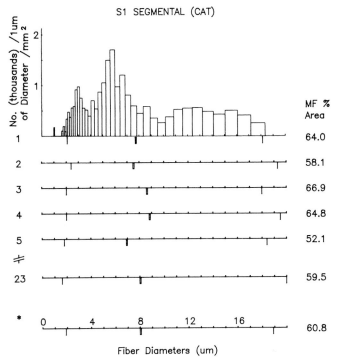

Fig. 2. See text for description.

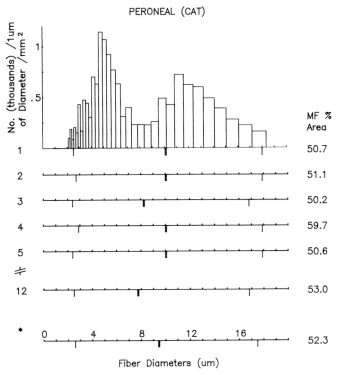

Fig. 3. See text for description.

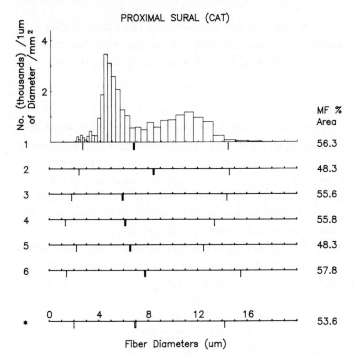

Fig. 4. See text for description.

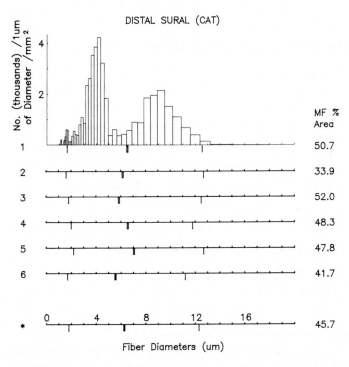

Fig. 5. See text for description.

range is higher proximally (10.5 and 14.2 μm, respectively) than distally (9.3 and 12.3 μm, respectively), evidence for axon tapering. Note also that the non-MF percentage area is lower for proximal (46.4%) than for distal nerve (54.3%), with obvious overlap of values.

Human nerves

The diameter histogram of human L5 VSR is different from that of cat in several important respects. The large diameter fibre peak and the P99 value of the diameter range of man (11.8 and 16.2 μm, respectively) are smaller than in cat (14.8 and 18.3 μm). In some, but not all, histograms 3 distinct peaks A_l (large), A_i (intermediate), and A_s (small) are seen, as illustrated in Fig. 6. The A_l peak is thought to be made up mostly of alpha motor neurone axons, A_i of gamma motor neurone axons and A_s of pre-ganglionic autonomic neurone axons.

The histograms for human L5 segmental nerve and peroneal nerve are quite similar to each other (Figs. 7 and 8). These and the other histograms of human nerves to follow are strikingly different from what has been found for other nerves of mammals and frogs in that they have a much higher non-MF percentage area.

The diameter histograms of sural nerves from midcalf and ankle levels are almost identical (Figs. 9 and 10). From proximal to distal along the length of nerves and ignoring nerves with different fibre classes the non-MF percentage area rises progressively from proximal to distal – 41.9%, 69.1%, 65.7%, 73.3% and 77.6%. The mean diameter of MFs decreases from 11.4 to 5.3, to 5.1, to 3.7 and to 4.1 μm.

Rat nerves

The diameter histograms of MFs of sural nerves of midcalf and ankle level are

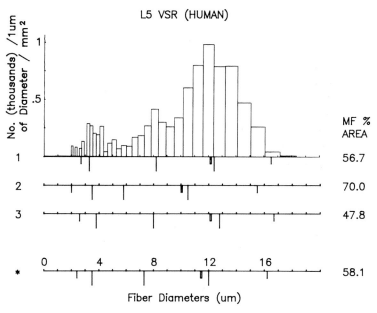

Fig. 6. See text for description.

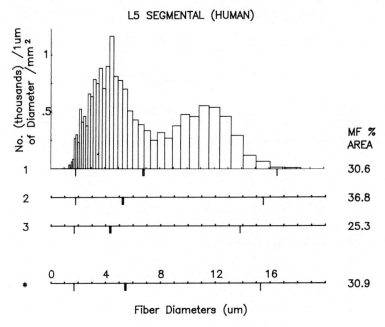

Fig. 7. See text for description.

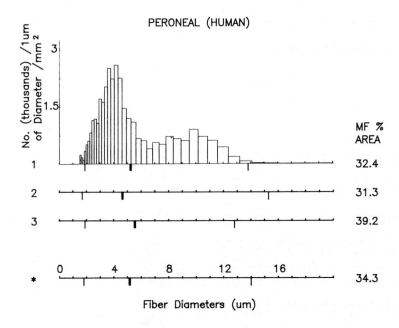

Fig. 8. See text for description.

almost identical (Figs. 11 and 12). The non-MF percentage area for the 2 levels is 46.8 and 50.4% respectively.

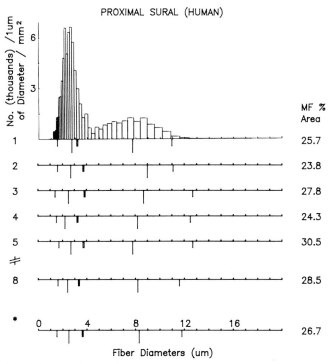

Fig. 9. See text for description.

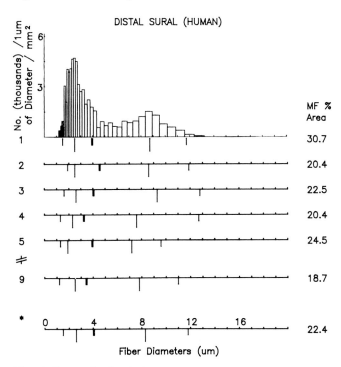

Fig. 10. See text for description.

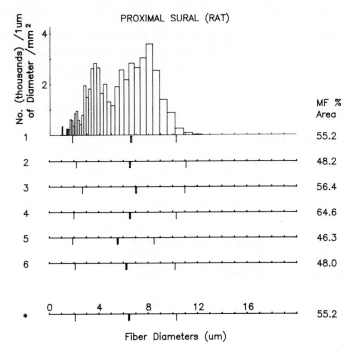

Fig. 11. See text for description.

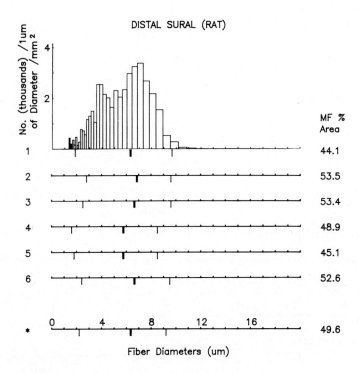

Fig. 12. See text for description.

Frog nerves

A few frog nerves were assessed because they share the prolonged resistance to ischaemia in vitro with human sural nerve. They did not have the small median diameter of MFs or the high non-MF percentage area of human sural nerve (Figs. 13–16).

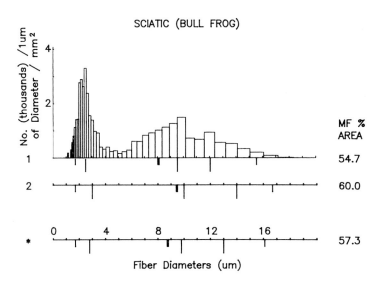

Fig. 13. See text for description.

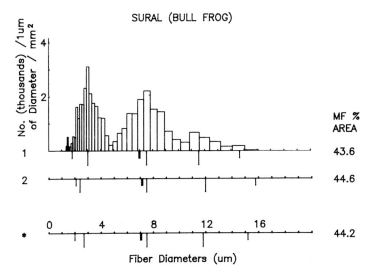

Fig. 14. See text for description.

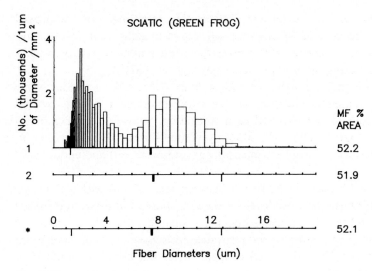

Fig. 15. See text for description.

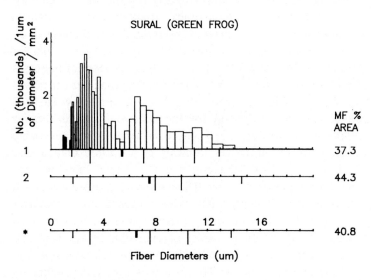

Fig. 16. See text for description.

(D) Discussion

The present work provides descriptive information on the number and size distribution of MFs of various nerves, of various proximal to distal levels of nerves, and of various species. These results show differences between nerves, between levels of nerve and between species in the number and size distributions (Erlander and Gasser 1933; Boyd and Davey 1968). These differences will not be discussed here or related to previously published data although the morphometric results provided should be as reliable as are now available because of the use of optimal histological processing, of extensive systematic sampling, of improved morphometric approaches, and of operator-interactive imaging. The results have provided histograms with reproducible peaks which are similar to our previously published histograms using other approaches (Dyck et al. 1971b).

The evaluation of the non-MF percentage area (NMFA%) provides some information, albeit imperfect, bearing on the nerve microenvironment. Several constituents contribute to the non-MF area, including: Schwann cell cytoplasm (SCC) outside of compact myelin, SCC of unmyelinated fibres (UF), UF, collagen, cells (endothelial, pericyte, fibroblast, macrophage and mast cell) and endoneurial fluid.

Our results show differences in NMFA% between species, and within the same species there are differences between levels of the same nerve and between different nerves. The large NMFA% in distal segments suggests that the increase in endoneurial space may be related to the resistance to ischaemic conduction block (RICB), perhaps by providing dissolved oxygen, better buffering of ionic pH or other physiological alterations.

The differences of NMFA% between species is clearly not the sole or a major mechanism of RICB. These mechanisms are complex; in addition to endoneurial buffering the following should also be considered. (1) Interspecies differences in O_2 consumption. Frog nerve resting O_2 consumption is only one-fourth that of mammalian nerves (Okada and McDougal 1971) and the time constant of increases and decreases in consumption with stress is far longer for frog than for rat nerves (Cranefield et al. 1957). Wright (1946) considered that the product of nerve survival time and oxygen uptake rate was a constant for the numerous species that he studied. (2) Differences in energy substrate stores. Glycogen levels in frog nerves are reported to be twice those of rabbit nerves (Stewart et al. 1965; Okada and McDougal 1971) and winter frogs, which have greater RICB than summer frogs (Fenn 1930), have much higher glycogen stores (Okada and McDougal 1971). (3) Alterations in energy utilization in ischaemic states. When power failure is imminent neuronal activity becomes greatly reduced before substrate stores are fully depleted (Stewart et al. 1965; Duffy et al. 1972). (4) Roles of anaerobic metabolism and pentose shunt. Peripheral nerve derives energy from anaerobic (Okada and McDougal 1971) as well as aerobic sources. The former is highly dependent on glycogen and glucose stores. The role of the pentose shunt in nerve is controversial but may contribute at least 16% of glucose metabolism at rest (Härkönen and Kauffman 1974). With a reduction in energy requirements in ischaemia such minor pathways may assume more important roles. (5) Electrolyte and pH alterations, especially potassium accumulation, have been considered to be important mechanisms in RICB (Shanes 1951). (6) Ionic gradients are maintained by the Na^+-K^+-ATPase enzyme system. There are major species differences. (7) Elimination mechanisms for K^+ accumulation have been studied in brain (Cordingley and Somjen 1978). Similar studies have not yet been performed on peripheral nerve. The elimination of metabolites in peripheral nerve may be of importance in RICB but no information is thus far available. (8) There appear to be important differences in lipid (or lipid-protein) compositions between frog and mammalian nerves (Chiu et al. 1979a). (9) There are entirely different distributions and densities of sodium and potassium channels in mammalian and amphibian nodes of Ranvier (Chiu et al. 1979b). (10) The blood-nerve barrier of frog peripheral nerve is markedly deficient compared to mammalian nerves (Krnjević 1954).

SUMMARY

An extensive morphometric evaluation of the number, density and diameter distribution of myelinated fibres (MFs) of different nerves, of different proximal-distal levels of nerves, and of different species is reported. The methodology used provides reliable estimates of number and size because of the use of optimal histological techniques, semi-thin sections, careful systematic sampling, non-subjective evaluation of transverse MF profiles using computerized imaging and evaluation of large numbers of MFs and nerves. The non-MF percentage of endoneurial area was also measured as an index of the amount of nerve microenvironment. We have confirmed that the MF composition is quite variable between nerves, between levels of nerves, and between species. In general the density of MFs is lower in the nerves of man than in the nerves of other animals evaluated, in distal than in proximal levels, in old age and in disease. Although increased endoneurial fluid may play a role in resistance to ischaemic block it appears that the intrinsic metabolic properties of the neural tissue itself are most important.

REFERENCES

Boyd, I.A. and Davey, M.R. Composition of Peripheral Nerves. Livingston, Edinburgh, 1968: 57 pp.

Chiu, S.Y., Mrose, H.E. and Ritchie, J.M. Anomalous temperature dependence of sodium conductance in rabbit nerve compared with frog nerve. Nature (Lond.), 1979a, 279: 327–328.

Chiu, S.Y., Ritchie, J.M., Rogart, R.B. and Stagg, D. A quantitative description of membrane currents in rabbit myelinated nerve. J. Physiol. (Lond.), 1979b, 292: 149–166.

Cordingley, G.E. and Somjen, G.G. The clearing of excess potassium from extracellular space in spinal cord and cerebral cortex. Brain Res., 1978, 151: 291–306.

Cranefield, P.F., Brink, F. and Bronk, D.W. The oxygen uptake of the peripheral nerve of the rat. J. Neurochem., 1957, 1: 245–249.

Duffy, T.E., Nelson, S.R. and Lowry, O.H. Cerebral carbohydrate metabolism during acute hypoxia and recovery. J. Neurochem., 1972, 19: 959–977.

Dyck, P.J. Inherited neuronal degeneration and atrophy affecting peripheral motor, sensory, and autonomic neurons. In: P.J. Dyck, P.K. Thomas and E.H. Lambert (Eds.), Peripheral Neuropathy. Saunders, Philadelphia, Pa., 1975: 825–867.

Dyck, P.J. and Karnes, J. Computer imaging for morphometry of neuron columns and fiber tracts in neurobiology and pathology. Trends Neurosci., 1981, 4: 138–141.

Dyck, P.J., Beahrs, O.H. and Miller, R.H. Peripheral nerves in hereditary neural atrophies: number and diameters of myelinated fibers. Paper presented at the 6th International Congress of Electroencephalography and Clinical Neurophysiology, Vienna, Austria, 1965.

Dyck, P.J., Gutrecht, J.A., Bastron, J.A., Karnes, W.E. and Dale, A.J.D. Histologic and teased fiber measurements of sural nerve in disorders of lower motor and primary sensory neurons. Mayo Clin. Proc., 1968, 43: 81–123.

Dyck, P.J., Johnson, W.J., Lambert, E.H. and O'Brien, P.C. Segmental demyelination secondary to axonal degeneration in uremic neuropathy. Mayo Clin. Proc., 1971a, 46: 400–431.

Dyck, P.J., Lambert, E.H. and Nichols, P.C. Quantitative measurement of sensation related to compound action potential and number and sizes of myelinated and unmyelinated fibers of sural nerves in health, Friedreich's ataxia, hereditary sensory neuropathy, and tabes dorsalis. In: A. Rémond (Ed.), Handbook of Electroencephalography and Clinical Neurophysiology, Vol. 9. Elsevier, Amsterdam, 1971b: 83–118.

Dyck, P.J., Windebank, A.J., Low, P.A. and Baumann, W.J. Blood nerve barrier in rat and cellular mechanisms of lead-induced segmental demyelination. J. Neuropath. exp. Neurol., 1980, 39: 700–709.

Dyck, P.J., Lambert, E.H., Windebank, A.J., Lais, A.C., Sparks, M.F., Karnes, J., Sherman, W.R., Hallcher, L.M., Low, P.A. and Service, F.J. Acute hyperosmolar hyperglycemia causes axonal shrinkage and reduced nerve conduction velocity. Exp. Neurol., 1981, 71: 507–514.

Erlander, J. and Gasser, H.S. Electrical Signs of Nervous Activity. University of Pennsylvania Press, Philadelphia, Pa., 1933.

Fenn, W.O. Anaerobic oxygen debt of frog nerve. Amer. J. Physiol., 1930, 92: 349–361.

Härkönen, M.H. and Kauffman, F.C. Metabolic alterations in the axotomized superior cervical ganglion of the rat. II. The pentose phosphate pathway. Brain Res., 1974, 65: 141–157.

Jacobs, J.M., Macfarlane, R.M. and Cavanagh, J.B. Vascular leakage in the dorsal root ganglia of the rat, studied with horseradish peroxidase. J. neurol. Sci., 1976, 29: 95–107.

Jakobsen, J. Axonal dwindling in early experimental diabetes. I. A study of cross sectioned nerves. Diabetologie, 1976, 12: 539–546.

Krnjević, K. The connective tissue of the frog sciatic nerve. Quart. J. exp. Physiol., 1954, 39: 55–72.

Krücke, W. Erkrankungen der peripheren Nerven. In: G. Doring, E. Herzog, W. Krücke and H. Orthner (Eds.), Handbuch der Speziellen Pathologischen Anatomie und Histologie, XII/5. Springer, Berlin, 1955: 1–203.

Lambert, E.H. and Dyck, P.J. Compound action potentials of sural nerve in vitro in peripheral neuropathy. In: P.J. Dyck, P.K. Thomas and E.H. Lambert (Eds.), Peripheral Neuropathy. Saunders, Philadelphia, Pa., 1975: 427–441.

Lasek, R.J. and Hoffman, P.N. The neuronal cytoskeleton, axonal transport, and axonal growth. In: R. Goldman, T. Pollard and J. Rosenbaum (Eds.), Cell Motility. Cold Spring Harbor Lab., Long Island, N.Y., 1976: 1021–1049.

Low, P.A. and Dyck, P.J. Increased endoneurial fluid pressure in experimental lead neuropathy. Nature (Lond.), 1977, 269: 427–428.

Low, P.A., McLeod, J.G., Turtle, J.R., Donelly, P. and Wright, R.A. Peripheral neuropathy in acromegaly. Brain, 1974, 97: 139–152.

Low, P., Marchand, G., Knox, F. and Dyck, P.J. Measurement of endoneurial fluid pressure with polyethylene matrix capsules. Brain Res., 1977, 122: 373–377.

Low, P.A., Dyck, P.J. and Schmelzer, J.D. Mammalian peripheral nerve sheath has unique responses to chronic elevations of endoneurial fluid pressure. Exp. Neurol., 1980, 70: 300–306.

Malmgren, L.T. and Olsson, Y. Differences between the peripheral and the central nervous system in permeability to sodium fluorescein. J. comp. Neurol., 1980, 191: 103–117.

Nichols, P.C., Dyck, P.J. and Miller, D.R. Experimental hypertrophic neuropathy: change in fascicular area and fiber spectrum after acute crush injury. Mayo Clin. Proc., 1968, 43: 297–305.

Nickel, S.N. and Frame, B. Neurologic manifestations of myxedema. Neurology (Minneap.), 1958, 8: 511.

Ochs, S. Axoplasmic transport. In: P.J. Dyck, P.K. Thomas and E.H. Lambert (Eds.), Peripheral Neuropathy. Saunders, Philadelphia, Pa., 1975: 213–230.

Ohnishi, A., Schilling, K., Brimijoin, W.S., Lambert, E.H., Fairbanks, V.F. and Dyck, P.J. Lead neuropathy. 1. Morphometry, nerve conduction and choline acetyltransferase transport: new findings of endoneurial edema associated with segmental demyelination. J. Neuropath. exp. Neurol., 1977, 36: 499–518.

Okada, Y. and McDougal, J.N.R. Physiological and biochemical changes in frog sciatic nerve during anoxia and recovery. J. Neurochem., 1971, 18: 2335–2353.

Olsson, Y. Topographical differences in the vascular permeability of the peripheral nervous system. Acta neuropath., 1968, 10: 26–33.

Olsson, Y. Vascular permeability in periheral nervous system. In: P.J. Dyck, P.K. Thomas and E.H. Lambert (Eds.), Peripheral Neuropathy. Saunders, Philadelphia, Pa., 1975: 190–200.

Powell, H.C. and Lampert, P.W. Hexachlorophene toxicity. In: P.J. Vinken and G.W. Bruyn (Eds.), Handbook of Clinical Neurology, Vol. 37, Part II. Elsevier/North-Holland, Amsterdam, 1979: Ch. 16.

Powell, H.C., Meyers, R.R., Costello, M.L. and Lampert, P.W. Endoneurial fluid pressure in Wallerian degeneration. Ann. Neurol., 1979a, 5: 550–557.

Powell, H.C., Meyers, R.R. and Costello, M.L. Endoneurial fluid pressure (EFP) and pathologic findings in galactose neuropathy. J. Neuropath. exp. Neurol., 1979b, 38: 335.

Shanes, A.M. Potassium movement in relation to nerve activity. J. gen. Physiol., 1951, 34: 795–807.

Sharma, A.K., Thomas, P.K. and Baker, R.W.R. Peripheral nerve abnormalities related to galactose administration in rats. J. Neurol. Neurosurg. Psychiat., 1976, 39: 794–802.

Spencer, P.S., Weinberg, H.J., Raine, C.S. and Prineas, J.W. The perineurial window – a model of focal demyelination and remyelination. Brain Res., 1975, 96: 323–329.

Stewart, M.A., Passonneau, J.V. and Lowry, O.H. Substrate changes in peripheral nerve during ischemia and Wallerian degeneration. J. Neurochem., 1965, 12: 719–727.

Thomas, P.K. and Eliasson, S.G. Diabetic neuropathy. In: P.J. Dyck, P.K. Thomas and E.H. Lambert (Eds.), Peripheral Neuropathy. Saunders, Philadelphia, Pa., 1975: 956–981.

Waksman, B.H. Experimental study of diphtheritic polyneuropathy in the rabbit and guinea pig. III. The blood nerve barrier in the rabbit. J. Neuropath., 1961, 20: 35.

Wright, E.B. A comparative study of the effects of oxygen lack on peripheral nerve. Amer. J. Physiol., 1946, 147: 78–89.

Zimmerman, I.R., Karnes, J.L., O'Brien, P.C. and Dyck, P.J. Imaging system for nerve and fiber tract morphometry: components, approaches, performance, and results. J. Neuropath. exp. Neurol., 1980, 39: 409–419.

Kyoto Symposia (EEG Suppl. No. 36)
Editors: P.A. Buser, W.A. Cobb and T. Okuma
© 1982, Elsevier Biomedical Press, Amsterdam

56

Immune-Mediated Demyelination – Immunopathological Basis for Electrophysiological Changes

TAKAHIKO SAIDA and KYOKO SAIDA

Department of Neurology and Clinical Research Center, Utano National Hospital, Kyoto 616 (Japan)

Local and generalized demyelinating neuropathies are important causes of human peripheral nerve disorders (Dyck et al. 1975). Diagnosis is frequently made by electromyographic demonstration of slowed conduction velocities or the presence of conduction block at the site of a lesion. Functional and electrophysiological recovery after a demyelinating neuropathy is usually very good, presumably because remyelination occurs around demyelinated but otherwise intact axons. However, the relationship between electrophysiological and morphological changes is incompletely understood. There are several studies concerning the relationship between electrophysiological and morphological changes in various experimental demyelinating neuropathies (Hall 1967; McDonald 1968; Morgan-Hughes 1968; Aguayo 1971; Fowler et al. 1972) on which information has been acquired from population studies on nerves with somewhat heterogeneous lesions. Although present experimental techniques do not allow study of both electrophysiological function and ultrastructural morphology in the same demyelinated axon, the focal demyelinating lesions induced by single injection of immune serum provide a better system for such correlative studies because the demyelinating lesions are homogenous and monophasic, progressing synchronously throughout the affected nerve. The time course of electrophysiological and morphological changes in this experimental model is predictable from animal to animal.

The present paper describes the sequential morphological evolution of demyelination resulting from subperineurial injection of serum from animals with experimental allergic neuritis (EAN), experimental allergic encephalomyelitis (EAE) and serum from animals sensitized with galactocerebroside (GC). The discussion concerns the immunopathological aspects of demyelination and chronologic evolution of demyelination in relation to electrophysiological changes.

MATERIALS AND METHODS

Male New Zealand albino rabbits weighing 2.3–2.7 kg were used to produce antisera. Sera were obtained from rabbits immunized with homogenized bovine white matter in complete Freund's adjuvant (CFA) to produce EAE (T. Saida et al. 1979a), with homogenized bovine peripheral nerve and CFA to produce EAN (K.

Address correspondence and reprint requests to Dr. T. Saida.

Saida et al. 1978a; T. Saida et al. 1978b), and with purified GC plus bovine serum albumin (BSA) in CFA (K. Saida et al. 1979; T. Saida et al. 1979b, 1981b) to produce anti-GC antibodies. Previous work demonstrated that the demyelinating activity in peripheral nerve induced by these sera correlated well with anti-GC antibody titre in each serum, and patterns of demyelination produced by the 3 sera could not be distinguished from one another (K. Saida et al. 1978a, 1979; T. Saida et al. 1978b, 1979a; Hahn et al. 1980). For this study we selected for injection 3 of each antiserum, all with anti-GC antibody titres of 1:128 or greater as measured by agglutination of liposomes containing GC (K. Saida et al. 1979; T. Saida et al. 1979b). Control sera were obtained from 8 rabbits inoculated with BSA, CFA, and saline (K. Saida et al. 1978a, 1979; T. Saida et al. 1979a).

Male Wistar rats weighing 200–350 g were used as recipients. Twenty to 50 μl of EAE serum, EAN serum, or anti-GC antiserum (subsequently referred to collectively as antiserum) were mixed with 20% fresh guinea pig serum (v/v) as a source of complement and were injected into the subperineurial portion of one sciatic nerve. An equal volume of control serum similarly mixed with guinea pig serum was injected into the opposite side. The method of injection is described elsewhere (K. Saida et al. 1978a). Injected rats were examined daily for signs of leg or foot weakness, and a quantitative assessment of the clinical state was recorded.

At least 2 animals were studied at each of the following times after injection: 20 min, 1 h, 3 h, 5 h, 8 h, 15 h, 1, 2, 3, 5, 7, 8, 10, 14, 21, 28, and 37 days. Following pentobarbital anaesthesia, rat sciatic nerves were fixed in situ for 5 min with 3.6% glutaraldehyde/phosphate buffered solution at pH 7.4. Some rats were perfused through the ascending aorta with physiological saline followed by 3.6% glutaraldehyde solution. The sciatic nerves were excised, dissected into 4 portions, fixed in 3.6% glutaraldehyde solution for 2 h, and washed overnight in phosphate buffered solution. Tissues were then postfixed with 2% osmium tetroxide for 2 h, dehydrated in graded ethanol and propylene oxide, and embedded in epoxy. Toluidine blue-stained cross-sections, 1 μm thick, were prepared and studied by light microscopy. Ultrathin sections were double stained with uranyl acetate and lead citrate and were examined with an electron microscope.

For single fibre studies, nerve segments were postfixed in 2% osmium tetroxide for 4 h, then placed in 66% glycerin solution and examined after 2 days. Fibres were teased onto glass slides in a droplet of creosote, overlaid with a Permount coverslip, and examined with the light microscope.

RESULTS

Clinical features

Most rats appeared normal on awakening from anaesthesia. After 2 or 3 h, slight weakness of feet and toes was noted on the side injected with antiserum. At 5 h all rats lost reflex toe spreading and developed paresis of toe abduction, adduction and flexion, instability of the ankle, and decreased response to pin prick on the antiserum-injected side. The disability persisted for at least 7 days following injection. Between days 7 and 14, all animals showed gradual daily improvement in toe and ankle movements. Reflex toe spreading returned about 10 days after injection. By 14 days, most rats walked normally with apparent full return of foot and ankle strength. By 16 days, all had attained complete clinical recovery. The control serum-injected hind limbs did not show evidence of weakness throughout the observation period.

Macroscopic features

Gross examination at the time of dissection revealed that the sciatic nerve segment early after injection of antiserum was slightly pink and swollen. No herniation of nerve through the perineurium was seen. In cross-section, antiserum-injected nerves appeared darker and more transparent than normal. Dilated vessels and punctate haemorrhages were not infrequent after 1 or 2 days of antiserum injection. Macroscopic observation 7 days after the injection revealed only a mild increase of epineurial connective tissue. The microscopic lesion within injected nerves ranged between 1 and 2 cm in length, extending both proximal and distal to the injection site. In most cases the lesion occupied 80–90% of the cross-sectional area of the fascicle, but at times the entire fascicle was affected (Fig. 1). At the proximal and distal ends of the lesion, demyelinated fibres were seen most frequently at the

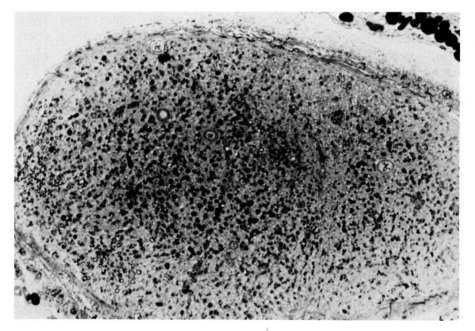

Fig. 1. Cross-section of rat sciatic nerve 10 days after intraneural injection of antiserum. The demyelinating lesion, identified by paleness of staining and numerous dark, punctate, lipid-filled macrophages, occupies all but the left portion of the fascicle (toluidine blue, ×230).

subperineurial portion of the fascicle. Control serum-injected nerves did not show demyelinating changes and generally appeared normal.

Despite unavoidable variations in injection technique, there was great uniformity in the extent and character of the demyelinating lesions among nerves from different animals killed on the same day.

General microscopic features

All injected nerve fascicles, both experimental and control, shared certain background changes. Small endoneurial haemorrhages were seen on occasion in association with separation of perineurium from the endoneurium. Along the needle track, several myelin sheaths were crushed, sometimes with aggregation or absence of axonal organelles. A few demyelinated axons were also present in the lesion. The area of the needle artifact generally occupied less than 10% of the fascicular area and extended proximally for only a few millimeters. Infiltration into endoneurium of a few polymorphonuclear cells and degranulation of mast cells were encountered on rare occasions. Endothelial cells of endoneurial vessels were found to be swollen after 8 h. At 2 days polymorphonuclear cells and monocytes infiltrated the epineurium to varying degrees.

Microscopic features of control serum-injected nerves

Schwann cells and nerve fibres were generally normal 20 min to 7 days after injection of control serum. On occasion we found minimal changes of Schwann cell cytoplasm, consisting of mild dilatation of ER and swelling of mitochondria, during the first 8 h after injection of control serum. Several demyelinated fibres were sometimes found on careful search.

Sequential morphological observations on nerves injected with antiserum

Twenty minutes

Twenty minutes after antiserum injection, the earliest time of pathological examination, ultrastructural changes of Schwann cells were identified in regions away from the injection site. Some Schwann cells associated with smaller myelinated fibres had mildly dilated endoplasmic reticulum (ER) and swollen mitochondria. Others showed slight opening of their external mesaxons. Occasionally, Schwann cells distant from the injection site showed mushroom-shaped or irregular outfoldings of their plasma membrane. Schwann cell processes surrounding unmyelinated fibres at times retracted from their basement membranes, and axons became bared over part of their circumferences.

One to five hours

Between 1 and 5 h after antiserum injection, the nerves had subtle changes that could be detected by light microscopy. Polymorphonuclear cells increasingly infiltrated the endoneurium. The cytoplasm of Schwann cells failed to stain with toluidine blue and their nuclei were pyknotic. Under the electron microscope Schwann cell cytoplasm was rarefied or occasionally electron dense. Myelin sheaths associated with these Schwann cells showed vesicular disruption starting at both the inner and outer myelin lamellae. In longitudinal sections, paranodal myelin was retracted and Schmidt-Lanterman (SL) clefts of nerve fibres were widened. Ultramicroscopically, outer myelin loops at paranodes were detached and cleft widenings consisted of myelin splitting, vacuolation and vesiculation. The frequency of Schwann cell and myelin changes was greatest around the site of injection and decreased in a graded fashion in areas remote from the injection site. By 5 h large mononuclear and polymorphonuclear cells had infiltrated into the perineurium, and there was oedema and destruction of perineurial lamellae. Despite the adjacent perineurial inflammation, mononuclear cells were rarely found in the endoneurium.

Eight hours

Extensive myelin vesiculation affected many nerve fibres (Fig. 2). This pattern of demyelination could be recognized on light microscopy as a gray halo surrounding individual axons. Phagocytic mononuclear cells were seldom found in the endoneurium and never in association with vesiculated myelin.

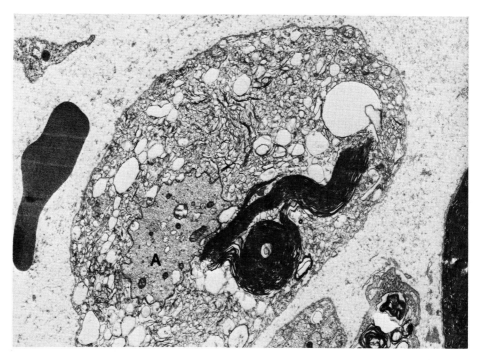

Fig. 2. Electron micrograph of cross-sectioned nerve fibre has extensive vesiculo-vacuolar degeneration of myelin sheath. Axon (A) is reduced in diameter. One day after antiserum injection ($\times$ 5000).

Fifteen hours to three days

Many large mononuclear cells with polysome-rich cytoplasm and pseudopodia appeared in the endoneurium at this time. They were present in and around endoneurial blood vessels and were considered to be monocytes. Macrophages also were seen, sometimes associated with demyelinating or normal-appearing myelinated nerves. The number of demyelinated axons increased during this period. By examining teased single fibres, we demonstrated that demyelination was segmental, usually extending over several internodes. Attachment of debris-laden macrophages was a frequent feature of the demyelinated segments in cross-section (Figs. 3 and 4). Schwann cells associated with nerve fibres which were invaded by macrophages usually had degenerative changes, consisting of amorphous granular and membranous profiles and swollen mitochondria (Fig. 4). However, Schwann cells in areas distant from the injection site showed only mild dilation of smooth ER and increased numbers of caveolae in their plasma membranes. Phagocytosis of myelin debris by Schwann cells was seldom observed. Unmyelinated fibres were frequently enclosed within a basement membrane but were unassociated with Schwann cell processes. Changes within axoplasm were observed rarely; axonal shrinkage of some demyelinating fibres was indicated by wrinkling and redundancy of axolemmal membranes (Fig. 2). Fibrinous exudates and extravasation of red cells were occasionally present around vessels. Subperineurial and endoneurial oedema was pronounced.

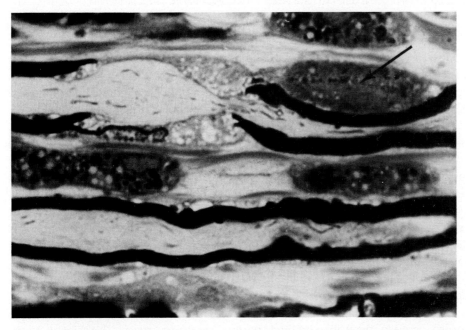

Fig. 3. Longitudinal section of a nerve 2 days after antiserum injection. Paranodal demyelination associated with vesicular disruption of myelin on the left heminode and detachment of outer myelin on the right heminode can be seen in association with phagocytic cell (arrow) (× 1170).

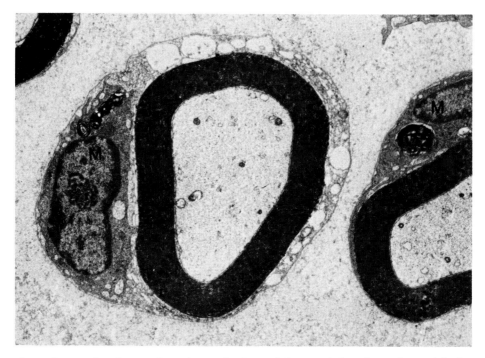

Fig. 4. Cross-section electron photomicrograph of rat sciatic nerve 1 day after antiserum injection. Myelin sheath appears normal, but Schwann cell cytoplasm shows vesiculo-vacuolar degeneration. Phagocytic mononuclear cells (M) have invaded underneath the basement membrane (×24,000).

Five to seven days

Most nerve fibres within the lesion were completely demyelinated and were associated with debris-laden macrophages after 5 days (Fig. 5). On occasion Schwann cell cytoplasm rich in polysomes and rough ER surrounded demyelinated axons. At 7 days, most demyelinated axons were encircled by Schwann cells (Fig. 6). Schwann cell cytoplasm had abundant polysomes, rough endoplasmic reticulum, and Golgi complexes. Degenerating Schwann cells, which are seen frequently in the acute phase of antiserum-mediated demyelination, were not observed. Axons surrounded by uncompacted myelin were infrequent despite careful search. In general, demyelinated axons were smaller than those still myelinated. Longitudinal sections demonstrated that this size reduction was an accompaniment of focal demyelination, as the diameter of individual axons was smaller at bare heminodes than at adjacent myelinated ones. On occasion, demyelinated axons contained abnormal membranous profiles, suggesting chronic axonal degeneration.

Eight to fourteen days

The earliest evidence of remyelination was found 8 days post injection at the border between demyelinated and normal-appearing zones. Occasional axons present in this region were encircled by a few turns of compacted myelin. Only a few had uncompacted myelin, and most axons remained unmyelinated at this time. By

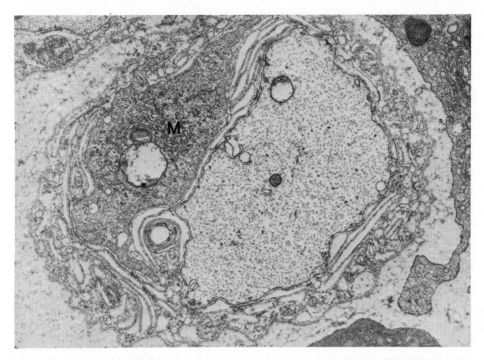

Fig. 5. Almost completely demyelinated axon is invaded by cytoplasmic process of phagocytic cell (M). Residual myelin lamella is loosened (×26,000).

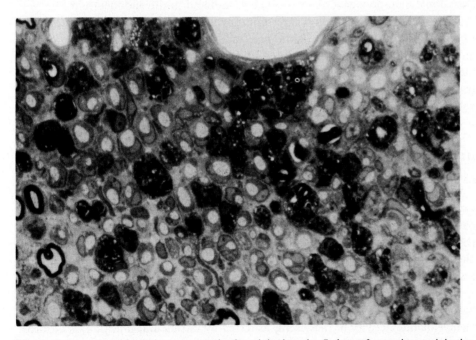

Fig. 6. Cross-section of sciatic nerve proximal to injection site 7 days after antiserum injection. Demyelinated axons are encircled by Schwann cell. Myelin formation is not seen in these fibres. Debris-laden macrophages are scattered in the endoneurium (×470).

10 days increasing numbers of axons at the periphery of the lesion were surrounded by compacted myelin. Myelination seemed to occur without relationship to axon size. Most axons located in the centre of the lesion remained unmyelinated; a few had uncompacted myelin. In distal portions of the demyelinated lesions, evidence of acute axonal degeneration with swollen, empty axons was observed, but usually less than 5 such fibres could be found per fascicle. Electron microscopy showed that most demyelinated axons in cross-section were surrounded by a single Schwann cell. Supernumerary Schwann cells and early remyelination by tunication were rarely seen around a central remyelinating axon, although concentric arrays of a few Schwann cell processes and redundant folds of basal lamina were sometimes present. Phagocytosis of myelin debris by Schwann cells and islands of small axons suggesting sprouts were occasionally encountered in the endoneurium.

By 14 days after the injection, both axon area and myelin thickness had increased in remyelinating fibres. Ultramicroscopically, remyelination progressed in a stereotyped way for the majority of axons.

Twenty-one days and thereafter

At 21 and 28 days, axon area and myelin thickness continued to enlarge. The density of macrophages within the endoneurium decreased. In longitudinal sections, short internodes with thinner than normal myelin sheaths were conspicuous. By 37 days, the last time examined, remyelinated nerve fibres appeared normal aside from myelin sheaths relatively thinner than would be expected for their axon size. Occasional macrophages were still evident scattered in the endoneurium.

Teased fibre studies 37 days after injection showed that most myelinated nerve fibres passing through the lesion had many short, faintly stained internodes intercalated between normally stained long internodes. At the centre of the lesion these continuously remyelinating segments were approximately 1 cm long. At the periphery the affected segments were shorter and were associated both proximally and distally with paranodal remyelination over several internodes.

DISCUSSION

Intraneural injection of sera from rabbits with EAN, EAE and rabbits sensitized with GC produces primary focal demyelination in recipient rat sciatic nerves. The patterns of demyelination and the evolution of demyelinative lesions induced by EAN, EAE and anti-GC sera are identical. Schwann cell changes, myelin splitting and vesiculation, macrophage phagocytosis of myelin, and the association of an acute inflammatory reaction are responses common to the 3 antisera.

Both EAN and EAE sera with in vivo PNS demyelinating activity have elevated anti-GC antibody titres (K. Saida et al. 1978b; T. Saida et al. 1978a, 1979a,c). Demyelinating activity in these sera, as tested by intraneural injection, is adsorbed with galactocerebroside but not with glucocerebroside or mixed gangliosides (K. Saida et al. 1978b; T. Saida et al. 1978a), as were the anti-GC serum (T. Saida et al.

1978a; K. Saida et al. 1979). Specific antibodies to GC from such sera, purified by using affinity binding to liposomes sensitized with synthetic galactocerebroside, also produced in vivo peripheral nerve demyelination (T. Saida 1981). It seems that anti-GC antibody is at least one major antibody responsible for the production of in vivo PNS demyelination in both EAN and EAE serum. In contrast, antiserum to CNS-BP does not produce significant myelinotoxicity when injected into peripheral nerve (K. Saida et al. 1978b) or in myelinated cultures of CNS tissue (T. Saida et al. 1978b, 1981a; Bornstein and Raine 1976), in spite of the well established encephalitogenicity of CNS-BP. Further, antiserum to P_2 myelin basic protein, which is known to induce EAN, does not show myelinotoxicity after intraneural injection (T. Saida et al. 1982). Activity is lost after heating serum at 56°C for 30 min. The demyelinating activity of antisera is therefore probably antibody-dependent, complement-mediated. The mechanism of myelinolysis or Schwann cell membrane lysis in this model could be postulated as follows. Antigenic determinant of membrane, probably galactose with some nearby ceramide structure, is first bound with complement fixing antibody. This binding initiates the activation of the complement cascade, and the activated last component of complement C9 produces holes in cell membranes, presumably by removing fatty acids from lecithin and thus making lysocompounds in the membrane (Müller-Eberhard 1976).

Table I summarizes the sequence of morphological changes and electrophysiological alterations after antiserum injection (K. Saida et al. 1980; Sumner et al. 1982). Serial recording of motor conduction through the demyelinating lesion in rat sciatic nerve revealed that focal conduction block begins 20–60 min after antiserum injection, when outer myelin loops at paranodes are detached and Schwann cell cytoplasm undergoes degenerative changes (K. Saida et al. 1978a, 1979; T. Saida et al. 1979a; Sumner et al. 1982). Focal conduction block progresses to completion within 3–4 h, when myelin sheaths at paranodes and Schmidt-Lantermann clefts reveal extensive vesiculo-vacuolar degeneration. While conduction block persists for approximately 7 days, myelin sheaths are phago-cytized by invaded macrophages, and axons become denuded. At around 8 days, when dispersed very low voltage muscle action potentials with long latency are detected, demyelinated axons are encircled with 2–8 turns of new myelin lamellae. As muscle action potentials increase and latencies shorten, myelin thickness of remyelinating axons increases. Functional recovery of the paralysed foot is achieved around 14–16 days after antiserum injection; electrophysiological recovery, around 25 days after injection, when the thickness of the myelin sheath is approximately one-third of normal (K. Saida et al. 1980). Rasminsky et al. (Rasminsky and Sumner 1980; Rasminsky et al. 1981; Lafontaine et al. 1982) studied precisely acute conduction block in single rat spinal root fibres following focal exposure to anti-GC serum. They reported that conduction block was preceded by a rise in internodal conduction time, block occurring within 1 h. Our recent study by ferric ion-ferrocyanide binding staining (Waxman 1980) showed that ferric-ion staining was localized at the nodal axolemma at 20 min after antiserum injection, when only several outer myelin loops were retracted from the axolemma of the node of

TABLE I

MORPHOLOGICAL AND ELECTROPHYSIOLOGICAL EVOLUTION OF ANTISERUM-MEDIATED DEMYELINATION

Hours or days after injection	Morphological findings	Electrophysiological findings
Pre-injection	Normal	Normal amplitude muscle action potentials
20 min	Schwann cell changes	Beginning of decrease in amplitude (partial conduction block)
1 h	Detachment of myelin terminal loops Widening of Schmidt-Lantermann clefts	Further decline of amplitude (partial conduction block)
3 h	Myelin retraction at paranodes Vesicular disruption of myelin at paranodes and S-L clefts	Disappearance of muscle response (complete conduction block)
1 day	Phagocytosis of myelin sheath by macrophages Denudation of myelinated axon Axon shrinkage	(complete conduction block)
5 days	Schwann cell proliferation	(complete conduction block)
8 days	Progressive remyelination Enlargement of axon size	Reappearance of delayed and dispersed muscle responses
>25 days	Remyelination progressed Establishment of short internodes	Regaining of normal response

Ranvier. One hour after antiserum injection when most lateral loops had been detached from the paranodal axolemma, the staining was less intense at the node and extended to the paranodal axolemma as well. After 5 h, when paranodal demyelination progressed mainly by vesiculation of myelin lamellae, staining was hardly present around the nodal area (T. Saida 1981). Using the freeze-fracture technique, Rosenbluth et al. (1981) found that intramembranous particle distribution at the node and adjacent axolemma was scattered sparsely in the nerve 6 days after anti-GC serum injection. These observations suggest the presence of cytochemical and ultrastructural dedifferentiation of the property of the axolemma and could be the morphological basis for the conduction slowing and block in the early phases of immune-mediated demyelination.

In acute inflammatory polyradiculoneuritis, the Guillain-Barré syndrome (GBS) of humans, 11 of 27 sera (41%) from GBS patients within 3 weeks of the onset of clinical illness had in vivo demyelinating capacity after intraneural injection into rat sciatic nerve (Feasby et al. 1980; T. Saida et al. 1982). The demyelinating activity of GBS sera was much less intense on average than that produced by sera from EAE or EAN animals. Sera obtained from multiple sclerosis patients in exacerbation did not show the similar demyelinative activity in peripheral nerve. Three of 40 (7.5%) sera obtained from normals and patients with other neurological diseases caused in vivo demyelination. Although the in vivo demyelinating activity of GBS sera is much less intense and only demonstrated by the careful morphological and quantitative studies (T. Saida et al. 1982) Sumner (1981) reported that electrophysiological techniques can bring out subtle changes produced by GBS sera. It is not yet known whether this model of antiserum-mediated demyelination has any relevance to human demyelinating disorders. However, it certainly brings us a new insight on the anatomico-electrophysiological relationship in demyelinating processes, and many interesting immunopathological and electrophysiological questions to solve.

SUMMARY

A focal immune-mediated demyelinating lesion of peripheral nerve was produced by intraneural injection of antiserum to galactocerebroside, a major glycosphingolipid hapten common in CNS and PNS myelin. This model provides an excellent system for correlative studies of physiological and pathological alterations in the processes of demyelination, because the time course of such changes is predictable from animal to animal. Twenty minutes after antiserum injection, Schwann cells showed focal cytoplasmic outpouching and their external mesaxons opened. Between 1 and 8 h after injection "melting," splitting, vesiculation and vacuolation of myelin became increasingly prominent at paranodal regions and Schmidt-Lantermann clefts, with concomitant degenerative changes in Schwann cell cytoplasm. Disruption of myelin in the paranodal region with detachment of the outermost paranodal myelin loops from paranodal axon resulted in an increase in nodal surface area. This seems to be the most critical anatomical alteration responsible for the early changes in propagation of nerve impulses in this antibody-mediated demyelinating lesion. Between 8 h and 3 days axons became demyelinated progressively over several internodes by macrophage phagocytosis. The onset of clinical and saltatory conduction recovery from the lesion corresponded to the appearance of 2–8 myelin lamellae around each remyelinating axon.

ACKNOWLEDGEMENTS

This study was supported in part by a grant from Neuroimmunological Disorders Research Committee and Grant No. 82-02 from the National Center for Nervous, Mental and Muscular Disorders of the Ministry of Health and Welfare, Japan.

REFERENCES

Aguayo, A., Nair, C.P.V. and Midgley, R. Experimental progressive compression neuropathy in the rabbit. Histologic and electrophysiologic studies. Arch. Neurol. (Chic.), 1971, 24: 358–364.
Bornstein, M.B. and Raine, C.S. The initial structural lesion in serum-induced demyelination in vitro. Lab. Invest. 1976, 35: 391–401.

Dyck, P.J., Thomas, P.K. and Lambert, E.H. Peripheral Neuropathy, Vols. 1 and 2. Saunders, Philadelphia, Pa., 1975.

Feasby, T.E., Habn, A.F. and Gilbert, J.J. Passive transfer of demyelinating activity in Guillain-Barré polyneuropathy. Neurology (Minneap.), 1980, 30: 363.

Fowler, T.J., Danta, G. and Gilliatt, R.W. Recovery of nerve conduction after a pneumatic tourniquet: observations on the hind-limb of the baboon. J. Neurol. Neurosurg. Psychiat. 1972, 35: 638–647.

Hahn, A.F., Gilbert, J.J. and Feasby, T.E. Passive transfer of demyelination by experimental allergic neuritis serum. Acta neuropath. (Berl.), 1980, 49: 169–176.

Hall, J.I. Studies on demyelinated peripheral nerves in guinea pigs with experimental allergic neuritis. A histological and electrophysiological study. Part II. Electrophysiological observations. Brain, 1967, 90: 313–332.

Lafontaine, S., Rasminsky, M., Saida, T. and Sumner, A.J. Conduction block in rat myelinated fibers following acute exposure to anti-galactocerebroside serum. J. Physiol. (Lond.), 1982, 323: 287–306.

McDonald, W.I. The effects of experimental demyelination on conduction in peripheral nerve: a histological and electrophysiological study. II. Electrophysiological observations. Brain, 1968, 86: 501–524.

Morgan-Hughes, J.A. Experimental diphtheritic neuropathy: a pathological and electrophysiological study. J. neurol. Sci., 1968, 7: 157–175.

Müller-Eberhard, H.J. The serum complement system. In: P.A. Miescher and H.J. Müller-Eberhard (Eds.), Textbook of Immunopathology, Vol. 1. Grune and Stratton, New York, 1976: 45.

Rasminsky, M. and Sumner, A.J. Development of conduction block in single rat spinal root fibers locally exposed to anti-galactocerebroside serum. Neurology (Minneap.), 1980, 30: 371.

Rasminsky, M., Sumner, A.J. and Lafontaine, S. Conduction block caused by anti-galactocerebroside serum is due to paranodal demyelination. Neurology (Minneap.), 1981, 31 (Suppl.): 65.

Rosenbluth, J., Sumner, A. and Saida, T. Dedifferentiation of the axolemma associated with demyelination. In: G.W. Bailey (Ed.), Proceedings of 39th Annual EMSA Meeting. Claitor Publ. Div., Baton Rouge, La., 1981: 496–497.

Saida, K., Saida, T., Brown, M.J. et al. Antiserum-mediated demyelination in vivo: a sequential study using intraneural injection of experimental allergic neuritis. Lab. Invest., 1978a, 39: 449–462.

Saida, K., Saida, T., Brown, M.J., Silberberg, D.H. and Asbury, A.K. Antiserum-mediated demyelination in vivo: Observations after intraneural injection of experimental allergic encephalomyelitis (EAE) and neuritis (EAN) serum. J. Neuropath. exp. Neurol., 1978b, 37: 684.

Saida, K., Saida, T., Brown, M.J. et al. In vivo demyelination induced by intraneural injection of anti-galactocerebroside serum: a morphologic study. Amer. J. Path., 1979, 95: 99–110.

Saida, K., Sumner, A.J., Saida, T., Brown, M.J. and Silberberg, D.H. Antiserum-mediated demyelination: Relationship between remyelination and functional recovery. Ann. Neurol., 1980, 3: 12–24.

Saida, T. Antiserum-mediated demyelination. In: Synopses of Symposia and Workshops, 10th International Congress of Electroencephalography and Clinical Neurophysiology. Jap. Soc. EEG and EMG, 1981: 114.

Saida, T., Saida, K., Alving, C., Brown, M.J., Silberberg, D.H. and Asbury, A.K. In vivo demyelination produced by purified antibodies to galactocerebroside. J. Neuropath. exp. Neurol 1978a, 38: 338.

Saida, T., Saida, K., Silberberg, D.H. et al. Transfer of demyelination with experimental allergic neuritis serum by intraneural injection. Nature (Lond.), 1978b 272: 639–641.

Saida, T., Saida, K., Brown, M.J. et al. Peripheral nerve demyelination induced by intraneural injection of experimental allergic encephalomyelitis serum. J. Neuropath. exp. Neurol., 1979a, 38: 498–518.

Saida, T., Saida, K., Dorfman, S.H. et al. Experimental allergic neuritis induced by sensitization with galactocerebroside. Science, 1979b, 204: 1103–1106.

Saida, T., Saida, K. and Silberberg, D.H. Demyelination produced by experimental allergic neuritis serum and antigalactocerebroside antiserum in CNS cultures: an ultrastructural study. Acta neuropath. (Berl.), 1979c, 48: 19–25.

Saida, T., Saida, K., Pleasure, D. and Nishitani, H. Demyelinative neuritis induced by P_2 protein and galactocerebroside: two distinctive diseases. In: Proceedings of 12th World Congress of Neurology. Excerpta Medica, Amsterdam, 1981a: 346–347.

Saida, T., Saida, K., Silberberg, D.H. and Brown, M.J. Galactocerebroside-induced experimental allergic neuritis. Ann. Neurol., 1981b, 9, Suppl.: 87–101.

Saida, T., Saida, K., Lisak, R.P., Brown, M.J. Silberberg, D.H. and Asbury, A.K. In vivo demyelinating activity of sera from patients with Guillain-Barré syndrome. Ann. Neurol., 1982, 11: 69–75.

Seil, F.J., Falk, G.A., Kies, M.W. and Alvord, Jr., E.C. The in vitro demyelinating activity of sera from guinea pigs sensitized with whole CNS and with purified encephalitogen. Exp. Neurol., 1968, 22: 545–555.

Sumner, A.J. Conduction block by intraneural injection of Guillain-Barré serum. In: Synopses of Symposia and Workshops, 10th International Congress of Electroencephalography and Clinical Neurophysiology. Jap. Soc. EEG and EMG, 1981: 112–113.

Sumner, A.J., Saida, K., Saida, T., Silberberg, D.H. and Asbury, A.K. Acute conduction block associated with experimental antiserum-mediated demyelination of peripheral nerve. Ann. Neurol., 1982, 11: 469–477.

Waxman, S.G. Variations in axonal morphology and their functional significance. In: S.G. Waxman (Ed.), Physiology and Pathobiology of Axons. Raven Press, New York, 1980: 169–190.

Kyoto Symposia (EEG Suppl. No. 36)
Editors: P.A. Buser, W.A. Cobb and T. Okuma
© 1982, Elsevier Biomedical Press, Amsterdam

Mechanisms for Preserved Nerve Function with Ischaemia in Peripheral Neuropathy

VIGGO KAMP NIELSEN*

Laboratory of Clinical Neurophysiology, Glostrup Hospital, University of Copenhagen, Copenhagen (Denmark)

In 1959, Steiness reported that diabetic nerves were abnormally resistant to the impairment of nerve function normally induced by ischaemia. For about 10 years this phenomenon was thought to be specific for diabetes mellitus, but it has since been shown that a similar resistance to ischaemia is present in patients with chronic renal failure (Christensen and Ørskov 1969; Castaigne et al. 1972; Nielsen 1978), chronic hepatic failure (Seneviratne and Peiris 1970b; Kardel and Nielsen 1974; Nielsen and Kardel 1975) and hypercalcaemia (Gregersen and Pilgaard 1971; Castaigne et al. 1972). These reports aroused a renewed interest in the study of physiological changes in normal nerves during ischaemia, and considerable variations have been disclosed in the normal response to ischaemia in different nerve segments (Nielsen and Kardel 1974, 1981; Nielsen and Stålberg 1978). Furthermore, there are observations suggesting that comparable nerve segments in various species may show differences in the ischaemic resistance pattern (Dyck, personal communication).

The present paper will review data reported in the literature and present additional unpublished observations pertinent to differences in the response to ischaemia in normal and pathological nerves. Various hypotheses have been advanced to account for the phenomenon, but to date there is little direct experimental evidence available to elucidate the underlying mechanism(s). Some possible models are discussed on the basis of published observations.

OBSERVATIONS

(I) Normal nerves

A few examples will be presented to illustrate that various segments of normal nerves may show quite marked differences in the resistance to ischaemia.

When the sural nerve is stimulated at the mid-calf level, purely sensory action potentials can be recorded proximally (upper calf) and distally (ankle) at the *same* distance from the site of stimulation. To produce ischaemia, a blood pressure cuff

---

*Present address: Department of Neurology, University of Pittsburgh, School of Medicine, 322 Scaife Hall, Pittsburgh, Pa. 15261, U.S.A.

around the thigh is inflated to well above the systolic blood pressure. Fig. 1, illustrating a typical experiment, shows that the latency increased at a faster rate in the proximal than in the distal segment, both measuring 15 cm. After 28 min the relative increases were 42% and 11%, respectively. Similarly, the potential amplitude at the upper calf decreased at a faster rate than at the ankle. After 28 min, when the upper calf potential was abolished, the potential at the ankle still had an amplitude of 50% of the pre-ischaemic value, and the potential was still present after 37 min of ischaemia.

In the median nerve, motor conduction velocity was measured in 2 segments of equal length, from elbow to forearm and from forearm to wrist. In 9 normal subjects the average conduction velocity decreased at a faster rate in the proximal than in the distal segment (Fig. 2). Conduction block was observed after 18 and

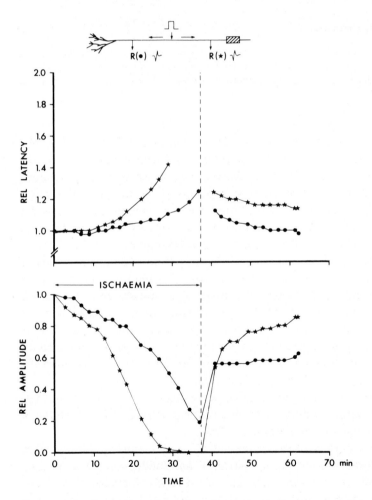

Fig. 1. Relative changes in latency and amplitude of evoked nerve action potentials at the upper calf (★) and ankle (•) during ischaemia. The sural nerve was stimulated at the mid-calf, midway between recording sites. Normal subject.

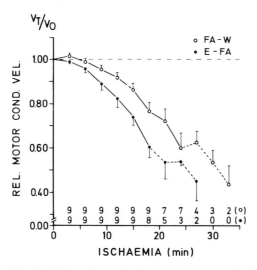

Fig. 2. Relative changes in the motor nerve conduction velocity in 2 segments of equal length in the median nerve during ischaemia. Numbers below curves indicate numbers of observations. E, elbow; FA, forearm; W, wrist; V_T, conduction velocity at T minutes of ischaemia; V_0 = pre-ischaemic conduction velocity. Mean ± S.E.M.

24 min of ischaemia in the proximal and distal segments, respectively. Despite slowing of the motor conduction, the amplitudes of action potentials in the abductor pollicis brevis muscle remained relatively well preserved, but eventually a rapid drop was seen within a few minutes. As shown in Fig. 3 the conduction block progressed in a distalward direction. Thus, after 30 min a potential could no longer be evoked from the elbow, and the amplitudes of potentials evoked at forearm and wrist were on average 6% and 55% of the pre-ischaemic value, respectively.

While the distal forearm-wrist segment was clearly more resistant to ischaemia than the proximal segment between elbow and forearm, the resistance was even more pronounced in the terminal segment between wrist and the abductor pollicis brevis muscle. The same was observed in a terminal motor nerve segment in the proximal part of the ischaemic limb. In the same experiments action potentials were recorded from the pronator teres muscle, stimulating the median nerve at the elbow (Fig. 3, right column). In this segment a conduction block was never observed in any of the 9 subjects during up to 40 min of ischaemia.

These findings from the compound median nerve could be reproduced in single undissected motor axons, recording single fibre action potentials from the abductor pollicis brevis muscle (Nielsen and Stålberg 1978).

Hence, as demonstrated by these experiments, it is a normal physiological response that the resistance to anoxic depolarization and conduction block increases in a peripheralward direction in the main trunk of the sural and median nerves, and that terminal motor nerve branches are highly resistant, irrespective of whether located distally or proximally in the ischaemic limb. This is not due to compression of the nerve beneath the blood pressure cuff, since the same sequence of events is

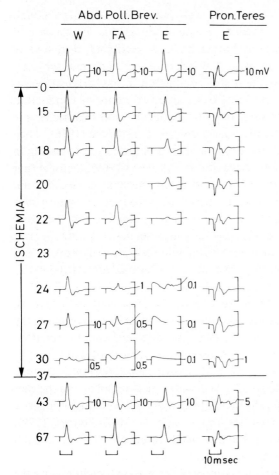

Fig. 3. Muscle action potentials recorded before, during and after ischaemia in the abductor pollicis brevis muscle and the pronator teres muscle (right column). The median nerve was stimulated at the wrist (W), forearm (FA) and elbow (E). A blood pressure cuff, with the lower edge 7 cm proximal to the elbow electrode, was inflated to 100 mm Hg above the systolic blood pressure for 37 min. Normal subject.

regularly observed in the tail nerve of rats after acute cardiac arrest. Furthermore, these findings are consistent with previous reports, showing that the centralward conduction of sensory action potentials is gradually slowed along the median nerve at any given time during the period of ischaemia (Nielsen and Kardel 1974, 1981).

(II) Pathological nerves

(A) Diabetes mellitus

Steiness (1959) originally observed that in diabetic patients the rise of the vibratory perception threshold during 30 min of ischaemia was either absent or considerably delayed as compared with normal controls. Later, Castaigne et al. (1966) showed that the sensory potential and motor and sensory conduction velocities in the ulnar nerve were abnormally well preserved. Gregersen (1968) extended the diabetic response to ischaemia to include thresholds for touch and pain, but made the important observation that temperature sensibility, mediated by unmyelinated fibres, was unaffected by 30 min of ischaemia, as in normal subjects. He also showed a delayed slowing of the motor conduction in the peroneal nerve. Seneviratne and Peiris (1968) made the same observations on sensory conduction distally in the median nerve and pointed out that ischaemic and post-ischaemic paraesthesiae were mild or absent, as previously described by Poole (1956). They were able to reproduce the increased ischaemic resistance pattern experimentally in the sciatic nerve of alloxan diabetic rats (Seneviratne and Peiris 1969), a model that was also used in their extensive study of the underlying mechanism (see below). Christensen and Ørskov (1969) noted that increased ischaemic resistance was demonstrable in newly diagnosed and untreated juvenile diabetics. On the other hand, mild glucose intolerance per se, as also seen in uraemics and chronic liver patients, was not accompanied by increased ischaemic resistance. Horowitz and Ginsberg-Fellner (1979) showed that the resistance to ischaemia affects the entire length of the ischaemic nerve in all types of diabetes.

Hence the "diabetic" ischaemic response can be demonstrated in nearly all patients with true diabetes mellitus. It has not been possible to correlate the phenomenon with signs of diabetic angiopathy, or with diabetic neuropathy. Neither does it appear to be influenced by the duration or severity of diabetes, e.g. as indicated by the insulin requirement. All patients with an abnormal ischaemic response have elevated concentrations of glycosylated haemoglobin component A_1C, but a direct correlation between the actual level and the severity of ischaemic resistance has not been demonstrated (Horowitz and Ginsberg-Fellner 1979). Increased ischaemic resistance cannot be provoked clinically by experimental hyperglycaemia in normal subjects (Steiness 1961a).

Steiness (1959, 1961b) observed that tight control of the diabetes might reverse the diabetic ischaemic response towards normal. This has been confirmed by others (Gregersen 1968; Terkildsen and Christensen 1971), but Christensen and Ørskov (1969) emphasized that the improvement lagged considerably behind normalization of the blood glucose level. In fact, it is still unsettled whether the improvement is actually due to correction of a metabolic disturbance in the nerves, or to a direct effect of insulin on the intra- and extracellular K^+ equilibrium. Thus, pretreatment of *normal* rats with insulin significantly shortens the ischaemic resistance period in the sciatic nerve (Seneviratne and Peiris 1970a), and the same effect has been demonstrated in vivo in normal human subjects (Castaigne et al. 1972).

(B) Uraemia

The nerve function is abnormally well preserved during ischaemia in patients with severe chronic renal failure (Christensen and Ørskov 1969; Castaigne et al. 1972; Nielsen 1978), while the response is normal in patients with mild to moderate renal insufficiency (Meilvang 1974). This does not seem to be related to impairment of the glucose tolerance, or to renal acidosis and electrolyte disturbances (Christensen and

Ørskov 1969). Several patients still exhibit increased ischaemic resistance during regular dialysis treatment, by which the degree of azotaemia is kept at a near normal level (Castaigne et al. 1972; Nielsen 1978). Single standard dialyses do not change the response, but is has been shown that hypovolaemia induced by dialysis markedly exaggerates the ischaemic resistance. This could be reversed to near normal by subsequent perfusion with Rheomacrodex (Castaigne et al. 1972).

It is not known whether the prolonged ischaemic resistance may eventually be reversed to normal during long-term dialysis treatment or after renal transplantation. In 2 patients, re-examined 3 and 6 months after a successful transplantation, the ischaemic resistance was still as severely prolonged as before the operation (Christensen and Ørskov 1969).

(C) Chronic hepatic failure

Increased resistance to ischaemia is not an uncommon finding in patients with chronic hepatic failure. In our material (Kardel and Nielsen 1974) it was present in 54% of 33 consecutive patients. In the study by Seneviratne and Peiris (1970b) it was seen in 7 out of 16 strictly selected patients, excluding all patients with an abnormal glucose tolerance test and with signs of neuropathy. However, we did not observe any relationship with glucose intolerance or electrophysiological evidence of neuropathy. Nor was the phenomenon related to the degree of liver failure.

In the median nerve, patients with preserved vibratory perception during ischaemia showed a very slow and uniform reduction of sensory potential amplitudes both at wrist and elbow (Nielsen and Kardel 1975). Sensory conduction velocity decreased slowly and in parallel in distal and proximal nerve segments for about 25 min, in contrast to the normal, but eventually the decrease took a more rapid course in the proximal than in the distal segment. Hence, except for a considerable delay in depolarization during ischaemia, the course of changes in nerve conduction was principally the same as in normal subjects.

(D) Hypercalcaemia

Patients with hypercalcaemia (hyperparathyroidism, neoplastic bone metastases, overtreatment with calciferol) show increased ischaemic resistance (Gregersen and Pilgaard 1971; Castaigne et al. 1972). Conversely, in hypocalcaemia after parathyroidectomy the resistance period is extremely shortened, sometimes down to a few minutes. It is noteworthy that in both situations, the ischaemic response can be normalized after serum Ca^{2+} has been reversed to normal levels. Pooled data showed a significant positive correlation between the ischaemic perception time for vibrations and serum Ca^{2+} concentrations (Gregersen and Pilgaard 1971).

(E) Miscellaneous

A few patients with *amyotrophic lateral sclerosis* have shown absence of ischaemic and post-ischaemic paraesthesia and abnormal preservation of sensory action potentials during ischaemia (Shahani and Russell 1969; Shahani et al. 1971; Horowitz and Ginsberg-Fellner 1979). This may be due to a previously reported endocrine and exocrine pancreatic insufficiency (Quick 1969) with an abnormally low insulin production (Steinke and Tyler 1964), influencing the K^+ equilibrium in nerves (ref. section II-A). On the contrary, 2 patients with *hyperinsulinism* have been reported, who showed a shortened or borderline low resistance to ischaemia (Castaigne et al. 1972; Horowitz and Ginsberg-Fellner 1979). Unfortunately, the actual level of serum insulin was not measured at the time of the examination.

From a pathophysiological point of view, it is of interest also to consider the few negative findings reported in the literature. A normal ischaemic response has been recorded in patients with severe demyelination (Charcot-Marie-Tooth's disease, hypertrophic type I) (Gregersen and Pilgaard 1971; Horowitz and Ginsberg-Fellner 1979). Castaigne et al. (1972) recorded a normal disappearance rate of sensory action potentials during ischaemia in 13 "non-diabetic patients with peripheral neuropathy." This was confirmed in the study by Horowitz and Ginsberg-Fellner (1979) comprising among others 11 patients with "non-metabolic" neuropathy of various aetiologies. If these observations can be reproduced in larger patient materials, the important practical implication would be that the ischaemic test might prove useful in the differentiation between metabolic and "non-metabolic" neuropathies.

MECHANISMS

Before going into a discussion of possible mechanisms of increased ischaemic resistance, a few general considerations are warranted. First, ischaemic resistance as described above only concerns myelinated fibres. Second, it is unlikely that a single pathogenetic factor can account for all the various conditions in which the phenomenon has been encountered. Third, increased ischaemic resistance indicates a delayed depolarization of nerves; this is the end result of several possible processes, which should be considered individually. Fourth, although several factors may be linked in a coherent process, isolated impairment of single steps may per se result in increased resistance.

(1) Metabolic energy reserve

The hypothesis of a surplus metabolic energy at disposal during ischaemia has attracted many investigators of diabetic neuropathy. However, the nature of this reserve fuel remains obscure. Normal rabbit sciatic whole-nerve subjected to 99% nitrogen is rapidly depleted of P-creatine, glycogen, glucose and ATP, with half-times of 3, 3, 8, and 20 min respectively, whereas depletion of fructose is very slow (Stewart et al. 1965). Alloxan diabetic rat nerves show an accumulation of fructose (Stewart et al. 1966). This is also found in the sural nerve of human diabetics (Dyck et al. 1980b). In vitro studies have shown that the ATP and O_2 uptakes can be maintained in endoneurial preparations for more than 1 h in a medium free of glucose, but containing DL-β-hydroxybutyrate (Greene and Winegrad 1979). Thus, possible candidates for an energy reserve might be high levels of fructose and ketone bodies in diabetic nerves, and possibly high creatine levels in uraemic nerves. Greene and Winegrad (1979) have emphasized that metabolic studies should be conducted on the endoneurial component of nerve in order to provide physiologically meaningful data. Such studies are not yet available in ischaemic nerves, and the significance of a metabolic energy reserve remains to be proved and specified.

(2) Calcium

Metabolic energy is not only required for the operation of the Na-K pump, but is equally important for the binding of Ca^{2+} at the nodal membrane. Extracellular $[Ca^{2+}]$ significantly influences the degree of membrane polarization (Maruhashi and Wright 1967). High $[Ca^{2+}]$ effectively "screens" the negative surface potential, creating a state equivalent to a hyperpolarization of the nodal membrane, and thereby increasing its resistance to any depolarizing action (Cahalan 1978), ischaemia included. Oppositely, low extramembrane $[Ca^{2+}]$ markedly increases the conductance of Na^+ and K^+ across the membrane, resulting in rapid depolarization during ischaemia. The study by Gregersen and Pilgaard (1971) provided direct evidence in favour of this concept (section II-D), but in addition raised levels of extramembrane Ca^{2+} may be suspected in uraemic patients with increased ischaemic resistance. Hypercalcaemia due to secondary hyperparathyroidism is a well known complication of terminal renal failure (Stanbury and Lumb 1966), which often manifests itself during long-term dialysis and also may be present after an otherwise successful transplantation (section II-B).

(3) Potassium

It is an old observation that anoxia depletes intracellular K^+ in a resting nerve. If nothing limits diffusion of expelled K^+ or if it is washed out of the surrounding medium, the nerve may continue to function, at least for a while. This suggests that the concomitant influx of Na^+ is less important, probably due to the relatively larger distribution volume intracellularly, which slows the rise time of intracellular $[Na^+]$. In normal myelinated nerve, K^+ accumulates in the perinodal space, bounded by a diffusion barrier. Provided that re-entry is impaired, as can be assumed during ischaemia, the rise time of extracellular $[K^+]$ is considerably faster than that of intracellular $[Na^+]$ due to the limited distribution volume of the perinodal space (dimension: nm^3). Hence, other things being equal, the rise time of $[K^+]$ becomes the determinant factor for depolarization and conduction block. Moreover, with a given volume of the perinodal space, the rise time may be influenced by the pre-existing intracellular K^+ concentration. This is suggested by the shortened duration of ischaemic resistance in normal rats (Seneviratne and Peiris 1970a) and normal human subjects (Castaigne et al. 1972) pretreated with insulin, promoting an influx of K^+ into the axon prior to the ischaemic test.

(4) Diffusion barrier

In a series of papers, Seneviratne et al. suggested that an increased permeability of the perinodal diffusion barrier with a subsequent slow rise time of extracellular

[K$^+$] might account for the increased ischaemic resistance in diabetes mellitus (Seneviratne and Weerasuriya 1974). However, their final demonstration of a reduced K$^+$ binding capacity of the nodal gap substance could not be confirmed by Sharma and Thomas (1974), and their hypothesis has not been critically tested by others.

(5) Volume of perinodal space

Any change in the volume of the perinodal space may affect the rise time of [K$^+$] during ischaemia. A widening of the space with a subsequent slower rise time would per se prolong the resistance period during ischaemia. An increased volume of the perinodal space could be the result of axonal shrinkage, as postulated in streptozotocin diabetic rats (Jakobsen 1976). Another possibility would be an interstitial oedema caused by acute or chronic hyperosmolality of the interstitial fluid (Dyck et al. 1980a). This mechanism might also account for the changes described after dialysis (Castaigne et al. 1972) (section II-B).

Furthermore, the volume of the perinodal space is probably influenced by the local *fibre density,* being smaller in segments with high fibre density and larger in segments with low fibre density. There are morphological data in support of a higher fibre density in proximal than in more distal segments of the same nerve trunk (Dyck, personal communication). Hence, it seems a reasonable assumption that this difference in fibre density may account for the difference in ischaemic resistance observed between proximal and distal nerve segments in normal nerves (Nielsen and Kardel 1974, 1981).

CONCLUSION

The clinical and electrophysiological features of increased resistance of peripheral nerve function to ischaemia are well established. Normal nerves show considerable variations in ischaemic resistance between proximal and distal segments, being greater in more distal segments. Increased ischaemic resistance is a pathological finding in diabetes mellitus and other metabolic diseases, while apparently a normal response can be expected in non-metabolic neuropathies with severe demyelination. Further clinical observations are desirable to confirm and supplement these observations. As regards the underlying mechanism of the phenomenon there is an obvious need for experimental studies to elucidate and extend the hypothetical possibilities presented in this paper. The ischaemic test is of interest in clinical neurology, since it may serve to distinguish between metabolic and non-metabolic neuropathies. In internal medicine, the test may prove useful in the control of treatment of metabolic diseases.

ACKNOWLEDGEMENT

This work was supported by a grant from the Danish Muscular Dystrophy Association.

REFERENCES

Cahalan, M. Voltage clamp studies on the node of Ranvier. In: S.G. Waxman (Ed.), Physiology and Pathobiology of Axons. Raven Press, New York, 1978: 155–168.

Castaigne, P., Cathala, H.-P., Dry, J. et al. Les réponses des nerfs et des muscles à des stimulations électriques au cours d'une épreuve de garrot ischémique chez l'homme normal et chez le diabétique. Rev. neurol., 1966, 115: 61–66.

Castaigne, P., Cathala, H.-P., Beaussart-Boulengé, L. and Petrover, M. Effect of ischaemia on peripheral nerve function in patients with chronic renal failure undergoing dialysis treatment. J. Neurol. Neurosurg. Psychiat., 1972, 35: 631–637.

Christensen, N.J. and Ørskov, H. Vibratory perception during ischemia in uremic patients and in subjects with mild carbohydrate intolerance. J. Neurol. Neurosurg. Psychiat., 1969, 32: 519–524.

Dyck, P.J., Low, P.A., Sparks, M.F. et al. Effect of serum hyperosmolality on morphometry of healthy human sural nerve. J. Neuropath. exp. Neurol., 1980a, 39: 285–295.

Dyck, P.J., Sherman, W.R., Loretta, M.H. et al. Human diabetic endoneurial sorbitol, fructose, and myo-inositol related to sural nerve morphometry. Ann. Neurol., 1980b, 8: 590–596.

Greene, D.A. and Winegrad, A.I. In vitro studies of the substrates for energy production and the effects of insulin on glucose utilization in the neural components of peripheral nerve. Diabetes, 1979, 28: 878–887.

Gregersen, G. A study of the peripheral nerve in diabetic subjects during ischemia. J. Neurol. Neurosurg. Psychiat., 1968, 31: 175–181.

Gregersen, G. and Pilgaard, S. The effect of ischemia on vibration sense in hypo- and hypercalcemia and in demyelinated nerves. Acta neurol. scand., 1971, 47: 71–79.

Horowitz, S.H. and Ginsberg-Fellner, F. Ischemia and sensory nerve conduction in diabetes mellitus. Neurology (Minneap.), 1979, 29: 695–704.

Jakobsen, J. Axonal dwindling in early experimental diabetes. I. A study of cross sectioned nerves. Diabetologia, 1976, 12: 539–546.

Kardel, T. and Nielsen, V.K. Hepatic neuropathy. A clinical and electrophysiological study. Acta neurol. scand., 1974, 50: 513–526.

Maruhashi, J. and Wright, E.B. Effect of oxygen lack on the single isolated mammalian (rat) nerve fiber. J. Neurophysiol., 1967, 30: 434–452.

Meilvang, S. Biothesiometri under iskaemi. Ugeskr. Laeg., 1974, 136: 1386–1389.

Nielsen, V.K. Pathophysiological aspects of uremic neuropathy. In: N. Canal and G. Pozza (Eds.), Peripheral Neuropathies. Elsevier/North-Holland Biomedical Press, Amsterdam, 1978: 197–210.

Nielsen, V.K. and Kardel, T. Decremental conduction in normal human nerves subjected to ischemia? Acta physiol. scand., 1974, 92: 249–262.

Nielsen, V.K. and Kardel, T. Delayed decrement of the nerve propagation during ischemia in chronic hepatic failure. J. Neurol. Neurosurg. Psychiat. 1975, 38: 966–976.

Nielsen, V.K. and Kardel, T. Temporo-spatial effects on orthodromic sensory potential propagation during ischemia. Ann. Neurol., 1981, 9: 597–604.

Nielsen, V.K. and Stålberg, E. Temporo-spatial slowing of conduction during ischemia in normal human nerves and single motor axons. In: A. Aguayo (Ed.), Proc. IVth International Congress on Neuromuscular Diseases, Montreal, 1978: Abstr. 390.

Poole, E.W. Ischemic and post-ischemic paresthesia in polyneuritis. J. Neurol. Neurosurg. Psychiat., 1956, 19: 148–154.

Quick, D.T. Pancreatic dysfunction in amyotrophic lateral sclerosis. In: F.H. Norris, Jr. and L.T. Kurland (Eds.), Motor Neurone Disease. Grune and Stratton, New York, 1969: 189–198.

Seneviratne, K.N. and Peiris, O.A. The effect of ischemia on the excitability of sensory nerves in diabetes mellitus. J. Neurol. Neurosurg. Psychiat., 1968, 31: 348–353.

Seneviratne, K.N. and Peiris, O.A. The effects of hypoxia on the excitability of the isolated peripheral nerves of the alloxan diabetic rats. J. Neurol. Neurosurg. Psychiat., 1969, 32: 462–469.

Seneviratne, K.N. and Peiris, O.A. The role of diffusion barriers in determining the excitability of peripheral nerve. J. Neurol. Neurosurg. Psychiat., 1970a, 33: 310–318.

Seneviratne, K.N. and Peiris, O.A. Peripheral nerve function in chronic liver disease. J. Neurol. Neurosurg. Psychiat., 1970b, 33: 609–614.

Seneviratne, K.N. and Weerasuriya, A. Nodal gap substance in diabetic nerve. J. Neurol. Neurosurg. Psychiat., 1974, 37: 502–513.

Shahani, B. and Russell, W.R. Motor neurone disease. An abnormality of nerve metabolism. J. Neurol. Neurosurg. Psychiat., 1969, 32: 1–5.

Shahani, B., Davies-Jones, G.A.B. and Russell, W.R. Motor neurone disease. Further evidence for an abnormality of nerve metabolism. J. Neurol. Neurosurg. Psychiat., 1971, 34: 185–191.

Sharma, A.K. and Thomas, P.K. Peripheral nerve structure and function in experimental diabetes. J. neurol. Sci., 1974, 23: 1–15.

Stanbury, S.W. and Lumb, G.A. Parathyroid function in chronic renal failure. A statistical survey of the plasma biochemistry in azotemic renal osteodystrophy. Quart. J. Med., 1966, 35: 1–23.

Steiness, I. Vibratory perception in diabetics during arrested blood flow to the limb. Acta med. scand., 1959, 163: 195–205.

Steiness, I. Vibratory perception in non-diabetic subjects during ischemia with special reference to the conditions in hyperglycemia, after carbohydrate starvation and after cortison administration. Acta med. scand., 1961a, 169: 17–26.

Steiness, I. Influence of diabetic status on vibratory perception during ischemia. Acta med. scand., 1961b, 170: 319–338.

Steinke, J. and Tyler, R.H. The association of amyotrophic lateral sclerosis (motor neurone disease) and carbohydrate intolerance, a clinical study. Metabolism, 1964, 13: 1376–1381.

Stewart, M.A., Passonneau, J.V. and Lowry, O.H. Substrate changes in peripheral nerve during ischemia and Wallerian degeneration. J. Neurochem., 1965, 12: 719–727.

Stewart, M.A., Sherman, W.R. and Anthony, F. Free sugars in alloxan diabetic rat nerve. Biochem. Biophys. Res. Commun., 1966, 22: 488–491.

Terkildsen, A.B. and Christensen, N.J. Reversible nervous abnormalities in juvenile diabetes with recently diagnosed diabetes. Diabetology, 1971, 7: 113–117.

Kyoto Symposia (EEG Suppl. No. 36)
Editors: P.A. Buser, W.A. Cobb and T. Okuma
© 1982, Elsevier Biomedical Press, Amsterdam

Electrophysiological Studies of Guillain-Barré Syndrome with Different Susceptibilities to Develop EAN Serum on 2 Strains of Rats*

PHILLIP A. LOW, JAMES SCHMELZER, PETER JAMES DYCK and JOHN J. KELLY

Neurophysiology Laboratory, Peripheral Nerve Center, Mayo Medical School and Foundation, Rochester, Minn. 55905 (U.S.A.)

The pathogenesis of acute inflammatory-demyelinative polyradiculoneuropathy (AIDP; Guillain-Barré syndrome) is not known, but inflammatory-immunological factors are thought to be involved and the blood-nerve barrier may be defective (Arnason 1975; Olsson 1975). Sera from patients with AIDP in the presence of complement were reported to demyelinate peripheral and central nervous system cultures (Yonezawa et al. 1968; Dubois-Dalcq et al. 1970; Cook et al. 1971; Hirano et al. 1971) and activity was found in both IgM and IgG fractions (Cook et al. 1971). Negative studies have also been reported (Arnason et al. 1969) and demyelinative activity of normal and abnormal control sera have been reported (Edgington and Dalessio 1970; Cook et al. 1971).

Recently, focal experimental allergic neuritis (EAN) has been produced in vivo by intraneural injection of EAN sera into rat sciatic nerve. Similar changes have been reported following intraneural injections of AIDP serum into rat nerve (Feasby et al. 1980).

Dyck et al. (1981) recently examined the rate of demyelination as a function of the depth of anaesthesia, the size of the needle, the rate of injection and the volume and constituents of the injectate. They concluded that all injections caused some demyelination and that hand-held injections using a 30 gauge needle ($\sim 300/150 \, \mu$m external/internal diameters) produced unacceptably high rates of demyelination. We report the results of AIDP sera injected into normal and demyelinated rat sciatic nerve using 33 and 34 gauge needles ($\sim 200/100 \, \mu$m respectively).

METHODS

(1) Patient sera

Clinical details are shown in Table I. All patients were treated at the Mayo Clinic and diagnosed by one of us as having AIDP. Criteria for diagnosis included an acute

---

* This investigation was supported in part by a Peripheral Neuropathy Center Grant from NINCDS (NS14304), a Center Grant from MDA (12), and Mayo, Borchard, and Gallagher Funds.

TABLE I

CLINICAL DETAILS OF PATIENTS WITH AIDP

Case	Age/sex	Onset to peak (days)	CSF	Phase	Modality	NDS	Cortico-steroids	Plasma exchange
1	35/M	17	N	I	S	76	Yes	No
2	29/M	10	N	P	M	66	No	No
3	19/F	10	N	I	M	61	No	No
4	79/F	10	Abn	P	M	140	No	No
5	64/M	3	Abn	W	M	109	Yes	No
6	57/F	2	N	P	M	160	Yes	No
7	58/M	4	Abn	W	M	134	Yes	Yes
8	36/F	16	Abn	P	M	144	No	No
9	13/F	8	Abn	W	M	82	No	No
10	67/M	12	Abn	W	M	140	Yes	Yes

I, improving; P, plateau; W, worsening; NDS, neurologic disability score (Dyck et al. 1980); M, S, predominantly motor, sensory; Abn, elevated CSF protein and/or immunoglobulin G; Phase, time point when serum was drawn.

monophasic polyradiculoneuropathy with onset to peak < 3 weeks and without another known cause for the neuropathy. CSF protein or IgG (usually both) were abnormal in 6/10 (protein, mean $= 125$ mg/dl, S.D. 182). Patients were severely to moderately affected and 6/10 were bed-ridden. The neurological disability scores (NDS) (Dyck et al. 1980) of < 50, $50-100$ and > 100 correspond approximately to mild, moderate and severe disabilities and patients with scores >100 are usually bed-ridden.

(2) Control sera

Control sera were obtained from healthy subjects free of neurological disease or recent immunization.

All sera (control and AIDP) were coded, stored in 0.5 ml quantities and stored at $-70°C$ until use. The code was not broken until all measurements had been completed.

(3) Electrophysiological methods

(i) Acute study of normal nerve (acute normal preparation)

300 g Sprague-Dawley rats were used. The animals were anaesthetized with intraperitoneal pentobarbital (50 mg/kg) and standard electrophysiological techniques were used to stimulate and record the compound muscle potential from the small foot muscles. The tibial division of sciatic nerve was stimulated at the hip and ankle levels. The peroneal division of sciatic nerve was sectioned, care being taken to preserve the blood supply to the sciatic nerve. The temperature of the limb

was monitored with subcutaneous thermistor probes at 2 sites (at the thigh level and below the knee) and maintained at 37°C with radiant heat.

The stimulus was a square wave of duration 0.1—0.2 msec and of amplitude 1.2 times that required to produce a maximal response. It was produced by a pulse generator (Model 830 interval generator, Model 832 "Preset" Control and Model 831 pulse delay, W-P Instruments, New Haven, Conn.), and isolated from ground by a photon-coupled stimulus isolation unit (Model 850 A, W-P Instruments, New Haven, Conn.). The evoked compound muscle action potential (CMAP) was led into an AC preamplifier set at × 1000 gain (DAM 5, W-P Instruments, New Haven, Conn.), displayed on a digital oscilloscope (Nicolet 1170, Nicolet Instrument Corp., Madison, Wis.), then stored on magnetic tape (Kennedy Model 9800, NIC-283B Magnetic Tape Control, Nicolet Instrument Corp., Madison, Wis.).

Following initial recording to ensure stability of the CMAP over 15—20 min, 10 μl of test solution was injected intraneurally under microscope and micromanipulator control into the tibial division of the sciatic nerve at the mid-sciatic level. Further records were made at 5 min intervals for 1 h. The electrophysiological recording was then terminated and the surgical wound repaired.

(ii) Acute study of focally demyelinated nerve (acute demyelinated preparation)

Focal demyelination was produced by the application of a 4 mm long polyethylene cuff over the left mid-sciatic nerve, secured by two 6-0 silk ties. The animal was then placed on a diet containing 40% w/w galactose to produce endoneurial oedema (Low 1982b). The rats were used 2 months after commencement of feeding and only if they showed the electrophysiological hallmarks of demyelination (conduction slowing and dispersion of CMAP). Otherwise the focally demyelinated preparation was studied in an identical fashion as the normal preparation.

(iii) One week study — part 1

Rats used in this study were microinjected as in (i) but not studied acutely. At 7 days electrophysiological records of conduction velocity and amplitude were made as in (i).

(iv) One week study — part 2: in vivo monophasic compound action potential (CAP) records in syngeneic Lewis rats

Syngeneic Lewis rats were microinjected as in (iii) but in this part of the study the peroneal nerve was not sectioned. The in vivo monophasic CAP records were made at 1 week, using the previously described techniques (Low and McLeod 1977; Smith and Hall 1980). The nerve had an intact blood supply. Stimulation and recording was done using platinum hook electrodes at the hip and midcalf levels respectively. The nerve was crushed between the pair of recording electrodes. The nerve and electrodes were bathed in temperature-controlled oxygenated mineral oil and maintained at 35°C. Records using this technique were very stable and the amplitude of the monophasic CAP at the end of the experiment was within 5% of that at the beginning.

As indices of dispersion width the CAP was measured from the onset to peak, onset to 50% (of the falling phase) and onset to 100% (when the falling phase had returned to baseline).

Paired stimuli with pulse intervals of 0.5, 1, 2, 3, 4, 5, 7 and 10 msec were used. The single response was subtracted from the paired response and the time integral (digitized area of the action potential) of the resultant was expressed as a percentage of the time integral of the unpaired response. This value provides an estimate of the number of myelinated fibres that have come out of the refractory period for the particular pulse interval.

(4) Statistical analysis

Data were graphically displayed and group values tested for skewness, kurtosis and outliers and a normal probability plot was displayed (Hewlett-Packard General Statistics program). Acceptable data were compared, using a 2-way Student's *t* test.

RESULTS

Qualitative results

Normal looking responses were often seen in both control and AIDP-injected nerves studied at 7 days (Fig. 1). In some AIDP-injected nerves the CMAP was greatly reduced on stimulation above the injection site (Fig. 2). Similar abnormalities were also seen in some control nerves (Fig. 2).

In the acute normal preparation only a small decrement of the CMAP appeared immediately following injection (Fig. 2, trace 2). In occasional control and AIDP nerves (Fig. 3) an appreciable reduction in CMAP amplitude was seen at 30 and 60 min (Fig. 3, traces 3 and 4).

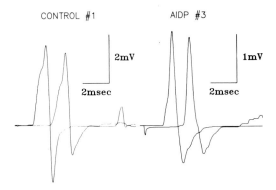

Fig. 1. Muscle action potential records from the small muscles of the foot on stimulating above and below the injection site. Temp. 37°C. Seven day preparation — part 1.

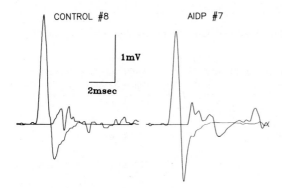

Fig. 2. Muscle action potentials showing a marked reduction in amplitude of compound muscle action potential in a control (Control No. 8) and an AIDP nerve (AIDP No. 7). Temp. 37°C. Seven day preparation — part 1.

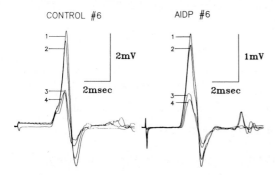

Fig. 3. Muscle action potentials recorded on stimulating the tibial division of sciatic nerve across the injection site. Responses 1, 2, 3, 4 refer to responses before and 2, 30, 60 min after microinjection, respectively. Temp. 37°C. Acute normal preparation.

Quantitative studies

Sera

Sera of control and AIDP patients were age-matched (controls, N = 10, mean age = 47.4, S.D. = 19.8; AIDP, N = 10, mean age = 45.7, S.D. = 22.2; difference n.s.).

Acute normal preparation (Table II)

Each serum was tested on 3 nerves from which a mean value was derived. At 30 min after injection, AIDP sera caused a slightly greater reduction of CMAP than did control sera but the difference was not significant ($P = 0.15$). At 60 min the difference between control and AIDP was significant ($P = 0.02$). When only severe AIDP cases (NDS > 100) were considered, AIDP CMAP was significantly reduced at both 30 min ($P = 0.03$) and 60 min ($P = 0.003$) although the differences were relatively small. When amplitude percentage was regressed against NDS scores, however, only a weak relationship was found ($y = 92.0 - 0.22x$, $R = 0.3$ at 30 min; $y = 109.4 - 0.42x$, $R = 0.4$ at 60 min).

TABLE II

SUMMARY OF ELECTROPHYSIOLOGICAL PARAMETERS FOLLOWING MICROINJECTION
OF AIDP AND NORMAL SERUM

	Conduction velocity (m/sec)	Amplitude % (injected/un-injected) segments
Electrophysiological studies for 7 day study — part 1 for ALL sera		
Control		
Mean (S.D.)	44.2 (4.0)	73.5 (8.0)
AIDP		
Mean (S.D.)	44.5 (3.1)	73.9 (7.9)
df	19	19
P	n.s.	n.s.
Electrophysiological studies for 7 day study — part 1 for subset of SEVERE cases (NDS > 100)		
Control		
Mean (S.D.)	44.2 (4.0)	73.5 (8.0)
AIDP		
Mean (S.D.)	45.0 (3.8)	72.8 (8.7)
df	15	15
P	n.s.	n.s.

	Normal nerve		Demyelinated nerve	
	30 min	60 min	30 min	60 min
Amplitude % (of preinjection amplitude) for acute study for ALL sera				
Control				
Mean (S.D.)	72.4 (9.4)	66.5 (10.9)	133 (114)	105.8 (46.9)
AIDP				
Mean (S.D.)	67.0 (12.3)	54.9 (11.2)	68.8 (30.4)	64.2 (38.8)
df	19	19	19	19
P	n.s.	0.02	n.s.	0.03
Amplitude % (of preinjection amplitude) for acute study for subset of SEVERE cases (NDS > 100)				
Control				
Mean (S.D.)	72.4 (9.4)	66.5 (10.9)	133 (114)	105.8 (46.9)
AIDP				
Mean (S.D.)	61.7 (11.2)	48.8 (9.3)	61.0 (38.4)	50.2 (36.6)
df	15	15	15	15
P	0.03	0.003	n.s.	0.02

Acute demyelinated preparation (Table II)

On the premise that demyelinated nerve fibres (with a reduced safety factor) may
be more suitable preparations to demonstrate a mild blocking factor than normal
nerves, control and AIDP sera were injected into focally demyelinated rat sciatic
nerve, as described under Methods. AIDP sera produced greater reduction in
CMAP at all time points. At 30 min AIDP sera did not cause a statistically
significant reduction ($P = 0.06$) when compared with controls. By 60 min AIDP
serum caused significantly greater reduction ($P = 0.03$) than control sera. If only
severe cases (NDS > 100) were considered the results were similar (Table II).

TABLE III

SUMMARY OF ELECTROPHYSIOLOGICAL PARAMETERS FOR 1 WEEK STUDY — IN VIVO MONOPHASIC CAP PREPARATION

	Conduction velocity (m/sec)	Amplitude (mV)
Control		
Mean (S.D.)	46.8 (4.0)	4.8 (1.9)
AIDP		
Mean (S.D.)	52.6 (7.3)	5.7 (2.3)
df	9	9
P	n.s.	n.s.

Monophasic compound action potential width (msec)

	Onset to peak	Onset to mid-point of falling phase	Full width
Control			
Mean (S.D.)	0.51 (0.02)	0.77 (0.03)	2.59 (0.25)
AIDP			
Mean (S.D.)	0.47 (0.06)	0.76 (0.12)	2.45 (0.39)
df	9	9	9
P	n.s.	n.s.	n.s.

Time integral % (paired response – single response/single response) for different pulse intervals

	0.5 msec	1 msec	2 msec	3 msec	4 msec	5 msec	7 msec	10 msec
Control								
Mean (S.D.)	13.7 (12.3)	50.6 (18.3)	71.9 (18.4)	82.3 (16.5)	87.3 (15.2)	89.6 (14.7)	92.2 (13.5)	92.7 (13.5)
AIDP								
Mean (S.D.)	13.2 (11.2)	54.5 (21.7)	78.9 (11.8)	88.0 (16.5)	92.4 (4.4)	94.2 (4.0)	96.6 (2.1)	97.2 (2.3)
df	9	9	9	9	9	9	9	9
P	n.s.	n.s.	n.s.	n.s.	n.s.	n.s.	n.s.	n.s.

Electrophysiological studies at day 7 (1 week study — part 1) (Table II)

Each control serum was injected into 6 nerves from which a mean value was derived. Each AIDP serum was identically treated with the exception of AIDP No. 8 (2 nerves harvested only since 2 animals died and there was inadequate serum for more injections). Control and AIDP conduction velocities or amplitude percentage (amplitude of CMAP on stimulating above the injected area/amplitude of CMAP on stimulating below the injected area, expressed as a percentage) were not significantly different. When only severe cases (NDS > 100) were considered the results were again not statistically different (Table II).

One week study — part 2: in vivo monophasic CAP preparation (Table III)

The conduction velocity, amplitude, indices of dispersion and time integral percentage of the resultant CAP (paired second response/single response) for pulse intervals from 0.5 to 10 msec for AIDP sera-injected nerves were statistically not different from those of control sera-injected nerves.

DISCUSSION

In the present study no significant difference in conduction velocity or amplitude (%) (1 week study — part 1) or any of the parameters from the in vivo monophasic CAP preparation (1 week study — part 2) was found following AIDP injection when compared with controls at 1 week. We have used coded sera, optimized the injection techniques, used an adequate number of nerves and rigorous statistical analysis. The time point of 1 week was chosen because demyelination is well established and repair is incomplete (Feasby et al. 1980; Dyck et al. 1981). The negative findings in 1 week study — part 1 could not be ascribed to non-specific nerve damage at the time of peroneal nerve section since identical results were obtained in 1 week study — part 2 when the nerve was left undisturbed. The acute normal preparation showed a small but significant effect of AIDP sera, and similar results were found in the acute demyelinated preparation.

We found clear electrophysiological abnormalities, usually seen in demyelinated nerves, with dispersion and the appearance of late components, following microinjection of both normal and AIDP sera in a few nerves. Factors that appear to accentuate these changes include large size of the needle, the rate of injection, movement of the needle, and constituents of the injectate (Dyck et al. 1981). Possible mechanisms are (1) a breach of nerve perineurium (Spencer et al. 1975; Pencek et al. 1980); (2) trauma due to the injection with breakdown of the blood-nerve barrier (Olsson 1975); (3) endoneurial oedema due to the high protein, high viscosity serum (Low 1982a); (4) chemical constituents such as lysolecithin, which occur in appreciable concentrations in normal serum (Yao and Dyck 1978); and (5) anti-nerve antibodies (Tse et al. 1971).

The negative findings at 1 week contrast with the clear-cut abnormalities in morphology and physiology following induction of EAN by passive transfer or by sensitization with galactocerebroside (Saida et al. 1978, 1979; Hahn et al. 1980). Sera used in the present study were used relatively soon after collection, came from patients with typical AIDP during the acute stage of the illness, mostly patients with severe disease, so that demyelinative activity directly against rat peripheral nerve should have been present if indeed it can be passively transferred by endoneural injection. Conceivably AIDP sera at 1 week produced demyelination that the 1 week preparation was not sensitive enough to detect. The absolute amplitudes of CMAP varied considerably among even normal nerves. For this reason, we chose the parameter of amplitude percentage relating amplitude across the demyelinated segment to that below the segment of the *same* nerve, reducing inter-nerve variability. The in vivo monophasic preparation studied with measurements of time integrals for different pulse intervals has been shown to be considerably more sensitive than studies of single responses (Smith and Hall 1980). Using these methods a large demyelinating effect should have been demonstrated.

Syngeneic Lewis rats have been used to minimize genetic heterogeneity of recipient rats. A second reason is that Lewis rats are much more susceptible to EAN than are Wistar or Sprague-Dawley rats (Hofmann et al. 1980). Even with parameters examined using this preparation, we were unable to find a difference between AIDP and control sera. We conclude that a pronounced demyelinating effect specific to AIDP serum on rat nerve fibres cannot be produced by endoneural injection using our methods. Our results are compatible with a small and early effect due to either conduction block or possibly demyelination.

SUMMARY

Sera from 10 patients with AIDP and 10 age-matched controls were microinjected into the tibial division of rat sciatic nerve using improved microinjection techniques and coded sera. No statistically significant changes in conduction velocity or amplitude of the compound muscle action potential (CMAP) or in the monophasic compound action potential (CAP) parameters was found at 1 week. In nerves studied with serial recording over 1 h a small but significantly greater reduction in CMAP amplitude was observed at 60 min in the AIDP group and at both 30 and 60 min when only sera from very severely affected (bed-ridden) patients were considered. A similar reduction was found following microinjection into focally demyelinated nerves. The finding of a small reduction in CMAP amplitude in the first hour suggests the presence in some AIDP patients of serum blocking or demyelinating factors but the clinical significance of this small reduction is uncertain.

REFERENCES

Arnason, B. Inflammatory polyradiculoneuropathies. In: P.J. Dyck, P.K. Thomas and E.H. Lambert (Eds.), Peripheral Neuropathy, Vol. 3. Saunders, Philadelphia, Pa., 1975: Ch. 56, 1104.

Arnason, B., Winkler, G.F. and Hadler, N.M. Cell-mediated demyelination of peripheral nerve in tissue culture. Lab. Invest., 1969, 21: 1.

Cook, S.D., Dowling, P.C., Murray, M.R. et al. Circulating factors in acute idiopathic polyneuropathy. Arch. Neurol. (Chic.), 1971, 24: 136–144.

Dubois-Dalcq, M., Niedieck, B. and Buyse, M. Action of anticerebroside sera on myelinated nervous tissue cultures. Path. Europ., 1970, 5: 331.

Dyck, P.J., Sherman, W.R., Hallcher, L.M., Service, F.J., O'Brien, P.C., Grina, L.A., Palumbo, P.J. and Swanson, C.J. Human diabetic endoneurial sorbital, fructose, and *myo*-inositol related to sural nerve morphometry. Ann. Neurol., 1980, 8: 590–596.

Dyck, P.J., Lais, A.C., Sparks, M.F. and Hansen, S.M. Technique assessment of demyelinating activity from endoneurially injected test solutions and sera: demyelinating activity of HMSN III sera. Neurology (Minneap.), 1981, 31: 154.

Edgington, T.S. and Dalessio, D.J. The assessment by immunofluorescence methods of humoral anti-myelin antibodies in man. J. Immunol., 1970, 105: 248–255.

Feasby, T.E., Hahn, A.F. and Gilbert, J.J. Passive transfer of demyelinating activity in Guillain-Barré polyneuropathy. Neurology (Minneap.), 1980, 30: 363.

Hahn, A.F., Gilbert, J.J. and Feasby, T.E. Passive transfer of demyelination by experimental allergic neuritis serum. Acta neuropath. (Berl.), 1980, 49: 169–176.

Hirano, A., Cook, S.D., Whitaker, J.N. et al. Fine structural aspects of demyelination in vitro: the effects of Guillain-Barré serum. J. Neuropath. exp. Neurol., 1971, 30: 249–264.

Hofmann, P., Powers, J., Weise, M.J. and Brostoff, S.W. Experimental allergic neuritis: I. Rat strain differences in the response to bovine myelin antigen. Brain Res., 1980, 195: 355–362.

Low, P.A. Endoneurial fluid pressure and microenvironment of nerve. In: P.J. Dyck, P.K. Thomas, E.H. Lambert and R. Bunge (Eds.), Peripheral Neuropathy. Saunders, Philadelphia, Pa., 1982a, in press.

Low, P.A. In vitro study of acute elevations of endoneurial pressure in mammalian peripheral nerve sheath. Exp. Neurol., 1982b, 74: 160–169.

Low, P.A. and McLeod, J.G. The refractory period, the effects of temperature and trains of stimuli on conduction in the hereditary hypertrophic neuropathy of the trembler mouse. J. Neurol. Neurosurg. Psychiat., 1977, 40: 434–447.

Olsson, Y. Vascular permeability in the peripheral nervous system. In: P.J. Dyck, P.K. Thomas and E.H. Lambert (Eds.), Peripheral Neuropathy, Vol. 3. Saunders, Philadelphia, Pa., 1975: Ch. 10, 190.

Pencek, T.L., Schauf, C.L., Low P.A., Eisenberg, B.R. and Davis, F.A. Morphological and physiological effects of disruption of the perineurium in amphibian peripheral nerve. Neurology (Minneap.), 1980, 30: 593–599.

Saida, T., Saida, K., Silverberg, D.H. and Brown, M.J. Transfer of demyelination with experimental allergic neuritis serum by intraneural injection. Nature (Lond.), 1978, 272: 639.

Saida, T., Saida, K., Dorfman, S.H. et al. Experimental allergic neuritis induced by sensitization with galactocerebroside. Science, 1979, 204: 1103–1106.

Smith, K.J. and Hall, S.M. Nerve conduction during peripheral demyelination and remyelination. J. neurol. Sci., 1980, 48: 201–219.

Spencer, P.S., Weinberg, H.J., Raine, C.S. and Prineas, J.W. The perineurial window – a new model of focal demyelination and remyelination. Brain Res., 1975, 96: 323–329.

Tse, K.S., Arbesman, C.E., Tomasi, T.B. and Tourville, D. Demonstration of antimyelin antibodies by immunofluorescence in Guillain-Barré syndrome. Clin. exp. Immunol., 1971, 8: 881–887.

Yao, J.K. and Dyck, P.J. Lipid abnormalities in hereditary neuropathy. J. neurol. Sci., 1978, 36: 225–236.

Yonezawa, T., Ishihara, Y. and Matsuyama, H. Studies on experimental allergic peripheral neuritis: I. Demyelinating patterns studied in vitro. J. Neuropath. exp. Neurol., 1968, 27: 453.

Kyoto Symposia (EEG Suppl. No. 36)
Editors: P.A. Buser, W.A. Cobb and T. Okuma
© 1982, Elsevier Biomedical Press, Amsterdam

Altered Nerve Conduction Studied by Reflex Methods

P. GUIHENEUC

Laboratoire de Physiologie, Université Nantes — U.E.R. Médecine, 44035-Nantes Cedex (France)

Determination of nerve conduction velocities has proved very useful in diagnosing the appearance of peripheral neuropathies and in following their course in humans. Yet, as these measurements are most often performed in distal segments of peripheral nerves, and, as biopsies are also taken from the distal ends of sensory nerves, functional alterations and pathological changes affecting the proximal segments and the largest myelinated fibres are at present relatively unknown.

However, reliable methods have been developed to explore conduction velocity (CV) in proximal segments of peripheral nerves. The study of the monosynaptic reflex response evoked in some muscles by electrical stimulation of primary afferents has proved quite interesting for the study of peripheral neuropathies. In 1965 the latency of the soleus H response was measured by Mawdsley and Mayer in alcoholic patients. The same year, Visser (1965) pointed out that this latency may increase following an acute L5-S1 disk prolapse.

Application of this method enabled us to explore proximal conduction velocity changes in several homogeneous populations of patients suffering from well defined neuropathies of mechanical (Descuns et al. 1973), metabolic (Bathien and Guiheneuc 1974; Guiheneuc and Bathien 1976) or toxic origin (Guiheneuc et al. 1980).

The present paper, based on work conducted in our laboratory from 1969 on, leads to the following conclusions: changes in proximal conduction velocity differ according to the cause, localization, severity and type of nerve lesion; proximal and distal conduction velocities may exhibit non-parallel modifications; studies of monosynaptic T and H response amplitudes, together with proximal CV determination, are very useful in discriminating the pattern of proximal nerve injury; a discrepancy between modifications of proximal conduction velocities and functional motor ability is frequently observed.

MATERIAL

Normal values for the H reflex were obtained from 68 normal subjects, aged between 19 and 54 years (mean: 32 ± 6 years).

The results presented in this paper were obtained from 103 patients suffering from terminal chronic renal insufficiency, examined before undergoing treatment by peritoneal or extracorporeal dialysis; from 125 patients hospitalized for complications of chronic alcoholic intoxication; from 27 subjects with Hodgkin's disease treated by vincristine; from 41 patients examined for acute L5-S1 disk prolapse which was later surgically confirmed; and from 36 subjects examined for sciatic pain due to a carcinomatous radiculopathy. For each patient, special care was taken to exclude any possible cause of neuropathy other than that under study.

METHODS

The H reflex was evoked by electrical stimulation of the popliteal branch of the sciatic nerve in the popliteal fossa (square wave shocks of 1.5 msec duration, at a frequency of 0.3 Hz) (Fig. 1). The soleus response was recorded by surface electrodes placed in line with the Achilles tendon, with the proximal electrode midway between the two extremities of the fibula and the other electrode 3 cm away distally. The maximal amplitudes of the reflex (H_{max}) and direct motor (M_{max}) responses were computed from at least 3 successive responses to constant stimulus intensity. The H_{max}/M_{max} ratio for normal subjects was 0.54 ± 0.10.

In addition, the time interval separating the M response from the H response was measured. This period corresponds to the time that the reflex impulse takes to complete the arc: popliteal fossa—spinal reflex level—popliteal fossa. Although the length of this arc cannot be measured directly, studies on cadavers have shown that it can be considered as a relatively constant fraction (80%) of the subject's height.

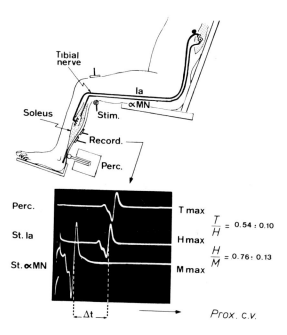

Fig. 1. Figure showing the position of the subject, the placement of stimulating and recording electrodes, typical T, H and M soleus responses displayed on an oscilloscope screen, and how the Δt time interval is measured to calculate proximal CV.

Thus, by estimating the time for passage through the spinal synapse as 1 msec, it is possible to compute an average conduction velocity (afferent and efferent) over the proximal segments of the sciatic nerve.

$$\text{Proximal NCV} = \frac{\text{height in mm} \times 0.8}{\Delta t \ (M \to H), \ - 1 \ \text{msec}}$$

The value of proximal NCV for normal subjects was 59.2 ± 2.6 m/sec.

Transformation of the preceding formula allows an H index to be calculated, offering the advantage of a useful expansion of the measuring scale into the zone of the usual variations in proximal NCV (between 60 and 35 m/sec, the relation between proximal NCV and the H index being almost linear).

$$\text{H index} = \left[\frac{\text{height in cm}}{\Delta t \ M \to H, \ \text{msec}} \right]^2 \times 2$$

The conduction value of the reflex pathway is therefore expressed in arbitrary units. The normal H index was approximately 100 (100.3 ± 7.1).

The soleus T response was evoked by maximal percussion of the Achilles tendon with an electromagnetic device at a frequency of 0.3 Hz, the mean amplitude of the 5 best out of 20 consecutive responses being measured. The T_{max}/M_{max} ratio (0.41 ± 0.14) makes it possible to estimate the percentage of motoneurones of the soleus muscle recruited by a maximal stimulus of the spindles, whereas the H_{max}/M_{max} ratio relates to the excitation of Ia fibres in the popliteal fossa. Consequently, the T_{max}/H_{max} ratio (0.76 ± 0.13) provides an indication of the functional value of the primary afferents (spindles + extremities of the Ia axons) between the soleus muscle and the popliteal fossa.

In some groups of patients, proximal NCV was compared with *distal motor CV* in the tibial nerve when stimulated in the popliteal fossa and at the ankle. The response of the flexor hallucis brevis muscle was recorded with surface electrodes.

Isometric twitch tension of extensor digitorum brevis muscle was measured using a special device with a strain gauge applied to the toes (article to be published). The peroneal nerve was maximally stimulated at the ankle with a shock 1 msec in duration.

Calculations and statistics. Linear correlations were carried out by the least square method. For non-linear correlations, the scattering of points of the graph was analysed by extracting successive means (cf. Guiheneuc and Bathien 1976). This method was employed to describe the relative changes of T and H responses with respect to proximal NCV.

RESULTS and DISCUSSION

(a) Proximal versus distal CV
   The proximal CV measured in a uraemic or alcoholic subject was plotted against

the tibial nerve motor CV obtained in the same subject. Thus the conduction velocity in proximal and distal segments of the same nerve trunk could be compared. In both uraemic and alcoholic subjects there was a linear relationship between the 2 parameters and the difference of slope of the 2 regression lines was not statistically significant (Fig. 2).

These results are consistent with the hypothesis that there are lesions diffused along the whole length of the peripheral nerves (proximal and distal parts). The existence of parallel changes in proximal and distal CV leads to the conclusion that these lesions are not only diffuse but are of similar magnitude all along the nerve.

Nevertheless, it is important to point out that the CV measured in the 2 cases does not refer to the same structures. The distal motor CV is related to the impulse propagation velocity in alpha motoneurones of the tibial nerve. On the other hand, the time interval between the M and H responses corresponds to a combined afferent and efferent conduction time. The changes in proximal CV may concern the Ia fibres, the intraspinal circuit or the motoneurones of the reflex arc.

The results we have obtained show that the conduction velocities (proximal and distal) are more markedly reduced in uraemic than in alcoholic patients. Many authors have described extensive lesions of Schwann cells and myelin sheaths in distal fibres of uraemic patients. So it seems logical to suppose that demyelinating lesions are also extensive in proximal segments of the peripheral nerves in uraemics. The more moderate reduction in proximal conduction velocities in alcoholics indicates more moderate alterations of the proximal nerve sheaths.

Results obtained in *patients suffering from pain in the region of the sciatic nerve* (Fig. 3) appear to be different according to the cause of nerve impairment. In the case of mechanical compression of the first sacral root by an acute L5-S1 disk prolapse, proximal CV is only slightly decreased, whereas distal motor CV is almost normal. When pain along the sciatic nerve is due to a carcinomatous radiculopathy (lymphopathies and lung, breast, kidney or intestinal cancers in our cases), proximal CV is sharply reduced, often much more than is distal CV. On several occasions

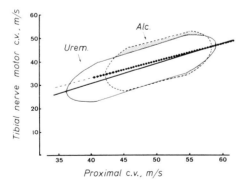

Fig. 2. Relationship between proximal nerve conduction velocity (abscissa) and tibial nerve motor CV (ordinate) in uraemic (clear area) and alcoholic (shaded area) subjects. For each group of patients the regression line and the area limited by the 95% tolerance ellipses and hyperbolas were obtained from individual values.

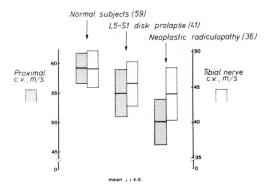

Fig. 3. Mean values ± S.D. of proximal CV (shaded columns) and tibial nerve motor CV (clear columns) in 3 groups of subjects.

such a discrepancy between proximal and distal CV led us to suggest complementary investigations which allowed a previously undetected malignant disease to be found in some patients.

(b) Proximal CV versus H/M ratio

The H_{max}/M_{max} ratio makes it possible to estimate the percentage of alpha motoneurones innervating the soleus muscle that can be recruited by stimulation of the Ia fibres in the popliteal fossa. Consequently, a decrease in this ratio indicates that a portion of the motoneurone pool remaining active (unimpaired) can no longer be affected by stimulation of the afferent pathway. If it is admitted that in peripheral neuropathies, at least at their onset, medullary synaptic transmissions are maintained intact (central controls and cutaneous polysynaptic reflexes evoke normal responses), diminution of the H/M ratio would thus signify that there are proximal lesions (between the popliteal fossa and the alpha motoneurones) of the primary afferent fibres.

In uraemic patients, the H/M ratio decreases only slightly when the H index is higher than 75 or 80 (Fig. 4). Below these values, H response amplitude decreases more rapidly, so that the curve (solid line) appears to be made up of 2 segments with different slopes. We venture to suggest that the early phase of this polyneuropathy is concerned with pure or almost pure demyelinating lesions. The slope of the upper segment of this curve would thus represent the physiological events related to demyelination, so that a 10% decrease of proximal CV corresponds to a very little diminution (about 5%) of reflex discharge.

When the lesions worsen, the slope of the curve changes. A 10% diminution of proximal CV is now accompanied by a 30% decrease of the H/M ratio. We postulate that axonal degeneration of Ia fibres, together with demyelination, is responsible for this more rapid decrease in amplitude of the H response.

In alcoholic patients, the H/M ratio, plotted against proximal CV, shows an early and very sharp decrease. A 10% diminution of proximal CV corresponds to an 80% decrease of the H/M ratio from its normal value. In chronic alcoholics, distal

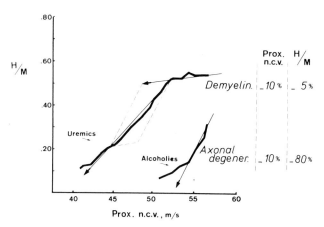

Fig. 4. Mean values of H/M ratio plotted against proximal CV for uraemic and alcoholic patients. Each curve is obtained by calculating recursive means from individual values (not shown here).

axonal lesions have been detected by electrophysiological examination and by histological examination based on a nerve biopsy (Walsh and McLeod 1970; Tackmann et al. 1977; Behse and Buchthal 1978). The diminution of the H response indicates that the main part of the motoneurone pool can no longer be recruited by the afferent fibres stimulated at the popliteal fossa. Thus, the diminution of the H/M ratio is to be related to important and early proximal lesions of Ia fibres. It seems that it would be more appropriate to describe this type of neuropathy as a diffuse axonal degeneration, and not as a uniquely distal axonal lesion.

The change of slope in the lower part of the H/M curve in alcoholics is due to the fact that in many patients no clear H response is found (when the polyneuritis becomes more severe).

(c) Proximal CV versus T/H ratio

The T/H ratio provides an indication of the functional value of the primary afferents between the soleus muscle and the popliteal fossa. It depends upon the state of excitability of annulo-spiral endings and the integrity of the distal segment of Ia fibres.

In uraemic patients (Fig. 5), the T/H ratio remains almost normal for a long time during the course of the neuropathy, thus indicating that lesions develop similarly in proximal and distal segments of Ia fibres.

During the *early phase of alcoholic neuropathy,* the T/H ratio is frequently above normal, sometimes equal to 1.5 or 2. However, the T response is decreased, but to a lesser degree than the H response, so that the T/H ratio is enhanced. We may suppose that axonal lesions predominate in fibres of larger diameter. Thus, the Ia fibres which remain functional have a diameter and a threshold comparable to those of motoneurones. Electrical stimulation cannot evoke an H response because the reflex impulse collides with the recurrent discharge on simultaneously excited motoneurones. But percussion of the Achilles tendon can evoke a discharge in these fibres, thus producing a T response larger than the H response.

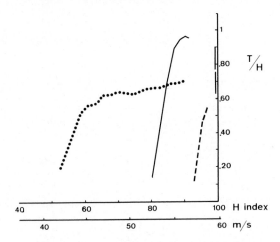

Fig. 5. Mean values of T/H ratio plotted against the proximal CV for uraemic (dotted line), alcoholic (solid line), and vincristine-treated patients (broken line).

In patients treated with vincristine, very rapid decrease of the T/H ratio is closely correlated with the dose of the drug administered. The T response disappears as the total dose of vincristine injected reaches 6—8 mg per square metre of body surface. This decrease of the T response occurs when, simultaneously, the H/M ratio is normal and proximal NCV not significantly modified. In a recent paper, we have shown that these results may be explained only by severe early lesions of the distal zones of Ia fibres, the proximal segments remaining unimpaired, and have indicated that the neuropathy induced by vincristine has all the features of a dying-back phenomenon (Guiheneuc et al. 1980).

(d) Proximal CV versus motor ability

Studies on peripheral neuropathies have to be planned not only to explore the cause or mechanisms of the nerve lesions but also to determine the sensory and motor defects the patients have to manage with. From this point of view, we have noted a frequent absence of correlation between the modifications of the proximal CV and the motor performance evaluated by measurement of muscle force or clinical testing. Fig. 6 is an example of such a discrepancy.

A patient with chronic renal insufficiency underwent haemodialysis, first at home for 6 months, where conditions of treatment were disastrous due to the social environment, then in our hospital where dialysis was strikingly improved.

The upper curves indicate the changes in proximal CV and distal motor CV of the peroneal nerve. In the lower part of the graph we have plotted the amplitude of the mechanical response of the extensor digitorum brevis muscle. The peroneal nerve was maximally stimulated at the ankle with a shock 1 msec in duration, and the twitch response of the muscle was measured using a special device with a strain gauge applied to the toes.

During the 6 months of poor dialysis at home, a considerable decrease of the

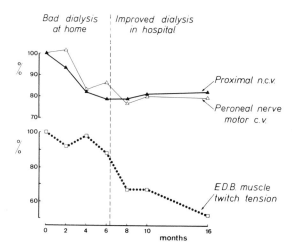

Fig. 6. Conduction velocity and distal muscle force changes in a patient undergoing haemodialysis.

proximal and distal CV occurred. Simultaneously, muscle twitch force remained almost normal. When treatment was improved, conduction velocities no longer decreased and seemed slightly enhanced. Yet, at the same time, muscle twitch amplitude decreased.

We conclude that measurement of proximal CV, though quite useful, must be complemented by other methods (amplitude of reflex responses, distal CV, EMG, measurement of muscle force, etc.) to perform meaningful investigations.

REFERENCES

Bathien, N. et Guiheneuc, P. L'exploration des polynévrites chroniques par la technique du réflexe H. Rev. E.E.G. Neurophysiol., 1974, 4: 587–595.

Behse, F. and Buchthal, F. Sensory action potentials and biopsy of the sural nerve in neuropathy. Brain, 1978, 101: 473–493.

Descuns, P., Collet, M., Resche, F. et Guiheneuc, P. Intérêt du réflexe H dans l'exploration des lésions radiculaires d'origine discale. Neurochirurgie, 1973, 19: 627–640.

Guiheneuc, P. and Bathien N. Two patterns of results in peripheral neuropathies explored by reflexological methods. Comparison between proximal and distal conduction velocities. J. neurol. Sci., 1976, 30: 83–94.

Guiheneuc, P., Ginet, J., Groleau, J.Y. and Rojouan, J. Early phase of vincristine neuropathy in man: electrophysiological evidence for a dying back phenomenon, with transitory enhancement of spinal transmission of the monosynaptic reflex. J. neurol. Sci., 1980, 45: 355–366.

Mawdsley, C. and Mayer, R.F. Nerve conduction in alcoholic neuropathy. Brain, 1965, 88: 335–356.

Tackmann, W., Minckenberg, R. and Strenge, H. Correlation of electrophysiological and quantitative histological findings in the sural nerve of man. Studies on alcoholic neuropathy. J. Neurol., 1977, 216: 289–299.

Visser, S.L. The significance of the Hoffmann reflex in the EMG examination of patients with herniation of the nucleus pulposus. Psychiat. Neurol. Neurochir. (Amst.), 1965, 68: 300–305.

Walsh, J.C. and McLeod, J.G. Alcoholic neuropathy. An electrophysiological and histological study. J. neurol. Sci., 1970, 10: 457–469.

Kyoto Symposia (EEG Suppl. No. 36)
Editors: P.A. Buser, W.A. Cobb and T. Okuma
© 1982, Elsevier Biomedical Press, Amsterdam

Physiological Properties of Dystrophic Mouse Spinal Root Axons

MICHAEL RASMINSKY

Neurosciences Unit, Montreal General Hospital, McGill University, 1650 Cedar Avenue, Montreal, Que. H3G 1A4 (Canada)

Our understanding of the nerve conduction abnormalities encountered in the setting of the clinical electrophysiology laboratory is based substantially on studies of experimentally induced demyelination and degeneration in animal preparations. However, abnormalities of nerve fibres may be genetic as well as acquired; this paper reviews recent studies of the physiological properties of the spinal root axons of dystrophic mice, one of several murine mutants in which myelination is congenitally abnormal.

ANATOMY

More than 15 years after the original description of the autosomal recessive dystrophic mouse mutation (dy/dy) (Michelson et al. 1955) as a putative model for muscular dystrophy, Bradley and Jenkison (1973) described major abnormalities of the cervical and lumbo-sacral spinal root axons of these mice. In these roots bundles of large diameter axons either lack Schwann cells and myelin sheaths or are invested with inappropriately thin myelin. The naked axonal segments, apposed to one another with virtually no intervening extracellular space, are concentrated at the mid root level of both dorsal and ventral roots, myelination being more normal near the spinal cord and exit from the spinal canal (Bray and Aguayo 1975). The internodes of many myelinated axons are inappropriately short and nodal gaps are frequently longer than normal (Rasminsky et al. 1978). Cytochemical staining with Fe^{3+}-ferrocyanide shows the bare axon membrane to have the cytochemical properties of normal C fibres (i.e., low sodium channel density membrane) rather than those of normal nodes of Ranvier (i.e., high sodium channel density membrane) (Waxman et al. 1978). This congenital abnormality of myelination does not appear to reflect a primary disorder of either axons or Schwann cells (Aguayo et al. 1979) but is perhaps due to absence of some extracellular element such as the collagen matrix (Bunge and Bunge 1978).

Address correspondence to: Dr. Michael Rasminsky, Division of Neurology, Montreal General Hospital, 1650 Cedar Ave., Montreal, Que. H3G 1A4, Canada.

CONDUCTION OF NERVE IMPULSES IN DYSTROPHIC MOUSE SPINAL ROOT AXONS

The conduction velocity of impulses propagating in dystrophic mouse spinal root axons is much less than in normal axons (Huizar et al. 1975; Rasminsky et al. 1978). Both saltatory and continuous conduction occur in the spinal root axons, saltatory conduction presumably occurring in the myelinated portions and continuous conduction in the bare portions of these axons (Rasminsky et al. 1978). The characterization of the mode of conduction as *continuous* implies the lack of significant spatial separation of sites of excitable membrane along the axon. The rigor of the demonstration of continuous conduction is dependent upon the spatial resolution of the recording system used to study conduction in single fibres. In recent experiments, we have re-examined conduction in dystrophic mouse spinal root fibres using records with improved spatial resolution, comparable to that used to demonstrate continuous conduction in rat spinal root fibres demyelinated with diphtheria toxin (Bostock and Sears 1978) and microsaltatory conduction (i.e., sites of excitation separated by as little as 125 μm) in rat spinal root fibres demyelinated with lysolecithin (Bostock et al. 1980). These new records (Rasminsky and Bostock, unpublished results) support our original conclusion that continuous conduction occurs in the bare axons. Continuous conduction in a bare axon implies a relatively uniform distribution of sodium channels within the axon membrane; we can thus tentatively conclude that the absence of effective axon-Schwann cell interaction in the dystrophic mouse bare axons allows sodium channels to be uniformly distributed throughout the axon membrane, rather than constrained to the axon membrane at nodes of Ranvier, as is the case in normal myelinated fibres (Ritchie and Rogart 1977).

ABNORMAL EXCITABILITY OF DYSTROPHIC MOUSE AXONS

A striking behavioural feature of the dystrophic mouse is the continuous muscle contraction or pseudomyotonia of the hind limbs. The abolition of this ongoing muscle activity by administration of curare (Eberstein et al. 1975) implies spontaneous activation of the motor unit proximal to the neuromuscular junction. Much, if not all, of this spontaneous excitation arises in the pathological lumbo-sacral spinal root fibres (Rasminsky 1978, 1980).

Spontaneous ectopic excitation

Sites of spontaneous ectopic excitation are found in mid root of dystrophic mouse spinal root fibres (Fig. 1). Such ectopic excitation may occur as single impulses, as uninterrupted continuous activity, or as bursts of impulses with an interimpulse frequency approaching 100 Hz (Rasminsky 1978).

Ephaptic interaction or cross-talk

Some impulses originate in mid root due to ephaptic excitation or cross-talk. Such an interaction between 2 fibres is illustrated in Fig. 1 in which records were made every 200 μm over a stretch of 4 mm straddling the site of cross-excitation. In this example, as in all of the others so far examined, cross-excitation was unidirectional and appeared, on the basis of conduction velocity criteria, to proceed from bare axon to myelinated axon (Rasminsky 1980). Ephaptic transmission is not necessarily dependent upon the direction of propagation of the impulse in the exciting fibre; Fig. 2 illustrates a pair of fibres in which the exciting impulse approached the ephapse from either the proximal or distal side of the site of interaction in mid root.

Autoexcitation

Huizar et al. (1975) and Kuno (1976) observed that intracellular stimulation of

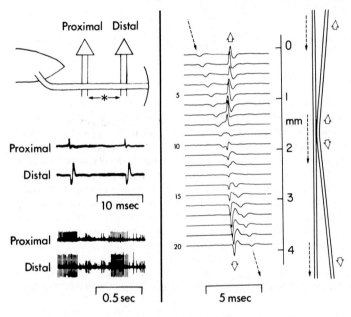

Fig. 1. Ectopic excitation and ephaptic transmission in dystrophic mouse ventral roots. Left: records of spontaneous activity are made biphasically from pairs of wire electrodes applied to the root; upward and downward deflections reflect impulses in single fibres propagating toward and away from the spinal cord, respectively. Impulses originating in mid root (*) travel in opposite directions and propagate past the 2 pairs of recording electrodes (upper traces). Bursting of the single unit shown in the upper traces is shown at slower sweep speed in the lower traces. Right: biphasic records are obtained at intervals of 200 μm along the root. From top to bottom, the records are progressively further away from the spinal cord. An impulse in one fibre propagates away from the spinal cord (downward deflection in record 1 with progressively greater latency at each successive recording site) (dashed arrows). A second fibre is ephaptically excited in mid root near recording site 9, and an impulse in this fibre (open arrows) is propagated back toward the spinal cord (upward deflections with progressively greater latencies in records 8–1) and towards the periphery (downward deflection with faster rise times and progressively greater latencies in records 10–20). See Rasminsky (1978, 1980) for details of recording procedures. Adapted from Rasminsky (1978, 1980) with permission of *Annals of Neurology* and the *Journal of Physiology*.

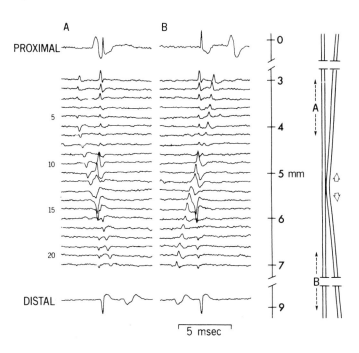

Fig. 2. Ephaptic transmission between 2 fibres in a dystrophic mouse ventral root for 2 directions of propagation in the exciting fibre. Simultaneous records were made from proximal and distal electrode pairs separated by almost 9 mm that remained fixed throughout and from a third pair of mobile electrodes (records 1–21) that were moved in steps of 200 μm. In sequence A an impulse arises ectopically in the exciting fibre at recording site 4 and is propagated toward the spinal cord (initial upward deflections in records 3–1 and proximal) and toward the periphery (downward deflections) in records 5–21 and distal). In sequence B an impulse arises ectopically in the exciting fibre between recording site 21 and the distal electrodes and is propagated towards the spinal cord (upward deflections in records 21–1 and proximal) and toward the periphery (initial downward deflection in distal). In both cases the second fibre is ephaptically excited between recording sites 12 and 13, giving rise to an impulse that propagates both centrifugally and centripetally. The position of the ephapse and the sites of origin of the exciting impulses are indicated in the diagram on the right, dashed and open arrows indicating the directions of propagation in the exciting and excited fibres, respectively. See Rasminsky (1980) for details of the recording procedure. Reproduced from Rasminsky (1980) with permission of the *Journal of Physiology*.

dystrophic mouse lumbar motoneurones or stimulation of peripheral nerve was frequently followed by repetitive antidromic invasion of lumbar motoneurones by impulses which must have originated in the periphery, either due to cross-excitation, re-excitation of the same axon (autoexcitation) or both. I subsequently showed that autoexcitation could indeed occur, a single impulse in a dystrophic mouse fibre priming a site of ectopic excitation to fire a burst of impulses some tens of milliseconds after the initial impulse had passed (Rasminsky 1980).

Mechanisms of abnormal excitability

Although the phenomenology of increased excitability of dystrophic mouse spinal root fibres has now been characterized in some detail, we have essentially no understanding of what underlies this increased excitability. The property of increased excitability is shared with other pathologically myelinated axons (see Rasminsky 1981, 1982 for review); it is possible that one aspect of disordered interaction between axons and myelin-forming cells is alteration in axon membrane properties which eventuate in a lower threshold for excitation.

A morphological observation may offer one clue as to how this might occur. Freeze fracture electron micrographs reveal occasional node-like accumulations of E face particles in dystrophic mouse bare spinal root axons (Bray et al. 1979; Ellisman 1979). Such focal accumulations of E face particles have been widely interpreted as reflecting high axonal densities of sodium channels (Rosenbluth 1976; Kristol et al. 1977, 1978). If these focal accumulations do indeed reflect aggregations of a large number of sodium channels, one can readily visualize their becoming sites of ectopic initiation of action potentials. Small membrane depolarizations (for whatever reason) will result in a slightly increased probability of opening of each sodium channel. At a site where sodium channels are densely aggregated, even a small increase in the probability of individual channels opening may thus result in opening of an adequate total number of sodium channels to permit sodium inflow sufficient to cause significant further depolarization and ultimately local generation of an action potential.

Other factors which might be of importance in the increased excitability of dystrophic mouse axons include the distribution of potassium channels, the passive membrane properties of the axons and their extracellular ionic milieu. We have preliminary evidence that potassium channel distribution is disordered in dystrophic mouse spinal root axons (Bostock and Rasminsky 1982). No information is yet available concerning the passive membrane properties of dystrophic mouse axons — any increase in membrane impedance would predispose towards increased excitability. Extracellular space between the closely apposed bare axons is probably much more restricted than in normal nerves and thus relatively small changes in total extracellular ions may give rise to relatively large changes in extracellular ion concentrations in comparison to normal roots.

A more detailed understanding of the increased excitability of pathologically myelinated axons will probably demand intracellular recording from sites of ectopic impulse generation. This will be a task of formidable technical difficulty.

SUMMARY AND CONCLUSIONS

In the spinal root axons of dystrophic mice conduction of nerve impulses is slow and either saltatory or continuous, presumably corresponding to areas of myelination and amyelination respectively. These abnormally myelinated axons contain foci of hyperexcitability manifested by spontaneous ectopic excitation, ephaptic excitation and autoexcitation. Similar phenomena in demyelinated central and peripheral nerve fibres may underlly positive neurological symptomatology in human peripheral and central demyelinating diseases (Rasminsky 1981, 1982).

ACKNOWLEDGEMENT

This investigation was supported by the Canadian Medical Research Council.

REFERENCES

Aguayo, A.J., Bray, G.M. and Perkins, S. Axon-Schwann cell relationships in neuropathies of mutant mice. Ann. N.Y. Acad. Sci., 1979, 317: 512–531.

Bostock, H. and Rasminsky, M. Potassium currents and "potassium nodes" in the spinal roots of dystrophic mice. J. Physiol. (Lond.), 1982, 325: 24P–25P.

Bostock, H. and Sears, T.A. The internodal axon membrane: electrical excitability and continuous conduction in segmental demyelination. J. Physiol. (Lond.), 1978, 280: 273–301.

Bostock, H., Hall, S.M. and Smith, K.L. Demyelinated axons can form "nodes" prior to remyelination. J. Physiol. (Lond.), 1980, 308: 21P–23P.

Bradley, W.G. and Jenkison, M. Abnormalities of peripheral nerve in murine muscular dystrophy. J. neurol. Sci., 1973, 18: 227–247.

Bray, G.M. and Aguayo, A.J. Quantitative ultrastructural studies of the axon-Schwann cell abnormality in spinal nerve roots from dystrophic mice. J. Neuropathol. exp. Neurol., 1975, 34: 517–530.

Bray, G.M., Cullen, J.M., Aguayo, A.J. and Rasminsky, M. Node-like areas of intramembranous particles in the unensheathed axons of dystrophic mice. Neurosci. Lett., 1979, 13: 203–208.

Bunge, R.P. and Bunge, M.B. Evidence that contact with connective tissue matrix is required for normal interaction between Schwann cells and nerve fibres. J. Cell Biol., 1978, 78: 943–950.

Eberstein, A., Goodgold, J. and Pechter, B.R. Effect of curare on EMG and contractile responses in the myotonic mouse. Exp. Neurol., 1975, 49: 612–616.

Ellisman, M.H. Molecular specializations at the axon membrane of nodes of Ranvier are not dependent on myelination. J. Neurocytol., 1979, 8: 719–735.

Huizar, P., Kuno, M. and Miyata, Y. Electrophysiological properties of spinal motorneurones of normal and dystrophic mice. J. Physiol. (Lond.), 1975, 248: 231–246.

Kristol, C., Akert, K., Sandri, C., Wyss, U.R., Bennett, M.V.L. and Moor, H. The Ranvier nodes in the neurogenic electric organ of the knifefish Sternarchus: A freeze-etching study on the distribution of membrane associated particles. Brain Res., 1977, 125: 197–212.

Kristol, C., Sandri, C. and Akert, K. Intramembranous particles at the nodes of Ranvier of the cat spinal cord: a morphometric study. Brain Res., 1978, 142: 391–400.

Kuno, M. Electrophysiological analyses of motoneuron properties in dystrophic mice. In: J.M. Andrews, R.T. Johnson and M.A.B. Brazier (Eds.), Amyotrophic Lateral Sclerosis. Academic Press, New York, 1976: 135–143.

Michelson, A.M., Russel, E.S. and Harman, P.J. Dystrophia muscularis: a hereditary primary myopathy in the house mouse. Proc. nat. Acad. Sci. (Wash.), 1955, 41: 1079–1084.

Rasminsky, M. Ectopic generation of impulses and cross-talk in spinal nerve roots of "dystrophic" mice. Ann. Neurol., 1978, 3: 351–357.

Rasminsky, M. Ephaptic transmission between single nerve fibers in the spinal nerve roots of dystrophic mice. J. Physiol. (Lond.), 1980, 305: 151–169.

Rasminsky, M. Hyperexcitability of pathologically myelinated axons and positive symptoms in multiple sclerosis. In: S.G. Waxman and J.M. Ritchie (Eds.), Demyelinating Disease: Basic and Clinical Electrophysiology. Raven Press, New York, 1981: 289–297.

Rasminsky, M. Ectopic excitation, ephaptic excitation and autoexcitation in peripheral nerve fibers of mutant mice. In: W. Culp and J. Ochoa (Eds.), Abnormal Nerves and Muscles as Impulse Generators. Oxford University Press, New York, 1982: 344–362.

Rasminsky, M., Kearney, R.E., Aguayo, A.J. and Bray, G.M. Conduction of nervous impulses in spinal roots and peripheral nerves of dystrophic mice. Brain Res., 1978, 143: 71–85.

Ritchie, J.M. and Rogart, R.B. The density of sodium channels in mammalian myelinated nerve fibres and nature of the axonal membrane under the myelin sheath. Proc. nat. Acad. Sci. (Wash.), 1977, 74: 211–215.

Rosenbluth, J. Intramembranous particle distribution at the node of Ranvier and adjacent axolemma in myelinated axons of the frog brain. J. Neurocytol., 1976, 5: 731–745.

Waxman, S.G., Bradley, W.C. and Hartwieg, E.A. Organization of the axolemma in amyelinated axons: a cytochemical study in dy/dy dystrophic mice. Proc. roy. Soc. B, 1978, 201: 301–308.

Kyoto Symposia (EEG Suppl. No. 36)
Editors: P.A. Buser, W.A. Cobb and T. Okuma
© 1982, Elsevier Biomedical Press, Amsterdam

Disorders of Conduction in the Somatosensory Pathway Studied by Averaged Cerebral Evoked Potentials in Man

JOHN E. DESMEDT

Brain Research Unit, University of Brussels Faculty of Medicine, 115 Boulevard de Waterloo, Brussels 1000 (Belgium)

The somatosensory evoked potentials (SEPs) recorded from the scalp provide invaluable data about clinical disorders involving either peripheral nerve or the central pathways (cf., Desmedt 1971, 1982; Desmedt and Noel 1973; Hume and Cant 1978; Anziska and Cracco 1980; Noel and Desmedt 1980). Diagnostic uses of SEPs emphasize the early components that can be reliably elicited by electrical stimulation of peripheral nerves or fingers or small skin areas. The method depends on an accurate estimation of the time of arrival of the corticopetal volley at the primary cortical projection in the contralateral parietal cortex. Recent evidence validates the onset time of component N20 as an estimate of the cortical SEP latency to stimulation of upper limb nerves in man (Desmedt and Cheron 1981b).

SEP components are designated by the polarity (N for negative, P for positive) and peak latency (cf. Donchin et al. 1977). Methods have been discussed in detail (Desmedt 1977). Current studies concur in distinguishing: (a) far-field components that are generated subcortically and are volume-conducted towards the entire scalp and the ear-lobes; and (b) cortical components generated by more or less restricted cortical regions. Far fields appear small or absent when using montages with a scalp reference electrode that is connected to grid 2 of the input amplifier (since such a reference also picks up the widespread far fields). Far fields are much larger and better delineated when using a non-cephalic (NC) reference such as the hand or shoulder. NC reference recording can admittedly raise problems of interference from the ECG and from muscle potentials in poorly relaxed patients; however, the method provides invaluable evidence about subcortical SEP activities, in conjunction with recording from the posterior neck (Cracco and Cracco 1976) and from prevertebral (oesophageal) sites (Desmedt and Cheron 1981a).

A first point is the precise identification of onset of the cortical SEP response for titration of afferent conduction. While subcortical far fields have usually been considered as of *positive* polarity (NC reference recording), recent data identified a widespread *negative* component N18 that must be distinguished from the more focally generated N20; the latter is confined to the postrolandic scalp contralateral to the upper limb stimulated (Desmedt and Cheron 1981b). No genuine N20 response occurs at the ipsilateral parietal scalp: therefore superimposition of records from the two parietal sides discloses a clear contralateral N20 that is riding on the widespread N18. Prerolandic records are also quite distinct in showing an early positive response P22 with a mean onset latency 0.6 msec later than that of the postrolandic N20. Superimposition of the pre- and postrolandic records thus allows another clear estimate of the onset of the N20 primary cortical response.

The time between the delivery of the peripheral stimulus and the arrival of the afferent volley at the cortex is made up of conduction times along several neurones. Current progress focusses on the analysis of transit times in these structures in an attempt to identify focal disorders of conduction. SEP studies appear indeed unique in providing access to the proximal part of the first sensory neurone, to the spinal roots and to the dorsal column and lemniscal pathway. New sets of pertinent issues should now become available for study, thereby extending the range of electrophysiological studies to the second and third neurones.

The recording of sensory nerve potentials (Gilliatt and Sears 1958), even when updated through electronic averaging, is rather vulnerable since slight desynchronization of the component action potentials of single nerve fibres (in neuropathy) reduces the sensory nerve potentials or even makes them unrecordable. The averaged SEPs from scalp are useful in such case: the peripheral nerve can be stimulated successively at two or more different levels and the latency difference of the corresponding cortical SEPs then serves to evaluate the peripheral sensory conduction. This method is based on the fact that, in patients with neuropathy, sizeable cortical SEP responses persist even for decimated and desynchronized afferent volleys that can be integrated through synaptic summation at the somatosensory relays (Desmedt 1971). For example, the sensory conduction velocity in different segments along the peripheral nerve can be estimated through the cortical SEPs, even though no sensory nerve potentials can be shown by standard techniques (Desmedt and Noel 1973).

Problems of interpretation of spinal potentials have recently been clarified by several sets of data. It is important in studies of neck SEP components to avoid a scalp reference electrode that will inject into grid 2 of the amplifier the positive scalp far-fields of fixed latency, thereby distorting the genuine spinal components (Desmedt and Cheron 1980). The time at which the sensory volley enters the spinal cord has been identified in normal subjects by comparison of latencies of sensory nerve potentials along the limb up to Erb's point (Fig. 1): extrapolation of these to the level of the appropriate spinal segments indicates that the onset of the first negative N11 response at the lower posterior neck (NC reference recording) indexes the spinal entry time (Desmedt and Cheron 1980). This also coincides with the onset of the P11 scalp far field (when this inconstant component is present) (Fig. 1). The mean conduction velocity in the median nerve afferents in normal adults is 71 m/sec. The N11 neck SEP component is normally preceded by a positive far-field P9 that reflects volume-conducted activity in the distal brachial plexus between axilla and Erb's point.

The posterior neck records disclose a second negative component N13 riding upon the N11 (Fig. 1F, G). This N13 has now been identified as reflecting a fixed generator in the dorsal horn of spinal segments C4 to C8: the main evidence for this stems from prevertebral (oesophageal) recording, disclosing a phase reversal of this component into a P13 with stable latency along the neck (Desmedt and Cheron

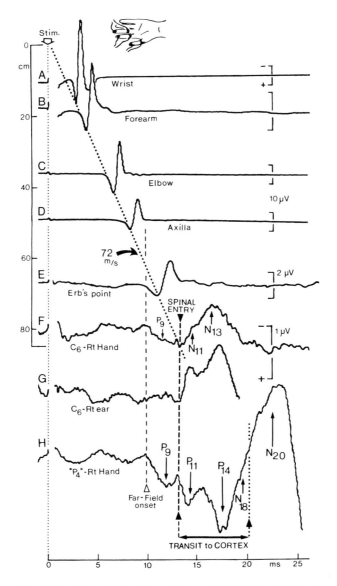

Fig. 1. Single shock stimulation of fingers I-II-III of the left hand. Sensory nerve potentials along the median nerve (A–E) and SEPs recorded from posterior neck (F, G) and contralateral parietal scalp (H) in a normal adult. (From Desmedt and Cheron 1980.)

1981a). By contrast the N11 indexes the volley ascending in the dorsal columns at a CV of about 58 m/sec, as suggested from the latency shift of N11 between levels C6 and 2 (NC reference recording).

Evidence from patients with lesions of various parts of the somatosensory pathway indicates that the early SEP components relate, not to the spinothalamic pathway, but to the lemniscal pathway (Halliday and Wakefield 1963; Noel and Desmedt 1975, 1980). The scalp P13-P14 far fields are preserved in patients with a thalamic vascular lesion that eliminates all subsequent SEP response (Nakanishi et al. 1978; Anziska and Cracco 1980; Mauguière and Courjon 1981). Analysis of central conduction times in normal adults actually suggests that the scalp-recorded P13-P14 are generated above foramen magnun, in the medial lemniscus (Desmedt and Cheron 1980).

Considering the mean maximum CV in dorsal columns and a synaptic delay of 0.5 msec in cuneate nucleus, initiation of conduction in lemniscal axons should start about 1.75 msec after spinal entry. This fits in remarkably with the recorded mean onset latency of the scalp far fields P13-P14 (1.75 ± 0.30 msec; Desmedt and Cheron 1981b, Table IV). A similar discussion of lemniscal conduction suggests that P13-P14 can be interpreted as the summation of volume-conducted travelling activities in medial lemniscus; the peak of P14 appears to reflect, to a first approximation, the time of arrival of the fastest lemniscal potentials at the thalamus.

Although the scalp far fields have a widespread distribution, they present a small but consistent amplitude difference on the two sides and this can be related to the anatomy of the pathway. Thus P11 is larger at the ipsilateral ear-lobe as it reflects the volume-conducted volley in the dorsal column ipsilateral to the stimulated median nerve. By contrast, P13-P14 are larger at the ear-lobe contralateral to the hand stimulated, as would be expected if they are generated above foramen magnum and after somatosensory decussation (Desmedt and Cheron 1980).

Difficult problems are raised by the analysis of subcortical SEP components in patients with various abnormalities of relative strength or time of activation of the different neural generators. It seems highly advisable to use in patients the (fairly neutral) non-cephalic reference connected to grid 2 of the input amplifier, because the scalp SEPs then display a remarkable sequence of widespread positive far fields that reflect volume-conducted activities in successive segments of the somatosensory pathway (Fig. 1H). However, when extraneous interference is excessive, as can happen in clinical patients who are inadequately relaxed, it may be necessary to accept the use of a scalp reference electrode instead. The far fields are then injected in both grid 1 and grid 2 of the input amplifier whereby they tend to cancel out. The scalp reference is even worse for neck SEP recording since the far fields injected into grid 2 then severely distort the genuine spinal SEP components injected into grid 1. Losing sight of the potentials contributed by such a reference electrode results in misleading interpretation of the wave forms (see Desmedt and Cheron 1980, 1981b).

This brief survey of recent SEP data indicates that we may be on the verge of important advances in the detailed study of patients with specific disorders of conduction in the first, second and third sensory neurones. Much remains to be done to establish further the data base in normals, and to design methods for circumventing special problems arising in the electrophysiological investigation of patients.

REFERENCES

Anziska, B. and Cracco, R.Q. Short latency somatosensory evoked potential studies in patients with focal neurological disease. Electroenceph. clin. Neurophysiol., 1980, 49: 227–239.

Cracco, R.Q. and Cracco, J.B. Somatosensory evoked potentials in man: far-field potentials. Electroenceph. clin. Neurophysiol., 1976, 41: 460–466.

Desmedt, J.E. Somatosensory cerebral evoked potentials in man. In: A. Rémond (Ed.), Handbook of Electroencephalography and Clinical Neurophysiology, Vol. 9. Elsevier, Amsterdam, 1971: 55–82.

Desmedt, J.E. Some observations on the methodology of cerebral evoked potentials in man. In: J.E. Desmedt (Ed.), Attention, Voluntary Contraction and Event-related Cerebral Potentials. Progress in Clinical Neurophysiology, Vol. 1. Karger, Basel, 1977: 12–29.

Desmedt, J.E. Cerebral evoked potentials. In: P.J. Dyck, P.K. Thomas and E.H. Lambert (Eds.), Peripheral Neuropathy, 2 edn. Saunders, Philadelphia, Pa., 1982.

Desmedt, J.E. and Cheron, G. Central somatosensory conduction in man: neural generators and interpeak latencies of the far-field components recorded from neck and right or left scalp and earlobes. Electroenceph. clin. Neurophysiol., 1980, 50: 382–403.

Desmedt, J.E. and Cheron, G. Prevertebral (oesophageal) recording of subcortical somatosensory evoked potentials in man: the spinal P_{13} component and the dual nature of the spinal generators. Electroenceph. clin. Neurophysiol., 1981a, 52: 257–275.

Desmedt, J.E. and Cheron, G. Non-cephalic reference recording of early somatosensory potentials to finger stimulation in adult or aging normal man: differentiation of widespread N18 and contralateral N20 from the prerolandic P22 and N30 components. Electroenceph. clin. Neurophysiol., 1981b, 52: 553–570.

Desmedt, J.E. and Noel, P. Average cerebral evoked potentials in the evaluation of lesions of the sensory nerves and of the central somatosensory pathway. In: J.E. Desmedt (Ed.), New Developments in Electromyography and Clinical Neurophysiology, Vol. 2. Karger, Basel, 1973: 352–371.

Donchin, E., Callaway, E., Cooper, R., Desmedt, J.E., Goff, W.R., Hillyard, S.A. and Sutton, S. Publication criteria for studies of evoked potentials: report of a Committee. In: J.E. Desmedt (Ed.), Attention, Voluntary Contraction and Event-related Cerebral Potentials. Progress in Clinical Neurophysiology, Vol. 1. Karger, Basel, 1977: 1–11.

Gilliatt, R.W. and Sears, T.A. Sensory nerve action potentials in patients with peripheral nerve lesions. J. Neurol. Neurosurg. Psychiat., 1958, 21: 109–118.

Halliday, A.M. and Wakefield, G.S. Cerebral evoked potentials with dissociated sensory loss. J. Neurol. Neurosurg. Psychiat., 1963, 26: 211–219.

Hume, A.L. and Cant, B.R. Conduction time in central somatosensory pathways in man. Electroenceph. clin. Neurophysiol., 1978, 45: 361–375.

Mauguière, F. and Courjon, J. The origin of short-latency somatosensory evoked potentials in man. A clinical contribution. Ann. Neurol., 1981, 9: 707–710.

Nakanishi, T., Shimada, Y., Sakuta, M. and Toyokura, Y. The initial positive component of the scalp-recorded somatosensory evoked potential in normal subjects and in patients with neurological disorders. Electroenceph. clin. Neurophysiol., 1978, 45: 26–34.

Noel, P. and Desmedt, J.E. Somatosensory cerebral evoked potentials after vascular lesions of the brainstem and diencephalon. Brain, 1975, 98: 113–128.

Noel, P. and Desmedt, J.E. Cerebral and far-field somatosensory evoked potentials in neurological disorders involving the cervical spinal cord, brainstem, thalamus and cortex. In: J.E. Desmedt (Ed.), Clinical Uses of Cerebral, Brainstem and Spinal Somatosensory Evoked Potentials. Progress in Clinical Neurophysiology, Vol. 7. Karger, Basel, 1980: 205–230.

Kyoto Symposia (EEG Suppl. No. 36)
Editors: P.A. Buser, W.A. Cobb and T. Okuma
© 1982, Elsevier Biomedical Press, Amsterdam

Features of Central and Peripheral Nerve Conduction in Demyelinating Diseases and Specific Neuropathies in Japan

HIROSHI SHIBASAKI, AKIO OHNISHI and YOSHIGORO KUROIWA

Departments of Neurology and Neuropathology, Neurological Institute, Faculty of Medicine, Kyushu University, 60 Fukuoka City 812 (Japan)

Multiple sclerosis (MS) is a chronic relapsing demyelinating disease of the central nervous system, but Japanese patients with MS are claimed to show acute, severe optic nerve and spinal cord involvement, presumably due to axonal lesions, more frequently than Caucasian patients (Kuroiwa et al. 1975, 1977; Shibasaki et al. 1978, 1981). Although many studies have been reported on the short latency somatosensory evoked potential (SEP) in Caucasian MS patients (Anziska et al. 1978; Small et al. 1978; Eisen et al. 1979; Eisen and Odusote 1980; Ganes 1980; Green 1980; Strenge et al. 1980; Abbruzzese et al. 1981), oriental patients have not been studied in the past.

Recently some neuropathies or myeloneuropathies have attracted special attention in Japan. One is "polyneuropathy with pigmentation, oedema, hypertrichosis and plasma cell dyscrasia (polyneuropathy with PEHP)." Approximately 50 cases have been reported in Japan since 1969. The hallmarks of this syndrome are severe motor and sensory polyneuropathy and skin pigmentation, frequently associated with dysglobulinaemia, oedema, gynecomastia and hypertrichosis (Iwashita et al. 1977). In half of the reported cases, myelomas, which are mostly solitary and osteosclerotic, have been documented.

The second is subacute myelo-optico-neuropathy (SMON). This disease had been endemic in Japan since 1955 (Sobue 1979), and was proved by Japanese neurologists to be due to clioquinol intoxication (Tsubaki 1974). Experiments on dogs fed with clioquinol by Tateishi et al. (1972) reproduced the characteristic pathological changes in the distal portion of the gracile fasciculus and also in the distal portion of the cortico-spinal tract, just as seen in human autopsy materials (Shiraki 1979).

In order to understand the pathophysiology of these neurological diseases, it has become increasingly important to study nerve conduction through individual portions of the peripheral as well as central nervous system. The short latency SEP, which has been studied by many investigators following the first report by Cracco in 1972, might be applicable to clinical investigation of the nerve conduction. But this would be so only if the generator source of each component of the short latency SEP were clarified.

The purpose of the present study is 3-fold; to elucidate the generator source of the short latency SEP, to confirm the usefulness of the short latency SEP in detecting subclinical lesions in Japanese MS patients, and to investigate the pathophysiology of the two specific neuropathies in Japan, with special emphasis being placed on the correlation with pathological findings.

SUBJECTS AND METHODS

Subjects studied were 14 patients with localized subcortical lesions, 27 Japanese patients with MS, 5 patients with "polyneuropathy with PEHP," and 5 patients with SMON. Patients with localized subcortical lesions consist of 3 with thalamic lesions, 2 with midbrain lesions, 4 with pontine lesions, 2 with medulla oblongata lesions and 3 with cervical cord lesions. Patients with MS were classified into 24 "MS probable," including one autopsy case and 3 "MS possible" according to the diagnostic criteria of the Japan MS Research Committee (Kuroiwa et al. 1975). Sixteen healthy adults served as controls for the SEP with median nerve stimulation, and 20 more for that with tibial nerve stimulation. In addition, several healthy young adults were used for investigating the normal distribution of the short latency SEP components.

To record SEP with hand stimulation, the median nerve was stimulated through a pair of surface electrodes placed on the wrist. Square wave pulses of 0.1 msec duration were generated twice a second for electrical stimulation. The stimulus strength was adjusted to 10–20% above the motor threshold.

Recording cup electrodes were placed on the supraclavicular region (Erb's point) on each side, over the spinous processes at C2 and C7 levels, and on the scalp corresponding to the somatosensory hand area (7 cm lateral to the midline on a line joining a point 2 cm posterior to the vertex to the external auditory meatus) on each side. Each electrode was referred to an electrode placed on the midline frontal scalp (Fz). In some of the normal subjects an electrode placed on the dorsum of the hand on the non-stimulated side was used as a reference. Resistance of all electrodes was reduced to below 5 kΩ. The amplifiers had a time constant of 0.3 sec and a high frequency cut-off less than 10% at 2000 Hz. 256–1024 samples were averaged by using a San-ei Signal Processor 7T08 with an ordinate period of 0.04 msec.

For SEPs with leg stimulation the tibial nerve was electrically stimulated at the ankle. Recording electrodes were placed in the popliteal fossa on each side, over the spinous processes at T12 and C2 levels, and on the scalp corresponding to the somatosensory foot area (2 cm posterior to the vertex). The popliteal and thoracic electrodes were referred to an electrode placed over the right scapula, and the cervical and scalp electrodes were referred to the Fz electrode. 512–2048 samples were averaged with an ordinate period of 0.08 or 0.12 msec.

Averaged data were plotted on an X-Y plotter. Measurement of the peak latency of each component was carried out by the computer. The amplitude of each component was measured by a ruler from the peak of the preceding component of the opposite polarity to the peak of the component. Values in excess of 3 standard deviations from the mean value of control subjects were judged abnormal.

Sural nerves were obtained by biopsy from 8 patients with "polyneuropathy with PEHP." In addition to the study of teased fibre preparations, the densities of myelinated fibres and their size distributions were evaluated on transverse sections embedded in Epon. In 4 autopsy cases of this disease, the densities of myelinated fibres and their fibre size distributions were evaluated in L5 dorsal and ventral roots and the gracile fasciculus at C3 and T5 segments on transverse sections embedded in Epon.

In an autopsy case of SMON (a 70-year-old woman), the sural nerve and the gracile fasciculus at the C8 segment were embedded in Epon, and the densities of myelinated fibres and their size distributions were evaluated in the transverse sections.

RESULTS

(1) Normal short latency SEP

(a) Median nerve stimulation

A large amplitude negative potential, occurring at a mean latency of 9.3 msec, was localized to the clavicular electrode. At the cervical electrodes a prominent negative potential occurred at a mean latency of 12.9 msec. With hand reference recording this component was maximal over the C4 to C7 electrodes, extending up to C2 with smaller amplitude. A negative potential occurring at a mean latency of 18.2 msec was localized to the somatosensory hand area contralateral to the stimulus. These 3 negative potentials were called $\overline{N9}$, $\overline{N13}$ and $\overline{N20}$, respectively, according to the terminology proposed by Jones (1977). The mean peak latency and interpeak latency, and their side-to-side differences are shown in Table I. There were positive correlations between the peak latency of each component and the arm length of subjects; $r = 0.41$ for $\overline{N9}$, 043 for $\overline{N13}$ and 0.49 for $\overline{N20}$. There was no correlation between 2 interpeak latencies and the arm length; $r = 0.04$ for $(\overline{N9}\text{-}\overline{N13})$ and 0.19 for $(\overline{N13}\text{-}\overline{N20})$.

(b) Tibial nerve stimulation

A negative potential was recorded from the popliteal electrode at a mean peak latency of 7.5 msec $(\overline{N7})$. From the spinal electrode at T12, a negative-positive, biphasic potential was recorded at a mean peak latency of the negative component of 20.1 msec $(\overline{N20})$. A positive peak occurred at a mean peak latency of 37.7 msec

TABLE I

LATENCY OF SEP (msec)

MN stim., normal control.

	R,L inclusive (n = 32)		R − L difference (n = 16)	
	Mean	S.D.	Mean	S.D.
$\overline{N9}$	9.3	0.50	0.11	0.31
$\overline{N13}$	12.9	0.52	0.14	0.41
N20	18.2	0.69	−0.01	0.40
$\overline{N9\text{-}N13}$	3.6	0.44	0.03	0.54
N13-N20	5.3	0.53	−0.13	0.62

at the somatosensory foot area ($\overline{P40}$). The details of this study will be reported elsewhere (Kakigi et al., Electroenceph. clin. Neurophysiol., 1982, 53: 602).

(2) Localized subcortical lesions (median nerve stimulation)

In all patients with lesions anywhere in the medulla oblongata or above, the cervical component $\overline{N13}$ was recognizable even if the affected hand showed complete loss of proprioceptive sensation and the cortical potential $\overline{N20}$ was absent. In a patient with a cervical cord lesion with normal proprioception in the hands, $\overline{N13}$ was normal. In 2 other patients with cervical cord lesions showing proprioceptive loss in the hands, $\overline{N13}$ and $\overline{N20}$ were totally absent, although $\overline{N9}$ was normal. One of them had cervical syringomyelia and her results are shown in Fig. 1. With stimulation of the right hand showing complete loss of pain and temperature sensation but normal proprioception, all components were recorded normally. With stimulation of the left hand, whose proprioception was also lost, only $\overline{N9}$ was recognized.

(3) Multiple sclerosis (MS)

The SEP with median nerve stimulation was abnormal in half the cases (Table II).

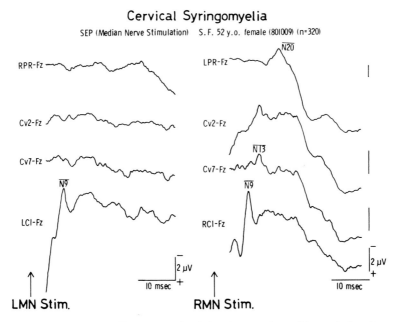

Fig. 1. SEPs with median nerve stimulation in a patient with cervical syringomyelia. Pain and temperature sensations were lost segmentally in both hands, and joint position and vibration sensations were also lost only in the left hand. Normal response with right hand stimulation (RMN Stim), but $\overline{N13}$ and $\overline{N20}$ are absent with left hand stimulation (LMN Stim). RPR and LPR, right and left post-rolandic areas; Cv2 and Cv7, 2nd and 7th cervical spines; LC1 and RC1, left and right clavicles; Fz, frontal midline.

TABLE II

SEP ABNORMALITIES IN JAPANESE MS PATIENTS

Median nerve stimulation; 12/24 cases (50%), 21/48 hands (43.8%).

	Absent or depressed	Delayed peak or interpeak latency	Asymmetry
$\overline{N9}$	0/43 (0%)	0/43 (0%)	0/21 (0%)
$\overline{N13}$	5/45 (11.1%)	3/45 (6.7%)	3/22 (13.6%)
$\overline{N20}$	6/48 (12.5%)	9/48 (18.8%)	8/24 (33.3%)
$\overline{N9}$-$\overline{N13}$		3/42 (7.1%)	2/19 (10.5%)
N13-N20		10/45 (22.2%)	3/23 (13.0%)

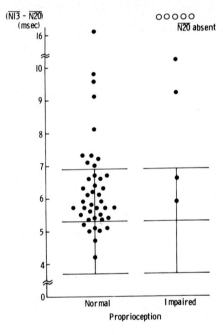

Fig. 2. Relationship between the interpeak latency ($\overline{N13}$-$\overline{N20}$) and sensory impairment in Japanese patients with MS. The interpeak latency is occasionally prolonged with stimulation of hands with normal sensation.

The most common abnormality was asymmetry of the $\overline{N20}$ peak latency, delayed interpeak latency ($\overline{N13}$-$\overline{N20}$) and delayed latency of $\overline{N20}$. Correlation with proprioceptive impairment of the hands is shown in Fig. 2. With stimulation of the clinically impaired hand, $\overline{N20}$ was absent in 5 out of 9 hands. In some hands with intact proprioception, the interpeak latency ($\overline{N13}$-$\overline{N20}$) was significantly prolonged. On the other hand, the interpeak latency ($\overline{N9}$-$\overline{N13}$) was mildly prolonged in a small

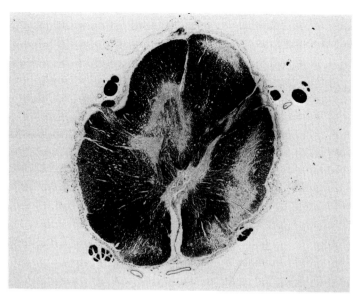

a

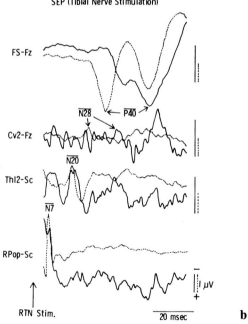

Multiple Sclerosis R.Y. 44 y.o. female (810267)

SEP (Tibial Nerve Stimulation)

FS-Fz

$\overline{\text{N28}}$ → $\overline{\text{P40}}$

Cv2-Fz

$\overline{\text{N20}}$

Th12-Sc

$\overline{\text{N7}}$

RPop-Sc

↑
RTN Stim.

|1 μV

20 msec

b

Fig. 3. a: spinal cord (T8) of a patient with MS, showing extensive demyelinating lesions. b: SEPs with right tibial nerve stimulation (RTN Stim) in the same patient as (a), recorded 2 months before death. Normal responses are shown in dotted lines. Note the significantly delayed peak latency of the cervical component $\overline{\text{N28}}$ and the cortical component $\overline{\text{P40}}$. FS, foot sensory area; Cv2, 2nd cervical spine; Th12, 12th thoracic spine; RPop, right poplitea; Fz, frontal midline; Sc, scapula.

proportion of hands with intact sensation. Among 6 hands with proprioceptive loss, however, $\overline{N13}$ was absent in 4 hands.

The SEP with tibial nerve stimulation was studied in 8 patients. It was found to be abnormal in 7 cases (87.5%). The most common abnormalities were prolonged interpeak latency ($\overline{N20}$-$\overline{P40}$) (72.7%), delayed peak latency of $\overline{P40}$ (71.4%) and absence or marked amplitude reduction of the component $\overline{P40}$ (42.9%). Even in 6 legs with normal proprioception, $\overline{P40}$ was absent in 1 and the interpeak latency ($\overline{N20}$-$\overline{P40}$) was significantly prolonged in 4.

In an autopsied case with an extensive demyelinating lesion in the thoracic cord (Fig. 3a), the components $\overline{N7}$ and $\overline{N20}$ were normal, but the cervical component $\overline{N28}$ and the cortical component $\overline{P40}$ were markedly delayed (Fig. 3b).

(4) Polyneuropathy with PEHP

(a) Physiological study

The amplitudes of components of the median nerve SEP were normal except for the component $\overline{N9}$, which was significantly reduced (Fig. 4). Latencies of all components were delayed in most patients, and the delay was most remarkable between $\overline{N9}$ and $\overline{N13}$, as revealed by a marked prolongation of the interpeak latency ($\overline{N9}$-$\overline{N13}$) (Fig. 5). The peak latency of $\overline{N9}$ was also moderately delayed in most

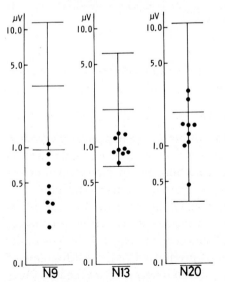

Fig. 4. Amplitude of SEP components with median nerve stimulation in 5 patients with "polyneuropathy with PEHP." Note the significant amplitude reduction of the clavicular component $\overline{N9}$, but not of the cervical component $\overline{N13}$ or of the cortical component $\overline{N20}$.

Peripheral and Central Conduction
in 'Polyneuropathy with P.E.H.P.'

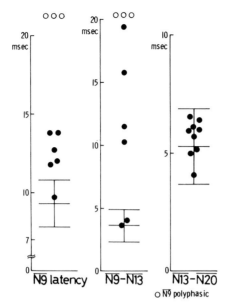

Polyneuropathy with P.E.H.P.

SEP (Median Nerve Stimulation)   N.T. 69 y.o. male

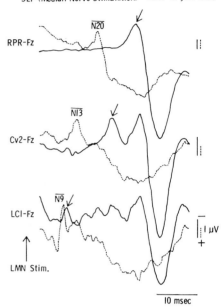

Fig. 5. Peak latency of $\overline{N9}$ and interpeak latencies $(\overline{N9}\text{-}\overline{N13})$ and $(\overline{N13}\text{-}\overline{N20})$ in 5 patients with "polyneuropathy with PEHP." The interpeak latency $(\overline{N9}\text{-}\overline{N13})$ is markedly prolonged, and the peak latency of the $\overline{N9}$ is moderately delayed, but the interpeak latency $(\overline{N13}\text{-}\overline{N20})$ is normal.

Fig. 6. SEP with left median nerve stimulation in a patient with "polyneuropathy with PEHP." $\overline{N9}$ is depressed in amplitude, but its latency is only mildly delayed. The interpeak latency is markedly prolonged between $\overline{N9}$ and $\overline{N13}$, but not between N13 and N20.

cases. The interpeak latency $(\overline{N13}\text{-}\overline{N20})$ was normal in all hands tested. An example of the typical abnormality is shown in Fig. 6.

(b) Pathological study

In the sural nerve there was an extensive loss of both large and small myelinated fibres. The teased fibre preparation of the sural nerve showed, in addition to axonal degeneration, segmental demyelination and remyelination. In the spinal root the myelin sheath was thin relative to the diameter of the axis cylinder. The number of myelinated fibres per root was decreased, mainly due to extensive segmental demyelination. In the teased fibre preparation of the spinal root, myelinated fibres showing segmental demyelination and remyelination were frequently found. In the posterior column there was no definite loss of myelinated fibres. Histograms of myelinated fibre diameters (Fig. 7) showed a marked decrease of myelinated fibres in the spinal root and in the sural nerve, but not in the posterior column.

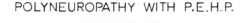

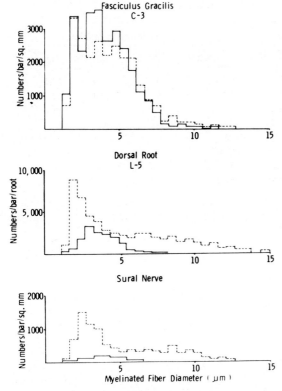

Fig. 7. Histogram of myelinated fibre diameters on transverse sections of the gracile fasciculus, spinal root and sural nerve in an autopsy case of "polyneuropathy with PEHP." Note a marked decrease of large myelinated fibres in the spinal root and in the sural nerve, but not in the gracile fasciculus. Control is shown in dotted lines.

(5) SMON

(a) Physiological study

SEPs with median nerve stimulation were normal in all cases (Table III). SEP with tibial nerve stimulation was studied in 3 patients. In 2 out of 3, the cortical component $\overline{P40}$ was markedly depressed and the interpeak latency ($\overline{N20}$-$\overline{P40}$) was significantly prolonged (Table III). But the peak latency of $\overline{N7}$ and the interpeak latency ($\overline{N7}$-$\overline{N20}$) were both normal. These 2 patients showed severe proprioceptive sensory loss in the legs. An example is shown in Fig. 8. In another patient with dysaesthesia but normal proprioception in the legs, all components were normal.

(b) Pathological study

A histogram from an autopsy case revealed a marked reduction of large myelinated fibres in the gracile fasciculus, but only slight reduction of large myelinated fibres in the sural nerve (Fig. 9).

TABLE III

PERIPHERAL AND CENTRAL CONDUCTION IN SMON (msec)

Case	Sex	Age (years)	Median nerve (wrist)			Tibial nerve (ankle)		
			N9	N9-N13	N13-N20	N7	N7-N20	N20-P40
1	F	50	8.6	3.3	6.2	6.5	11.9	27.8
2	F	80	8.8	3.1	6.7	6.7	9.4	33.7
3	M	73	9.6	4.3	5.9	7.7	13.5	19.0
4	M	61	10.2	3.8	5.9	—	—	—
5	F	77	7.8	3.6	6.4	—	—	—
Control		Mean	9.3	3.6	5.3	7.5	12.6	17.7
		S.D.	0.50	0.44	0.53	0.67	0.63	1.50

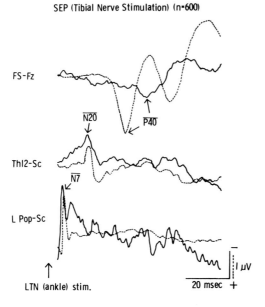

Fig. 8. SEPs with tibial nerve stimulation in a patient with SMON. The popliteal potential $\overline{N7}$ and the thoracic component $\overline{N20}$ are normal, but the cortical component $\overline{P40}$ is depressed in amplitude and significantly delayed.

DISCUSSION

It is generally agreed that the $\overline{N9}$ component (by Jones' terminology) of the SEP with median nerve stimulation reflects the propagating action potential through the brachial plexus (Jones 1977). Likewise, $\overline{N20}$ recorded from the somatosensory hand area is believed to be generated in the postcentral gyrus (Goff et al. 1962; Giblin

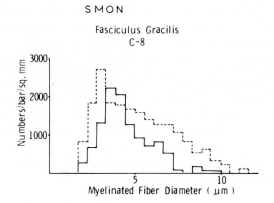

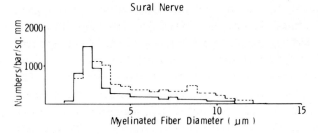

Fig. 9. Histogram of myelinated fibre diameters on transverse sections of the gracile fasciculus and sural nerve in an autopsy case of SMON. Note a marked reduction of large myelinated fibres in the gracile fasciculus, but only slight reduction in the sural nerve. Control is shown in dotted lines.

1964). But the origin of the component $\overline{N13}$ is still controversial (Jones 1977; El-Negamy and Sedgwick 1978; Hume and Cant 1978; Sances et al. 1978; Desmedt and Cheron 1980; Yamada et al. 1980). $\overline{N13}$ recorded over the cervical spine with the Fz reference appears to be complex, as Desmedt and Cheron (1980) pointed out, because it is the result of subtraction of the far-field components at Fz from the cervical negativity.

Nevertheless, results of our present study suggest the cervical cord origin of this component. In normal subjects it was maximally recorded from electrodes placed at the C4 to C7 spinous processes. The $\overline{N13}$ component was absent in cases with localized lesions in the cervical cord only when proprioception was markedly impaired in the hand. Hence it seems reasonable to take the interpeak latency ($\overline{N13}$-$\overline{N20}$) as an index of central conduction from the cervical cord to the somatosensory cortex. It is also conceivable that the interpeak latency ($\overline{N9}$-$\overline{N13}$) might reflect nerve conduction through the dorsal roots.

The present study in Japanese patients with MS revealed that, as in western cases (Anziska et al. 1978; Small et al. 1978; Eisen et al. 1979; Eisen and Odusote 1980; Ganes 1980; Green 1980; Strenge et al. 1980; Abbruzzese et al. 1981), the short latency SEP is useful in detecting subclinical demyelinating lesions. This was more so with tibial nerve stimulation than with median nerve stimulation. This difference is considered to be due to the existence of a larger number of, or more severe, demyelinating plaques in the spinal cord than in the brain stem or cerebral hemisphere. Studies with leg stimulation have been few (Terao et al. 1979).

In view of clinical findings suggesting that oriental MS cases show more frequent and more severe involvement of the optic nerves and spinal cord than Caucasians (Kuroiwa et al. 1975, 1977; Shibasaki et al. 1978, 1981), it was expected that absence or amplitude reduction of the components might be seen relatively more frequently in Japanese patients; but absence or amplitude reduction of SEP components, either $\overline{N13}$ or $\overline{N20}$, has been reported not infrequently in Caucasian MS patients, too (Anziska et al. 1978; Small et al. 1978; Green and McLeod 1979; Eisen and Odusote 1980; Ganes 1980). A conclusion, however, awaits a study based on a larger number of oriental cases.

Pathogenesis of the peripheral nerve involvement in "polyneuropathy with PEHP" has not been elucidated, but the present physiological and pathological studies revealed quite clear findings. Among the physiological findings, a marked amplitude reduction and moderately delayed peak latency of the $\overline{N9}$ component with median nerve stimulation could be interpreted to suggest the presence of severe axonal degeneration and some segmental demyelination in the peripheral nerve. The most conspicuous finding was a marked prolongation of the interpeak latency from the clavicular component $\overline{N9}$ to the cervical component $\overline{N13}$, suggesting an extensive segmental demyelination in the dorsal root. These findings were in conformity with pathological findings consisting of an extensive fibre loss and segmental demyelination and remyelination in the sural nerve and remarkable segmental demyelination and remyelination in the spinal root. The interpeak latency from $\overline{N13}$ to $\overline{N20}$ was normal, suggesting normal central conduction. There was no definite loss of myelinated fibres in the posterior column. Therefore, the primary neurological involvement in this disease appears to be segmental demyelination of the peripheral nerve, especially of the spinal root (Fig. 10).

With regard to SMON, both autopsied human material (Shiraki 1979) and animal experiments (Tateishi et al. 1972) revealed the main neuropathological involvement in the distal portion of the gracile fasciculus and also in the distal portion of the cortico-spinal tract. The present physiological findings, consisting of amplitude reduction of the cortical component $\overline{P40}$ with tibial nerve stimulation and the prolonged interpeak latency from $\overline{N20}$ to $\overline{P40}$, are consistent with the extensive fibre loss seen in the gracile fasciculus (Fig. 11). Normal conduction up to the $\overline{N20}$ component recorded from T12 spine appears to be compatible with the pathological finding of slight, if any, involvement of the peripheral nerve. Sensory impairment of the upper extremities is usually very mild in SMON (Sobue 1979). This clinical finding is reflected by normal SEPs with median nerve stimulation. Therefore, SMON seems to be characterized by primary involvement of longer fibres in the posterior column.

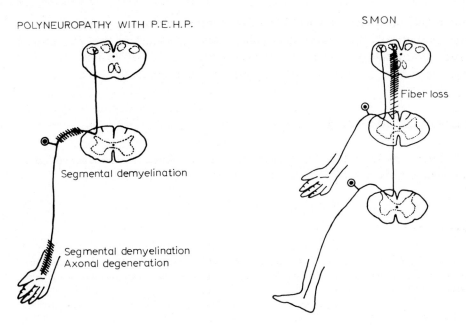

POLYNEUROPATHY WITH P.E.H.P.   SMON

Fig. 10. Schematic illustration of the main sites of lesions and pathophysiology in "polyneuropathy with PEHP."

Fig. 11. Schematic illustration of the main sites of lesions and pathophysiology in SMON.

SUMMARY

Short latency SEPs, either with median nerve stimulation at the wrist or with tibial nerve stimulation at the ankle, were recorded in 14 patients with localized subcortical lesions, 27 Japanese patients with multiple sclerosis (MS), 5 patients each of "polyneuropathy with pigmentation, oedema, hypertrichosis and plasma cell dyscrasia (polyneuropathy with PEHP)" and subacute myelo-optico-neuropathy (SMON), and healthy adults for controls.

The component $\overline{N13}$ with median nerve stimulation was localized at C4 to C7 electrodes, and was absent in cases with cervical cord lesions but present in cases with lesions anywhere in the medulla or above. $\overline{N13}$ was concluded to be generated in the cervical cord.

Short latency SEP was found applicable to clinical investigation of the peripheral and central conduction. It was found useful for detecting subclinical demyelinating lesion in MS, and this was especially so with tibial nerve stimulation.

In "polyneuropathy with PEHP," the present physiological findings (prolonged interpeak latency from $\overline{N9}$ to $\overline{N13}$, and amplitude reduction and delayed peak latency of $\overline{N9}$ with median nerve stimulation) were in conformity with neuropathological findings consisting of an extensive segmental demyelination in the spinal root, and axonal degeneration and segmental demyelination in the peripheral nerve.

In SMON, the primary involvement of the central conduction, exclusively in the distal portion of the gracile fasciculus, was substantiated by the present physiological findings (prolonged interpeak latency from $\overline{N20}$ to $\overline{P40}$ with tibial nerve stimulation, but normal SEP with median nerve stimulation).

ACKNOWLEDGEMENTS

Dr. Sadatoshi Tsuji and Dr. Ryusuke Kakigi contributed to the study of SEPs with median nerve and tibial nerve stimulation, respectively.

REFERENCES

Abbruzzese, G., Cocito, L., Ratto, S., Abbruzzese, M., Leandri, M. and Favale, E. A reassessment of sensory evoked potential parameters in multiple sclerosis: a discriminant analysis approach. J. Neurol. Neurosurg. Psychiat., 1981, 44: 133–139.

Anziska, B., Cracco, R.Q., Cook, A.W. and Feld, E.W. Somatosensory far field potentials: Studies in normal subjects and patients with multiple sclerosis. Electroenceph. clin. Neurophysiol., 1978, 45: 602–610.

Cracco, R.Q. The initial positive potential of the human scalp-recorded somatosensory evoked response. Electroenceph. clin. Neurophysiol., 1972, 32: 623–629.

Desmedt, J.E. and Cheron, G. Central somatosensory conduction in man: Neural generators and interpeak latencies of the far-field components recorded from neck and right or left scalp and earlobes. Electroenceph. clin. Neurophysiol., 1980, 50: 382–403.

Eisen, A. and Odusote, K. Central and peripheral conduction times in multiple sclerosis. Electroenceph. clin. Neurophysiol., 1980, 48: 253–265.

Eisen, A., Stewart, J., Nudleman, K. and Cosgrove, J.B.R. Short-latency somatosensory responses in multiple sclerosis. Neurology (Minneap.), 1979, 29: 827–834.

El-Negamy, E. and Sedgwick, E.M. Properties of a spinal somatosensory evoked potential recorded in man. J. Neurol. Neurosurg. Psychiat., 1978, 41: 762–768.

Ganes, T. Somatosensory evoked responses and central afferent conduction times in patients with multiple sclerosis. J. Neurol. Neurosurg. Psychiat., 1980, 43: 948–953.

Giblin, D.R. Somatosensory evoked potentials in healthy subjects and in patients with lesions of the nervous system. Ann. N.Y. Acad. Sci., 1964, 112: 93–142.

Goff, W.R., Rosner, B.S. and Allison, T. Distribution of cerebral somatosensory evoked responses in normal man. Electroenceph. clin. Neurophysiol., 1962, 14: 697–713.

Green J.B. Short-latency somatosensory evoked potentials in multiple sclerosis. Arch. Neurol. (Chic.), 1980, 37: 630–633.

Green, J.B. and McLeod, S. Short latency somatosensory evoked potentials in patients with neurological lesions. Arch. Neurol. (Chic.), 1979, 36: 846–851.

Hume, A.L. and Cant, B.R. Conduction time in central somatosensory pathways in man. Electroenceph. clin. Neurophysiol., 1978, 45: 361–375.

Iwashita, H., Ohnishi, A., Asada, M., Kanazawa, Y. and Kuroiwa, Y. Polyneuropathy, skin hyperpigmentation, edema, and hypertrichosis in localized osteosclerotic myeloma. Neurology (Minneap.), 1977, 27: 675–681.

Jones, S.J. Short latency potentials recorded from the neck and scalp following median nerve stimulation in man. Electroenceph. clin. Neurophysiol., 1977, 43: 853–863.

Kuroiwa, Y., Igata, A., Itahara, K., Koshijima, S., Tsubaki, T., Toyokura, Y. and Shibasaki, H. Nationwide survey of multiple sclerosis in Japan. Clinical analysis of 1,084 cases. Neurology (Minneap.), 1975, 25: 845–851.

Kuroiwa, Y., Hung, T.-P., Landsborough, D., Park, C.S., Singhal, B.S., Soemargo, S., Vejjajiva, A. and Shibasaki, H. Multiple sclerosis in Asia. Neurology (Minneap.), 1977, 27: 188–192.

Sances, Jr., A., Larson, S.J., Cusick, J.F., Myklebust, J., Ewing, C.L., Jodat, R., Ackmann, J.J. and Walsh, P. Early somatosensory evoked potentials. Electroenceph. clin. Neurophysiol., 1978, 45: 505–514.

Shibasaki, H., Okihiro, M.M. and Kuroiwa, Y. Multiple sclerosis among Orientals and Caucasians in Hawaii: A reappraisal. Neurology (Minneap.), 1978, 28: 113–118.

Shibasaki, H., McDonald, W.I. and Kuroiwa, Y. Racial modification of clinical picture of multiple sclerosis: Comparison between British and Japanese patients. J. neurol. Sci., 1981, 49: 253–271.

Shiraki, H. Neuropathological aspects of the etiopathogenesis of subacute myelo-optico-neuropathy (SMON). In: P.J. Vinken and G.W. Bruyn (Eds.), Handbook of Clinical Neurology, Vol. 37, Intoxications of the Nervous System, Part II. North-Holland, Amsterdam, 1979: pp 141–198.

Small, D.G., Matthews, W.B. and Small, M. The cervical somatosensory evoked potentials (SEP) in the diagnosis of multiple sclerosis. J. neurol. Sci., 1978, 35: 211–224.

Sobue, I. Clinical aspects of subacute myelo-optico-neuropathy (SMON). In: P.J. Vinken and G.W. Bruyn (Eds.), Handbook of Clinical Neurology, Vol. 37, Intoxications of the Nervous System, Part II. North-Holland, Amsterdam, 1979: 115–139.

Strenge, H., Tackmann, W., Barth, R. and Sojka-Raytscheff, A. Central somatosensory conduction time in diagnosis of multiple sclerosis. Europ. Neurol., 1980, 19: 402–408.

Tateishi, J., Ikeda, H., Saito, A., Kuroda, S. and Otsuki, S. Myeloneuropathy in dogs induced by iodoxyquinoline. Neurology (Minneap.), 1972, 22: 702–709.

Terao, A., Nomura, N., Fukunaga, H. and Matsuda, E. Detection of spinal cord lesion using skin electrode recordings of spinal evoked potential. Folia psychiat. neurol. jap., 1979, 33: 525–531.

Tsubaki, T. Aetiological and clinical study on subacute myelo-optico-neuropathy (SMON). J. Jap. Soc. intern. Med., 1974, 63: 1–17.

Yamada, T., Kimura, J. and Nitz, D.M. Short latency somatosensory evoked potentials following median nerve stimulation in man. Electroenceph. clin. Neurophysiol., 1980, 48: 367–376.

3. Neuroplasticity and Functional Compensation

Kyoto Symposia (EEG Suppl. No. 36)
Editors: P.A. Buser, W.A. Cobb and T. Okuma
© 1982, Elsevier Biomedical Press, Amsterdam

Repair Processes in Relation to Spinal Motoneurones: a Brief Review

J.K.S. JANSEN and R. DING

Institute of Physiology, University of Oslo, Oslo (Norway)

The repair and functional compensation after damage to the nervous system depends on several different factors. Some of these are reasonably well known and have been examined experimentally in some detail, others are still very vague and not yet firmly established within the repertoire of behaviour of nerve cells and neuronal circuits. The papers selected for the present discussion of neuroplasticity and functional compensation were intended to illustrate such repair processes at different levels of the nervous system. This should give some indication of the range of processes involved, and the problems we are facing in attempts to explain the compensatory mechanisms.

The spinal motoneurones have long been favourites for the study of repair processes. This is largely because their function is unambiguous and easy to determine and their target tissue, the skeletal muscles, is homogeneous and innervated according to a few simple rules. In the present review we shall consider some of the properties of motoneurones of potential importance for long-term functional changes. The relevant behaviour of the motor axon terminals in the muscle has been most intensely studied, and is dealt with initially. Some corresponding functional changes of the soma-dendritic region of the cells and their synaptic inputs are discussed in the second part. The total material available is very extensive and there is no attempt to make the account comprehensive in this brief review.

RECEPTIVITY TO INNERVATION AND AXONAL REGENERATION

Muscle fibres will not normally accept additional innervation from other motor axons in functionally intact muscles. After denervation, however, several of the properties of the muscle fibres are dramatically changed. Most important in the present context is the induction of receptivity to innervation. After a few days such denervated muscle fibres can be reinnervated by any available cholinergic motor axon (see Jansen et al. 1978). After denervation due to nerve crush or section, regrowing motor axons from the proximal stump are guided by the Schwann cell sheaths that are left after distal degeneration of the injured nerve (Ramón y Cajal 1959). The guidance, however, is not muscle specific. The regenerating axons will essentially follow the first Schwann cell sheath they encounter in the distal stump.

This explains the great difference in the efficiency of functional repair which one finds after nerve damage with maintained continuity of the nerve sheath (such as after nerve crush) and complete transection of the nerve. In the latter case, many of the regenerating axons end up in inappropriate nerve fascicles and are guided to wrong targets. Functionally, such misguided axons are often useless and can even be detrimental. Once established the inappropriate connections are permanent, at least in mammals (Sperry 1945).

The guidance of the regenerating motor axons usually leads to the reformation of synapses at the original end-plate sites (Gutmann and Young 1944). However, the receptivity to innervation of the denervated muscle is not always restricted to the original sites, but may spread over the entire surface of the muscle fibre. This can be shown by transplanting a foreign motor nerve to an extrajunctional region of a muscle (Frank et al. 1975). Subsequent denervation allows ectopic, new end-plates to form on virgin regions of the muscle fibres. The ectopic receptivity to innervation can be prevented by direct electrical stimulation of the denervated muscle. In contrast, the receptivity of the denervated original end-plate sites is largely independent of muscle activity. Thus, the level of activity in the muscle and the availability of vacant synaptic space determine the receptivity of the target to synapse formation.

SPROUTING OF MOTOR AXONS

In addition to regenerating after axotomy, axon terminals can be induced to grow in partially denervated muscle. In this case, remaining intact axons sprout to reinnervate neighbouring muscle fibres (Edds 1953). Thus, the peripheral fields of innervation of the remaining motoneurones are increased and the function of the muscle partly or fully restored. There are, however, limits to the extent of sprouting of the remaining motoneurones. In partially denervated rat muscles the remaining motor units can innervate 4–5 times as many muscle fibres as they do normally, but appear unable to sprout further even in the presence of remaining denervated muscle fibres as potential targets (Thompson and Jansen 1977).

Morphologically, the axonal sprouts in partially denervated muscle are of two types: terminal sprouts arising from existing axon terminals at the end-plates and collateral sprouts from the nodes of Ranvier in the preterminal region of the motor axon. To some extent the terminal and the collateral sprouting are separately induced in the partially denervated muscle (Brown et al. 1981). The terminal sprouting appears to depend upon the presence of inactive muscle fibres: it occurs in chemically paralysed muscles with otherwise intact innervation, and it can be prevented by maintained electrical stimulation of the muscle. In contrast, collateral sprouting is not prevented by muscle activity and appears to be induced by the presence of degenerating nerve fibres in partially denervated muscles. This is shown most elegantly by the collateral sprouting found in muscles with sensory nerve degeneration, but intact motor nerve supply (Brown et al. 1978).

MOTONEURONAL GROWTH FACTORS

The actual substance or substances which stimulate axonal growth and terminal differentiation have not been identified. The prevention of ectopic innervation and terminal sprouting by maintained muscle activity suggests that one such factor is produced by inactive muscle fibres. An appealing model is derived from studies on the nerve growth factor. Besides being produced in target tissues according to their level of activity (Ebendal et al. 1980), this substance enhances the survival of sympathetic motoneurones and stimulates and directs the growth of their axons (Patterson 1978). An analogous substance acting on somatic motoneurones could explain aspects of the behaviour of regenerating and sprouting motor axons. Attempts to identify such a substance are currently in progress at several laboratories (Patrick et al. 1978; Nishi and Berg 1979; Henderson et al. 1981).

Once the regenerating motor axons reach the vacant end-plate sites on the denervated muscle fibres, their further growth is guided by the remaining synaptic gutters with an amazing precision (Letinsky et al. 1976). In addition, the terminal axons differentiate and develop the machinery required for synaptic function. Presumably this differentiation is induced by contact with the target. Again the specific factor involved has not been identified. It appears, however, to be a constituent of the basal lamina in the end-plate region of the muscle fibre, since a comparable differentiation takes place when remaining basal lamina ghosts are reinnervated after complete degeneration of the muscle fibre and its plasma membrane (Sanes et al. 1978). This appears to be a particularly favourable possibility for the identification of one of the factors involved in the formation of synapses in muscle.

CONTROL OF DENSITY OF MUSCLE INNERVATION

Mature mammalian skeletal muscle fibres are usually innervated only by a single motor axon. The traditional explanation for this striking pattern was that the axon which first established contact with a fibre during development quickly rendered the fibre refractory to further innervation. It came as a surprise, therefore, when Redfern reported, about a decade ago, that the muscle fibres just after birth were innervated by terminal branches of several different motor axons (Redfern 1970). This has since been confirmed in many different preparations and appears to be a general feature in the development of innervation of skeletal muscle. In the newborn rat soleus muscle, for instance, there are as many as 5 different axon terminals innervating each muscle fibre. These terminals are all located within one discrete end-plate region on the muscle fibre, and all but one of them is lost during the first few weeks of postnatal development (Brown et al. 1976). Morphologically, the loss appears to be due to retraction of terminal axonal branches (Korneliussen and Jansen 1976).

A rather comparable situation is found after reinnervation of denervated adult mammalian muscles. Initially, each muscle fibre is reinnervated by several different motor axons (McArdle 1975; Kuffler et al. 1980). As the innervation matures, many of the initially formed synapses are eliminated, and the pattern approaches that of the normal muscle. It is as if the muscle has a limited capacity for maintaining innervation, and this capacity is higher in immature and denervated muscle than in the adult, fully functional muscle.

It is not yet known how this constancy in the pattern of innervation is brought about. However, since it is of considerable general interest, we shall outline the current views and some of the relevant experimental observations. The idea of a competitive interaction between nerve fibres for synaptic territory is a central concept in these considerations. This is appealing from a consideration of the end result of the developmental process, a single surviving terminal axon supplying each muscle fibre. There is also experimental support for competitive interactions. A muscle may be fully cross-innervated by a foreign nerve, and this is a stable situation. If, however, the original nerve, or another foreign nerve is permitted to superinnervate the muscle, the second nerve will establish its exclusive field of innervation in the muscle at the expense of that of the first nerve (Dennis and Yip 1978; Grinnell et al. 1979). Similarly, Betz et al. (1980) emphasized competitive interactions between motor units for the neonatal elimination of synapses. The competitive process applies to axon terminals which innervate the same muscle fibre. It affects not only terminals which are located together in the same end-plate region, but acts also between terminals that are spatially separate along the muscle fibre. This indicates that the competitive process is somehow mediated by the same muscle fibre. There is, however, a limit to the effective extension of the process along the fibre. Close synapses are strongly exposed, while synapses separated by some millimetres along the same fibre may be able to coexist and function for prolonged periods (Kuffler et al. 1977). The extent of the competitive process probably varies between muscles, and this may explain the rather constant distance between end-plates seen on many slow muscle fibres with the distributed nerve supply common in lower vertebrates.

The intensity of the competition appears to vary with the level of activity in the target muscle fibres. Inactivity, for instance, due to a block of impulse conduction in the muscle nerve, delays the elimination of redundant synapses (Thompson et al. 1979), whereas additional activity, caused by stimulation of the muscle nerve, accelerates their removal (O'Brian et al. 1978).

There have been several suggestions for the nature of the competitive advantage of the favoured terminals. It has been postulated that certain terminals may be better "matched" for a particular muscle fibre. This has been used to explain situations where the original nerve appears to be favoured in a competitive reinnervation with a foreign muscle nerve (Dennis and Yip 1978). Some of the results have, however, recently been questioned (Wigston 1980), and in the case of mammalian muscle there is not much evidence for a preference for the original muscle nerve. More support has accumulated for the importance of motor unit size in their competitive interactions (see Jansen et al. 1978). The central notion is that each motoneurone has a certain limited capacity for maintaining synaptic terminal arborizations, which determines the size of the motor unit. The actual size of the motor unit determines its competitive vigor, so that the terminals of a relatively small motor unit have a competitive advantage over those belonging to a motor unit which has expanded beyond its optimal size. This view appealingly explains a common finding in partially denervated muscle. Initially, the remaining intact motoneurones sprout and may innervate the entire muscle. Eventually, the injured motor axons regenerate and regain control over part of the muscle as the sprouted terminals are disfavoured in the competitive interaction (Brown and Ironton 1978; Thompson 1978).

Several suggestions have been made for the actual mechanism of the competitive process. So far, these are largely speculative and the available evidence does not permit a critical distinction between the various proposals. Here it is probably enough to mention that a motoneuronal growth substance of the type proposed in the preceding section could, by being available in limiting amounts, serve as the vehicle for the competitive process. At present, one should point out that the various proposals are only of heuristic value, and that the final description may well turn out to be more complicated than now commonly imagined.

INTRASPINAL PROPERTIES OF MOTONEURONES

Besides the peripheral effects, motoneurones also undergo changes centrally after injury or alteration of their functional state. This is probably not entirely surprising, but the interpretation of the changes raises intriguing questions. Axotomy has dramatic effects on the properties of neurones, and it has been examined repeatedly in motoneurones. In addition to the chromatolytic, morphological and biochemical changes, there are clear effects on the membrane properties of the cells (Huizar et al. 1977). Among the membrane effects which have been demonstrated are a reduced axonal conduction velocity, an increased overshoot of the action potential, a small reduction in membrane potential and a marked reduction of the duration of the after-hyperpolarization of slow motoneurones. In addition, increased electrical excitability of the dendritic membrane has frequently been described. Some of these changes are apparently due to direct injury of the neurone, while others may be caused by the separation of the cell body from the target tissue. In general, the rationale for the latter notion is that some of the properties of the motoneurone are maintained by virtue of its contact with the muscle and through retrograde axonal transport of a postulated "trophic" factor originating in the target tissue. Such trophic effects have not been directly demonstrated, but rather inferred from the imitation of the effects of axotomy and colchicine block of axonal transport (Pilar and Landmesser 1972; Purves 1976a,b).

The after-hyperpolarization of slow motoneurones has been examined in particular detail by Kuno and his group. They found that the reduced duration of the after-hyperpolarization was also present in intact motoneurones of a partially

denervated muscle and the degree of reduction in after-hyperpolarization was
related to the extent of denervation of the muscle (Huizar et al. 1977). In line with
this, they report that the duration of the after-hyperpolarization is progressively
normalized with increasing reinnervation of the muscle, but apparently independent
of whether or not the particular motoneurone has re-established functional
connections with the muscle fibres (Kuno et al. 1974). Of equal interest is the further
demonstration that comparable changes in the duration of the after-hyperpolarization can be induced by reducing the level of activity in the muscle. For instance,
7 days after a maintained conduction block of the muscle nerve, the duration
of the after-hyperpolarization is reduced to about the same extent as it is a week
after nerve section. The effect of inactivity is probably related to the inactivity
of the muscle, since it can be prevented by nerve stimulation distal to, but not
central to the conduction block (Czéh et al. 1978). In attempting to explain these
observations, it is appealing to think in terms of a neurotrophic factor released by
the muscle according to its level of activity. It could well be the same as that
presumably involved in the induction of terminal sprouting in the muscle (see
above).

THE SYNAPTIC INPUT TO MOTONEURONES

Axotomy, changes in functional state and deprivation of input also lead to
changes in the synaptic input to motoneurones. Along with the chromolytic reaction
following axotomy there is a striking reduction in the amplitude of the
monosynaptic EPSP in the motoneurones (Eccles et al. 1958; Kuno and Llinás
1970a,b). Morphologically, there is at the same time a reduction in the number of
synaptic contacts on the cells. Synaptic boutons appear to be retracted and
separated from the postsynaptic membrane by glial cell processes. These changes are
largely reversed after restoration of the innervation of the target (Cull 1974).

Section of peripheral muscle nerves leads to depression of their monosynaptic
effects on motoneurones. The effect is largely independent of a response to axotomy
of motoneurones, since it takes place also in the input to synergistic motoneurones
which are intact. After 6–8 months, virtually all monosynaptic input from the
sectioned nerve to motoneurones has been lost (Goldring et al. 1980). If, however,
the muscle nerve is allowed to reinnervate the muscle, the monosynaptic input
recovers and goes through a hypernormal period before it settles at a moderately
subnormal level (Gallego et al. 1980). The restoration and the enhancement of
transmission is related to the reinnervation of the muscle by the sensory axons.
Surprisingly, however, the synaptic effects of the spindle afferents with restored
function is not enhanced, and the authors suggest that the transiently enhanced
transmission is due to signals in sensory fibres which have reached the muscle
without regaining normal function. This interpretation is supported by their finding
that a reversible impulse conduction block also leads to an enhancement of the
monosynaptic EPSPs from the blocked nerve (Gallego et al. 1979). Apparently, lack

of impulse activity in these afferent fibres may lead to enhanced synaptic efficiency at their central terminals on motoneurones. The way this is brought about is still open.

Elimination of part of the input to motoneurones may also lead to qualitative changes in their synaptic connectivity. There are reports of sprouting and expansion of remaining dorsal root fibres after section of neighbouring roots in adult cats (Liu and Chambers 1958). It is not known, however, to what extent this affects the motoneurones directly.

Recently, comparable experiments have been performed on very young animals and have given some interesting results. In frogs, virtually the entire sensory innervation of the forelimb is derived from the second dorsal ganglion, and muscle afferents produce monosynaptic EPSPs on homonymous motoneurones, rather like the well established pattern in mammals (Frank and Westerfield 1982a). After surgical removal of the second dorsal root ganglion in tadpoles at early limb bud stages, the sensory ganglion cells of the third ganglion will sprout both peripherally to invade the forelimb and centrally to the terminal territory of the deleted second ganglion. Some of the sprouting ganglion cells establish monosynaptic connections with the motoneurones of the deafferented second segment. The interesting point is that these novel central connections are specific in the sense that the afferents which terminate on a particular motoneurone provide the peripheral sensory innervation of the corresponding muscle. Thus, after lesions in very young tadpoles, neighbouring ganglion cells are able to re-establish functional connections between the periphery and the motoneurones so that the appropriate pathways are largely restored (Frank and Westerfield 1982b). Similar segmental defects in slightly older tadpoles are not repaired in this way.

Rather comparable experiments have been performed in embryonic chickens. In these studies, the segmental sensory lesions were performed in the neural crest even before all the sensory ganglion cells were born (Eide et al. 1982). Surprisingly, the remaining sensory ganglion cells in chickens were largely unable to compensate for this early defect. However, if the afferents from a particular muscle had been only partly deleted, there was some moderate enhancement of the monosynaptic EPSPs from the remaining ones. Inappropriate afferents did not establish monosynaptic connections with motoneurones, even when the motoneurones had lost their entire monosynaptic input from the dorsal roots. This suggests that in the chicken the developmental fate of the sensory ganglion cells has been permanently determined already at a very early embryonic stage. Furthermore, a comparison with the frog experiments illustrates that even the same class of neurones may have strikingly different properties in different species. Considerable caution is obviously required for the extrapolation of neuronal behaviour between species.

These investigations of the central properties of the motoneurones show that even these, presumably hard-wired, systems can undergo appreciable long-term changes after injury and during changes in the level of activity of the system. The cellular mechanisms behind these changes are at present not well understood. Neither do we know the extent to which such changes contribute to the disturbances of motor function and possibly the recovery of purposeful movements seen after damage to the spinal cord.

CONCLUDING REMARKS

The motoneurones and their afferents provide a series of well documented examples of neuronal responses to injury and to abnormal levels of activity. Growth and axonal sprouting in the periphery have been particularly well examined. These processes are of obvious importance for the repair and restoration of function after peripheral nerve injury. In addition they illustrate some of the more general principles of axonal growth and formation of synaptic connections.

The notion of cellular interactions, often loosely called "trophic effects," between neurones and target cells, figures prominently in present attempts to account for the behaviour of motoneurones in these respects. So far, however, the molecular bases of these interactions have not been established and remain a major challenge for future neurobiology. The study of the motoneurones will probably continue to contribute to our understanding of these fundamental properties of neurones.

REFERENCES

Betz, W.J., Caldwell, J.H. and Ribchester, R.R. The effects of partial denervation at birth on the development of muscle fibres and motor units in rat lumbrical muscles. J. Physiol. (Lond.), 1980, 303: 265–280.

Brown, M.C. and Ironton, R. Sprouting and regression of neuromuscular synapses in partially denervated mammalian muscles. J. Physiol. (Lond.), 1978, 278: 325–348.

Brown, M.C., Jansen, J.K.S. and Van Essen, D. Polyneuronal innervation of skeletal muscle in newborn rats and its elimination during maturation. J. Physiol. (Lond.), 1976, 261: 387–422.

Brown, M.C., Holland, R.L. and Ironton, R. Degenerating nerve products affect innervated muscle fibres. Nature (Lond.), 1978, 275: 652–654.

Brown, M.C., Holland, R.A. and Hopkins, W.G. Motor nerve sprouting. Ann. Rev. Neurosci., 1981, 4: 17–41.

Cull, R.E. Role of nerve-muscle contact in maintaining synaptic connections. Exp. Brain Res., 1974, 20: 307–310.

Czéh, G., Gallego, R., Kudo, N. and Kuno, M. Evidence for the maintenance of motoneurone properties by muscle activity. J. Physiol. (Lond.), 1978, 281: 239–252.

Dennis, M.J. and Yip, J.W. Formation and elimination of foreign synapses on adult salamander muscle. J. Physiol. (Lond.), 1978, 274: 299–310.

Ebendal, T., Olson, L., Seiger, Å. and Hedlund, K.O. Nerve growth factors in the rat iris. Nature (Lond.), 1980, 286: 25–28.

Eccles, J.C., Libet, B. and Young, R.R. The behaviour of chromatolyzed motoneurones studied by intracellular recording. J. Physiol. (Lond.), 1958, 143: 11–40.

Edds, Jr., M.V. Collateral nerve regeneration. Quart. Rev. Biol., 1953, 28: 260–276.

Eide, A.-L., Jansen, J.K.S. and Ribchester, R.R. The effect of lesions in the neural crest on the formation of synaptic connections in the embryonic chick spinal cord. J. Physiol. (Lond.), 1982, in press.

Frank, E. and Westerfield, M. Synaptic organization of sensory and motor neurones innervating the triceps brachii muscles in the bullfrog. J. Physiol. (Lond.), 1982a, 324: 479–494.

Frank, E. and Westerfield, M. The formation of appropriate central and peripheral connexions by foreign sensory ganglion neurones of the bullfrog. J. Physiol. (Lond.), 1982b, 324: 495–505.

Frank, E., Jansen, J.K.S., Lømo, T. and Westgaard, R.H. The interaction between foreign and original motor nerve innervating the soleus muscle of rats. J. Physiol. (Lond.), 1975, 247: 725–743.

Gallego, R., Kuno, M., Nuñez, R. and Snider, W.D. Disuse enhances synaptic efficacy in spinal motoneurones. J. Physiol. (Lond.), 1979, 279: 191–205.

Gallego, R., Kuno, M., Nuñez, R. and Snider, W.D. Enhancement of synaptic function in cat motoneurones during peripheral sensory regeneration. J. Physiol. (Lond.), 1980, 306: 205–218.

Goldring, J.M., Kuno, M., Nuñez, R. and Snider, W.D. Reaction of synapses on motoneurones to section and restoration of peripheral sensory connexions in the cat. J. Physiol. (Lond.), 1980, 309: 185–198.

Grinnell, A.D., Letinsky, M.S. and Rheuben, M.B. Competitive interaction between foreign nerves innervating frog skeletal muscle. J. Physiol. (Lond.), 1979, 289: 241–262.

Gutmann, E. and Young, J.Z. The reinnervation of muscle after various periods of atrophy. J. Anat. (Lond.), 1944, 78: 15–43.

Henderson, C.E., Huchet, M. and Changeux, J.-P. Neurite outgrowth from embryonic chicken spinal neurons is promoted by media conditioned by muscle cells. Proc. nat. Acad. Sci. (Wash.), 1981, 78: 2625–2629.

Huizar, P., Kudo, N., Kuno, M. and Miyata, Y. Reaction of intact spinal motoneurones to partial denervation of the muscle. J. Physiol. (Lond.), 1977, 265: 175–191.

Jansen, J.K.S. and Lømo, T. Development of neuromuscular connections. Trends Neurosci., 1981, 4: 178–181.

Jansen, J.K.S., Thompson, W., Kuffler, D.P. The formation and maintenance of synaptic connections as illustrated by studies of the neuromuscular junction. Progr. Brain Res., 1978, 48: 3–18.

Korneliussen, H. and Jansen, J.K.S. Morphological aspects of the elimination of polyneuronal innervation of skeletal muscle fibres in newborn rats. J. Neurocytol., 1976, 5: 591–604.

Kuffler, D., Thompson, W. and Jansen, J.K.S. The elimination of synapses in multiply-innervated skeletal muscle fibres of the rat: Dependence on distance between end-plates. Brain Res., 1977, 138: 353–358.

Kuffler, D.P., Thompson, W. and Jansen, J.K.S. The fate of foreign end-plates in cross-innervated rat soleus muscle. Proc. roy. Soc. B, 1980, 208: 189–222.

Kuno, M. and Llinás, R. Enhancement of synaptic transmission by dendritic potentials in chromatolysed motoneurones of the cat. J. Physiol. (Lond.), 1970a, 210: 807–821.

Kuno, M. and Llinás, R. Alterations of synaptic action in chromatolysed motoneurones of the cat. J. Physiol. (Lond.), 1970b, 210: 823–838.

Kuno, M., Miyata, Y. and Muños-Martinez, E.J. Properties of fast and slow alpha motoneurones following motor reinnervation. J. Physiol. (Lond.), 1974, 242: 273–288.

Letinsky, M.S., Fischbeck, K.H. and McMahan, V.J. Precision of reinnervation of original post-synaptic sites in frog muscle after nerve crush. J. Neurocytol., 1976, 5: 691–718.

Liu, C.N. and Chambers, W. Intraspinal sprouting of dorsal root axons. Arch. Neurol. Psychiat. (Chic.), 1958, 79: 46–61.

Lømo, T. and Jansen, J.K.S. Requirements for the formation and maintenance of neuromuscular connections. Curr. Top. Develop. Biol., 1980, 16: 253–281.

McArdle, J.J. Complex endplate potentials at the regenerating neuromuscular junction of the rat. Exp. Neurol., 1975, 49: 629–638.

Nishi, R. and Berg, D.K. Survival and development of ciliary ganglion neurones grown alone in cell culture. Nature (Lond.), 1979, 277: 232–234.

O'Brain, R.A.D., Østberg, A.J.C. and Vrbová, G. Observations on the elimination of polyneuronal innervation in developing mammalian skeletal muscle. J. Physiol. (Lond.), 1978, 282: 571–582.

Patrick, J., Heinemann, S. and Schubert, D. Biology of cultured nerve and muscle. Ann. Rev. Neurosci., 1978, 1: 417–443.

Patterson, P.H. Environmental determination of autonomic neurotransmitter function. Ann. Rev. Neurosci., 1978, 1: 1–17.

Pilar, G. and Landmesser, L. Axotomy mimicked by localized colchicine application. Science, 1972, 177: 1116–1118.

Purves, D. Functional and structural changes in mammalian sympathetic neurones following colchicine application to postganglionic nerves. J. Physiol. (Lond.), 1976a, 259: 159–175.

Purves, D. Long-term regulation in the vertebrate peripheral nervous system. Int. Rev. Physiol. Neurophysiol. II, 1976b, 10: 125–177.

Purves, D. and Lichtman, J.W. Formation and maintenance of synaptic connections in autonomic ganglia. Physiol. Rev., 1978, 58: 821–862.

Purves, D. and Njå, A. Trophic maintenance of synaptic connections in autonomic ganglia. In: C.W. Cotman (Ed.), Neuronal Plasticity. Raven Press, New York, 1978: 27–47.

Ramón y Cajal, S. Degeneration and Regeneration of the Nervous System. Hafner, New York, 1959.

Redfern, P.A. Neuromuscular transmission in newborn rats. J. Physiol. (Lond.), 1970, 209: 701–709.

Sanes, J.R., Marshall, L.M. and McMahan, W.J. Reinnervation of muscle fiber basas lamina after removal of myofibers. Differentiation of regenerating axons at original synaptic sites. J. Cell Biol., 1978, 78: 176–198.

Sperry, R.W. The problem of central nervous reorganization after nerve regeneration and muscle transposition. Quart. Rev. Biol., 1945, 20: 311–369.

Thompson, W. Reinnervation of partially denervated rat soleus muscle. Acta physiol. scand., 1978, 103: 81–91.

Thompson, W. and Jansen, J.K.S. The extent of sprouting of remaining motor units in partly denervated immature and adult rat soleus muscles. Neuroscience, 1977, 2: 523–535.

Thompson, W., Kuffler, D.P. and Jansen, J.K.S. The effect of prolonged, reversible block of nerve impulses on the elimination of polyneuronal innervation of new-born rat skeletal muscle fibers. Neuroscience, 1979, 4: 271–281.

Wigston, D.J. Suppression of sprouted synapses in axolotl muscle by transplanted foreign nerves. J. Physiol. (Lond.), 1980, 307: 355–366.

Kyoto Symposia (EEG Suppl. No. 36)
Editors: P.A. Buser, W.A. Cobb and T. Okuma
© 1982, Elsevier Biomedical Press, Amsterdam

Modifiability of Cerebellar Neuronal Networks Related to Adaptive Control of Vestibulo-Ocular Reflex

MASAO ITO

Department of Physiology, Faculty of Medicine, University of Tokyo, Bunkyo-ku, Tokyo 113 (Japan)

That cerebellar tissues have plasticity was suggested by the classic experiments of Flourens (1842) and Luciani (1891) and also by the more recent works of Moruzzi's school (Batini and Pompeiano 1957; Batini et al. 1957). Though only conceptually, this plasticity has been considered as the basis for compensatory action of the cerebellum for various motor deficiencies and also for learning capabilities involved in practising and acquiring motor skills. In recent years, new light has been shed on this problem from two lines of approach. First, on the basis of ample experimental data on neuronal circuit structures of the cerebellum (cf. Eccles et al. 1967), possible learning mechanisms in the cerebellum have been explored by theorists, as represented by Marr (1969) and Albus (1971), who built a learning machine model of the cerebellum. Second, several concrete examples of adaptative phenomena have been shown to imply a simple form of cerebellar plasticity. An example is the adaptive modification of the vestibulo-ocular reflex (VOR) under visual-vestibular interactions, first demonstrated by Gonshor and Melvill-Jones (1976a,b). This adaptive modification of the VOR has been related to the learning capability of the cerebellar flocculus, conceived from a neuronal circuitry analysis of the flocculo-vestibulo-ocular system (Ito 1970, 1972, 1974). Thus an interesting situation has been born for experimental examination of cerebellar plasticity, using the flocculus as material and the Marr-Albus model as a guide.

MARR-ALBUS MODEL OF THE CEREBELLUM

The cerebellar cortex receives two distinctively different afferents, mossy fibres and climbing fibres. In 1969 Marr proposed an ingenious hypothesis that these two types of afferent play essentially different functional roles. Mossy fibres provide major inputs to the cerebellar cortex which are eventually converted to Purkinje cell outputs, while climbing fibres carry "instruction" signals for reorganizing the relationship between mossy fibre inputs and Purkinje cell outputs (Fig. 1). The model is based on a plasticity assumption that the transmission efficacy of a parallel fibre synapse which mediates mossy fibre signals to a Purkinje cell is modified when impulses of that parallel fibre and those in a climbing fibre converge simultaneously on the same Purkinje cell dendrites (Fig. 1). The model assumes that this heterosynaptic interaction from a climbing fibre to a parallel fibre synapse causes

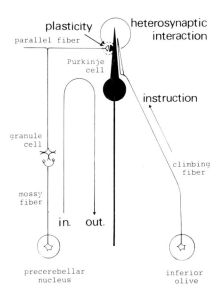

Fig. 1. Diagram of Marr-Albus model of the cerebellum. In this as well as Fig. 2, inhibitory neurones are filled in black, while excitatory neurones are represented by hollow structures.

modification of transmission efficacy at the latter synapse. Marr (1969) suggested an enhancement of the transmission efficacy, but Albus (1971) preferred the opposite, i.e., depression of the parallel fibre-Purkinje cell transmission. These two diagonally opposed postulates are similar in theoretical implications, but they differ from each other in practical implications such as the stability of the system and applicability to actual situations of cerebellar learning in animals (Albus 1971).

FLOCCULUS HYPOTHESIS OF THE VOR CONTROL

The basic connections for the Marr-Albus model (Fig. 1) have been found to be complete in the system which involves the flocculus in association with the VOR arc (Fig. 2). The primary vestibular fibres project to the flocculus as a mossy fibre input, while flocculus Purkinje cells in turn project to vestibular nuclei and supply inhibitory synapses to relay cells of the VOR (Ito et al. 1970; Baker et al. 1972; Fukuda et al. 1972); thus the flocculus is incorporated in the VOR system as a sidepath to the major VOR arc. The flocculus also receives climbing fibres which convey visual signals (Maekawa and Simpson 1973). From these structural aspects, the flocculus hypothesis of VOR control was formulated to propose that the flocculus adaptively controls the VOR, referring to retinal error signals (Ito 1970, 1972, 1974). Since retinal error signals imply "instruction" concerning the performance of the VOR, the hypothesis is in accordance with the Marr-Albus hypothesis. Retinal error signals conveyed by climbing fibres would modify parallel fibre-Purkinje cell synapses in the flocculus and thereby alter the signal transfer

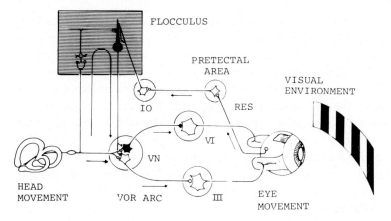

Fig. 2. Diagram of the flocculo-vestibulo-ocular system. Flocculus sidepath is shaded to indicate its similarity to the Marr-Albus model in Fig. 1. RES, retinal error signals; IO, inferior olive, VN, vestibular nuclei.

characteristics across the flocculus sidepath, which eventually would lead to adaptive modification of the VOR.

An important issue related to the flocculus-VOR arc relationship was the finding of a microzonal structure in the flocculus. The flocculus in rabbits has been separated into at least 5 longitudinal zones projecting differentially to the vestibular nuclear complex and the lateral cerebellar nucleus (Yamamoto and Shimoyama 1977; Yamamoto 1978). Only one (zone II) of these 5 zones is involved in control of the horizontal VOR. The flocculus in Fig. 2 thus represents only this zone II, but not others which are to be involved in other types of the VOR or in other functions than the VOR.

SUPPORT FOR THE FLOCCULUS HYPOTHESIS OF THE VOR CONTROL

The flocculus hypothesis of VOR control has been supported by lesion experiments. The adaptability of the VOR was abolished by ablation of the flocculus (Ito et al. 1974) or the vestibulo-cerebellum including the flocculus (Robinson 1976). Ablation of the flocculus caused a serious retrograde degeneration of the inferior olive neurones (Barmack and Simpson 1980). This complication, however, could be avoided by using chemical destruction with kainic acid (Ito et al. 1980), which still removed the VOR adaptability (Ito et al. 1982a). Destruction of the dorsal cap of the inferior olive, which mediates the visual climbing fibre pathway to the flocculus, also abolished VOR adaptability (Ito and Miyashita 1975; Haddad et al. 1980). Death of olivary neurones caused a complication, i.e., attenuation of inhibitory action of flocculus Purkinje cells deprived of climbing fibres on relay cells of the VOR (Dufossé et al. 1978a, b). This was avoided by interrupting the visual pathway entering the dorsal cap, without involving dorsal cap neurones, which still abolished the VOR adaptability (Ito and Miyashita 1975).

The flocculus hypothesis of VOR control has also been supported by recording impulse discharges from flocculus Purkinje cells. In rabbits, responsiveness of these cells to vestibular mossy fibre inputs during head rotation was altered in amplitude in parallel with the VOR adaptation (Dufossé et al. 1978). In monkeys, however, changes observed in Purkinje cell responsiveness to vestibular stimuli were in the opposite direction to the theoretical prediction, and therefore were ascribed to secondary effects of VOR adaptation (Miles et al. 1980). Microzonal structures have not yet been worked out in monkey flocculus, and there is no firm basis for assuming that flocculus Purkinje cells sensitive to horizontal gaze velocity, sampled by Miles et al. (1980), are really involved in control of the VOR. This situation makes it difficult to interpret the monkey data immediately against the flocculus hypothesis of the VOR control.

PLASTICITY OF PARALLEL FIBRE-PURKINJE CELL SYNAPSES

A more direct test of the Marr-Albus plasticity assumption has recently been performed by substituting electrical pulse stimulation of a vestibular nerve and the inferior olive in high decerebrate rabbits for natural vestibular and visual stimulation of alert rabbits (Ito 1981, 1982b). Purkinje cells were sampled extracellularly from the rostral flocculus and identified by their characteristic responses to stimulation of the contralateral inferior olive. Basket cells were also sampled and identified by absence of olivary responses and also by their location in the molecular layer adjacent to identified Purkinje cells. Single pulse stimulation of a vestibular nerve, either ipsilateral or contralateral, at a rate of 2/sec excited Purkinje cells with a latency of 3–6 msec. This early excitation represents activation through vestibular mossy fibres, granule cells and their axons (Fig. 2). Similar excitation was commonly seen in putative basket cells as well. Conjunctive stimulation of a vestibular nerve at 20/sec and the inferior olive at 4/sec, for 25 sec per trial, effectively depressed the early excitation of Purkinje cells by that nerve, without an associated change in spontaneous discharge. The depression recovered in about 10 min, but it was followed by the onset of a slow depression lasting for an hour (Fig. 3).

Conjunctive vestibular-olivary stimulation produced no such depression in other responses: early excitation in Purkinje cells induced from the vestibular nerve not involved in the conjunctive stimulation; early excitation in putative basket cells from either vestibular nerve; inhibition or rebound facilitation in Purkinje cells following the early excitation; vestibular nerve-evoked field potentials in the granular layer and white matter of the flocculus. These responses represent impulse transmission in mossy fibres and cortical networks except for the parallel fibre-Purkinje cell synapses. Hence, it is concluded that the depression occurs specifically at parallel fibre-Purkinje cell synapses involved in conjunctive stimulation.

Iontophoretic application of glutamate, i.e., the putative neurotransmitter of parallel fibres (Sandoval and Cotman 1978; Hacket et al. 1979), in conjunction with

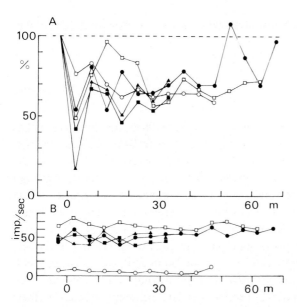

Fig. 3. Long-term recovery after conjunctive vestibular-olivary stimulation. A: ordinate: values of the firing index of rabbit's flocculus Purkinje cells activated by electrical stimulation of a vestibular nerve. The plotted values of the firing index are normalized by control values before conjunctive stimulation, which happened at zero time. B: spontaneous discharge rates. Measurements from 5 different Purkinje cells (Ito et al. 1982b).

4/sec olivary stimulation, was found to depress very effectively the glutamate sensitivity of Purkinje cells; aspartate sensitivity was depressed to a much lesser degree. The depression diminished in about 10 min, but this recovery was succeeded by a slow depression lasting for an hour. The depression was seen only when glutamate sensitivity was relatively high, suggesting that the microelectrode was located on a Purkinje cell dendrite. These observations suggest that subsynaptic chemosensitivity of Purkinje cells to the putative neurotransmitter of parallel fibres is involved in the depression observed after conjunctive stimulation of a vestibular nerve and the inferior olive. The possible mechanism for climbing fibre impulses to depress the transmitter sensitivity of Purkinje cell dendrites may be speculated to be as follows. Since climbing fibre activation of Purkinje cells appears to involve a voltage dependent increase of calcium permeability of the dendritic membrane (Llinás and Sugimori 1980), Ekerot and Oscarsson (1981) suggested that an increased intradendritic calcium concentration affects subsynaptic receptors of Purkinje cell dendrites, just as intracellular calcium is supposed to desensitize acetylcholine receptors in muscle end-plates (Miledi 1980). An alternative possibility is that climbing fibres liberate a chemical substance(s) which reacts with subsynaptic receptor molecules at parallel fibre-Purkinje cell synapses together with the parallel fibre neurotransmitter, thereby rendering the receptors insensitive to the parallel fibre neurotransmitter. An analogous phenomenon has been reported in cerebral cortical cells in which application of thyrotropin-releasing hormone (TRH) causes a reduction in glutamate sensitivity without affecting aspartate sensitivity (Renaud et al. 1979).

CONCLUSION

The modifiable neuronal network hypothesis of Marr (1969) and Albus (1971) has been tested by work on the flocculo-vestibulo-ocular system. Results from neuronal circuitry analysis, eye movement studies and recording from flocculus Purkinje cells all support the hypothesis that signal transfer from mossy fibre afferents through granule cells, and parallel fibres to Purkinje cells, is reorganized by modification at parallel fibre-Purkinje cell synapses, according to conjunctive instruction signals from climbing fibre afferents. Recent observation that electrical conjunctive stimulation of vestibular mossy fibres and climbing fibres induces a long lasting depression in parallel fibre-Purkinje cell synapses in the flocculus is consistent with Albus' (1971) assumption. The appropriateness of this assumption has already been indicated by observations of Purkinje cell activity in alert, behaving animals (Gilbert and Thach 1977; Ito 1977). The long lasting depression would thus account for modification of mossy fibre responsiveness of Purkinje cells underlying cerebellar adaptation. However, the long-term course of this depression has yet to be investigated, as it is not yet clear whether the recovery of the depression involves a still slower process analogous to a permanent memory. It is also an important future problem to determine molecular processes involved in the long lasting depression of parallel fibre-Purkinje cell transmission.

REFERENCES

Albus, J.S. A theory of cerebellar functions. Math. Biosci., 1971, 10: 25–61.

Baker, R.G., Precht, W. and Llinás, R. Cerebellar modulatory action on the vestibulo-trochlear pathway in the cat. Exp. Brain Res., 1972, 15: 364–385.

Barmack, N.J. and Simpson, J.I. Effects of microlesions of dorsal cap of inferior olive of rabbits on optokinetic and vestibulo-ocular reflexes. J. Neurophysiol., 1980, 43: 182–206.

Batini, C. and Pompeiano, O. Chronic fastigial lesions and their compensation in the cat. Arch. ital. Biol., 1957, 95: 147–165.

Batini, C., Moruzzi, G. and Pompeiano, O. Cerebellar release phenomena. Arch. ital. Biol., 1957, 95: 71–95.

Dufossé, M., Ito, M., Jastreboff, P.J. and Miyashita, Y. A neuronal correlate in rabbit's cerebellum to adaptive modification of the vestibulo-ocular reflex. Brain Res., 1978a, 150: 511–616.

Dufossé, M., Ito, M. and Miyashita, Y. Diminution and reversal of eye movements induced by local stimulation of rabbit cerebellar flocculus after partial destruction of the inferior olive. Exp. Brain Res., 1978b, 33: 139–141.

Eccles, J.C., Ito, M. and Szentágothai, J. The Cerebellum as a Neuronal Machine. Springer, New York, 1967.

Ekerot, C.-F. and Oscarsson, O. Prolonged depolarization elicited in Purkinje cell dendrites by climbing fibre impulses in the cat. J. Physiol. (Lond.), 1981, 318: 207–221.

Flourens, P. Recherches Expérimentales sur les Propriétés et les Fonctions du Système Nerveux dans les Animaux Vertébrés. Baillière, Paris, 1842.

Fukuda, J., Highstein, S.M. and Ito, M. Cerebellar inhibitory control of the vestibulo-ocular reflex investigated in rabbit IIIrd nucleus. Exp. Brain Res., 1972, 14: 511–526.

Gilbert, P.F.C. and Thach, W.T. Purkinje cell activity during motor learning. Brain Res., 1977, 128: 309–328.

Gonshor, A. and Melvill-Jones, G. Short-term adaptive changes in the human vestibulo-ocular reflex arc. J. Physiol. (Lond.), 1976a, 265: 361–379.

Gonshor, A. and Melvill-Jones, G. Extreme vestibulo-ocular adaptation induced by prolonged optical reversal of vision. J. Physiol. (Lond.), 1976b, 256: 381–414.

Hacket, J.T., Hou, S.-M. and Cochran, S.L. Glutamate and synaptic depolarization of Purkinje cells evoked by parallel fibers and by climbing fibers. Brain Res., 1979, 170: 377–380.

Haddad, G.M., Demer, J.L. and Robinson, D.A. The effect of lesions of the dorsal cap of the inferior olive on the vestibulo-ocular and optokinetic systems of the cats. Brain Res., 1980, 185: 265–275.

Ito, M. Neurophysiological aspects of the cerebellar motor control system. Int. J. Neurol., 1970, 7: 162–176.

Ito, M. Neural design of the cerebellar motor control system. Brain Res., 1972, 40: 81–84.

Ito, M. The control mechanisms of cerebellar motor system. In: F.O. Schmitt and F.G. Worden (Eds.), The Neurosciences, Third Study Program. MIT Press, Cambridge, Mass., 1974: 293–303.

Ito, M. Neuronal events in the cerebellar flocculus associated with an adaptive modification of the vestibulo-ocular reflex of the rabbit. In: R.G. Baker and A. Berthoz (Eds.), Control of Gaze by Brain Stem Neurons. Elsevier, Amsterdam, 1977: 391–398.

Ito, M. and Miyashita, Y. The effects of chronic destruction of inferior olive upon visual modification of the horizontal vestibulo-ocular reflex of rabbits. Proc. Jap. Acad., 1975, 51: 716–760.

Ito, M., Highstein, S.M. and Fukuda, J. Cerebellar inhibition of the vestibulo-ocular reflex in rabbit and cat and its blockage by picrotoxin. Brain Res., 1970, 17: 524–526.

Ito, M., Shiida, T., Yagi, N. and Yamamoto, M. The cerebellar modification of rabbit's horizontal vestibulo-ocular reflex induced by sustained head rotation combined with visual stimulation. Proc. Jap. Acad., 1974, 50: 85–89.

Ito, M., Jastreboff, P.J. and Miyashita, Y. Retrograde influence of surgical and chemical flocculectomy upon dorsal cap neurons of the inferior olive. Neurosci. Lett., 1980, 20: 45–48.

Ito, M., Sakurai, M. and Togroach, P. Evidence for modifiability of parallel fiber-Purkinje cell synapses. In: J. Szentágothai, J. Hámori and M. Palkovits (Eds.), Advances in Physiological Sciences 2. Pergamon, Oxford, 1981: 97–105.

Ito, M., Jastreboff, P.J. and Miyashita, Y. Specific effects of unilateral lesions in the flocculus upon eye movements of rabbits. Exp. Brain Res., 1982a, 45: 233–242.

Ito, M., Sakurai, M. and Togroach, P. Climbing fibre induced depression of both mossy fibre responsiveness and glutamate sensitivity of cerebellar Purkinje cells. J. Physiol. (Lond.), 1982b, 324: 113–134.

Llinás, R. and Sugimori, M. Electrophysiological properties of in vitro Purkinje cell dendrites in mammalian cerebellar slices. J. Physiol. (Lond.), 1980, 305: 197–213.

Luciani, L. Il Cervelletto: Nuovi Studi di Fisiologia Normale e Pathologica. Le Monnier, Florence, 1891.

Maekawa, K. and Simpson, J.I. Climbing fiber responses evoked in vestibulocerebellum of rabbit from visual system. J. Neurophysiol., 1973, 36: 649–666.

Marr, D. A theory of cerebellar cortex. J. Physiol. (Lond.), 1969, 202: 437–470.

Miledi, R. Intracellular calcium and desensitization of acetylcholine receptors. Proc. roy. Soc. B, 1980, 209: 447–452.

Miles, F.A., Braitman, D.J. and Dow, B.M. Long-term adaptive changes in primate vestibulo-ocular reflex. IV. Electrophysiological observations in flocculus of adapted monkeys. J. Neurophysiol., 1980, 43: 1477–1493.

Renaud, L.P., Blume, H.W., Pittman, Q.J., Lamour, Y. and Tan, A.T. Thyrotropin-releasing hormone selectively depressed glutamate excitation of cerebral cortical neurons. Science, 1979, 205: 1275–1277.

Robinson, D.A. Adaptive gain control of vestibulo-ocular reflex by the cerebellum. J. Neurophysiol., 1976, 39: 954–969.

Sandoval, M.E. and Cotman, C.W. Evaluation of glutamate as a neurotransmitter of cerebellar parallel fibers. Neuroscience, 1978, 3: 199–206.

Yamamoto, M. Localization of rabbit's flocculus Purkinje cells projecting to the cerebellar lateral nucleus and the nucleus prepositus hypoglossi, investigated by means of the horseradish peroxidase retrograde axonal transport. Neurosci. Lett., 1978, 12: 29–34.

Yamamoto, M. and Shimoyama, I. Differential localization of rabbit's flocculus Purkinje cells projecting to the medial and superior vestibular nuclei, investigated by means of the horseradish peroxidase retrograde axonal transport. Neurosci. Lett., 1977, 5: 279–283.

Kyoto Symposia (EEG Suppl. No. 36)
Editors: P.A. Buser, W.A. Cobb and T. Okuma
© 1982, Elsevier Biomedical Press, Amsterdam

Pyramidal Tract Neurones and Mechanisms for Recovery of Function Following Lesions of Motor Cortex

EDWARD V. EVARTS

Laboratory of Neurophysiology, National Institute of Mental Health, Bethesda, Md. 20205 (U.S.A.)

This review will consider anatomical and physiological studies on pyramidal tract neurones (PTNs) in precentral motor cortex (MI) and postcentral sensory cortex (SI), and discuss the implications of these studies for an understanding of recovery of function following MI lesions. The physiological studies to be reviewed have involved recording the activity of individual PTNs during voluntary movement as well as investigations in anaesthetized animals using cortical and spinal cord electrical stimulation and recording from spinal cord motoneurones and cortical PTNs. The anatomical studies have involved the use of retrograde transport of horseradish peroxidase (HRP) to mark PTN cell bodies and orthograde transport of intra-axonally injected HRP to identify the distribution of the terminals of individual PTNs.

Before proceeding with the substance of this review, however, it should be pointed out that the review will focus on only one of the several major output systems arising from MI. It goes without saying that these additional output systems (cortico-striatal, cortico-pontine, cortico-olivary, cortico-rubral and others) destroyed by MI lesions are of at least as much significance as the single output system — the PTNs — to be dealt with in this report. It is hoped, however, that some of the general principles emerging from consideration of PTNs may be applicable to these other systems as well.

DISTRIBUTION OF PTN SYNAPTIC TERMINALS IN SPINAL CORD AND OF PTN CELL BODIES IN CEREBRAL CORTEX

Any understanding of the mechanisms of recovery of function following MI lesions depends on knowledge of the projections from MI to lower centres, and this review will therefore begin by considering the spinal cord distribution of the synaptic terminals of single pyramidal tract neurones (PTNs) as revealed by orthograde transport of horseradish peroxidase (HRP) following intra-axonal HRP injection (cf. Shinoda 1978). Knowledge of the distribution of PTN synaptic terminals in spinal cord is of critical importance to an understanding of the functional role of PTNs, since the role of any neurone (PTN or otherwise) is to influence those additional neurones (or effectors) with which it has synaptic interconnections. It is in the light of this fact that Shinoda's results on the distribution of PTN terminals assume such great significance. First of all, they make it clear that, rather than confining its terminals to the motoneurones of a single muscle, a single PTN projects to motoneurones of several different muscles. Furthermore, a PTN axon descending on one side of the spinal cord and terminating primarily on this same side may also send some branches across to terminate on the opposite side of the cord. When we combine this widespread spinal cord distribution of the synaptic terminals of a single PTN with the widespread distribution of its collateral supraspinal branches (e.g., to pontine nuclei and red nucleus), we see that the functions of a given PTN are indeed numerous: a single PTN influences spinal cord motoneurones of different muscles over a number of segments and on both sides of the spinal cord, influences Ia inhibitory interneurones and other interneurones in the spinal cord, sends "efference copy" signals to cerebellum via the pontine nuclei, and at the same time interacts with neurones in the red nucleus.

The results of anatomical studies on terminal distribution of single PTNs complement the results of physiological studies on the projections of PTNs to alpha motoneurones in the monkey (Jankowska et al. 1975). These studies dealt with the spatial organization of monosynaptic cortico-spinal projections to hind limb motoneurones, using near threshold stimulation of the surface of the precentral gyrus to activate PTNs and recording intracellular EPSPs from motoneurones. Cortical areas from which monosynaptic EPSPs were evoked in individual motoneurones were remarkably large, most often between 3 and 7 mm^2. Several motoneurones appeared to receive excitatory inputs from 2 or 3 separate areas within the hind limb division of the motor cortex. The areas containing PTNs projecting to various motoneurones innervating one muscle were usually not identical, and they overlapped only partially or not at all. These results gave strong evidence for multiple representations of muscles with overlapping areas of cortical projections to motoneurones.

Shinoda et al. (1979) have employed a third technique to demonstrate spinal branching of PTNs in the monkey. This involved activating PTNs antidromically from within motor nuclei of the spinal cord. These studies, like those already cited, led to the conclusion that some PTNs in MI send multiple axon branches to different levels of the spinal gray matter.

Additional information on multiple representation of muscles in MI has been provided by the work of Strick and Preston (1978a,b). These authors used intracortical microstimulation to explore the possibility of multiple representation within the MI forearm zone. It was shown that there were two anatomically separate hand-wrist representations in MI. Furthermore, stimulation of forelimb sensory receptors during unit recording demonstrated that different patterns of afferent input projected to these two different representations. Neurones driven by cutaneous input were concentrated in the caudal motor representation while neurones driven by deep input were concentrated in the rostral representation. Strick and Preston suggested that the two different representations might be involved in different sorts of movements, pointing out that the concentration of cutaneous input in the caudal motor representation might allow it to play a special role in control of movements which use tactile input for their guidance. In contrast, the concentration of deep input in the rostral motor representation suggested that it might be preferentially involved in movements requiring kinaesthetic feedback. Thus, Strick and Preston proposed that the double motor representation in MI reflects two motor control systems that deal with different components of motor behaviour.

An additional body of data relevant to pathways that may play a role in recovery of function following cortical lesions has been provided by studies using retrograde transport of HRP following intraspinal injections to identify the cortical loci in which PTN cell bodies are located (Jones and Wise 1977; Murray and Coulter 1981). It was found that 60% of the cortical cells labelled by HRP injections in spinal cord were located outside the traditional "motor" areas 4 and 6, with 40% of the axons in the pyramidal tract arising from the parietal lobe. This means that even extensive motor cortex lesions spare about half of the pyramidal tract, and that these residual fibres provide one possible pathway over which the cerebral cortex output (from the parietal lobe) can play a role in voluntary movement.

ACTIVITY OF PTNs IN ASSOCIATION WITH VOLUNTARY MOVEMENT

The anatomical studies that have now been reviewed have shown that PTNs are widely distributed not only in MI (area 4) and SI (areas 3a, 3b, 1 and 2), but in area 5 of the parietal lobe and in parts of the premotor cortex (area 6) as well: injections of HRP into spinal cord are followed by retrograde transport to PTN cell bodies throughout the sensorimotor cortex. Furthermore, electrical stimulation of SI (as well as of MI) can elicit muscular contractions. Therefore, the question arises as to the functional grounds on which MI can be distinguished from SI. Among the physiological criteria used to designate a given cortical area as "motor" or "sensory" are the following: (1) threshold and latency of spinal cord motoneurone responses to cortical electrical stimulation; (2) threshold and latency of cortical neurone responses to peripheral receptor stimulation; (3) effects of cortical lesions on production of motor output as compared to detection of sensory input.

Comparisons of MI and SI in the monkey show that: (1) MI has lower threshold and shorter latency for generation of muscle responses to cortical electrical stimulation; (2) SI has lower threshold and shorter latency cortical neuronal responses to peripheral receptor stimulation; (3) MI lesions produce relatively greater impairments of movement; (4) SI lesions produce relatively greater impairments of signal detection.

But these distinctions between MI and SI are relative and none are as sharp as the distinctions between the dorsal and ventral roots. Differences in effects of dorsal and ventral root lesions are unequivocal. In contrast, the losses of signal detection following total SI lesions do not approach the anaesthesia which follows dorsal root section, and the losses of movement following total MI lesions do not approach the total paralysis that follows ventral root section.

In seeking to identify the distinct functional roles of the different areas (6, 4, 3a, 3b, 1, 2 and 5) within the cerebral sensorimotor cortical complex, it is therefore important to have information as to how the neurones of these areas are related to sensory input and motor output during natural movement. Some of the early records of the activity of sensorimotor cortex neurones in association with limb movements in a visual reaction time paradigm showed that MI neurones discharge in advance of muscular contraction, whereas SI neurones discharge about 60 msec later, presumably as a result of sensory feedback (Evarts 1974). Furthermore, Bioulac and Lamarre (1979) showed that limb deafferentation eliminates SI discharge in association with ballistic limb movements, whereas MI discharge continues to occur. Both of these studies seemed to indicate that SI discharge with movement was caused by the influx of sensory feedback resulting from movement.

However, newer studies by Soso and Fetz (1980), confirmed by Evarts and Fromm (1981), indicate that under other circumstances SI neurones may indeed discharge prior to feedback associated with movement. Additional experiments on SI (Fromm and Evarts 1982) have been aimed at characterizing the properties of SI PTNs. In these studies, antidromically identified PTNs in MI and SI were contrasted according to three features: (1) timing with respect to onset of motor activity, (2) discharge frequencies as a function of level of muscular activity, and (3) responses to afferent input. It was found that postcentral PTNs receive central inputs prior to movement as well as inputs from the periphery once receptors have been activated in the course of movement. Indeed, the onset of activity in area 3a occurred even earlier than that in area 4 prior to voluntary movement. The fact that the discharge of postcentral PTNs occurs in advance of muscular contraction means that outputs from the postcentral gyrus to the spinal cord can play a role in motor control well in advance of muscular contraction. It remains for further studies to obtain additional data contrasting the targets and functional roles of these pre- and postcentral PTNs. Finally it should be emphasized that the postcentral gyrus itself is far from homogeneous, and that certain areas (3a and 2) that are in receipt of input from deep receptors seem to differ in many significant respects from those regions that receive inputs from cutaneous receptors.

At present we can only speculate as to the functional significance of outputs via SI PTNs prior to movement onset. Evidence favouring the view that sensory cortex might have a motor output prior to movement has been summarized by Woolsey (1958), who pointed out that "afferent" cortical areas are not strictly sensory. Studies by Woolsey showed that cortical somatic areas SI and SII have well organized motor outflows which remain functional months after removal of the precentral motor area. Even granting the higher thresholds of SI for elicitation of movements by electrical stimulation, the occurrence of SI PTN outputs prior to muscular contraction and the relation of SI PTN discharge frequencies to magnitude of muscular contraction point to a very significant potential within SI for assumption of motor control functions following MI damage.

IMPLICATIONS FOR MECHANISMS OF RECOVERY OF FUNCTION FOLLOWING MOTOR CORTEX LESIONS

Glees and Cole (1950) studied the recovery of function following MI lesions in monkey and showed that a small restricted lesion of the hand area results in an impairment which is followed by rather rapid recovery. A second lesion of the remaining adjacent MI tissue following recovery from the first lesion reinstates the deficit, implying that MI cortex adjacent to the first lesion played a role in recovery. Even following total MI destruction within a given hemisphere, there is considerable recovery of proximal movements of the contralateral limb, though individual finger movements of the contralateral hand are permanently abolished. If such a total lesion of MI within a given hemisphere is followed by a lesion of MI in the opposite (previously intact) hemisphere, impairments will be produced in *both* limbs.

These results on effects of sequential lesions point to the role of remaining cortex in taking over functions of MI tissue lost as a result of brain damage. The anatomical studies summarized in this report suggest that PTNs in intact MI or SI cortex adjacent to an MI lesion can control spinal cord motoneurones which were, in part at least, controlled by the MI tissue destroyed by the lesion. Furthermore, studies of SI PTNs in association with volitional movements show that these PTNs can become active prior to movement. Reorganization of the synaptic contacts of these SI PTNs within the spinal cord might be an important mechanism of recovery.

REFERENCES

Bioulac, B. and Lamarre, Y. Activity of postcentral cortical neurons of the monkey during conditioned movements of a deafferented limb. Brain Res., 1979, 172: 427–437.

Evarts, E.V. Precentral and postcentral cortical activity in association with visually triggered movement. J. Neurophysiol., 1974, 37: 373–381.

Evarts, E.V. and Fromm, C. Transcortical reflexes and servo control of movement. Canad. J. Physiol. Pharmacol., 1981, 59: 757–775.

Fromm, C. and Evarts, E.V. Pyramidal tract neurons in somatosensory cortex: central and peripheral inputs during voluntary movement. Brain Res., 1982, 238: 186–191.

Glees, P. and Cole, J. Recovery of skilled motor functions after small repeated lesions of motor cortex in macaque. J. Neurophysiol., 1950, 13: 137–148.

Jankowska, E., Padel, Y. and Tanaka, R. Projections of pyramidal tract cells to α-motoneurones innervating hind-limb muscles in the monkey. J. Physiol. (Lond.), 1975, 249: 637–667.

Jones, E.G. and Wise, S.P. Size, laminar and columnar distribution of efferent cells in the sensory-motor cortex of monkeys. J. comp. Neurol., 1977, 175: 391–438.

Murray, E.A. and Coulter, J.D. Organization of corticospinal neurons in the monkey. J. comp. Neurol., 1981, 195: 339–365.

Shinoda, Y. Intraspinal multiple projections of single corticospinal neurons in the cat and monkey. In: M. Ito (Ed.), Integrative Control Functions of the Brain, Vol. 1. Kodansha-Scientific Co., Tokyo, 1978: 137–151.

Shinoda, Y., Zarzecki, P. and Asanuma, H. Spinal branching of pyramidal tract neurons in the monkey. Exp. Brain Res., 1979, 34: 59–72.

Soso, M.J. and Fetz, E.E. Responses of identified cells in postcentral cortex of awake monkeys during comparable active and passive joint movements. J. Neurophysiol., 1980, 43: 1090–1110.

Strick, P.L. and Preston, J.B. Multiple representation in the primate motor cortex. Brain Res., 1978a, 154: 336–370.

Strick, P.L. and Preston, J.B. Sorting of somatosensory afferent information in primate motor cortex. Brain Res., 1978b, 156: 364–368.

Woolsey, C.N. Organization of somatic sensory and motor areas of the cerebral cortex. In: H.F. Harlow and C.N. Woolsey (Eds.), Biological and Biochemical Bases of Behavior. University of Wisconsin Press, Madison, Wis., 1958: 63–81.

Kyoto Symposia (EEG Suppl. No. 36)
Editors: P.A. Buser, W.A. Cobb and T. Okuma
© 1982, Elsevier Biomedical Press, Amsterdam

Plasticity and Specificity in the Red Nucleus

N. TSUKAHARA

Department of Biophysical Engineering, Faculty of Engineering Science, Osaka University, Toyonaka, and National Institute for Physiological Sciences, Okazaki (Japan)

The red nucleus (RN) offers several advantages for the study of neuronal plasticity and functional compensation because of the prominent plasticity of the cortico-rubral inputs. In normal kittens, as in adult cats, the cortico-rubral projection to the rubro-spinal (RN) neurones is unilateral and somatotopically organized. After chronic lesions of this projection at early developmental stages, new functional connections are formed from the contralateral cerebral cortex. Although there is morphological evidence that sprouting occurs from the remaining contralateral cortex (Nah and Leong 1976a,b), the details of the nature of sprouting are far from clear. We asked two questions. First, whether the newly formed connections are functional and, secondly, how specific are the newly formed connections?

Kittens from 17 to 149 days after birth were used. They were anaesthetized with pentobarbital sodium and ablation of the left cerebral sensorimotor cortex was performed under direct vision in aseptic conditions. Procedures for intracellular recording from RN neurones were essentially the same as those reported previously (Tsukahara and Kosaka 1968) with consideration of the size of the brain. RN neurones were identified antidromically by stimulating the contralateral C_1 and L_1 spinal segments; RN neurones activated antidromically from C_1 and L_1 were designated "L cells" and those activated only from C_1, "C cells." Cortico-rubral fibres were stimulated at two levels: within the sensorimotor cortex (SM) and the cerebral peduncle (CP).

Fig. 1 shows synaptic potentials recorded intracellularly in normal kitten RN neurones. Such potentials at 2–3 months after birth are virtually the same as those recorded in adults. Stimulation of the contralateral nucleus interpositus (IP) produces a fast rising EPSP (Fig. 1A,E). This EPSP was only produced by stimulation of the contralateral IP and not of the ipsilateral IP, as shown in Fig. 1B. Stimulation of the ipsilateral cerebral sensorimotor cortex (SM) or its fibres at the cerebral peduncle (CP) produced a slowly rising dendritic EPSP as in normal adult cats (Fig. 1C,F). Stimulation of the contralateral CP did not produce any postsynaptic potentials, as shown in Fig. 1D.

Cerebral lesions destroying the cortico-rubral fibres were found to induce sprouting from three sources: (1) most importantly from the contralateral cerebral cortex via the contralateral CP (Nah and Leong 1976a,b); (2) contralateral IP; and (3) ipsilateral IP. As shown in Fig. 2A, stimulation of contralateral CP produces a slowly rising EPSP with a latency of 1.4 msec in kittens in which the ipsilateral

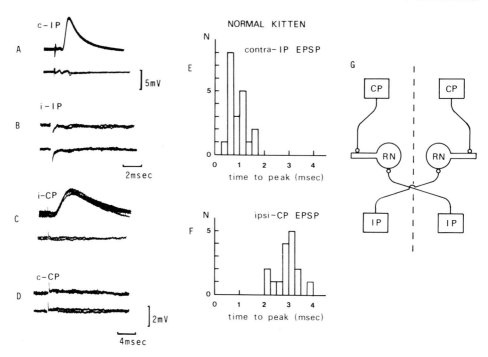

Fig. 1. A–G: EPSPs produced in normal kitten red nucleus neurones. A: EPSPs elicited in an RN cell by stimulating the contralateral nucleus interpositus of the cerebellum (c-IP) (upper trace). Corresponding extracellular traces just outside the cell are illustrated in the lower traces of A–D. B: same as A but by stimulating the ipsilateral IP (i-IP). C: EPSPs induced by stimulation of the ipsilateral cerebral peduncle (i-CP). D: same as C, but by stimulating the contralateral cerebral peduncle (c-CP). E, F: frequency distribution of the time to peak of the EPSPs elicited in kitten red nucleus 80 days after birth. E: c-IP, F: i-CP. G: connections of the red nucleus (RN). The broken line indicates the midline.

cerebral sensorimotor cortex was ablated at the 17th day after birth. Similar slowly rising EPSPs were also produced by stimulating contralateral SM, but with a longer latency of 2.6 msec. Assuming the conduction distance from SM to CP as 25 mm, the conduction velocity of fibres for the newly appeared EPSPs is about 20 m/sec. This is in the range of that of the normal cortico-rubral fibres or slowly conducting pyramidal tract. EPSPs were followed in some cases by an IPSP with longer latency, as was found by stimulating the ipsilateral CP in normal cats.

Stimulation of the bilateral IP produced in some cases slowly rising EPSPs (Fig. 2B,C). There are interesting features on the possible sources of sprouting following cerebral lesions in kittens. Although three possible sources exist, as described above, sprouting does not seem to take place from these sources simultaneously on the same cell. Most frequently, only one source gave sprouting in 20 out of 29 RN cells tested. Less frequently, simultaneous sprouting from two independent inputs occurred, in 7 out of 29 RN cells. Simultaneous sprouting from three independent sources occurred in 2 out of 29 RN cells (Fig. 2F). As for the frequency of occurrence of these three sprouting sources, the contralateral cerebral cortex was most predominant (18 out of 29 RN cells); second was the contralateral IP (15 out

IPSILATERAL HEMISPHERECTOMIZED KITTEN

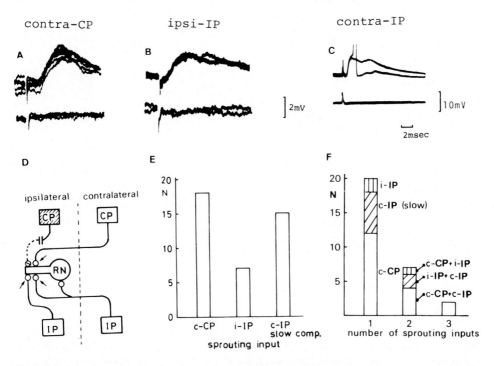

Fig. 2. Sprouting in kitten red nucleus after destruction of the cortico-rubral input. A: newly appeared EPSPs induced in an RN cell by stimulating the contralateral cerebral peduncle in a cat in which ipsilateral cortico-rubral input was destroyed at the 27th day after birth. B: same as A but stimulation of the ipsilateral nucleus interpositus. C: newly appeared slow component superimposed on the fast rising IP-EPSP by stimulation of the contralateral IP. B,C: from a cat operated at the 67th day postnatally. D: diagram of three sources of sprouting after ablation of ipsilateral cortico-rubral input. Midline shown by vertical interrupted line. E: frequency distribution of the newly appeared EPSPs. c-CP, contralateral CP-EPSPs; i-IP, ipsilateral IP-EPSPs; c-IP slow comp., slowly rising component of contralateral IP-EPSPs. F: frequency distribution of number of sprouting sources.

of 29 RN cells), and the last possibility was the ipsilateral IP (7 out of 29 RN cells) (Fig. 2E). Although the chance of reaching the denervated synaptic sites seems to be equal for the three input fibres, it is likely that one of them would suppress the connection of the others on the denervated synaptic sites. There is evidence showing that sprouting and functional synaptic formation occurs on the distal dendrites of RN cells, as diagrammatically illustrated in Fig. 2D. This indicates that it might be a good model to answer the question of how specifically the newly formed connections are organized.

It is well known that the ipsilateral cortico-rubral projection is somatotopically organized (Tsukahara and Kosaka 1968). We investigated whether somatotopic organization is preserved in the newly formed crossed cortico-rubral projection or not. The forelimb cortical area projects to the contralateral RN neurones

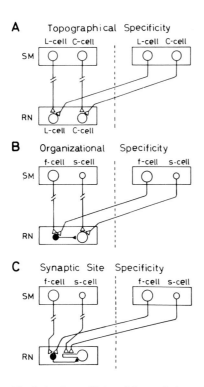

Fig. 3. A–C: specificity of the newly formed cortico-rubral projection. A: SM, sensorimotor cortex; RN, red nucleus; L cell, cells innervating lumbo-sacral spinal cord; C cell, cells innervating cervico-thoracic spinal cord. Dotted vertical line, midline. B: f cell, fast conducting pyramidal tract cells; s cell, slowly conducting pyramidal tract and cortico-rubral cells. C: same as B. Open circles, excitatory neurones; filled circles, inhibitory neurones.

innervating the forelimb and the hind limb cortical area projects to RN neurones innervating the hind limb. Thus, the newly formed crossed cortico-rubral projections have *topographical specificity*. However, this specificity is modified after additional lesions in the intact contralateral sensorimotor cortex. After chronic ablation of the forelimb area of the contralateral sensorimotor cortex in addition to the ipsilateral sensorimotor cortical lesions, new connections were formed from the remaining hind limb area even to RN neurones innervating the forelimb, as well as to RN neurones innervating the hind limb, suggesting expansion of the projection from the remaining cortex.

In normal cats, RN neurones receive inhibition from fast conducting pyramidal tract fibres and excitation from slowly conducting pyramidal and cortico-rubral fibres. After chronic lesions of the ipsilateral cerebral cortex, inhibitory postsynaptic potentials (IPSPs) could be induced by a train of stimuli applied to the contralateral corticofugal fibres. The IPSPs were considered to be mediated by the fast conducting pyramidal tract fibres because the threshold was lower for the IPSPs than for the EPSPs to stimuli applied to the contralateral corticofugal fibres. In addition, the conduction velocities of fibres responsible for the EPSPs belonged to those of slowly conducting pyramidal tract fibres.

Thus, the newly formed crossed cortico-rubral projections have *organizational specificity* as to the polarity of connections: fast conducting fibres inhibit whereas slowly conducting fibres excite the RN neurones. Finally, the *specificity of synaptic location* seems to be preserved for the sprouting after neonatal ipsilateral cerebral lesions, as diagrammatically illustrated in Fig. 3. The present studies on the newly formed cerebro-rubral map thus seem to have given some insight into hitherto unasked questions in similar experiments. It is likely that sprouting and formation of functional synapses account, at least in some part, for the behavioural recovery that cats show after brain lesions.

REFERENCES

Nah, S.H. and Leong, S.K. Bilateral corticofugal projection to the red nucleus after neonatal lesions in the albino rat. Brain Res., 1976a, 107: 433–436.

Nah, S.H. and Leong, S.K. An ultrastructural study of the anomalous corticorubral projection following neonatal lesions in the albino rat. Brain Res., 1976b, 111: 162–166.

Tsukahara, N. Synaptic plasticity in the mammalian central nervous system. Ann. Rev. Neurosci., 1981, 4: 351–379.

Tsukahara, N. and Fujito, Y. Neuronal plasticity in the newborn and adult feline red nucleus. In: H. Flohr and W. Precht (Eds.), Lesion-Induced Neuronal Plasticity in Sensorimotor Systems. Springer, Berlin, 1981: 64–74.

Tsukahara, N. and Kosaka, K. The mode of cerebral excitation of red nucleus neurons. Exp. Brain Res., 1968, 5: 102–117.

4. Electrophysiological Evaluation of Muscle Relaxants

Kyoto Symposia (EEG Suppl. No. 36)
Editors: P.A. Buser, W.A. Cobb and T. Okuma
© 1982, Elsevier Biomedical Press, Amsterdam

Muscle Restraint in Speed Controlled Voluntary and Passive Movements

E. KNUTSSON

Department of Clinical Neurophysiology, Karolinska Sjukhuset, 10401 Stockholm (Sweden)

Antispastic therapy is based on the concept that reflex depression can result in relief from some of the restraint imposed upon movement by spastic muscles and also reduce disturbing clonus and spasms. The mechanisms involved in spasms are not well defined and the estimation of depressive effects on these has been limited to subjective ratings and quantification by taped long-term records of integrated EMG (Knutsson et al. 1973). The restraint of movement by spastic muscles and clonus is intimately related to enhanced muscle stretch reflexes. Therefore, the estimation of depressive effects upon these has been regarded as a cornerstone in the evaluation of antispastic therapy.

Various procedures have been used to test effects on stretch reflexes. They include studies of the influence on phasic reflexes such as tendon jerks and H reflexes as well as on tonic vibration reflexes. These reflexes have the advantage of being available for quite well defined testing of specific functions (Delwaide et al. 1980). Problems arise when trying to relate the effects on these reflexes to the changes in clinical symptoms. The reflex activations that appear in movements are quite different from those experimentally induced with regard to the mode of generation, patterns of sensory input and efferent discharge. Therefore, studies on these experimentally elicited reflexes cannot readily be used for the evaluation of therapeutic efficacy, although they are fundamental in the analysis of mode of action.

Thus, passive movements at speeds corresponding to those of the movements of daily living appear more relevant for the evaluation of antispastic therapy. Passive movements are made manually or enforced by electric or hydraulic motors. They can also be tested in pendular movements (Boczko and Mumenthaler 1958).

Reliability in the evaluation of depressive effects on stretch reflexes with this type of movement depends on the possibility of eliminating the influence of posture-related and "spontaneous" variations in reflex tone, as well as on precision in repeating identical test movements. Posture-related variation in muscle tone is minimal when the body can be kept in a well defined position during testing. Spontaneous variations can usually be kept small during tests when these do not occur during periods directly following a posture change or skin touch with limb adaptor or hand.

The use of a motor to enforce passive movements is a good basis for reproducing identical movements. Tests of restraint of ankle movements are usually performed with sinusoidal dorsal and plantar foot flexions, obtained with a motor-driven excentric wheel (Herman 1970). Other passive joint movements are commonly enforced by hydraulic (Knutsson et al. 1973; Sahrmann et al. 1974) or electric systems (Hagbarth and Eklund 1968) with linear or near linear angular rotations. There are problems in all systems with the adaptation to sudden spasms and movements to exclude the risk of injury, especially in full-range movements at high speeds.

Manually produced movements are safer in this respect, but the repetition of identical movements is not easy unless monitored by angular displacement records (Jones et al. 1970). Combining manually produced movements with speed control from a motor diminishes the risk of injury while maintaining a high degree of precision in the reproduction of identical movements at different pre-selected speeds.

This type of speed-controlled passive movement can be obtained by using an isokinetic dynamometer which acts by braking the movement at a pre-set speed of angular rotation. Fig. 1 gives a schematic representation of the dynamometer. The motor rotates an axle at pre-selected speed, kept constant by servo control. After alignment of the joint axis, the limb segment to be moved is attached to a rotational lever arm connected to the motor-driven axle by a clutch coupling. This coupling allows free movement of the lever arm at low speeds but when the speed reaches that pre-set, the coupling becomes engaged and the movement is inhibited from rotating faster than the selected speed. Thus, in voluntary movements, which are those usually tested with the isokinetic dynamometer (Perinne 1968), after a phase of acceleration, the movement proceeds at a constant angular rotation.

To determine restraint to passive movements, the lever arm is equipped with a high precision transducer (Fig. 2). The movement is enforced manually by the examiner with an optional lever arm in direct connection with the speed-controlled axis of the dynamometer. The force applied is not recorded by the transducer. Only the torque of the other lever arm (active) will be recorded by gauges on the two wings of the transducer. The torque thus recorded in a passive movement is the sum of gravitational force and muscle restraint, when present. Thus, passive muscle restraint in a movement is obtained by correcting the recorded torque by subtracting or adding the gravitational force that is a cosine function of the joint angle.

Fig. 3 gives the passive restraint to foot dorsal flexion at 3 different speeds of

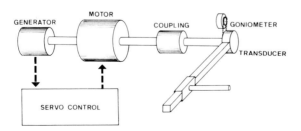

Fig. 1. Schematic representation of isokinetic dynamometer with transducer for torque record. (From Knutsson and Mårtensson 1980.)

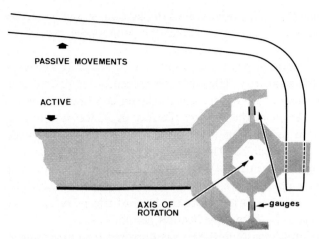

Fig. 2. Strain gauge transducer for records of torque in passive and voluntary movements. Passive movements enforced via lever arm (passive) acting directly on rotational axis. Resistance to passive movements and force in voluntary movements recorded by gauges on metal wings connecting rotational axis with "active" lever arm to which limb is attached. (From Knutsson and Mårtensson 1980.)

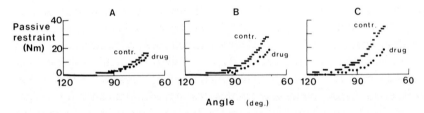

Fig. 3. Passive restraint to foot dorsal flexion in patient with spastic paraparesis during pre-medication control (contr.) and medication (drug) period (tizanidine, 32 mg/day). Speeds of movement in A, B and C were 30, 60 and 120 deg/sec, respectively. Movements started at 120 deg between foot and leg. Each curve gives the average of 3 tests with torque corrected for gravitation. (From Knutsson et al. 1982.)

motion in a patient with spastic paraparesis. Restraint is given in torque (Nm) for different angular positions of the movement. Three speeds were used (30, 60 and 120 deg/sec). Each curve gives torque for different angular positions of the movement corrected for gravitational force as obtained from 3 tests of each movement. The collection and processing of the approx. 30,000 measurements summarized in the figure were made with a previously described computer system (Gransberg et al. 1980). The movement started at 120° (foot plantar flexed) and continued to a dorsal flexed position. As seen in the records, restraint increases successively in all movements. By comparing the curves at slow and fast speed, a marked increase in restraint with speed of movement is seen.

In the pre-medication period (contr.), the restraint at the highest speed (120 deg/sec) reached a level of about 35 Nm. It corresponded to a tension in the Achilles tendon of about 700 N, well above that needed to lift the body. After medication (drug) with a recently introduced antispastic drug, tizanidine (Ringwald et al. 1977), the restraint in the two fastest movements (B and C) decreased markedly but only slightly in the slowest movement (A). Apparently, tests of passive restraint had to be made at a relatively high speed of motion to reveal the pronounced depressive effects on spastic reflexes.

Concomitant with the depression of passive restraint seen in Fig. 3, there was a marked improvement in walking capacity. Thus, in the pre-medication period, gait computer analysis with movement and EMG records (Isaksson and Knutsson 1980) indicated strong restraint to the tilt of the leg over the foot in stance, resulting in short strides and slow forward progression. During medication, the stride length and the progression velocity were doubled. These changes appeared to be due to a lessened restraint of the triceps surae muscles that allowed the leg a larger forward tilt over the foot in the stance phase of walking. Thus, the angular displacement between leg and foot became twice as large before the level of triceps surae EMG activity reached the same level as in the pre-medication period.

In this example, a depression of spastic reflexes was mirrored by a pronounced improvement in functional capacity. This is not always true. In fact, depression of spastic reflexes in many patients does not result in any apparent improvement of function. In some it can even lead to deterioration. The lack of favourable effects on motor capacity despite reduction of spastic reflexes can usually be referred to one of the following factors: (1) the use of spastic reflexes to achieve function; (2) the difference of the restraint of spastic muscles in passive and voluntary movements; (3) the individual relation between muscle strength and passive restraint.

The first of these is commonly recognized as the ''spastic crutch'' which implies that exaggerated stretch reflexes are used to obtain stability in standing and walking. In gait analyses of a few patients with this feature, the activation of weight supporting muscles (hip abductor, quadriceps) at the end of the swing to prepare the leg for weight acceptance was found to be low or lacking (Knutsson 1982). Activation appeared first after start of load and was probably supported by the muscle stretch imposed. With the time needed to build up contractile tension in the muscles, the stability of the leg would be critical in the early part of the stance phase. A drug-induced lowering of the stretch reflex activation will further compromise weight support and seems to be experienced by the patients as muscle weakness.

Evaluation of restraint in voluntary movement and the relation between muscle strength and passive restraint calls for records of voluntary muscle strength and EMG activity in agonistic and antagonistic muscles. Isometric strength determinations are usually of little value since they mirror neither prime mover activation in shortening nor restraint in antagonists during their lengthening. Dynamic strength determinations are more appropriate. They will disclose the capacity to produce tension at different speeds of motion. Incapacitation due to prime mover dysfunction or to antagonist restraint is commonly more marked in fast than in slow motion (Knutsson and Mårtensson 1980).

Differences in restraint by spastic muscles during passive and voluntary movements of equal range and speed have been seen in cyclical tracking movements (McLellan 1977) and isokinetic movements (Knutsson and Mårtensson 1977). The activation of the antagonistic muscles stretched by a voluntary motion may be smaller or larger than during similar stretch in passive motion. Inhibition of stretch reflexes during voluntary effort seems to be relatively frequent in mild spasticity and at submaximal effort. In severe spasticity and at vigorous effort, enhancement of the restraint to stretch during voluntary movement is more common.

Fig. 4 illustrates an enhancement of restraint of this type. It was observed in a paraparetic patient with strong spasticity during maximal voluntary knee flexion. As seen in the figure, the EMG activity in the antagonistic quadriceps muscle was much larger in the voluntary than in the passive movements. There is no precise method to determine the increase in tension corresponding to the increased EMG activity. However, if the tension is supposed to be roughly proportional to the EMG activity it would mean that the restraint to knee flexion given by the quadriceps in the voluntary movements was increased several times compared to the restraint in the passive movements at equal pre-set speed. The restraint reached levels of about 20 and 30 Nm respectively in the passive movements at 30 and 90 deg/sec. Thus, it seems probable that the antagonist restraint in voluntary movement can have reached levels of 60–120 Nm. This is not far from the peak tension produced in knee flexion of healthy subjects. It explains the low capacity for knee flexion despite forceful activation of the prime mover muscles.

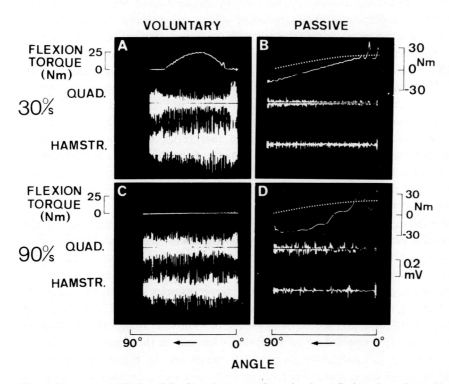

Fig. 4. Torque and EMG activity in voluntary and passive knee flexions in patient with spastic paraparesis. Interrupted lines in B and D indicate torque expected from gravitation. Deviations from these curves give spastic restraint. (From Knutsson et al. 1982.)

The mechanisms behind the change of restraint during voluntary movement are not fully understood. Reciprocal inhibition may be operative in the depression of restraint seen in some patients. In patients displaying enhanced restraint during voluntary movements, the reason could be misdirected supraspinal commands or stretch reflex facilitation by the voluntary effort. The latter concept is supported by two observations. First, peak restraint appears in the same phase of passive and voluntary movements (McLellan 1977). Secondly, the antagonist restraint in voluntary movement increases markedly with speed of movement and thus with the speed of stretch (Knutsson and Mårtensson 1980). A speed dependence of this type suggests activation via a phasic reflex loop and cannot readily be expected from supraspinal commands. This does not, of course, exclude that misdirected commands also play a role.

Irrespective of the mechanisms constituting enhanced antagonist restraint in voluntary movements it is important to find out whether or not this restraint can be damped by antispastic therapy. There is scant information on this subject due to the relatively complex examination procedures needed to estimate restraint in voluntary movements. It was first studied by McLellan (1977) by determining the change of antagonist EMG activity in voluntary tracking of cyclical knee flexions and extensions after a single dose of baclofen. The study showed that depressive effects on the antagonist co-activation were infrequent, despite high plasma concentrations of the drug and despite marked depressive effects on restraint of equal passive movements. Furthermore, during therapy with tizanidine, depression of restraint of passive movements seems to be much more common than depression of antagonist restraint in equal isokinetic movements at maximal voluntary effort (Knutsson et al. 1982). Thus, damping of the stretch reflexes elicited by passive movements cannot be used to evaluate the restraint opposing voluntary movements in daily life.

The third reason for lack of favourable effect on motor disability by reduced stretch reflexes is quite obvious. It implies that reflex depression, even when considerable, has no chance to improve a motor function that is not limited by spastic reflexes. It includes situations where the strength is too low to attain function whether or not the restraint is depressed. It also includes situations in which spastic restraint is easily outbalanced by strong prime movers.

Besides the depressive effects seen on restraint of movement, antispastic therapy can result in reduction of prime mover dysfunction. This effect was first observed in response to tizanidine therapy (Knutsson et al. 1982), but has later been seen in response to other forms of therapy in some of the cases so far studied. It consists of an improved capacity to activate the prime mover muscles at maximal voluntary effort. Fig. 5 gives an illustration; it shows torque and averaged EMG activity in voluntary knee flexion at 3 speeds of isokinetic movement at maximal effort before (A) and after (B) a single dose of tizanidine. As seen in the figure, there was a marked increase in contraction strength. It could not be related to depressed restraint but there was a marked rise of the EMG activity in the hamstring muscles that acted as prime movers. In isokinetic movements, the maximal voluntary capacity can be assessed with a high degree of precision providing a minimal

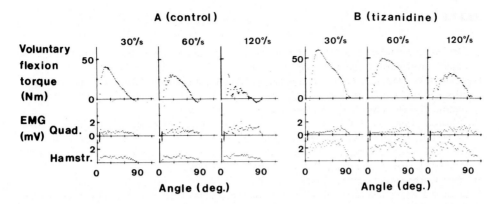

Fig. 5. Torque and EMG activity in isokinetic voluntary knee flexion in patient with spastic paraparesis before (A) and 1 h after (B) a single dose of tizanidine (12 mg). Each curve averaged from 3 tests. Torque corrected for gravitational force. EMG given in amplitude of rectified time-averaged records with electrodes unchanged between records in A and B. Records taken at 3 speeds of motion as indicated. Negative torque in fast flexion in A indicates antagonist restraint by the quadriceps muscle was larger than the flexion force produced by the prime movers. (From Knutsson et al. 1982.)

variation of torque in repeated tests is used as criterion of maximal effort (Gransberg et al. 1980). This holds true especially for fast movements, showing a mean difference of less than 1% in tests on 2 successive days in healthy subjects. In patients with spasticity, mean torque was unchanged after administration of placebo or ineffectively low doses of tizanidine. Thus, the marked increase in strength seen in Fig. 5 after drug administration can be regarded as a true increase in strength.

The cause of an enhanced capacity for activation of the prime mover muscles has not yet been analysed in detail. It seems to occur together with depression of the stretch reflexes elicited by passive movement. Thus, it can be related to a deprivation of reciprocal inhibition from stretch receptors in the antagonists but its explanation has to await the results of further studies.

The complex disorganization of motor control in muscular hypertonias and the variation in response to therapy imply that the evaluation of antispastic therapy cannot be based solely on determinations of the influence on passive stretch reflexes. It requires also information on the functions of agonists and antagonists during performance of different motor tasks and how they are influenced by therapy. Methods so far tested provide information only on a few of the many motor tasks disturbed by lesions of the central nervous system. To generalize from this information can be misleading. Different types of movement have highly different features for control. Thus, there remains a challenging field for further studies of the disorganization of motor control and its therapeutic approach.

REFERENCES

Boczko, M. and Mumenthaler, M. Modified pendulousness test to assess tonus of thigh muscles in spasticity. Neurology (Minneap.), 1958, 8: 846–851.

Delwaide, P.J., Martinelli, M.D. and Crenna, P. Clinical neurophysiological measurement of spinal reflex activity. In: R.G. Feldman, R.R. Young and W.P. Koella (Eds.), Spasticity: Disordered Motor Control. Year Book Medical Publishers, Chicago, Ill., 1980: 345–371.

Gransberg, L., Knutsson, E. and Litton, J.-E. A computer programmed system for the analysis of active and passive isokinetic movements. IEEE, 1980: 292–295.

Hagbarth, K.-E. and Eklund, G. The effects of muscle vibration in spasticity, rigidity and cerebellar disorders. J. Neurol. Neurosurg. Psychiat., 1968, 31: 207–213.

Herman, R. The myotatic reflex. Brain, 1970, 93: 273–312.

Isaksson, A.I. and Knutsson, E. Microcomputer implementation of gait examination in clinical routine. IEEE, 1980: 42–45.

Jones, R.F., Burke, D., Marosszeky, J.E. and Gillies, J.D. A new agent for the control of spasticity. J. Neurol. Neurosurg. Psychiat., 1970, 33: 464–468.

Knutsson, E. Analysis of isokinetic movements and gait in the evaluation of antispastic therapy. In: J.E. Desmedt (Ed.), Motor Control Mechanisms in Man. Electrophysiological Methods and Clinical Applications. Raven Press, New York, 1982, in press.

Knutsson, E. and Mårtensson, A. Activation patterns in spastic muscles stretched by passive and active movements. Electroenceph. clin. Neurophysiol., 1977, 43: 605.

Knutsson, E. and Mårtensson, A. Dynamic motor capacity in spastic paresis and its relation to prime mover dysfunction, spastic restraint and antagonist co-activation. Scand. J. rehab. Med., 1980, 12: 93–106.

Knutsson, E., Lindblom, U. and Mårtensson, A. Differences in effects in gamma and alpha spasticity induced by the GABA derivative baclofen (Lioresal). Brain, 1973, 96: 26–46.

Knutsson, E., Mårtensson, A. and Gransberg, L. Antiparetic and antispastic effects induced by tizanidine in patients with spastic paresis. J. neurol. Sci., 1982, 53: 187–204.

McLellan, D.L. Co-contraction and stretch reflexes in spasticity during treatment with baclofen. J. Neurol. Neurosurg. Psychiat., 1977, 40: 30–38.

Perinne, J.J. Isokinetic exercise in the mechanical energy potentials of muscle. J. Hlth Phys. Educ. Recreat., 1968, 39: 40.

Ringwald, E., Campean, F., Gerstenbrand, P., Lörinez, P. und Ludin, H.P. Klinische Erfahrungen mit DS 103-282, ein neuartiges Myotonolytikum. Nervenarzt, 1977, 48: 355–358.

Sahrmann, S.A., Norton, B.J., Bomze, H.A. and Eliasson, S.G. Influence of the site of lesion and muscle length on spasticity in man. Phys. Ther., 1974, 54: 1290–1296.

Kyoto Symposia (EEG Suppl. No. 36)
Editors: P.A. Buser, W.A. Cobb and T. Okuma
© 1982, Elsevier Biomedical Press, Amsterdam

The Use of Electromyograms to Assess Impaired Voluntary Movement Associated with Increased Muscle Tone

D.L. McLELLAN and N.H. HASSAN

Wessex Neurological Centre, University of Southampton, Southampton SO9 4XY (England)

Stretch responses are normally regarded as an important source of inappropriate muscle contraction in spasticity and suppression with drugs is accepted as one of the aims of treatment. By recording surface electromyograms, muscle activity during passive movement can be compared with the patterns that occur during various types of voluntary movement in such a way as to identify the components of inappropriate activity that can be attributed to stretch responses.

The patterns of muscle activity induced by passive sinusoidal movements around a joint in spasticity were first described by Burke et al. in 1971. By integrating the electromyographic activity in flexor and extensor muscles during passive and voluntary sinusoidal movements of the knee, McLellan (1977) expressed the amount of activity occurring in each muscle as it was passively stretched, and also the amount of inappropriate activity occurring during voluntary movement, as indices of stretch response activity and co-activation. Patients with mild spasticity were found to suppress their stretch responses during voluntary movement, while in some patients with more severe spasticity a peak of inappropriate activity was seen in the quadriceps muscle during voluntary movements at a point in the cycle suggesting that it was due to a released stretch response. However, abolition of the passive stretch responses with Baclofen did not alter abnormal co-activation during voluntary movement. Similar results were obtained under different conditions by Knutsson and Mårtensson (1980).

In order to test the hypothesis that abnormal co-activation during voluntary movement is due to released spastic stretch responses, the technique has been extended to examine patterns of muscle activity during 2 sinusoidal tracking tasks. The upper limb is placed in a comfortable light plastic splint, supported horizontally with a pivot at the elbow that allows the elbow to flex and extend in the horizontal plane. The angle of the elbow is recorded with a potentiometer fixed to the rig and the subject uses the signal from the potentiometer to track a sine wave target displayed in front of him on an oscilloscope. This task is called position tracking. Alternatively, the rig is locked by a strain gauge and the subject tracks simply by pressing against the rig in the direction of flexion or extension, without any movement taking place. This isometric task is called force tracking.

It is necessary to set up and control the conditions of the 2 tasks in such a way that when a normal subject is position tracking, the muscles are active only when they are actually shortening and are silent when they are lengthening. In addition, similar amplitudes and similar profiles of electromyographic activity need to be generated in both position tracking and force tracking modes. After many empirical trials in volunteers, springs have been fitted to the rig to increase the similarity of the 2 tasks and we have chosen a repetition rate of 0.64 Hz for a 45° arc of elbow movement, from 90 to 135° at the elbow. Such a task in normal subjects gives reasonably similar electromyographic profiles during force tracking and position tracking in the biceps, triceps and brachioradialis muscles. The accuracy of the subject's performance can be measured by integrating the error − that is the electrical difference between the target signal and the tracking signal − over a set period of time.

Normal subjects rapidly learn how to do these tasks with the minimum of co-activation. The task is rather fast for many severely spastic subjects and even in the milder ones it takes the patient at least half an hour of practice, preferably spread over several days, before the co-activation that characterizes the early stages of learning begins to diminish and reveals consistent patterns of activity that are characteristic and repeatable for that individual.

Provided that the subject tracks the target well, 30 or more cycles of movement can be averaged and a profile of electromyographic activity during the cycle can be obtained. We have examined performance in these tasks in 18 spastic subjects but only 8 of these showed evidence of abnormal co-activation during tracking. More severely affected patients were unable to follow the target at the necessary speed. All the subjects so far studied have suffered from cerebral lesions due to stroke, head injury or cerebral palsy. Patients with mild spasticity have been shown to have passive stretch responses, and sometimes passive shortening responses in the triceps muscle, which appear to be suppressed during voluntary movement. This is in agreement with the previous studies already mentioned. Eight of the more severe patients showed abnormal peaks of activity in the biceps and brachioradialis muscle during position tracking. Despite this, all subjects except one showed a greater tracking error when force tracking than when position tracking, in the same way as normal subjects. Analysis of the profile of electromyographic activity during force tracking showed that identical peaks of co-activation occurred in the biceps and brachioradialis muscles even though no movement had taken place. This activity could not therefore have been due to stretch responses in the muscles, since the muscles were not stretched during force tracking.

When the records from the flexor muscles were superimposed upon the records from the triceps, it became clear that the burst of co-activation in the flexor muscles coincided precisely with the burst of voluntary activity in the triceps muscle. This was not due to artifactual spread of the electrical signal from the triceps, since stretch responses in triceps could be recorded without any activity being detected by the electrodes over the flexor muscles.

This evidence suggests that the abnormal co-activation seen in the flexor muscles is not stretch induced, but is part of a centrally programmed pattern of co-activation during attempts voluntarily to extend the limb. Seven patients were able to activate the flexors without activating the extensors, but could not voluntarily activate the extensors without activating the flexors also. Although antispastic drugs can be shown to reduce the frequency of spasms during the recording session, and this improves overall tracking performance, these peaks of co-activation have not been affected by antispastic treatment. In retrospect, it seems likely that the explanation originally offered for the peak of activity seen in quadriceps muscles during tracking movement was incorrect (McLellan 1977). It seems likely that a similar disorder of central co-activation occurs in the lower limbs in spasticity and that this could explain the failure of some patients to respond to antispastic medication.

REFERENCES

Burke, D., Andrews, C.J. and Gillies, J.D. The reflex response to sinusoidal stretching in spastic man. Brain, 1971, 94: 455.

Knutsson, E. and Mårtensson, A. Dynamic motor capacity and its relation to prime mover dysfunction, spastic reflexes and antagonist co-activation. Scand. J. rehab. Med., 1980, 12: 93–106.

McLellan, D.L. Co-contraction and stretch reflexes in spasticity during treatment with Baclofen. J. Neurol. Neurosurg. Psychiat., 1977, 40: 30–38.

Kyoto Symposia (EEG Suppl. No. 36)
Editors: P.A. Buser, W.A. Cobb and T. Okuma
© 1982, Elsevier Biomedical Press, Amsterdam

172

Stretch Reflex Activity in the Spastic Patient

DAVID BURKE

Unit of Clinical Neurophysiology, Department of Neurology, The Prince Henry Hospital, and School of Medicine, University of New South Wales, Sydney 2036 (Australia)

Spasticity is a disorder of spinal proprioceptive (stretch) reflexes, manifested by tendon jerk hyperreflexia and an increase in muscle tone that is dependent on the speed of joint rotation (see Feldman et al. 1980). Spasticity is a symptom not a disease: many factors may combine to produce the typical clinical manifestations and the factors may differ in importance in different patients. The goal of electrophysiological tests on a patient is to understand the factors responsible for that patient's symptom complex. In assessing medication there are two further goals: to establish efficacy and to define the mode of action of the drug. The ultimate aim is that a patient's medication be tailored to his disability.

Spasticity constitutes only 1 of the 5 major manifestations of the upper motoneurone syndrome (Table I). In the majority of patients, the most important manifestations are: weakness, loss of manual dexterity and, in some hemiplegic patients, an abnormal posture. Unfortunately these manifestations are the ones least responsive to therapy. Disturbances of spinal reflex mechanisms commonly respond well to drug therapy but they are generally a problem only in patients with spinal or brain stem lesions; they usually contribute little to the disability of the patient with a cerebral lesion, such as capsular hemiplegia. The hemiplegic posture, with relatively fixed flexion and adduction of the upper limb and extension of the lower limb, is best considered a dystonic manifestation of the upper motoneurone syndrome, not the result of spasticity, and unlikely to be influenced by medication directed at spinal reflex circuits.

The most important test that can be performed in a spastic patient is a proper clinical examination to assess which of the manifestations of the upper motoneurone

TABLE I

MANIFESTATIONS OF THE UPPER MOTONEURONE SYNDROME

1.	Weakness
2.	Loss of dexterity
3.	Abnormal posture
4.	"Spasticity" – increased muscle tone – exaggerated tendon jerks, clonus, reflex irradiation
5.	"Release" of flexor reflexes – flexor spasms – clasp-knife inhibition – extensor plantar response

syndrome contributes to the patient's disability. Electrophysiological testing may help in this respect but it cannot replace clinical skills. Too often spastic patients are treated vigorously for their spasticity when it is responsible for little disability and may even provide a degree of reflex stiffness to support a paretic muscle group. Under such circumstances therapy which is effective may not be efficacious.

There are many sophisticated electrophysiological tests that can be used in the human subject. Care should be taken to apply the same degree of sophistication to the interpretation of data as to its collection. Interpretations are often based on data from animal experiments without consideration of size and other anatomical peculiarities of the human subject. These points will be illustrated in the second half of this paper. In the first, 2 relatively simple methods for assessing stretch reflex activity will be described. Neither method is ideal, but they are relatively simple and do not require complicated equipment so that they can be used in departments which possess only basic facilities. Both methods were developed primarily to help analyse motor mechanisms (see Burke and Lance 1973; Neilson and Lance 1978), but have proved useful in assessing therapy.

(1) The aim of the first method is to assess stretch reflex activity under conditions comparable to the clinical assessment of muscle tone. The patient lies prone on a bed, as completely relaxed as possible. Surface EMG electrodes are fixed to the skin over the quadriceps and hamstring muscle groups at standard measured positions, after abrasion of the skin to reduce electrode impedance to below 5 kΩ (Fig. 1). The leg is moved manually by the experimenter through approximately 100° from full extension into flexion, the extent of movement being recorded by a goniometer at the knee. The parameters recorded are joint position and the EMG activity of the two muscle groups. The joint angle signal is differentiated to provide a signal proportional to angular velocity. The EMG activity is integrated using an RC low pass filter with the time constant set so that it integrates the response to the stretching movement but not activity occurring after movement has ceased.

Fig. 2A shows the responses from the quadriceps muscle of a spastic patient. The knee joint has been flexed from the fully extended position to approximately 100° 4 times, at increasing velocity for successive movements. In the spastic patient, slow stretching movements may produce little or no reflex response, faster movements being required before the typical increase in muscle tone becomes apparent. With the subject in Fig. 2A, the first movement was so slow that it did not produce any

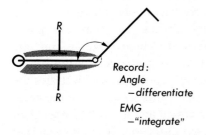

Fig. 1. The experimental design.

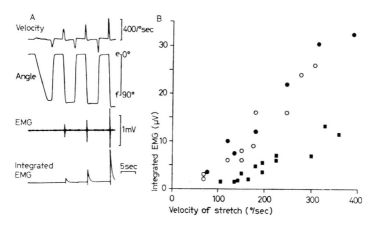

Fig. 2. Reflex responses to ramp stretch. A: original data, showing a larger reflex EMG response with faster stretching movements, and subsidence of EMG activity on cessation of movement. B: for 3 patients, the size of the reflex EMG burst is plotted against the velocity of joint movement. Each relationship approximates a straight line. (From Burke and Lance 1973.)

reflex EMG activity, but with the subsequent movements a reflex response appeared, and built up with the increase in the velocity of movement. In Fig. 2B, the velocity of stretch is plotted against the size of the reflex EMG burst for 3 different patients. Each relationship approximates a straight line. For each subject, the intensity of stretch reflex activity can be quantitated in terms of the velocity of joint movement that had to be exceeded before reflex EMG appeared, and the slope of the EMG/velocity relationship.

Changes in the degree of spasticity, be they spontaneous, due to the passage of time, due to some change in the disease process, or due to drug therapy, are reflected in parallel changes in the relationship between EMG and velocity of stretch. The lower the threshold velocity that has to be exceeded before reflex activity appears, the worse the spasticity. The greater the slope of the EMG/velocity relationship, the worse the spasticity. Fig. 3 shows the dramatic effect on stretch reflex activity produced by clinically effective drug therapy.

Essentially similar techniques can be used to study the reflex response to continuous sinusoidal stretching instead of the response to ramp stretch. To produce the sinusoidal movement the experimenter tracks a sine wave produced by a function generator and displayed on an oscilloscope screen. With training the experimenter can quite easily move the patient's leg backwards and forwards in a highly reproducible way, and it then becomes possible to study the phase relationships of the stretch reflex with sinusoidal stretching (Fig. 4). Fig. 4A illustrates the response from the quadriceps muscle, with stretch (flexion of the knee) as an upward movement on the averaged angle record. Fig. 4B illustrates the response from the hamstrings, with stretch of the hamstrings (extension of the knee) upwards. The EMG activity has been full wave rectified and averaged rather than integrated because a low pass filter introduces phase distortion. It can be seen that the EMG activities of the 2 muscle groups occur at quite different phases of their

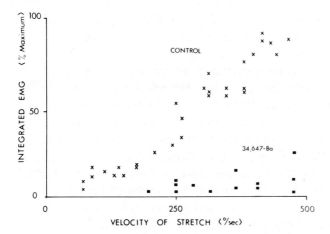

Fig. 3. Effect of drug therapy on stretch reflex activity. Treatment resulted in a clinically obvious decrease in the degree of spasticity with parallel changes in the EMG/velocity relationship.

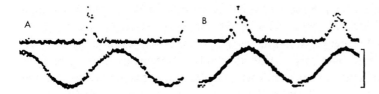

Fig. 4. Reflex responses to sinusoidal stretch at 0.5 Hz. A, quadriceps; B, hamstrings, with rectified and averaged EMG in the upper traces and averaged knee joint position in the lower traces, stretch for each muscle group being an upward deflection of the angle records. Forty stretching cycles have been averaged in A and B. The amplitude of joint movement (cf. calibration) was 100° from full extension. (From Burke and Lance 1973.)

respective stretching cycles. Studies such as this have been used not to demonstrate the efficacy of drug therapy but to analyse the underlying mechanisms in spasticity and the effects of medication on them.

The techniques just described measure reflex activity when the subject is relaxed; the resulting measures correlate quite well with muscle tone felt by a neurologist when he is examining a spastic patient clinically. However, reflex activity as tested in a relaxed patient may not reflect reflex behaviour during voluntary movement. If stretch reflex disturbances can disrupt movement, then reflex studies carried out during a background voluntary contraction should reveal a reflex contribution to the disability of the patient better than studies performed when the patient is relaxed. This is the rationale for the second technique, developed and used in our department by Dr. P.D. Neilson.

The subject performs a steady background contraction of biceps brachii of between 10 and 30% maximum and a sinusoidally varying perturbation is applied through a spring to the forearm. The EMG activity of biceps brachii is recorded by surface electrodes, and is then rectified and filtered, much as already described.

Power spectra of elbow angle and of "integrated" EMG are computed. By calculating the EMG power correlated to the perturbation it is possible to extract the power attributable to reflex activity from the overall EMG activity.

Changes in reflex activity can be quantitated by looking at changes in the proportion of total EMG power that is correlated with the perturbation. For example, it is relatively easy in one experimental session to train normal subjects, using biofeedback techniques, to suppress completely the reflex response to a perturbation while maintaining the same degree of steady voluntary contraction (Neilson and Lance 1978). Dr. Neilson has now subjected 4 patients with spastic cerebral palsy to daily biofeedback training for approximately 18 months. These 4 patients have gained the ability to control voluntarily the strength of their reflex pathways, much as normal subjects can do. The data are still being analysed but the result is very exciting because of its obvious therapeutic implications.

(2) The goal of developing and using different tests in patients is ultimately the prescription of the most appropriate treatment for each individual. Basic neuronal circuitry and synaptic connectivity may well not differ significantly in man and animals, such as the cat, but the size difference constitutes a factor which can make it difficult to generalize from cat to man. While the use of different tests in patients is to be encouraged, such tests should be interpreted with caution. It is rarely possible to make more than rather general qualified statements about effects on specific neuronal circuits or mechanisms. To illustrate this point, two widely believed assumptions will be discussed. These assumptions are considered in greater detail elsewhere (Burke 1982): (i) that the tendon jerk and the H reflex are essentially identical reflexes for which fusimotor activity is the only significant difference; (ii) that the tendon jerk and the H reflex are exclusively monosynaptic reflexes.

There are in fact 7 other differences apart from fusimotor activity between the H reflex and the tendon jerk (Table II). The major ones are probably: (i) ankle dorsiflexion inhibits the H reflex but may facilitate the tendon jerk; (ii) with the H

TABLE II

DIFFERENCES BETWEEN H REFLEX AND TENDON JERK APART FROM FUSIMOTOR ACTIVITY

	H reflex	Tendon jerk
Distribution	Relatively restricted	Widespread
Dorsiflexion	Inhibits	Potentiates (then suppresses)
Afferents	Ia, Ib	Ia, cutaneous, Pacinian
Source of afferents	Calf muscles	Calf muscles
	Intrinsic muscles of the foot	Pretibial muscles
		Skin at percussion and fixation points
Pattern of discharge	Single impulse	Repeated impulses
Dispersion of Ia volley at motoneurone pool	About 7.5 msec	Much greater
Activated motoneurones	Small	Small, but large not excluded

reflex, the electrical stimulus will excite Ia and Ib afferents in similar proportions, but tendon percussion will excite Ia, cutaneous and Pacinian afferents; (iii) with the H reflex the activated afferents will come mainly from the calf muscles and the intrinsic muscles of the foot, but with the tendon jerk the afferents will be from the calf muscles, their antagonists, skin at the percussion site, etc.; (iv) with the H reflex, the stimulus produces a single impulse in each afferent, but with tendon percussion there may be multiple discharges at high frequency in individual afferents; (v) with an electrical stimulus, the slowest Ia afferent will reach the motoneurone pool approximately 7.5 msec after the fastest Ia afferent, but with the tendon tap the dispersion will be much greater because of the mechanical properties of the muscle, the different sites of each spindle in the muscle, and the different conduction distances to the popliteal fossa.

The degree of dispersion of the afferent volleys is much greater in man than in the cat, and this has important consequences. The rise time of the composite EPSP is believed to be very long in man (Ashby and Labelle 1977; Noguchi et al. 1979), and this is probably due to the dispersion of the afferent volley. So long can the EPSP be that there is more than adequate time for disynaptic, trisynaptic and even polysynaptic EPSPs to be generated in motoneurones by the fastest Ia afferents − and such pathways are now known to exist (Watt et al. 1976). The motoneurones of lowest threshold may well discharge just in response to the monosynaptic input if the stimulus is strong and the composite EPSP has an abrupt onset. However, motoneurones of higher threshold will receive disynaptic and trisynaptic inputs before they fire. Hence, although the H reflex and tendon jerk are both presumably oligosynaptic, neither reflex can be considered exclusively monosynaptic in man. Furthermore, with the H reflex volley, the EPSP lasts long enough for Ib disynaptic inhibitory effects to occur, and with the tendon jerk volley there is adequate time for second impulses in the fastest Ia afferents to reach the motoneurone pool before the first impulses in slow Ia afferents. With both volleys, particularly the tendon jerk volley, the EPSP lasts long enough for Renshaw inhibition set up by the first recruited motoneurones to affect high threshold motoneurones.

Thus, it may be concluded first, that comparing the H reflex with the tendon jerk is like comparing apples with oranges: it is clearly unwise to use such comparisons as a measure of fusimotor activity; secondly, that changes in the tendon jerk and H reflex do not necessarily reflect changes in the monosynaptic pathway.

REFERENCES

Ashby, P. and Labelle, K. Effects of extensor and flexor group I afferent volleys on the excitability of individual soleus motoneurones in man. J. Neurol. Neurosurg. Psychiat., 1977, 40: 910–919.

Burke, D. A critical examination of the case for and against fusimotor involvement in disorders of muscle tone. In: J.E. Desmedt (Ed.), Motor Control in Man. Raven Press, New York, 1982: in press.

Burke, D. and Lance, J.W. Studies of the reflex effects of primary and secondary spindle endings in spasticity. In: J.E. Desmedt (Ed.), New Developments in Electromyography and Clinical Neurophysiology, Vol. 3. Karger, Basel, 1973: 475–495.

Feldman, R.G., Young, R.R. and Koella, W.P. (Eds.). Spasticity: Disordered Motor Control. Year Book Publishers, Chicago, Ill., 1980.

Neilson, P.D. and Lance, J.W. Reflex transmission characteristics during voluntary activity in normal man and patients with motor disorders. In: J.E. Desmedt (Ed.), Cerebral Motor Control in Man: Long Loop Mechanisms. Progr. clin. Neurophysiol., Vol. 4. Karger, Basel, 1978: 263–299.

Noguchi, T., Homma, S. and Nakajima, Y. Measurements of excitatory postsynaptic potentials in the stretch reflex of normal subjects and spastic patients. J. Neurol. Neurosurg. Psychiat., 1979, 42: 1100–1105.

Watt, D.G.D., Stauffer, E.K., Taylor, A., Reinking, R.M. and Stuart, D.G. Analysis of muscle receptor connections by spike-triggered averaging. 1. Spindle primary and tendon organ afferents. J. Neurophysiol., 1976, 39: 1375–1392.

Kyoto Symposia (EEG Suppl. No. 36)
Editors: P.A. Buser, W.A. Cobb and T. Okuma

Discriminative Electrophysiological Tests to Study the Mode of Action of Myorelaxant Drugs*

P.J. DELWAIDE

Section of Neurology and Clinical Neurophysiology, Department of Internal Medicine, University of Liège, Liège (Belgium)

MODES OF EVALUATION OF A MYORELAXANT

The study of myorelaxant drugs should not be limited to pharmacological data, since extrapolations from animals to man are even more hazardous for these products than for other classes of drugs. In fact, current pharmacological tests remain distant from the pathophysiological defects because, even in primates, no good experimental model of spastic paresis is available. Laboratory results must necessarily be complemented by studies performed in spastic patients, in whom two types of investigation deserve to be performed: clinical evaluations and electrophysiological analysis of the effect.

Table I compares the advantages and limitations of each of these complementary approaches.

Double blind clinical studies are the only satisfactory means to evaluate therapeutic effectiveness provided that the subjective and objective improvement of patients are correctly scored. The results can lead to drug selection as a function of the clinical picture: duration and severity of the handicap, type of complaint, site of the lesion and so on. Clinical studies also give information on long term effects and can, for example, establish whether a drug remains active over a long period of time. They can also reveal side effects and, finally, they define the precise indications for a drug in therapeutics.

On the other hand, electrophysiological studies, often performed on only a single occasion, provide different information. They can disclose that a drug has the property of modifying an electrophysiological parameter of spasticity. Usually, the modification can be easily quantified, allowing comparisons between different drugs or between equivalent doses of chemically related drugs. However, the test influenced by a drug does not necessarily have a close relationship with the therapeutic efficacy, and it cannot be inferred, from an electrophysiological result, that a drug has useful therapeutic myorelaxant properties. But the electrophysiological study has other objectives: it can be unique in allowing an analysis of the mode of action of a myorelaxant, it can reveal — or at least suggest — the pathophysiological mechanism sensitive to medication if the test has been proven to

* This work was supported by the INSERM, France (Prot. 120054) and the FRSM, Belgium (cred. 3.4565.81).

TABLE I

COMPARISON BETWEEN CLINICAL AND ELECTROPHYSIOLOGICAL EVALUATIONS OF A
MYORELAXANT

Controlled clinical evaluations of treatment	Electrophysiological evaluations of the drug
Precise evaluation of the effectiveness	Objective evaluation by syndrome-related tests
	Quantification of the effect
Characterization of the drug-responsive symptoms or signs	
Effectiveness in long term treatments	
Acceptability of the drug	
	Analysis of the mode of drug action (pathophysiological mechanism)
	Measurement of latency and duration of effects on CNS after single administration

explore a well defined neuronal circuit. Finally, an added advantage of the electrophysiological study is the potential for pharmacokinetic measurements inside the
central nervous system, that is, to determine the delay, the intensity and the duration
of drug effects. These specificities of the electrophysiological study make it worth-
while, and justify that it should complement the clinical studies.

THE DEVELOPMENT OF THE ELECTROPHYSIOLOGICAL EVALUATION
OF MYORELAXANTS

The advantages of the electrophysiological study have long been recognized and
the first experiments demonstrating modifications of reflexes after giving a
myorelaxant are at least 20 years old (Paillard et al. 1961).

Until 1970, the research workers involved in these studies usually limited
themselves to the use of the Hoffmann reflex and, in some instances, to the ratio
between the H reflex and the maximal response recorded in the soleus after
stimulation of the tibial nerve (Matthews 1966). This ratio is considered to reflect
the excitability of the soleus motor nucleus and is increased in patients suffering
from spasticity. Thus, it was reasonable to hypothesize that a myorelaxant would
reduce this ratio. However, the results so far obtained were somewhat disappointing
and there was no clear correlation between the lowering of this value and the clinical
picture, a conclusion already reached by Matthews in 1966. Over the years, new
techniques were developed with more specific physiopathological meaning and were
applied to the study of myorelaxants.

In 1971, during our study on vibratory inhibition of the monosynaptic reflexes in
spastic patients (Delwaide 1971), we were able to show that diazepam distinctly
reinforces this inhibition. Since the latter is reduced in spasticity, diazepam brings
values closer to normal. Fig. 1 illustrates an example of the action of diazepam. In
the upper part are recruitment curves of the H reflex recorded in a spastic subject.

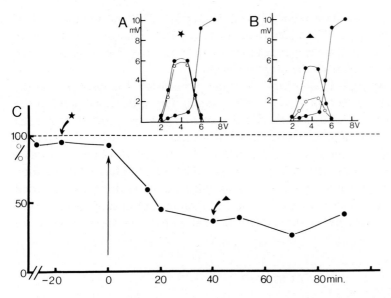

Fig. 1. Vibratory inhibition in a 32-year-old spastic patient. A: recruitment curves of the H reflex in control conditions. Filled circles: without conditioning; empty circles: under vibration. B: recruitment curves 40 min after an injection of 10 mg of diazepam. The values recorded under vibration (empty circles) are lower than without conditioning (filled circles). C: evolution of the $H_{vibrated}/H_{max}$ ratio × 100 (in ordinate) after i.m. injection (arrow) of 10 mg diazepam. The star corresponds to the values of A and the triangle to the values of B.

The filled circles indicate the values of the H reflex at different stimulation intensities; the empty circles, the values obtained when a vibrator stimulates the Achilles tendon. In the control conditions, on the left, the vibration has a very limited effect and the 2 curves are more or less similar. Such a result is usually observed in spastic patients. On the right, the 2 curves are obtained 40 min after an i.m. injection of 10 mg diazepam. The amplitudes of the H reflexes (filled circles) are only slightly reduced but the vibration is definitely more effective and produces a clear depression of the reflex. The greatest difference observed under diazepam is this reinforcement of vibratory inhibition. In the lower part of the figure the curve indicates the time course of the vibratory inhibition, the star indicating inhibition under control conditions, and the triangle, under medication. It can be seen that the reinforcement of vibratory inhibition occurs soon after the injection and lasts in this particular case for more than 100 min. Clonus, hyperreflexia and hypertonicity were reduced during the same period of time, so we concluded that the vibratory inhibition test was better correlated with the clinical improvement than the H_{max}/M_{max} ratio.

Some years later we tried electrophysiologically to objectify the effects of baclofen, whose chemical structure is related to that of GABA. Of course, we were expecting that the vibratory inhibition test would be modified by this drug. To our great disappointment, vibratory inhibition was not reinforced by an i.m. injection of 20 mg of baclofen, even though the clinical picture was improved. Some conflicting results have been reported (Pedersen et al. 1974) but the majority of authors (Castaigne et al. 1973) failed to observe significant change in the vibratory inhibition. At that point, we concluded that no one test is capable of reflecting the myorelaxant properties of all the drugs available.

After various attempts to objectify the action of baclofen, we observed that the recovery curve of the Hoffmann reflex after stimulation of the tibial nerve at the ankle was clearly modified by an i.m. injection of 20 mg of that product. In normal subjects, the H reflex amplitude is depressed by medication to a delay of 1000 msec after the electrical conditioning (Fig. 2A) (Delwaide 1971; Martinelli and Delwaide 1980). In spastic patients, after a brief period of inhibition, a phase of facilitation is observed which reaches its maximum around 100 msec. After this phase, a second period of inhibition is observed but less marked than in control subjects (Delwaide 1971). The differences between the curves in normal subjects and spastic patients are

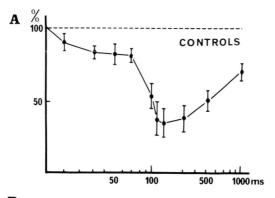

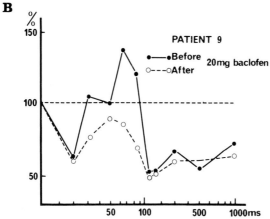

Fig. 2. A: recovery curve of the H reflex amplitude in normal subjects after non-painful stimulation (3 shocks of 1 msec; 300/sec) of the tibial nerve at the ankle. In abscissa, delays in msec separating the conditioning stimulus and the evocation of the H reflex. In ordinate, H reflex amplitude expressed as a percentage of the control values. The vertical bars correspond to 2 S.D. B: recovery curves of the H reflex amplitude after the same conditioning as in A observed in a spastic patient. Filled circles: without drug the curve is definitely distinct from the normal aspect (see A). 30 min after an i.m. injection of 20 mg baclofen, the curve is modified (empty circles) and is closer to the control curve (A).

thus clearly definable. After 20 mg of baclofen, the curve drawn from the responses of a spastic patient is modified (Fig. 2B). The facilitation is clearly reduced and in some instances the following inhibition is more marked. Under baclofen, the recovery curve is thus closer to normal values. After this finding, we went back to diazepam and tested its effect on the recovery curve of a patient in whom baclofen was very effective. Even 20 mg of the drug did not produce a modification.

This step by step review clearly indicates that a myorelaxant drug can specifically modify one electrophysiological test while having no effect on another: *a battery of complementary tests is thus necessary if one expects to reflect, by electrophysiological data, the activity of a given myorelaxant drug.* This opinion received confirmation recently when we conducted a comparative study in 51 spastic patients using 4 different myorelaxants: diazepam, baclofen, tizanidine and LCB 29. The effects were evaluated on the following tests: H_{max}/M_{max}, T_{max}/M_{max}, vibratory inhibition and the recovery curve of the H reflex after stimulation of the tibial nerve at the ankle. The results confirmed the preliminary observations. Diazepam moderately reduced the H_{max}/M_{max} and T_{max}/M_{max} ratios. It reinforced vibratory inhibition of the monosynaptic reflexes but did not modify the recovery curves. Tizanidine had the same effects although less marked, probably due to the dosage used. Baclofen did not alter the vibratory inhibition but it corrected anomalies of the recovery curves. LCB 29 acted similarly. It thus appears that there are 2 different types of electrophysiological modification induced by the myorelaxants. When the same patient is studied under diazepam and baclofen respectively, the tests are modified according to the drug, irrespective of the site of the lesion, the duration of the illness, the intensity of the motor handicap and so on (Fig. 3).

At the present time, we propose 2 reference drugs as far as their ability to modify electrophysiological tests is concerned: diazepam on the one hand and baclofen on the other.

WHAT IS THE VALUE OF ELECTROPHYSIOLOGICAL TESTING?

The result of a single test is not necessarily well correlated with the myorelaxant effect. Depending on the drug, a test can be specifically modified or remain unchanged. The meaning of this observation deserves investigation. The results indicate, first, that the ways in which myorelaxants improve spasticity differ: in one group, the presynaptic inhibition appears to be reinforced on Ia afferents thus leading to a decrease in the excitability of the myotatic arc; in the second, the mechanism seems to involve a reduction of impaired excitability of the spinal interneurones. Thus, electrophysiological testing permits dissociation of different modes of action of the myorelaxants.

Secondly, each type of modification might be correlated with a specific pharmacological mechanism. The reinforcement of vibratory inhibition leads to postulation of a strengthened effect of GABA, which is assumed to be the

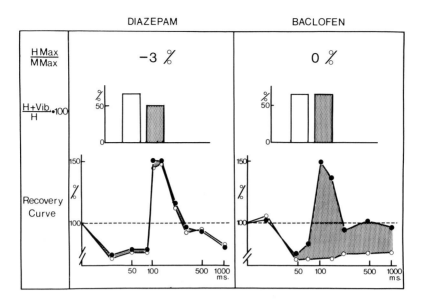

Fig. 3. Comparisons of the modifications of 3 electrophysiological tests performed in the same spastic patient after 10 mg diazepam and 20 mg baclofen respectively. After diazepam, the ratio H_{max}/M_{max} is reduced by 3%; the index reflecting the vibratory inhibition $((H + vib/H) \times 100)$ is 70% in control conditions and 50% 30 min after the injection (hatched column); the recovery curve is not modified. After baclofen, the H_{max}/M_{max} is unchanged, as well as the vibratory inhibition. The recovery curve, on the contrary, is clearly depressed, the differences being indicated by the hatched area.

neurotransmitter for presynaptic inhibition: this is exactly the function attributed to diazepam by pharmacological methods (Davidoff 1978). In contrast, the correction of the recovery curve alterations suggests a predominant action at the level of interneurones and a reduction of their activity. Baclofen could thus interfere with the release of an excitatory neurotransmitter. Here, too, there is a good correlation with the mode of action proposed by pharmacologists (Koella 1980; Krnjević 1980). A practical conclusion derives from the previous observations: if the two most commonly used myorelaxants, diazepam and baclofen, have different modes of action, it would appear logical to prescribe them in combination in order to correct the largest number of pathophysiological defects.

Once a test selectively modified by a myorelaxant has been defined, a valuable tool becomes available for the clinical pharmacology of the central nervous system. The delay of action of the drug can be measured. In this way, it is not necessary to perform lumbar punctures to establish that a drug is acting beyond the blood brain barrier. Fig. 1, for example, illustrates the delay after which vibratory inhibition is modified. It also indicates how long this effect lasts. We have shown in other experiments that a dose-response relationship has been established: the intensity of vibratory inhibition is increased with progressive doses of diazepam. With the same test in the same patient, it becomes possible to compare the efficacy of identical doses of drugs within one chemical class, namely the benzodiazepines. As shown in Fig. 4, the effects of 10 mg of diazepam are compared with the same dose of the

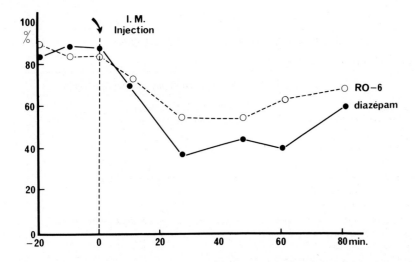

Fig. 4. Evolution of vibratory inhibition ((H vib/H) × 100) measured in a spastic patient after 10 mg diazepam and 10 mg of RO6-9098 respectively. The latter product appears to be less active in reinforcing the vibratory inhibition.

TABLE II

CRITERIA FOR THE DESIGN OF A SPINAL ELECTROPHYSIOLOGICAL TEST

An ideal test should be:

(1)   ethically admissible
(2)   simple and rapid
(3)   possible with limited patient participation
(4)   stable in controls
(5)   sensitive
(6)   specifically correlated with a well defined pathophysiological mechanism

compound RO6-9098 in a given patient. The second drug appears to be less potent than diazepam in reinforcing vibratory inhibition. On the other hand, clinical studies have shown that RO6-9098 is less effective than diazepam as a myorelaxant, a result thus in agreement with the electrophysiological data.

A new field combining reflex studies and pharmacology is now opening. It is becoming possible to determine, in man, the point of impact of drugs; to establish the pathophysiological mechanism they are able to correct; and to study the pharmacokinetics inside the CNS. In the future, a variety of neuroactive drugs other than myorelaxants may be studied by electrophysiological techniques.

TOWARDS THE IDEAL BATTERY OF TESTS!

However, the last point is more a perspective than acquired fact. Until now 2 tests have proved to have discriminative properties and they seem sufficient to make a

TABLE III

PROPOSED BATTERY OF TESTS FOR THE STUDY OF A MYORELAXANT

Electrophysiological study of a myorelaxant.

Proposed tests	Assumed pathophysiological correlation
(1) Ratio H_{max}/M_{max}	Motor nucleus excitability
(2) Degree of vibratory inhibition of the monosynaptic reflex	Presynaptic inhibition
(3) Inhibition of H reflex (sol.) by dorsiflexion of the foot	Reciprocal inhibition
(4) Pattern reflex responses evoked in short biceps femoris and tibialis anterior after sural nerve stimulation	Study of interneuronal circuits
(5) EMG recording of antagonistic muscles (sol. and tib. ant.) voluntary activity: number of bursts for 30 sec	Quality of descending motor control
(6) Maximum isometric torque of the ankle	Force

clear-cut distinction between diazepam and baclofen. However, due to the multiple pathophysiological mechanisms responsible for spasticity, it is not certain that the two tests will be enough to disclose the properties of a new product. Moreover, if one expects to broaden the spectrum of possible applications, an effort must be made to define a battery of useful tests. An ideal technique should fulfil the criteria indicated in Table II. Of course, it is not simple to design a test satisfying all these requirements, some of which are sometimes contradictory. Compromises have to be made and the selection has to be regularly re-evaluated as soon as improved techniques are reported or better correlations with pathophysiological mechanisms are demonstrated. With these restrictions, a battery of complementary tests, as shown in Table III, can be proposed because it reflects the state of the current knowledge in reflexology in 1981.

REFERENCES

Castaigne, P., Held, J.P., Laplane, D., Pierrot-Deseilligny, E., Bussel, B. et Macquart-Moulin, J. Etude de l'effet du Lioresal® dans la spasticité. Rev. neurol., 1973, 128: 245–250.

Davidoff, R.A. Pharmacology of spasticity. Neurology (Minneap.), 1978, 28: 46–51.

Delwaide, P.J. Etude Expérimentale de l'Hyperréflexie Tendineuse en Clinique Neurologique. Editions Arscia, Brussels, 1971: 324 pp.

Koella, W.P. Baclofen: Its general pharmacology and neuropharmacology. In: R. Feldman, R.R. Young and W.P. Koella (Eds.), Spasticity: Disordered Motor Control. Year Book Medical Publishers, Chicago, Ill., 1980: 383–396.

Krnjević, K. Mechanisms of drug action on spinal and supraspinal reflexes, with special reference to the action. In: R. Feldman, R.R. Young and W.P. Koella (Eds.), Spasticity: Disordered Motor Control. Year Book Medical Publishers, Chicago, Ill., 1980: 397–416.

Martinelli, P. and Delwaide, P.J. Complementary techniques in the study of the soleus motor nucleus by an exteroceptive reflex. Electroenceph. clin. Neurophysiol., 1980, 50: 3–4.

Matthews, W.B. Ratio of maximum H reflex to maximum M response as a measure of spasticity. J. Neurol. Neurosurg. Psychiat., 1966, 29: 201–204.

Paillard, J., Bert, J., Zwingelstein, J. et Giudicelli, P. Recherche d'une méthode d'approche de l'action neurophysiologique de diverses drogues. Rev. neurol., 1961, 104: 227–228.

Pedersen, E., Arlien-Soborg, P. and Mai, J. The mode of action of the GABA derivative baclofen in human spasticity. Acta neurol. scand., 1974, 50: 665–680.

Kyoto Symposia (EEG Suppl. No. 36)
Editors: P.A. Buser, W.A. Cobb and T. Okuma

Enhancement of GABAergic Inhibition: A Mechanism of Action of Benzodiazepines, Phenobarbital, Valproate and L-Cycloserine in the Cat Spinal Cord

P. POLC

Pharmaceutical Research Department, F. Hoffmann-La Roche and Co. Ltd., CH-4002 Basle (Switzerland)

Convincing evidence suggests that γ-aminobutyric acid (GABA) is a transmitter released at axo-axonal synapses on primary afferents to motoneurones, supposed to be the morphological basis of presynaptic inhibition (Eccles 1964; Nicoll and Alger 1979) and associated primary afferent depolarization (PAD) (Levy 1977; Nicoll and Alger 1979). It is unknown to what extent the reduced efficacy of this GABA-mediated presynaptic inhibition contributes to spasticity. However, increased spinal GABA levels in paraplegic dogs, which were correlated with the development of spasticity, have been attributed to a diminished release of GABA from the interneurones mediating presynaptic inhibition (Smith et al. 1976). In conditions of reduced presynaptic inhibition, such as in chronic spinal dogs and cats (Naftchi and Lowman 1977; Naftchi et al. 1979) as well as in spastic patients (Delwaide 1970; Verrier et al. 1975), diazepam, known to augment GABAergic presynaptic inhibition in cats (Polc et al. 1974), concurrently reduced spasticity and enhanced presynaptic inhibition. Studies with epidural electrodes in neurologically normal humans revealed an increased PAD after i.v. injections of diazepam (Kaieda et al. 1981) and the anaesthetic thiamylal (Shimoji and Kano 1975); the effect of thiamylal is in agreement with the facilitating effect of barbiturates on GABAergic presynaptic inhibition in animals (Nicoll and Alger 1979).

A potentiation of GABA mechanisms by inhibition of the GABA degradating enzyme, GABA-transaminase, in nerve terminal/synaptosomes, has been proposed to underly the anticonvulsant action of valproate (Iadarola and Gale 1979) and L-cycloserine (Wood et al. 1980).

The present investigation was undertaken to study the effects of valproate and L-cycloserine on spinal activities and to compare them with those of benzodiazepines and barbiturates.

MATERIALS AND METHODS

Mongrel cats, weighing 2.5–3.5 kg, were used. The spinal cord was transected under ether anaesthesia at the level of C1, the medulla oblongata, including the caudal trigeminal nucleus, being destroyed to avoid painful stimulation from the head. The animals were ventilated artificially and the end-tidal pCO_2 was held at 3.5–4 vol.%. Gallamine triethiodide was given when necessary to avoid movement artifacts. The arterial blood pressure was monitored in the femoral artery. Body temperature was maintained at 37°C. The lumbo-sacral spinal cord was exposed by laminectomy and covered with warm mineral oil (kept at 36–37°C), which was also used to cover the exposed peripheral nerves in the left hind limb.

The general experimental arrangement is schematically drawn in Fig. 1. The central end of the cut left ventral root (VR) S1 was mounted on a bipolar platinum electrode for recording of monosynaptic and polysynaptic ventral root reflexes (VRR). From the VR S1 filaments containing a spontaneously active gamma motoneurone, identified by the conduction velocity (15–45 m/sec), were isolated and placed on a fine bipolar platinum electrode. A left dorsal rootlet L7 was mounted on a bipolar Ag-AgCl electrode for the DC recording of dorsal root potentials (DRP). The central ends of the severed nerves to the gastrocnemius muscle (nGC) and the biceps femoris muscle (nBF) as well as the cutaneous sural nerve in the left hind limb were mounted on a bipolar electrode for supramaximal stimulation to elicit DRPs and VRRs (5–10 mA single 0.05 msec shocks at 0.5 Hz). The excitability of primary afferent endings was assessed by the technique of Wall (1958) (not shown in the figure). Submaximal single shocks delivered through a coaxial stainless steel semimicroelectrode (0.1 mm in diameter) inserted in the left dorsal horn L7 elicited action potentials in a fraction of afferent terminals which were conducted antidromically and recorded in the ipsilateral dorsal rootlet L7. The increase in excitability of primary afferents which occurs during PAD due to the release of GABA at axo-axonal synapses was measured by the increased size of the antidromic responses. PAD was induced by single conditioning supramaximal volleys in the nBF, delivered at intervals of 10, 20, 30, 50, 70, 90/100, 200 and 500 msec prior to the test stimuli applied to the semimicroelectrode. Presynaptic inhibition of monosynaptic VRRs was assessed by a similar procedure of conditioning test stimuli applied to nBF and nGC, respectively, and delivered at the

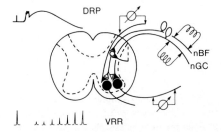

Fig. 1. Schematic diagram of the experiment. Simplified neuronal circuitry within the spinal cord shows the last-order GABAergic interneurone (open circle) mediating depolarization of group I afferents (dorsal root potential, DRP) and presynaptic inhibition of motoneurones (solid circles). Interneurones are activated disynaptically by stimulation of afferents from the biceps femoris muscle (nBF). The first order interneurone exciting the GABAergic interneurone is not shown. Motoneurones are activated monosynaptically (monosynaptic ventral root reflex, VRR) by stimulation of afferents from the gastrocnemius (nGC).

same intervals as in the case of PAD. In 8 cats, a tungsten microelectrode (1 μm tip diameter, 5 MΩ impedance) was inserted in the ventral horn S1 to record extracellular action potentials from single Renshaw cells, identified by their characteristic high frequency response to antidromic single shock stimulation of a part of the VR S1 (Eccles et al. 1954). Mass and unit potentials were amplified, displayed on an oscilloscope and recorded photographically. Eight consecutive DRPs were averaged.

GABA content in the lumbo-sacral spinal cord was measured by a method described elsewhere (Polc et al. 1974).

RESULTS

(1) Interaction of benzodiazepines with GABA transmission

Diazepam (0.1–1 mg/kg i.v.), within 5 min after its injection, consistently enhanced DRPs and presynaptic inhibition of monosynaptic VRRs, but only marginally reduced the size of unconditioned monosynaptic VRRs (Fig. 2). These effects were accompanied by a depression of polysynaptic VRRs and a marked reduction of the spontaneous firing of single gamma motoneurones. Injected at the top of the diazepam action, the GABA receptor antagonist bicuculline (0.5 mg/kg

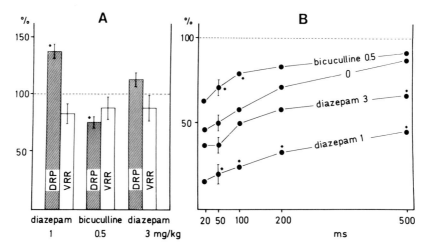

Fig. 2. Interaction between diazepam and bicuculline on (A) DRP and monosynaptic VRR, and on (B) presynaptic inhibition of monosynaptic VRR in 12 cats. Values are the means ± S.E., asterisks indicate statistically significant differences ($P < 0.05$, paired t test) from pre-drug values. A: columns are the areas of DRP and the amplitudes of monosynaptic VRR (expressed in percentages of controls) in response to a first dose of diazepam (1 mg/kg i.v.), followed 5 min later by bicuculline (0.5 mg/kg i.v.) and 10 min later by a second dose of diazepam (3 mg/kg i.v.). B: on the ordinate are the amplitudes of monosynaptic VRR in percentages of the unconditioned control VRR (evoked by stimulation of nGC). On the abscissa is the time interval between conditioning volleys (applied to nBF) and test stimuli. The pre-drug curve is marked by O. The sequence of drug injections is the same as in A. (From Polc et al. 1974.)

i.v.) reversed the effects of diazepam on DRPs and presynaptic inhibition, reducing both phenomena even below the control levels (Fig. 2), without consistently affecting other effects of diazepam. Since the bicuculline-induced effects appeared 3–5 min after the administration and typically declined within the next 30 min, the next diazepam dose was injected immediately after the recording of bicuculline effects. A higher dose of diazepam (3 mg/kg i.v.) then overcame the afore mentioned effects of bicuculline (Fig. 2), pointing to a surmountable antagonism between diazepam and the GABA receptor blockade on presynaptic inhibition.

The recently discovered specific benzodiazepine antagonists (Hunkeler et al. 1981) prompted us to re-investigate the action of benzodiazepines on the spinal cord. A low dose of the potent benzodiazepine, 3-methylclonazepam (0.1 mg/kg i.v.), enhanced DRPs, depressed polysynaptic VRRs and reduced the number of VR-evoked Renshaw cell spikes as well as those of a spontaneously active gamma motoneurone (Fig. 3). In contrast to the previously shown "selective" mutual antagonism between diazepam and bicuculline on presynaptic inhibition, the specific benzodiazepine antagonist Ro 15-1788 (ethyl-8-fluoro-5,6-dihydro-5-methyl-6-oxo-4H-imidazo[1,5-a[1,4] benzodiazepine-3-carboxylate) almost abolished all effects of 3-methylclonazepam (Fig. 3). The effect of Ro 15-1788 (1 mg/kg i.v.)

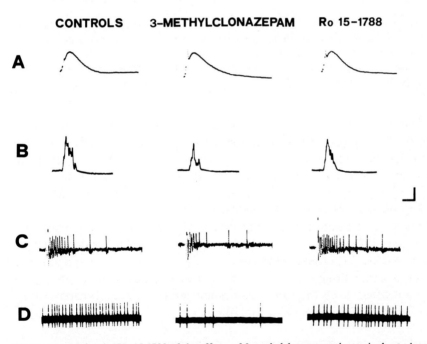

Fig. 3. Antagonism by Ro 15-1788 of the effects of 3-methylclonazepam in a spinal cat. A and B: DRPs and polysynaptic VRRs elicited by sural nerve stimulation, respectively. C: VR-evoked Renshaw cell discharge. D: spontaneous activity of a gamma motoneurone. After the recording of pre-drug potentials in the left-hand vertical row, the potentials are shown 5 min following 0.1 mg/kg 3-methylclonazepam i.v., followed by responses obtained 5 min after 1 mg/kg Ro 15-1788 i.v. injected 10 min after 3-methylclonazepam. Calibration: (A) 100 μV and 50 msec, (B) 100 μV and 5 msec, (C) 200 μV and 10 msec, (D) 50 μV and 200 msec. (From Polc et al. 1981b.)

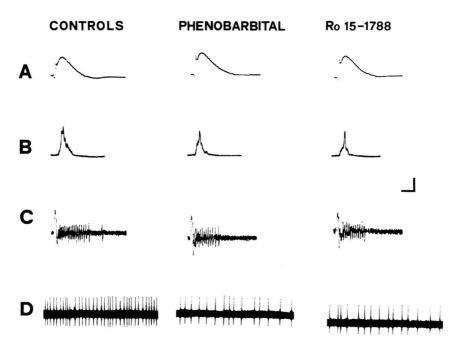

CONTROLS   PHENOBARBITAL   Ro 15-1788

A

B

C

D

Fig. 4. Lack of antagonism by Ro 15-1788 of the effects of phenobarbital on the same activities as those recorded in Fig. 3, in another spinal cat. The left-hand vertical row shows pre-drug potentials. Potentials obtained 10 min after 10 mg/kg phenobarbital i.v. are followed by responses recorded 5 min after 1 mg/kg Ro 15-1788 i.v. administered 20 min following phenobarbital. Calibrations are the same as in Fig. 3. (From Polc et al. 1981b.)

appeared within 2–3 min after injection and lasted 70–80 min. When Ro 15-1788 (1–10 mg/kg i.v.) was given at the beginning of an experiment, it failed to affect spinal activities (in contrast to bicuculline which alone markedly affected spinal neurones), but prevented the usual effects of 3-methylclonazepam to appear.

(2) Effects of phenobarbital on spinal activities

Barbiturates, like benzodiazepines, facilitate GABAergic presynaptic inhibition (Nicoll and Alger 1979). However, the increase of DRPs as well as the depression of polysynaptic VRRs, VR-evoked Renshaw cell response and of the spontaneous gamma motoneurone firing, observed 5–10 min after phenobarbital (10 mg/kg i.v.), were not affected by the subsequent administration of the benzodiazepine antagonist Ro 15-1788 (1 mg/kg i.v., Fig. 4).

(3) Interaction of valproate with GABAergic inhibition

High doses of valproate were necessary to influence the spinal activities studied here. The following effects were obtained 5–10 min after 100 mg/kg valproate i.v.: enhancement of DRPs, depression of polysynaptic VRRs and reduction of spontaneous gamma motoneurone discharge, accompanied by a slight augmentation of presynaptic inhibition and an increase in excitability of primary

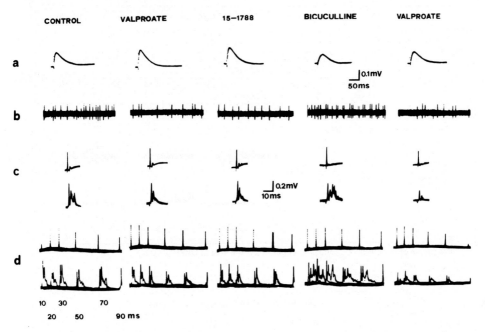

Fig. 5. Effects of valproate and its mutual antagonism with bicuculline in a spinal cat. a: sural nerve-evoked DRPs. b: spontaneous firing of a gamma motoneurone. c: antidromic responses to stimulation of the primary afferent terminals in the upper trace and mono- and polysynaptic VRRs induced by volleys in nGC in the lower trace. d: potentials as in c but now elicited at intervals given below after a conditioning volley in nBF. Pre-drug records in the left-hand vertical row are followed by potentials obtained 10 min after valproate (100 mg/kg i.v.) and those taken 5 min after Ro 15-1788 administered 15 min after valproate; the responses to bicuculline (0.5 mg/kg i.v.), injected 20 min after valproate, are followed by responses to valproate (300 mg/kg i.v.) obtained 10 min after its injection and 15 min following the administration of bicuculline.

afferents (Fig. 5). The unconditioned VRR and the excitability of primary afferents in the absence of conditioning stimuli were unaffected (Fig. 5). The effect of valproate lasted 50–60 min. While the benzodiazepine antagonist Ro 15-1788 (1 mg/kg i.v.) did not change the valproate effects, bicuculline (0.5 mg/kg i.v.), injected 5 min after Ro 15-1788 and 15 min after valproate, reversed all effects of valproate (Fig. 5). The next higher dose of valproate (300 mg/kg i.v.) overcame the bicuculline-induced effects within 10 min after its administration (Fig. 5).

(4) Interaction of L-cycloserine with GABA transmission

L-Cycloserine induced changes in spinal activities which were correlated in time with elevated GABA levels in the spinal cord. One hour after 10 mg/kg L-cycloserine i.v. DRPs started to increase and the maximal enhancement was achieved 1.5–2 h after the injection, when the GABA content was more than doubled (Fig. 6). Interestingly, DRPs increased only in amplitude, but not in duration, and in addition ''spontaneous'' DRPs appeared (Fig. 6). A simultaneous reduction of the spontaneous gamma motoneurone activity, but no obvious alteration in excitability

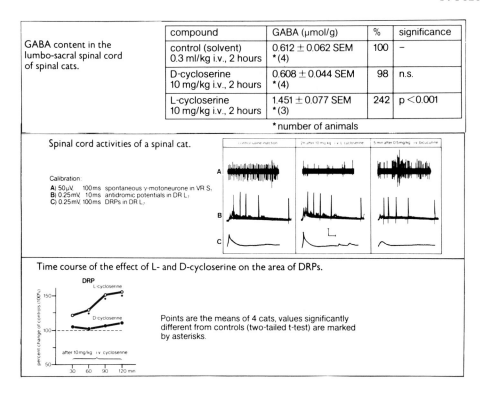

GABA content in the lumbo-sacral spinal cord of spinal cats.	compound	GABA (μmol/g)	%	significance
	control (solvent) 0.3 ml/kg i.v., 2 hours	0.612 ± 0.062 SEM *(4)	100	–
	D-cycloserine 10 mg/kg i.v., 2 hours	0.608 ± 0.044 SEM *(4)	98	n.s.
	L-cycloserine 10 mg/kg i.v., 2 hours	1.451 ± 0.077 SEM *(3)	242	p < 0.001

* number of animals

Fig. 6. Effects of L- and D-cycloserine on the GABA content (above) and DRPs (below) in 7 and 8 cats, respectively. The middle part of the figure shows original records from a cat given 10 mg/kg L-cycloserine and 2 h later 0.5 mg/kg bicuculline.

of primary afferents, was observed 2 h after L-cycloserine. Bicuculline (0.5 mg/kg i.v.), administered at that time, within 5 min antagonized the effects of L-cycloserine (Fig. 6).

The stereoisomer of L-cycloserine, D-cycloserine (10 mg/kg i.v.) neither elevated GABA nor induced any change in spinal activities (Fig. 6).

DISCUSSION

Although all compounds in the present study facilitate GABA-mediated presynaptic inhibition, they do so by involvement of different mechanisms.

(1) The difference in the blockade by bicuculline (only the potentiating effect of diazepam on presynaptic inhibitory phenomena is antagonized) and by the selective benzodiazepine antagonist Ro 15-1788 (all effects of 3-methylclonazepam are nearly abolished) indicates a complex relationship between benzodiazepines and GABA in the spinal cord. Since the high affinity benzodiazepine binding sites are considered to be pharmacologically relevant (Möhler and Okada 1977; Squires and Braestrup 1977), the interaction between Ro 15-1788 and 3-methylclonazepam should have

occurred at the benzodiazepine receptors. Autoradiographic studies indicate that benzodiazepine receptors and glutamic acid decarboxylase (GAD) immunore-activity, the latter being the marker of GABA neurones, show similar distributions in the rat spinal cord, with the highest density in the dorsal horn (Young and Kuhar 1979). This suggests that the benzodiazepine recognition site within the GABA-benzodiazepine-barbiturate receptor complex (Olsen 1981) might be responsible, at least partly, for the muscle relaxant action of benzodiazepines. The most direct evidence for this assumption comes from the recent observation that in a spastic mouse strain, where the muscle relaxant effect of benzodiazepine is prominent (Biscoe and Fry 1980), an increase in the binding of [^{3}H]diazepam and [^{3}H]muscimol (a GABA receptor ligand) in the mouse spinal cord is accompanied by a defect in the coupling between GABA and benzodiazepine binding sites (Biscoe et al. 1981).

(2) Phenobarbital-induced effects are unaffected by the benzodiazepine antagonist Ro 15-1788. Therefore, the enhancement of PAD by barbiturates must be due to a site different from the benzodiazepine recognition site within the GABA-benzodiazepine-barbiturate receptor complex; barbiturates act presumably directly at the Cl$^-$ ionophore where they may prolong the mean open time of Cl$^-$ channels activated by GABA (Study and Barker 1981).

(3) The enhancement of PAD, observed within minutes after valproate, cannot be explained by an inhibition of GABA-transaminase or other enzymes of the GABA catabolism (Turner and Whittle 1980), as the accumulation of GABA in the synaptic cleft leading to an increased GABAergic inhibition would require a much longer period of time. In contrast, an inhibition of GABA re-uptake (Hackman et al. 1981) might account for the fast GABA potentiating effect found here and in other investigations (Macdonald and Bergey 1979; Kerwin et al. 1980; Baldino and Geller 1981; Hackman et al. 1981). Lack of antagonism by Ro 15-1788 to valproate effects in the present study agrees well with the failure of valproate to affect the [^{3}H]diazepam binding in vitro (Ticku and Davis 1981) and suggests no involvement of benzodiazepine receptors in the effect of valproate. However, valproate inhibits [^{3}H]dihydropicrotoxin binding sites indicating a possible action on the Cl$^-$ ionophore as a GABA potentiating mechanism of valproate (Ticku and Davis 1981).

(4) The increase of PAD and the concomitant parallel elevation of GABA in the spinal cord, found 2 h after the injection of L-cycloserine, are the effects which one would expect to occur if the inhibition of GABA-transaminase should cause an increased amount of GABA at GABAergic synapses. Lack of effect of the stereoisomer D-cycloserine substantiates the selective facilitating effect of L-cycloserine on GABA-mediated processes in the spinal cord. Other GABA-transaminase inhibitors, as in amino-oxyacetic acid and γ-acetylenic GABA, seem to be rather unspecific agents (Iadarola and Gale 1979; Rumigny et al. 1981) and have inconsistent effects on GABA-mediated presynaptic inhibition (Davidoff et al. 1973; Bell and Anderson 1974; Polc et al. 1974; Larson and Anderson 1979). Assuming the specificity of action of L-cycloserine, it would be worth while to test this compound in brain dysfunctions supposed to be related to a GABA deficiency,

like epilepsy (Roberts 1980), and to evaluate a possible role of GABA in conditions of reduced presynaptic inhibition, as in spasticity (Davidoff 1978).

Some questions remain unresolved. Are all effects of the drugs tested in the present study due to an enhancement of GABAergic inhibition? To what extent is GABA involved in postsynaptic inhibition? What is the role of gamma motoneurones in the development of spasticity? On the one hand, pharmacological manipulation of the GABA system has indicated that the effects of benzodiazepines on presynaptic inhibition depend on the presence of GABA (Polc et al. 1974) and, in addition, the late bicuculline sensitive part of the postsynaptic recurrent inhibition seems to be enhanced by benzodiazepines (Polc and Haefely 1982). On the other hand, the depressant action of benzodiazepines on the gamma system, polysynaptic VRRs and the Renshaw cell discharge is not related in a simple way to GABA (Polc et al. 1981a, b) since in preliminary experiments some of these depressant effects were unaffected after inhibition of GABA synthesis by the GAD blocking agents, semi- and thiosemicarbazide. In particular, the depression by benzodiazepines of the gamma system, which is probably overactive in spasticity, may in part explain the alleviation by diazepam of spastic symptoms in patients with complete spinal cord transection (Cook and Nathan 1967), where diazepam has been unable to increase presynaptic inhibition (Verrier et al. 1975).

SUMMARY

Unanaesthetized spinal cats were used to assess the effects of several central depressant drugs on GABA-mediated presynaptic inhibition. Benzodiazepines enhance GABAergic inhibition by interaction with specific receptors in the spinal cord. Phenobarbital facilitates GABAergic inhibition by a mechanism unrelated to that of benzodiazepines, perhaps by an effect on the Cl^- ionophore within the GABA-benzodiazepine-barbiturate receptor complex. A similar mechanism or the inhibition of GABA re-uptake might be responsible for the facilitating effect of valproate on GABA transmission. By selectively inhibiting GABA transaminase, L-cycloserine presumably increases the amount of GABA available for release.

ACKNOWLEDGMENT

The author thanks Dr. Haefely for critical reading of the manuscript.

REFERENCES

Baldino, Jr., F. and Geller, H.M. Sodium valproate enhancement of γ-aminobutyric acid (GABA) inhibition: electrophysiological evidence for anticonvulsant activity. J. Pharmacol. exp. Ther., 1981, 217: 445–450.

Bell, J.A. and Anderson, G. Dissociation between amino-oxyacetic acid-induced depression of spinal reflexes and the rise in cord GABA levels. Neuropharmacology, 1974, 13: 885–894.

Biscoe, T.J. and Fry, J.P. Pharmacological studies of the spastic mouse. J. Physiol. (Lond.), 1980, 308: 38–39P.

Biscoe, T.J., Fry, J.P., Martin, I.L. and Rickets, C. Binding of GABA and benzodiazepine receptor ligands in the spinal cord of the spastic mouse. J. Physiol. (Lond.), 1981, 317: 32–33P.

Cook, J.B. and Nathan, P.W. On the site of action of diazepam in spasticity in man. J. neurol. Sci., 1967, 5: 33–37.

Davidoff, R.A. Pharmacology of spasticity. Neurology (Minneap.), 1978, 28: 46–51.

Davidoff, R.A., Grayson, V. and Adair, R. GABA-transaminase inhibitors and presynaptic inhibition in the amphibian spinal cord. Amer. J. Physiol., 1973, 224: 1230–1234.

Delwaide, P.J. Etude Expérimentale de l'Hyperréflexie Tendineuse en Clinique Neurologique, Thèse. Arscia, Bruxelles, 1970.

Eccles, J.C. Presynaptic inhibition in the spinal cord. In: J.C. Eccles and J.P. Schadé (Eds.), Progress in Brain Research, Vol. 12. Elsevier, Amsterdam, 1964: 65–91.

Eccles, J.C., Fatt, P. and Koketsu, K. Cholinergic and inhibitory synapses in a pathway from motor-axon collaterals to motoneurones. J. Physiol. (Lond.), 1954, 126: 524–562.

Hackman, J.C., Grayson, V. and Davidoff, R.A. The presynaptic effects of valproic acid in the isolated frog spinal cord. Brain Res., 1981, 220: 269–285.

Hunkeler, W., Möhler, H., Pieri, L., Polc, P., Bonetti, E.P., Cumin, R., Schaffner, R. and Haefely, W. Selective antagonists of benzodiazepines. Nature (Lond.), 1981, 290: 514–516.

Iadarola, M.J. and Gale, K. Dissociation between drug-induced increases in nerve terminal and non-nerve terminal pools of GABA in vivo. Europ. J. Pharmacol., 1979, 59: 125–129.

Kaieda, R., Maekawa, T., Takeshita, H., Maruyama, Y., Shimizu, H. and Shimoji, K. Effects of diazepam on evoked electrospinogram and evoked electromyogram in man. Anesth. Analg. Curr. Res., 1981, 60: 197–200.

Kerwin, R.W., Olpe, H.-R. and Schmutz, M. The effect of sodium-n-dipropyl acetate on γ-aminobutyric acid-dependent inhibition in the rat cortex and substantia nigra in relation to its anticonvulsant activity. Brit. J. Pharmacol., 1980, 71: 545–551.

Larson, A.A. and Anderson, E.G. Changes in primary afferent depolarization after administration of γ-acetylenic γ-aminobutyric acid (GAG), a γ-aminobutyric acid (GABA) transaminase inhibitor. J. Pharmacol. exp. Ther., 1979, 211: 326–330.

Levy, R.A. The role of GABA in primary afferent depolarization. Progr. Neurobiol., 1977, 9: 211–267.

Macdonald, R.L. and Bergey, G.K. Valproic acid augments GABA-mediated postsynaptic inhibition in cultured mammalian neurons. Brain Res., 1979, 170: 558–562.

Möhler, H. and Okada, T. Benzodiazepine receptors: demonstration in the central nervous system. Science, 1977, 198: 849–851.

Naftchi, N.E. and Lowman, E.W. The effect of diazepam on presynaptic inhibition. Scient. Exhibit. Amer. Acad. rehab. Med., Miami Beach, Fla., 1977: 1–15.

Naftchi, N.E., Schlosser, W. and Horst, W.D. Changes in the GABA system with development of spasticity in paraplegic cats. In: P. Mandel and F. De Feudis (Eds.), GABA-Biochemistry and CNS Functions. Raven Press, New York, 1979: 431–450.

Nicoll, R.A. and Alger, B.E. Presynaptic inhibition: transmitter and ionic mechanisms. Int. Rev. Neurobiol., 1979, 21: 217–258.

Olsen, R.W. GABA-benzodiazepine-barbiturate receptor interactions. J. Neurochem., 1981, 37: 1–13.

Polc, P. and Haefely, W. Benzodiazepines enhance the bicuculline-sensitive part of recurrent Renshaw inhibition in the cat spinal cord. Neurosci. Lett., 1982, 28: 193–197.

Polc, P., Möhler, H. and Haefely, W. The effect of diazepam on spinal cord activities: possible sites and mechanisms of action. Naunyn-Schmiedeberg's Arch. exp. Path. Pharmak., 1974, 284: 319–337.

Polc, P., Bonetti, E.P., Pieri, L., Cumin, R., Angioi, R.-M., Möhler, H. and Haefely, W. Caffeine antagonizes several central effects of diazepam. Life Sci., 1981a, 28: 2265–2275.

Polc, P., Laurent, J.-P., Scherschlicht, R. and Haefely, W. Electrophysiological studies on the specific benzodiazepine antagonist Ro 15-1788. Naunyn-Schmiedeberg's Arch. exp. Path. Pharmak., 1981b, 316: 317–325.

Roberts, E. Prospectus. Epilepsy and antiepileptic drugs: a speculative synthesis. In: G.H. Glaser, J.K. Penry and D.M. Woodbury (Eds.), Antiepileptic Drugs: Mechanisms of Action. Raven Press, New York, 1980: 667–713.

Rumigny, J.-F., Maitre, M., Recasens, M., Blindermann, J.-M. and Mandel, P. Multiple effects of repeated administration of γ-acetylenic GABA on rat brain metabolism. Biochem. Pharmacol., 1981, 30: 305–312.

Shimoji, K. and Kano, T. Evoked electrospinogram: interpretation of origin and effects of anesthetics. Int. Anesthesiol. Clin., 1975, 13: 171–189.

Smith, J.E., Hall, P.V., Campbell, R.L., Jones, A.R. and Aprison, M.H. Levels of γ-aminobutyric acid in the dorsal grey lumbar spinal cord during the development of experimental spinal spasticity. Life Sci., 1976, 19: 1525–1530.

Squires, R.F. and Braestrup, C. Benzodiazepine receptors in rat brain. Nature (Lond.), 1977, 266: 732–734.

Study, R.E. and Barker, J.L. Diazepam and (−)pentobarbital: fluctuation analysis reveals different mechanisms for potentiation of GABA responses in cultured central neurons. Proc. nat. Acad. Sci. (Wash.), 1981, 78: 7180–7184.

Ticku, M.K. and Davis, W.C. Effect of valproic acid on [^{3}H]diazepam and [^{3}H]dihydropicrotoxinin binding sites at the benzodiazepine-GABA receptor-ionophore complex. Brain Res., 1981, 223: 218–222.

Turner, A.J. and Whittle, S.R. Sodium valproate, GABA and epilepsy. Trends pharmacol. Sci., 1980, 2: 257–260.

Verrier, M., Macleod, S. and Ashby, P. The effect of diazepam on presynaptic inhibition in patients with complete and incomplete spinal cord lesions. Canad. J. neurol. Sci., 1975, 2: 179–184.

Wall, P.D. Excitability changes in afferent fibre terminations and their relation to slow potentials. J. Physiol. (Lond.), 1958, 142: 1–21.

Wood, J.D., Russell, M.P. and Kurylo, E. The γ-aminobutyrate content of nerve endings (synaptosomes) in mice after the intramuscular injection of γ-aminobutyrate-elevating agents: a possible role in anticonvulsant activity. J. Neurochem., 1980, 35: 125–130.

Young, W.S. and Kuhar, M.J. Autoradiographic localisation of benzodiazepines receptors in the brain of humans and animals. Nature (Lond.), 1979, 280: 393–395.

Kyoto Symposia (EEG Suppl. No. 36)
Editors: P.A. Buser, W.A. Cobb and T. Okuma
© 1982, Elsevier Biomedical Press, Amsterdam

Animal Techniques for Evaluating Muscle Relaxants

HIDEKI ONO

Department of Toxicology and Pharmacology, Faculty of Pharmaceutical Sciences, The University of Tokyo, Hongo 7-3-1, Bunkyo-Ku, Tokyo 113 (Japan)

For the evaluation of muscle relaxants, alpha and gamma rigidities and spinal reflexes in cats have been used. However, these experiments are not suitable for preliminary screening. Because rats are usually used in behavioural and neurochemical studies for their ease of handling, our laboratory has been using rats in electrophysiological studies in an attempt to compare the electrophysiological, behavioural and neurochemical results. In the present paper, evaluations of muscle relaxants in rats, done in our laboratory, are reviewed (Fukuda et al. 1974a, 1979; Togari et al. 1978; Ono et al. 1979).

(1) RIGIDITY IN RATS DUE TO ANAEMIC DECEREBRATION AND EFFECTS OF DRUGS

Rigidity produced by anaemic decerebration is thought to be dependent on the hyperactivity of alpha motoneurones and has been the subject of neuropharmacological study (Maxwell and Read 1972), as have intercollicular decerebrate rigidity (so-called gamma rigidity) (Keary and Maxwell 1967; Fukuda et al. 1974b) and ischaemic spinal rigidity. Anaemic decerebrate rigidity in cats was originally reported by Pollock and Davis (1930), who succeeded in producing rigidity by means of ligation of the basilar and the common carotid arteries. Because of the ease of using rats as experimental animals, an attempt was made to produce anaemic decerebrate rigidity in these animals (Fukuda et al. 1974a). In the anaemic decerebrate rats, phasic tension of the rigid forelimbs was obtained by mechanical stimulation of the hind limbs, and it was expected that such rigid animals would provide a good experimental model for some type of spasticity. The purpose of the present study is to examine the effects of some centrally acting muscle relaxants on muscle tension in the rigid forelimbs (tonic response) and the phasic tension of the forelimbs induced by mechanical stimulation of the hind limbs (phasic response), and to classify such drugs on the basis of their effectiveness on the tonic and phasic responses (Togari et al. 1978).

Results and Discussion

Rats were anaesthetized with ether and the common carotid arteries were ligated.

After a trephine opening (diameter 5 mm) had been made in the central part of the occipital bone, the basilar artery was cauterized using bipolar tweezer electrodes of a coagulator, and then anaesthesia was stopped. Marked extension of the forelimbs and rigidity of the neck occurred within 30 min after the operation and lasted for more than 2 h. Blood circulation of the smaller inferior part of the cerebellum, the medulla and the spinal cord was intact in the anaemic decerebrate rat. The difference between the anaemic and intercollicular decerebrate rigidities in rats was that, in the former, a greater part of the cerebellum and all of the pons were decerebrated. The rigidity was not reduced by previous section of dorsal roots C4-C8 (2–3 weeks), and not abolished by high doses of chlorpromazine. Such observations suggest that this type of rigidity does not involve a gamma loop.

The rat with sustained rigidity was placed on its back, and the forelimb tension was measured by a semi-isotonic transducer (Fig. 1). The tonic tension of the forelimbs (about 20 g) was termed the tonic response. The hind limbs were fixed at the ankle and the feet were stretched mechanically (rostrally 5 mm, for 3 sec, once every 45 sec). The mechanical stimulation augmented the forelimb tension, and this increase was termed the phasic response (Fig. 2B–D). The modality of the afferent fibres which caused the phasic response was studied. The effect of muscle stretch of triceps surae was not clear; on the other hand, the phasic response caused by pinching, pricking or puffing on the skin near an ankle was marked and regular (Fig. 2A). These results indicate that the phasic response of forelimb rigidity is caused by cutaneous afferents, but not by muscle afferents. Both tonic and phasic responses were abolished by spinal section at C1 level.

On the basis of their effects on the tonic and phasic responses of rigidity, the drugs examined were classified into 3 types of groups (Figs. 2 and 3): (1) drugs which depressed both tonic and phasic responses (mephenesin (20–80 mg/kg, i.v.), tolperisone-HCl (5–20 mg/kg, i.v.) and baclofen (1.25–5 mg/kg, i.v.)); (2) drugs which depressed tonic and augmented phasic responses (orphenadrine-HCl (2.5–10 mg/kg, i.v.) and chlorpromazine-HCl (0.625–2.5 mg/kg, i.v.)); and (3) drugs which depressed phasic but had almost no effect on the tonic responses (diazepam,

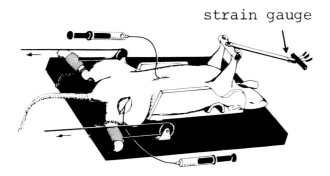

Fig. 1. Diagram of arrangements for recording rigid forelimb tension and stimulating hind limbs to elicit the phasic response to tension in anaemic decerebrate rats. (From Togari et al. 1978.)

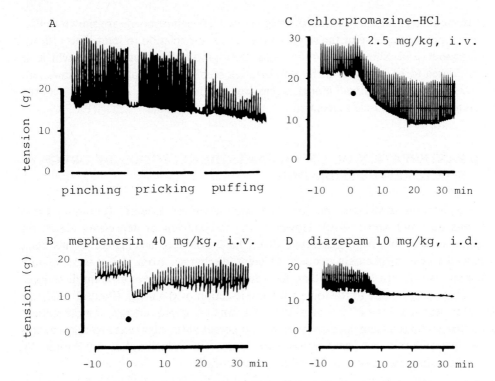

Fig. 2. Effects of stimulation and drugs on the rigid forelimb tension in anaemic decerebrate rats. A: tonic response (baseline) and phasic response (upward deflection) induced by pinching, pricking or puffing of the skin near an ankle. B–D: effects of drugs on tonic response and phasic response induced by stretching the hind feet. (Reconstructed from Togari et al. 1978.)

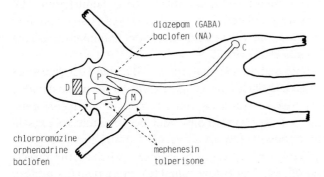

Fig. 3. Speculative sites of drug action on anaemic decerebrate rigidity in rats. D, decerebrated area; T, pathway of tonic response; P, pathway of phasic response; M, spinal motoneurone; C, cutaneous afferent.

nitrazepam and clonazepam (2.5–40 mg/kg, intraduodenally)). The depressant action of baclofen on the phasic response was selectively abolished by noradrenalin depletion, and the depressant action of diazepam on the phasic response was reduced by GABA depletion and increased by the elevation of GABA level (Fukuda et al. 1979).

In summary, speculative sites of drug actions on each response are shown in Fig. 3. The phasic response of the rigidity may have some relation to inter-limb reflexes (Gernandt and Shimamura 1961) and the spino-bulbo-spinal reflex which is considered to be involved in the startle reflex seen in spastic patients (Shimamura 1973). Thus, this animal model is easy to produce and is convenient for the classification of muscle relaxants.

(2) PARTICIPATION OF LOCAL ANAESTHETIC ACTION OF DRUGS IN SPINAL REFLEX INHIBITION

Mephenesin depresses mono- and polysynaptic reflexes (Latimer 1956; Crankshaw and Raper 1970). However, the mechanisms of depressant action on spinal reflexes by mephenesin-type drugs have not been elucidated. It has been reported that mephenesin reduces afferent discharges from the muscle spindle (Grossie and Smith 1966) and that the reduction of frequency of afferent discharges by drugs may be due to the local anaesthetic action of the drugs (Paintal 1964). In the present study the effects of muscle relaxants on spinal reflexes, muscle spindle discharges (in situ) and conduction of action potential (in vitro) were compared, and the participation of local anaesthetic action in spinal reflex inhibition by mephenesin-type drugs was examined (unpublished).

Results and Discussion

Rats were anaesthetized with urethane and α-chloralose. After laminectomy, L4 and L5 dorsal and ventral roots were isolated, and ventral root reflexes (mono- and polysynaptic) were recorded from the L5 ventral root after stimulation of the ipsilateral dorsal root L5 (Fukuda et al. 1977).

As shown in Fig. 4, mephenesin and a local anaesthetic, lidocaine-HCl depressed mono- and polysynaptic reflexes, and baclofen strongly depressed the monosynaptic reflex. These drugs depressed the ventral root reflexes also in C1 spinal rats. Tolperisone-HCl (10 mg/kg, i.v.) depressed mono- and polysynaptic reflexes in non-spinal and spinal rats (not shown). Orphenadrine-HCl, more than 5 mg/kg, i.v., produced a transient increase in ventral root reflexes, whereas the effects disappeared in spinal rats (Fig. 4E, F). Chlorpromazine-HCl, more than 0.1 mg/kg, i.v., prolongedly depressed ventral root reflexes in non-spinal rats. In spinal rats, however, a higher dose of chlorpromazine-HCl (10 mg/kg, i.v.) did not reduce the ventral root reflexes (Fig. 4G, H). It has been reported that orphenadrine and chlorpromazine act on a supraspinal structure and affect descending influences to the spinal cord (Ginzel 1966; Hudson 1968). Diazepam 0.1–2 mg/kg, i.v. markedly enhanced the dorsal root reflex without affecting the ventral root reflexes in non-spinal (Fig. 4D) and spinal rats. It has been suggested that diazepam increases presynaptic inhibition (cf. Haefely et al. 1979).

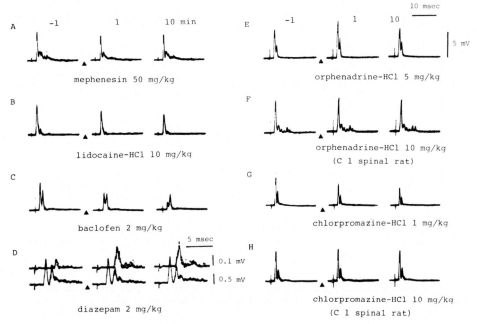

Fig. 4. Effects of drugs on ventral root reflexes (A–H) and dorsal root reflexes (D) in rats. A–E and G: non-spinal rats. F and H: spinal rats (C1). (Unpublished.)

Afferent impulses from the de-efferented triceps surae muscle were recorded from the medial or lateral gastrocnemius nerve in anaesthetized rats (Fukuda et al. 1974c). The depressant activity of drugs on afferent discharges was regarded as the local anaesthetic action of drugs in situ. Recorded afferent discharges were considered to be of muscle spindle origin, because the larger amplitude impulses were integrated. As shown in Fig. 5, lidocaine-HCl (2.5–20 mg/kg, i.v.), tolperisone-HCl (10–40 mg/kg, i.v.) and mephenesin (20–80 mg/kg, i.v.) reduced the afferent activity and the same doses of the drugs depressed the ventral root reflexes. Although baclofen 1–2 mg/kg, i.v. strongly depressed the monosynaptic reflex, the afferent discharges were not reduced by a higher dose of baclofen (10 mg/kg, i.v.). Very high dose of chlorpromazine-HCl (20 mg/kg, i.v.) reduced the frequency of discharge. Orphenadrine-HCl (5–20 mg/kg, i.v.) reduced the afferent discharge, whereas the same doses of orphenadrine-HCl did not depress ventral root reflexes. On the contrary, higher doses of diazepam (2.5–10 mg/kg, i.v.) increased the afferent discharges.

The order of reducing afferent discharges by drugs except diazepam and chlorpromazine in situ (Fig. 5) corresponded to that of their conduction blocking activities in the isolated sciatic nerve of rats (Fig. 6). From the results, it was indicated that mephenesin, tolperisone and lidocaine depress muscle spindle discharges as well as spinal reflexes at the same dose range. This suggests the participation of a membrane stabilizing action of the drugs in spinal reflex inhibition by mephenesin-type drugs. Baclofen did not show any membrane stabilizing action.

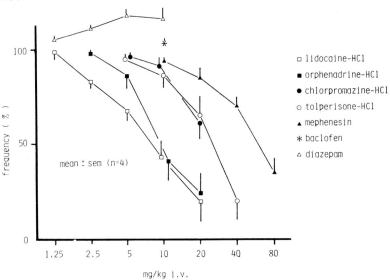

Fig. 5. Dose-response relationships of the effects of drugs on resting afferent discharges from the triceps surae muscle in rats. The muscle was continuously loaded with 10 g tension. Abscissa: doses of drugs. Ordinate: means of frequencies of afferent discharges in percentage of controls, with the S.E.M. indicated. (Unpublished.)

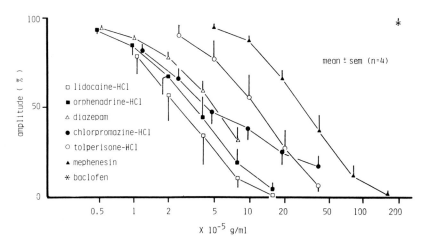

Fig. 6. Dose-response relationships of the effects of drugs on action potential conduction in isolated sciatic nerve of the rat (in vitro). Abscissa: concentration of drugs. Ordinate: means of relative amplitudes of compound action potentials in percentage of controls, with the S.E.M. indicated. (Unpublished.)

(3) MECHANISMS OF DEPRESSANT ACTIONS OF BACLOFEN AND MEPHENESIN

The mechanisms of depressant actions of baclofen and mephenesin were studied in detail in spinal rats (Ono et al. 1979).

Results and Discussion

To detect the change of membrane potential or the stabilization of the membrane by the drugs, the excitability of primary afferent fibres (PAFs) and motoneurone somata (MN) was measured by Wall's method (Wall 1958) of stimulating a motoneurone pool (Løyning et al. 1964). The monosynaptic response (MS) caused by transmitter release was also recorded from the ventral root.

Baclofen did not affect the primary afferent fibre excitability, and produced a small reduction in the motoneurone soma excitability, although the monosynaptic response was strongly depressed (Fig. 7A). These results indicate that baclofen does not alter the resting membrane potential or exert a membrane stabilizing action. In contrast, mephenesin significantly reduced the excitability of the primary afferent fibre and motoneurone soma and strongly reduced the monosynaptic response (Fig. 7A). Thus, it seems likely that mephenesin produces a hyperpolarizing action or a membrane stabilizing action on the primary afferent fibre and the motoneurone soma.

The effects of drugs on the focal synaptic potential were studied by means of

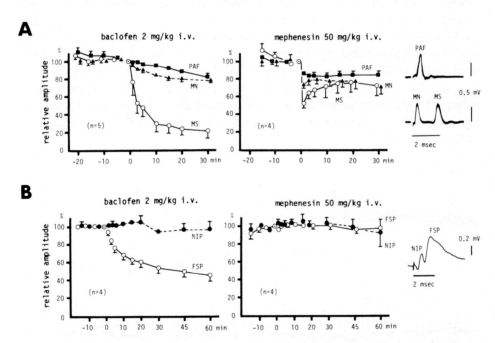

Fig. 7. A: effects of baclofen and mephenesin on excitability of primary afferent fibre and motoneurone soma. Abscissae: time in minutes after the drug injection. Ordinates: means of relative response amplitudes of evoked potentials in percentage of controls, with the S.E.M. indicated. PAF, excitability of an afferent fibre; MN, excitability of a motoneurone soma; MS, monosynaptic response produced in the ventral root. B: effects of baclofen and mephenesin on focal potentials. Focal potentials were evoked by stimulation applied to the dorsal rootlet. Ordinates: mean of potential amplitudes in percentage of control. NIP, negative initial potential; FSP, focal synaptic potential. (Reconstructed from Ono et al. 1979.)

extracellular recording from a dorsal horn. The negative initial potential and the focal synaptic potential reflect the presynaptic impulse and mass EPSP respectively (Løyning et al. 1964). Baclofen produced a long lasting depressant action on the focal synaptic potential without affecting the negative initial potential. Mephenesin affected neither the negative initial potential nor the focal synaptic potential (Fig. 7B). Thus, primary afferent fibre conduction is not affected by baclofen or mephenesin, and the EPSP is reduced by baclofen, but not by mephenesin.

It was suggested that mephenesin hyperpolarizes or stabilizes the presynaptic and motoneuronal membranes. Therefore, the effects of drugs on the resting potential of the dorsal or ventral root were studied. In preliminary experiments, muscimol, a GABA agonist, selectively depolarized the dorsal root. As shown in Fig. 8, baclofen did not affect the resting potential of the ventral root. Mephenesin slightly hyperpolarized the ventral root, although the effect was not significant (unpublished). Baclofen did not affect the resting potential of the dorsal root; mephenesin slightly hyperpolarized it, although the effect was not significant.

In summary, mephenesin depressed the ventral root reflexes and the excitability of the motoneurone soma and the primary afferent fibre, but did not affect the resting potential of the dorsal root, or mass EPSP. From these results, it was suggested that the depression of spinal reflexes by mephenesin is due to membrane stabilization of the initial segment. The conduction of the action potential may be more resistant to membrane stabilization than the generation of the action potential from the EPSP, because the conduction of action potentials has a high safety factor. Baclofen did not show any membrane stabilization and it was suggested that baclofen antagonizes the primary afferent transmitter, or suppresses the release of primary afferent transmitter in the spinal cord (Ono et al. 1979; cf. Curtis et al. 1981; Davies 1981).

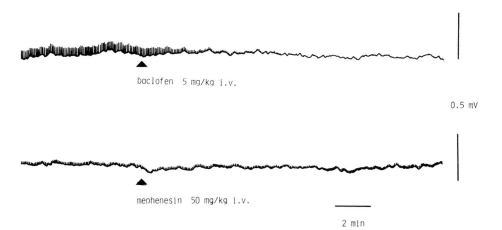

baclofen 5 mg/kg i.v.

0.5 mV

mephenesin 50 mg/kg i.v.

2 min

Fig. 8. Effects of baclofen and mephenesin on resting ventral root potential. Upward deflections do not represent the true amplitude of DR-VRP, because a low frequency DC recorder was used for recording. (Unpublished.)

SUMMARY

Studies in our laboratory on the depressant actions of muscle relaxants on rigidity and spinal reflexes in rats are reviewed.

Anaemic decerebrate rigidity (alpha type) of the forelimbs was obtained by ligation of both basilar and common carotid arteries. In addition to the rigidity developed in the forelimbs (tonic response), phasic tension (phasic response) was induced by mechanical stimulation of the hind limbs. Mephenesin, tolperisone and baclofen depressed both tonic and phasic responses. Orphenadrine and chlorpromazine depressed tonic and augmented phasic responses. Diazepam, nitrazepam and clonazepam depressed phasic but had almost no effect on tonic responses.

The participation of local anaesthetic action in spinal reflex inhibition by mephenesin-type drugs was examined by comparing the depressant actions on spinal reflexes, muscle afferent discharges (in situ) and action potential conduction (in vitro). At doses producing depression of spinal reflexes, mephenesin, tolperisone and a local anaesthetic, lidocaine, reduced the frequency of afferent discharges, suggesting the participation of a membrane stabilizing action in spinal reflex inhibition. Although baclofen depressed spinal reflexes, the drug did not show any membrane stabilizing action.

To examine the above possibility, the effects of drugs on the excitability of the motoneurone pool and the focal potentials were studied. Mephenesin reduced the excitability of the primary afferent fibre and the motoneurone soma but did not change the focal synaptic potential which reflects the mass EPSP, suggesting the participation of membrane stabilization of the initial segment in spinal reflex inhibition. On the contrary, baclofen produced a significant reduction in the focal synaptic potential without affecting the excitability of the primary afferent fibre and the motoneurone soma, suggesting the inhibition of transmitter release or antagonism toward the transmitter released from the afferent terminal. Mephenesin and baclofen did not produce any significant change of resting potential of the ventral or dorsal root.

ACKNOWLEDGEMENT

I wish to thank Dr. H. Fukuda, the professor of the Department of Toxicology and Pharmacology, for his kind suggestions and a critical reading of the manuscript.

REFERENCES

Crankshaw, D.P. and Raper, C. Mephenesin, methocarbamol, chlordiazepoxide and diazepam: actions on spinal reflexes and ventral root potentials. Brit. J. Pharmacol., 1970, 38: 148–156.

Curtis, D.R., Lodge, D., Bornstein, J.C. and Peet, M.J. Selective effects of (−)-baclofen on spinal synaptic transmission in the cat. Exp. Brain Res., 1981, 42: 158–170.

Davies, J. Selective depression of synaptic excitation in cat spinal neurones by baclofen: an iontophoretic study. Brit. J. Pharmacol., 1981, 72: 373–384.

Fukuda, H., Ito, T., Hashimoto, S. and Kudo, Y. Rigidity in rats due to anemic decerebration and the effect of chlorpromazine. Jap. J. Pharmacol., 1974a, 24: 810–813.

Fukuda, H., Ito, T. and Kokubo, M. Effects of some antiparkinsonism drugs and centrally acting muscle relaxants on the intercollicular decerebrate rigidity in rats. Chem. pharm. Bull., 1974b, 22: 2883–2888.

Fukuda, H., Kudo, Y. and Ono, H. Excitation of rat muscle spindle afferents by lyoniol-A. Europ. J. Pharmacol., 1974c, 26: 136–142.

Fukuda, H., Kudo, Y. and Ono, H. Effects of β-(p-chlorophenyl)-γ-aminobutyric acid (Baclofen) on spinal synaptic activity. Europ. J. Pharmacol., 1977, 44: 17–24.

Fukuda, H., Kudo, Y. and Togari, A. Effects of diazepam and baclofen on the anemic decerebrate rigidity in rats (in Japanese). Folia pharmacol. jap., 1979, 75: 535–542.

Gernandt, B.E. and Shimamura, M. Mechanisms of interlimb reflexes in cat. J. Neurophysiol., 1961, 24: 665–676.

Ginzel, K.H. The blockade of reticular and spinal facilitation of motor function by orphenadrine. J. Pharmacol. exp. Ther., 1966, 154: 128–141.

Grossie, J. and Smith, C.M. Depression of afferent activity originating in muscle spindles induced by mephenesin, procaine and caramiphen. Arch. int. Pharmacodyn., 1966, 159: 288–298.

Haefely, W., Polc, P., Schaffner, R., Keller, H.H., Pieri, L. and Möhler, H. Facilitation of GABA-ergic transmission by drugs. In: P. Krogsgaard-Larsen, J. Scheel-Krüger and H. Kofod (Eds.), GABA-Neurotransmitters. Munksgaard, Copenhagen, 1979: 357–375.

Hudson, R.D. Effects of chlorpromazine on motor reflexes of the chronic spinal cat. Arch. int. Pharmacodyn., 1968, 174: 442–450.

Keary, E.M. and Maxwell, D.R. A comparison of the effects of chlorpromazine and some related phenothiazines in reducing the rigidity of the decerebrate cat and in some other central actions. Brit. J. Pharmacol., 1967, 29: 400–416.

Latimer, C.N. The action of mephenesin upon three monosynaptic pathways of the cat. J. Pharmacol. exp. Ther., 1956, 118: 309–317.

Løyning, Y., Oshima, T. and Yokota, T. Site of action of thiamylal sodium on the monosynaptic spinal reflex pathway in cats. J. Neurophysiol., 1964, 27: 408–428.

Maxwell, D.R. and Read, M.A. The effects of some drugs on the rigidity of the cat due to ischaemic or intercollicular decerebration. Neuropharmacology, 1972, 11: 849–855.

Ono, H., Fukuda, H. and Kudo, Y. Mechanisms of depressant action of baclofen on the spinal reflex in the rat. Neuropharmacology, 1979, 18: 647–653.

Paintal, A.S. Effects of drugs on vertebrate mechanoreceptors. Pharmacol. Rev., 1964, 16: 341–380.

Pollock, L.J. and Davis, L. The reflex activities of a decerebrate animal. J. comp. Neurol., 1930, 50: 377–411.

Shimamura, M. Neuronal mechanisms of the startle reflex in cerebral palsy, with special reference to its relationship with spino-bulbo-spinal reflexes. In: J.E. Desmedt (Ed.), New Developments in EMG and Clinical Neurophysiology. Karger, Basel, 1973: 761–766.

Togari, A., Kudo, Y. and Fukuda, H. Effects of centrally acting muscle relaxants on the anemic decerebrate rigidity in rats. J. Pharm. Dyn., 1978, 1: 332–337.

Wall, P.D. Excitability change in afferent fibre terminations and their relation to slow potentials. J. Physiol. (Lond.), 1958, 142: 1–21.

Kyoto Symposia (EEG Suppl. No. 36)
Editors: P.A. Buser, W.A. Cobb and T. Okuma
© 1982, Elsevier Biomedical Press, Amsterdam

Several Methods for the Evaluation of Muscle Relaxants in Gamma Motor Activity

KOHSI TAKANO

Department of Physiology, University of Göttingen, Humboldtallee 7, D-3400 Göttingen (F.R.G.)

In this article a short review of several methods for evaluating central muscle relaxants is presented, concerning the effects of diazepam, for an example which has been well documented.

(1) ACTIVE TENSION-EXTENSION DIAGRAM (a-TED)

A method for analysing the integrated (true or pseudo*), actions of alpha and gamma motoneurone pools is recording of the TED. The total tension which a muscle with intact innervation develops during a progressive stretch consists of 2 components: one is the passive tension, due to the viscoelastic properties of the muscle; the other is the active tension produced by neuromuscular activity. Active tension alone is obtained by subtracting the amount of passive tension from the total tension. In the classical study the passive tension or passive (p)-TED was obtained at the end of each experiment, in the denervated or totally inhibited muscle preparation. Then the a-TED was obtained by subtracting the p-TED from the total TED. This was a rather tedious graphical procedure. Takano and Henatsch (1971) have described an electrical compensation method which allows immediate recording of the a-TED during the ongoing extension.

The muscle under study is stretched together with the homonymous contralateral muscle, which is denervated. The mechanical conditions should be carefully equalized for the two muscles, so that the p-TEDs on both sides are practically identical. The transduced electrical equivalents could be cancelled in a Wheatstone's bridge. Today such a process could also be done using a computer.

Granit (1958) and others (e.g. Koella et al. 1956) considered the slope constants of a-TED as indicators of the overall gain of the stretch reflex. Pompeiano (1960) investigated the slope increases of a-TED due to disinhibition of the alpha motoneurones. Parallel shifts of the a-TED, on the other hand, were mainly studied by Matthews (1959a, b), who interpreted them as being predominantly caused by changes of the gamma bias.

---

* A pseudo reflex is a tension response of the muscle in the activated state from alpha motor activity during muscle stretch, but without any afferent input to the alpha motoneurones from the muscle spindles.

Our groups have used model experiments and confirmed that those procedures which enhance the gain, either at the peripheral muscular, or at the spinal motoneurone pool, will lead to an increased slope of a-TED. In vivo this is most commonly, but not exclusively, done by recruitment of further motor units or by higher density of impulses reaching the muscle. On the other hand, a bias change will cause a parallel shift of the a-TED. It is certainly true that in vivo modulation of the efferent gamma control is predominantly the means of changing the bias. It is possible that some other stretch-dependent changes of the input could cause the parallel shift. Excluding the latter cases, we can interpret a parallel shift of the a-TED as a sign of gamma bias change (Henatsch et al. 1976).

The gamma motor system was activated progressively in the early period of local tetanus (Kano and Takano 1969; Takano and Kano 1973). The development of symptoms typical of local tetanus proceeded rather rapidly after the first visible signs. The changes of TED curves were followed during this period (Fig. 1a). The triceps surae muscle of the cat was freed from the surrounding tissue and the Achilles tendon was cut and connected to a stretch machine. The TED was recorded during stretching of the muscle at constant velocity (2 mm/sec). Within 3.25 h the total TED shifted parallel to the left side of the graph without any change of slope, which means a pure change of bias, or stretch reflex threshold. In this record total TEDs were recorded instead of the active TED. During the recording period some kind of inhibitory action on the alpha motoneurones still exists (Takano and Henatsch 1973). Therefore, this parallel shift of the curves, namely the increase of reflex tension, is predominantly due to an augmented gamma bias.

Matthews and Rushworth (1957) have demonstrated that bathing the muscle

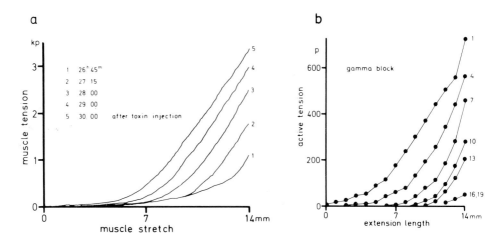

Fig. 1. a: change of the total TED of the triceps surae muscle of the cat during the early period of local tetanus. b: change of a-TED during the development of selective block of gamma fibre conduction by procaine. The numbers at the end of each curve show the time after procaine bath. At 16 and 19 min, 80% of the alpha fibres were still intact. The curves were plotted after the calculation, because direct recording in tetanus of the intoxicated muscle is very difficult. Note the parallel shifts of the curves in both a and b (Takano and Henatsch 1973).

nerve with procaine can selectively block the conduction of the gamma fibres without impairing the alpha fibres. In Fig. 1b, a-TED of a muscle intoxicated by tetanus toxin was plotted by a classical method during the procaine bath. The a-TEDs show clearly the parallel shift to the right. During this experiment supramaximal single electrical stimuli were applied to the nerves supplying the muscle at a site proximal to the area of the procaine bath, in order to test the excitability of the alpha fibres. Twitch response to the stimuli remained almost constant until 13 min after the beginning of procaine local anaesthesia.

There are many clinical reports of extensive use of benzodiazepines in tetanus therapy. First choice of medication is mostly diazepam in developing countries, and even in the industrial countries where intensive care could be used when necessary. Diazepam in doses larger than 0.01 mg/kg causes a parallel shift of the active TED. In Fig. 2 a-TEDs, resulting from 10 stretching trials at intervals of 3 min before (1) and after (2) administration of diazepam, were superimposed on the same sheet of paper. The first curve in (2) was recorded 45 min after the drug administration.

(2) SPINDLE AFFERENTS

The effects of central muscle relaxants on the gamma motor system can be observed in functionally isolated group Ia fibres and also in the "integrated" afferent discharges of a whole (or a part) of the dorsal root in response to stretching of the triceps surae of the decerebrate cat.

The muscle was stretched 10, 12 or 14 mm in a ramp-and-hold manner at the constant rate of 10 mm/sec (Fig. 3, lower graph). The muscle stretches were repeated at intervals of 30 or 60 sec in order to avoid post-tetanic potentiation in the development of reflex tension and of gamma activity by frequent stretching of the

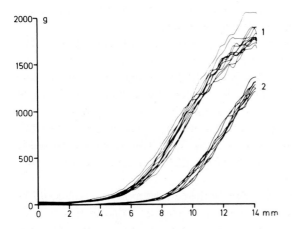

Fig. 2. a-TED before (1) and after (2) diazepam (0.5 mg/kg i.v.). Triceps surae muscle of the decerebrate cat. (Brausch et al. 1973, reprinted with permission from "The Benzodiazepines", copyright Raven Press.)

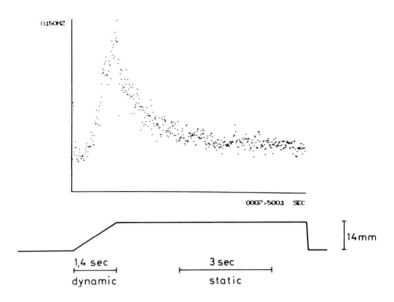

Fig. 3. Upper graph: computer plotted frequency (ordinate) diagram of the muscle spindle discharge. Lower: muscle stretch (14 mm). Same time scale for both graphs. Horizontal bar indicates the time range over which the mean static or dynamic frequencies from a single group Ia fibre have been calculated (Takano and Student 1978).

muscle. A mean frequency can be calculated both for the dynamic and static periods (see Fig. 3). In this communication only the responses during the static phase are shown in Fig. 4. The number of spikes from the primary ending of the muscle spindle was counted and monitored during each stretch period. The mean discharge frequency was analogically computed by an operational amplifier. The instantaneous frequency of the spindle discharge was also calculated by a laboratory computer (Fig. 3, upper graph). The instantaneous frequency is defined as the reciprocal value of the interval between successive spikes.

Fig. 4 shows the effects of procaine and diazepam on the static phase. The discharge frequency of the Ia fibre decreases toward a minimum during procaine administration. In this period gamma fibres were totally blocked. The final blocking of discharges occurs abruptly, when the Ia fibre under study is anaesthetised (see time 21–22 min marked by arrow). After removing the procaine by washing with Ringer's solution the spindle discharge returned to nearly control levels. Thereafter, diazepam (0.2 mg/kg) was administered i.v.; the discharge frequency promptly decreased to values obtained after the blocking of the gamma efferents with procaine.

Thus the effect of central muscle relaxants on the gamma motor system could be compared to the "zero gamma level" obtained also by procaine in this type of experiment. When the muscle spindle under study showed strong dynamic properties the measurement could be easier when the responses in the dynamic (i.e. during the ongoing stretch) period were used. The second method, in which the

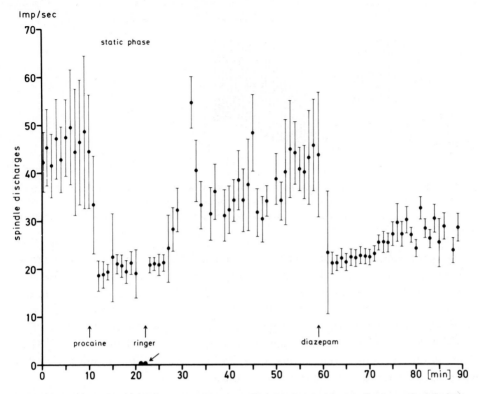

Fig. 4. Effect of procaine and diazepam on spindle discharges. Vertical bars indicate standard deviation. Decerebrate cat (Takano and Student 1978).

integrated afferent discharges from the whole nerve are recorded, has statistically far more value than recording from the isolated Ia fibre. Further, this method permits long lasting recording of the afferent input to the spinal cord. In these experiments a nerve fibre bundle of the dorsal root S1 was placed on the recording electrodes and the afferent mass discharges from muscle spindles and other muscle receptors in the triceps surae (all nerves in the hind leg under investigation were cut except that to triceps surae muscle) were amplified, rectified and integrated. The integrated mass activity was recorded by a pen recorder.

Diazepam had no effect on the de-efferented muscle afferents and no receptor in the hind leg, other than the muscle spindle, had efferent innervation, therefore the change of the integrated mass activity must be a change of the gamma activity (for this chapter see Takano and Student 1978).

(3) "ALPHA MUSCLE"

The sciatic nerve at the middle part of the thigh of the cat was denervated by freezing with dry ice (10 mm wide, 10 min). About 60 days after the denervation the cat moved normally and one could hardly distinguish between the operated and non-operated sides.

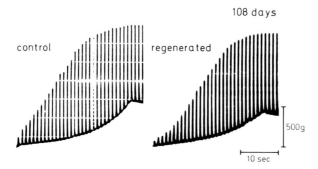

Fig. 5. Tension (ordinate) and extension and/or time relation of the triceps surae muscles, 108 days after operation. Left non-operated, right operated sides. The muscles were stretched 14 mm with a constant velocity (0.5 mm/sec). The muscle nerves were stimulated with maximal intensity at 1/sec repetition rate.

The twitch tension at longer lengths of the muscle was practically not different between the control and operated sides after about 90 days. Fig. 5 shows the oscilloscopic picture of the tension change. The muscle nerve was stimulated during progressive extension (constant rate, 0.5 mm/sec) with maximal intensity at 1/sec. Total TED was lower on the operated than on the control side. This was most probably due to the low level of gamma activity, when the difference in physical properties of the muscle could be excluded. Twitch tension at longer muscle lengths was practically not different in the two muscles.

By measuring the conduction velocity of the afferent and efferent fibres to the muscle, it could be concluded that the afferent fibres of groups I, II and III had well regenerated, while of the efferent fibres the alpha and gamma groups had scarcely regenerated 6 (Takano 1976) or even 18 months after the operation (unpublished data). Since the reinnervated muscles lacked the support of a functional gamma innervation, the muscle was called an ''alpha muscle''.

Neither diazepam nor procaine had any effect on the muscle spindle discharges in the alpha muscle. The spindle discharges were only changed by pinna stimulation when the muscle contracted (Takano 1976). The rigidity after an intercollicular decerebration did not appear in the alpha muscle (unpublished observation). The effect of muscle relaxants exclusively on the alpha motor system could be evaluated using an ''alpha muscle''. Care must be taken in preparing such an alpha muscle, because there are some contradictory results (e.g. De Santis et al. 1972). The length of reinnervation may play an important role in obtaining an alpha muscle. (For further details of this chapter see Takano 1976.)

SUMMARY

(1) The active tension-extension diagram of slowly (2 mm/sec) stretched triceps surae muscle of the decerebrate cat has been shown to be a sensitive indicator of spinal motor activity. For example, diazepam at doses larger than 0.01 mg/kg shifted the diagram parallel to the right.

(2) The effects of central muscle relaxants on the gamma system can be observed in functionally isolated group Ia fibres but also in the "integrated" afferent discharges of the whole (or a part of) S1 dorsal root in response to stretching of the triceps surae muscle. The latter has statistically more value than the former recording. The effect of diazepam could block the gamma fibres selectively. Diazepam at doses larger than 0.1 mg/kg could block the gamma activity totally.

(3) More than 3 months after degeneration with dry ice, the reinnervated muscle shows a fully recovered twitch tension but fails to show gamma activity (alpha muscle). Diazepam has no effect on the discharge from the muscle spindles in the alpha muscle.

REFERENCES

Brausch, U., Henatsch, H.-D., Student, J.C. and Takano, K. Effect of diazepam on development of stretch reflex tension. In: S. Garattini, E. Mussini and L.O. Randall (Eds.), The Benzodiazepines. Raven Press, New York, 1973: 531–543.

De Santis, M., Whetsell, W.O.J.R. and Francis, K. Localization of normal and reinnervated mammalian muscle spindles for microscopy. Brain Res., 1972, 39: 240–244.

Granit, R. Neuromuscular interaction in postural tone of the cat's isometric soleus muscle. J. Physiol. (Lond.), 1958, 143: 387–402.

Henatsch, H.-D., Student, C., Student, U. and Takano, K. Controlled variations of input-output parameters affecting the active tension-extension diagram during muscle stretch. In: S. Homma (Ed.), Understanding the Stretch Reflex, Progress in Brain Research, Vol. 44. Elsevier, Amsterdam, 1976: 403–412.

Kano, M. and Takano, K. Gamma activity of rigid cat in tetanus intoxication. Jap. J. Physiol., 1969, 19: 1–10.

Koella, W.P., Nakao, H., Evans, R.L. and Wada, J. Interaction of vestibular and proprioceptive reflexes in the decerebrate cat. Amer. J. Physiol., 1956, 185: 607–613.

Matthews, P.B.C. The dependence of tension upon extension in the stretch reflex of the soleus muscle of the decerebrate cat. J. Physiol. (Lond.), 1959a, 147: 521–546.

Matthews, P.B.C. A study of certain factors influencing the stretch reflex of the decerebrate cat. J. Physiol. (Lond.), 1959b, 147: 547–564.

Matthews, P.B.C. and Rushworth, G. The selective effect of procaine on the stretch reflex and tendon jerk of soleus muscle when applied to its nerve. J. Physiol. (Lond.), 1957, 135: 246–262.

Pompeiano, O. Alpha types of "release" studied in tension-extension diagrams from cat's forelimb triceps muscle. Arch. ital. Biol., 1960, 98: 91–117.

Takano, K. Absence of the gamma spindle loop in the reinnervated hind leg muscles of the cat: "alpha-muscle". Exp. Brain Res., 1976, 26: 343–354.

Takano, K. und Henatsch, H.-D. Direkte Aufnahme von längen Reflex-spannungs Diagrammen einzelner Muskeln in situ. Pflügers Arch. ges. Physiol., 1964, 281: 105.

Takano, K. and Henatsch, H.-D. The effect of the rate of stretch upon the development of active reflex tension in hind limb muscles of the decerebrate cat. Exp. Brain Res., 1971, 12: 422–434.

Takano, K. and Henatsch, H.-D. Tension-extension diagram of the tetanus-intoxicated muscle of the cat. Naunyn-Schmiedeberg's Arch. exp. Path. Pharmak., 1973, 276: 421–436.

Takano, K. and Kano, M. Gamma-bias of the muscle poisoned by tetanus toxin. Naunyn-Schmiedeberg's Arch. exp. Path. Pharmak., 1973, 276: 413–420.

Takano, K. and Student, J.C. Effect of diazepam on the gamma motor system indicated by the responses of the muscle spindle of the triceps surae muscle of the decerebrate cat to the muscle stretch. Naunyn-Schmiedeberg's Arch. exp. Path. Pharmak., 1978, 302: 91–101.

Kyoto Symposia (EEG Suppl. No. 36)
Editors: P.A. Buser, W.A. Cobb and T. Okuma
© 1982, Elsevier Biomedical Press, Amsterdam

216

Mechanism of Action of Dantrolene Sodium, a Peripherally Acting Muscle Relaxant

MAKOTO ENDO and SHINOBU YAGI

Department of Pharmacology, Tohoku University School of Medicine, Sendai 980 (Japan)

Much of the discussion at this symposium is confined to muscle relaxants that exert their action by influencing events within the central nervous system. There is, however, another class of muscle relaxants, i.e., peripherally acting. As one of the objectives of this symposium is to help in understanding the mechanism of action of muscle relaxants, it may well be worth mentioning here the mechanism of a peripherally acting one, dantrolene sodium, which has recently been proved to be clinically useful.

CLASSIFICATION OF PERIPHERALLY ACTING MUSCLE RELAXANTS

There are 2 types of peripherally acting muscle relaxants, one blocking neuromuscular transmission and the other excitation-contraction coupling. Since neuromuscular transmission blockers inhibit muscle contraction by finally inhibiting action potential production of muscle cells this is an all-or-none process; the inhibition of contraction obtained by this group of drugs tends also to be all-or-none as far as contraction of individual muscle cells is concerned, and hence when muscle relaxation is obtained, the inhibition of respiratory muscles, for example, can be too strong. This type of drug is, therefore, mainly used to obtain complete muscle relaxation during general anaesthesia. On the other hand, excitation-contraction coupling is a graded process and, therefore, inhibition of muscle contraction by excitation-contraction coupling blockers can be graded and the magnitude of the action of the drugs can, at least theoretically, be adjusted by varying the dose.

Among excitation-contraction coupling blockers, there are 2 representative agents, heavy water (Kaminer 1960; Yagi and Endo 1976a) and dantrolene sodium (Ellis and Bryant 1972; Ellis and Carpenter 1972; Hainaut and Desmedt 1974; Putney and Bianchi 1974). Replacement of water in external solution by heavy water has a very similar inhibitory action on excitation-contraction coupling to that of dantrolene sodium. To obtain a sufficient magnitude of inhibition, however, most of the water must be replaced by heavy water, which can, therefore hardly be a clinically useful agent. The following discussion is confined to the mechanism of action of dantrolene sodium.

CHARACTERISTICS OF ACTION OF DANTROLENE SODIUM

One of the characteristics of the inhibition by dantrolene is that whereas inhibition of twitch is strong, inhibition of tetanus is rather weak. For example, Putney and Bianchi (1974) have shown that 8.3 μM dantrolene sodium depresses twitch tension by about 80%, but tetanus tension only by 25%. Similarly, if muscle fibres are stimulated by a depolarizing current pulse of rectangular form, dantrolene sodium strongly inhibits contraction evoked by a short pulse but that evoked by a long pulse only very weakly (Morgan and Bryant 1977). It is conceivable that some of the steps in excitation-contraction coupling are slowed down by the drug, but, if time is allowed, it eventually reaches a level not too much suppressed, even in the presence of the drug. Such a dependence of magnitude of inhibition on firing frequency of muscle cells may well be related to a clinically useful aspect of the effect of this drug on patients with spastic paralysis: while spasticity is very much relieved by dantrolene sodium, their voluntary contractions are not much impaired.

MECHANISM OF ACTION OF DANTROLENE SODIUM

In Fig. 1, the events occurring during excitation-contraction coupling are listed. Which of these steps are affected by dantrolene sodium? Action potentials are not affected by the drug at all when twitch is strongly inhibited (Ellis and Bryant 1972). In order to examine the effects of this drug on intracellular structures, we have used skinned muscle fibres. Single fibres were dissected from skeletal muscles of *Xenopus laevis*, and skinned in a relaxing solution. Experimental methods and procedures were as previously described (Endo and Nakajima 1973). As shown in Fig. 2, the relation between free Ca ion concentration and tension developed was not altered at all by 50 μM dantrolene sodium that suppressed twitch tension very strongly. This indicates that even under the influence of the drug, if the same number of Ca ions were released, contractions of the same magnitude should occur. The fact that contraction was strongly inhibited in this condition, therefore, indicates that the amount of Ca acting on the contractile proteins is somehow reduced. In fact,

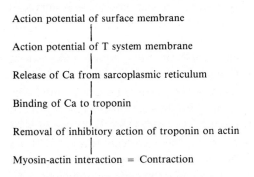

Fig. 1. Events occurring during excitation-contraction coupling (cf. Ebashi et al. 1969).

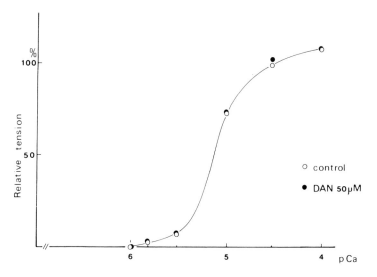

Fig. 2. Absence of effect of 50 μM dantrolene sodium on the relation between free Ca ion concentration and isometric tension developed by a skinned skeletal muscle fibre. Mechanically skinned fast twitch fibre from *Xenopus* iliofibularis muscle. Free Ca ion concentration in the medium, expressed as minus logarithm of its molar concentration (pCa), was buffered with 10 mM EGTA (ethyleneglycol-bis-(β-aminoethylether)-N,N′-tetraacetic acid) and an appropriate amount of Ca and calculated by assuming an apparent binding constant of $10^{5.7}$ M^{-1} for Ca-EGTA. In the presence of 4 mM Mg and 4 mM ATP, at pH 6.8 and 15°C. Other experimental details were as previously described (Endo and Nakajima 1973).

Hainaut and Desmedt (1974) showed a reduction in aequorin luminescence of barnacle muscle fibres.

Fig. 3 shows absence of effect of 50 μM dantrolene on Ca uptake by the SR in skinned muscle fibres. If the Ca uptake process of the SR were stimulated by the drug, even when the same amount of Ca was released, contraction would be inhibited, but this was not the case. These results confirm that described by Brocklehurst (1975), who demonstrated the two properties shown in Figs. 2 and 3 in a combined experiment. She showed that contraction-relaxation cycles of skinned fibres in oil, produced by direct application of Ca by means of a light touch of a Ca^{2+}-gel pipette, were not changed at all by dantrolene sodium. These results lead us to the conclusion that dantrolene sodium inhibits contraction by reducing the amount of Ca released from the SR.

The mechanism of physiological Ca release from the SR is totally unknown at present. Therefore, further details of the mechanism of action of dantrolene sodium are also unknown. However, a few experiments in the literature that might be relevant will be briefly described. The drug weakly inhibits caffeine- and Ca-induced Ca release (Ellis and Carpenter 1972; Yagi and Endo 1976b), but since this type of Ca release does not seem to play a role in physiological Ca release (Endo 1977), no conclusion can be drawn from it about the mechanism of twitch inhibition. Ca release from the SR by "depolarization" of the SR membrane is not inhibited at all by this drug (Yagi and Endo 1976b). Charge movement, which might be an

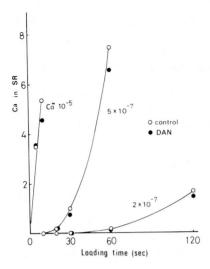

Fig. 3. Absence of effect of 50 μM dantrolene sodium (DAN) on the rate of Ca uptake by the SR of a skinned fibre. Ca in SR, expressed in arbitrary units, was estimated by releasing it almost completely by applying 25 mM caffeine and measuring the area under the resulting transient tension response of the fibre. Ca was then reloaded to the SR in a solution containing various free Ca ion concentrations for various periods of time (loading time), as indicated in the figure, and the amount accumulated in the SR was estimated again as above. Other experimental conditions were similar to those of Fig. 2.

indication of the first step between the action potential of the T system membrane and Ca release from the SR, is reported to be not appreciably inhibited by the drug (Morgan and Bryant 1977).

ELECTROPHYSIOLOGICAL EVALUATION OF THE EFFECTIVENESS OF DANTROLENE SODIUM

Since dantrolene sodium does not inhibit action potential production by muscle cells, it is obvious that the electrophysiological method, which is the main theme of this symposium, is useless in evaluating the efficacy of this class of muscle relaxants. Some method of determining muscle contractility directly should be introduced for the evaluation of this class of drugs.

SUMMARY

The mechanism of action of dantrolene sodium, a peripherally acting muscle relaxant, is reviewed. It does not alter action potentials or responses of the contractile proteins to Ca. The amount of Ca acting on the contractile proteins during twitch must, therefore, be reduced, but since Ca uptake by the SR is not altered, Ca release from the SR must be reduced by the drug. Other characteristics of this drug and their clinical implications are discussed.

REFERENCES

Brocklehurst, L. Dantrolene sodium and "skinned" muscle fibres. Nature (Lond.), 1975, 254: 364.

Ebashi, S., Endo, M. and Ohtsuki, I. Control of muscle contraction. Quart. Rev. Biophys., 1969, 2: 351–384.

Ellis, K.O. and Bryant, S.H. Excitation contraction uncoupling in skeletal muscle by dantrolene sodium. Naunyn Schmiedeberg's Arch. exp. Path. Pharmak., 1972, 274: 107–109.

Ellis, K.O. and Carpenter, J.F. Studies on the mechanism of action of dantrolene sodium. Naunyn Schmiedeberg's Arch. exp. Path. Pharmak., 1972, 275: 83–94.

Endo, M. Calcium release from the sarcoplasmic reticulum. Physiol. Rev., 1977, 57: 71–108.

Endo, M. and Nakajima, Y. Release of calcium induced by "depolarisation" of the sarcoplasmic reticulum membrane. Nature New Biol., 1973, 246: 216–218.

Hainaut, K. and Desmedt, J.E. Effects of dantrolene sodium on calcium movements in single muscle fibers. Nature (Lond.), 1974, 252: 728–729.

Kaminer, B. Effect of heavy water on different types of muscle and on glycerol-extracted psoas fibres. Nature (Lond.), 1960, 185: 172–173.

Morgan, K.G. and Bryant, S.H. The mechanism of action of dantrolene sodium. J. Pharmacol. exp. Ther., 1977, 201: 138–147.

Putney, J.W. and Bianchi, C.P. Site of action of dantrolene in frog sartorius muscle. J. Pharmacol. exp. Ther., 1974, 189: 202–212.

Yagi, S. and Endo, M. Effect of deuterium oxide (D_2O) on excitation-contraction coupling of skeletal muscle. J. physiol. Soc. Jap., 1976a, 38: 298–300.

Yagi, S. and Endo, M. Effect of dantrolene on excitation-contraction coupling of skeletal muscle. Jap. J. Pharmacol., 1976b, 26: 164P.

Kyoto Symposia (EEG Suppl. No. 36)
Editors: P.A. Buser, W.A. Cobb and T. Okuma
© 1982, Elsevier Biomedical Press, Amsterdam

Effect of Dantrolene Sodium on Skeletal Muscles and Stretch Reflexes

YASUHIKO TAMAI

Department of Physiology, Wakayama Medical College, 9-Kyubancho, Wakayama 640 (Japan)

Dantrolene sodium was first reported as a unique muscle relaxant (Snyder et al. 1967) which acted peripherally beyond the neuromuscular junction (Honkomp et al. 1970; Ellis and Carpenter 1971, 1972; Heald and Matsumoto 1971) by a direct action on excitation-contraction coupling (Ellis and Bryant 1972; Nott and Bowman 1974; Takauji and Nagai 1977), perhaps by interference with calcium availability (Zorychta et al. 1971; Putney and Bianch 1974; Von Winkle 1976).

Dantrolene sodium decreased the force of electrically induced isometric twitch in man without altering the muscle action potential, and it reduced reflex more than voluntary contraction (Herman et al. 1972). The isometric twitch tension was affected more than the tetanic tension and fast muscle was more sensitive than slow muscle (Tamai et al. 1973; Monster et al. 1974; Wendt and Barclay 1980). Further, the drug prevented the increase of spindle discharge during fusimotor stimulation (Zorychta et al. 1971) and the effect on the intrafusal muscle fibre resulted in varied EMG activity in the stretch reflex of the decerebrate cat in connection with the effect on the extrafusal muscle fibre (Tamai et al. 1974a).

This paper summarises the effect of dantrolene sodium on the intrafusal and extrafusal muscle fibres in the decerebrate cat and makes clear the relations between the primary effect on these muscle fibres and the secondary effect on the afferent discharges caused by the muscle relaxing effect of the drug. These results in animal experiments may be useful for the evaluation of muscle relaxants and clinical observations in patients with spasticity (Herman et al. 1972; Monster et al. 1973; Monster 1974; Knutsson and Mårtensson 1976).

The analysis of the stretch reflex is based upon single unit recording from muscle spindle afferents in the dorsal root of the decerebrate cat. The recording technique and the system for data collection and processing have been described in detail in other reports (Tamai et al. 1973, 1974a, b).

EFFECT OF DANTROLENE SODIUM ON ISOMETRIC TWITCH AND TETANIC TENSIONS

The percentage reductions of the twitch and tetanic tensions of the gastrocnemius medialis and soleus were investigated at various times after dantrolene sodium administration in doses of 2 mg/kg, i.v., as shown in Fig. 1. The tension fell

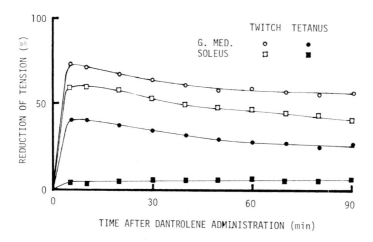

Fig. 1. Percentage reduction of isometric twitch (open symbols) and tetanic tension (closed symbols) at various times after the administration of dantrolene sodium (2 mg/kg, i.v.) in gastrocnemius medialis (circle) and soleus (square) of the cat. The lengthening of the muscle was 6 mm in both muscles and the tetanic tension was measured at 1 sec after initiation of the tetanic stimuli (100 Hz, 0.5 msec) for 1.5 sec. Note that the twitch tension was affected more than the tetanic tension and gastrocnemius medialis was more sensitive than soleus.

immediately after the drug injection and reached its minimum within 10 min, then began to recover gradually but did not improve completely within 90 min. The twitch tension was reduced by 68–76% (mean 70%) in the gastrocnemius medialis and 50–75% (mean 60%) in the soleus of 6 cats at 10 min after the drug injection. The tetanic tension was, however, reduced only by 29–56% (mean 41%) in the gastrocnemius medialis and 2–6% (mean 4%) in the soleus. The tension was not completely reduced by larger doses of 4 mg/kg, i.v., but the recovery was further delayed (cf. Kotsias and Muchnik 1978).

The reduction of tension in drug-treated preparations was dependent on the frequency of stimulation, as shown in the left picture of Fig. 2 (cf. Herman et al. 1972). The percentage reduction of tension in the drug-treated preparation became small with increasing frequency of stimulation, up to 100 Hz in gastrocnemius medialis and 30 Hz in soleus. This indicates that the effect of the drug is smaller in complete tetanus than in incomplete tetanus.

The length dependency of tension reduction was also observed in the drug-treated preparation, as shown in the right picture of Fig. 2. The percentage reduction of tension was decreased by elongating the muscles, especially in the tetanic tension of gastrocnemius medialis.

Fig. 3 shows the effect of dantrolene sodium on the time course of the active state in gastrocnemius medialis and soleus. The most pronounced effect was that the rate of rise was decreased and its decay was remarkably accelerated. The short duration of the active state in treated muscles may support the result that the tetanic fusion frequency was increased by the drug (Ellis and Carpenter 1972). Further, the large effect on the decaying phase of the active state may account for the large reduction

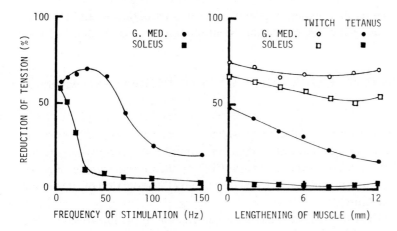

Fig. 2. Left: percentage reduction of tension produced by various frequencies of stimulation of gastrocnemius medialis (closed circle) and soleus (closed square) in the dantrolene-treated preparation (2 mg/kg, i.v.). The lengthening was 6 mm in both muscles. Note that complete tetanic tension was not so much affected by the drug as the incomplete tetanic tension. Right: percentage reduction of isometric twitch (open symbols) and tetanic tension (closed symbols) at various lengths of dantrolene-treated muscles (2 mg/kg, i.v.). The resting tension was subtracted at each length of the muscle. Note the length dependency of the percentage reduction, especially in the tetanus of gastrocnemius medialis.

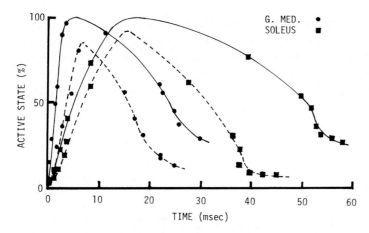

Fig. 3. Time course of active state in gastrocnemius medialis (closed circle) and soleus (closed square). The solid and broken lines show the active state before and after dantrolene sodium administration (2 mg/kg, i.v.), respectively. Note the change in the rising and decaying speed of the active state in the drug-treated preparation.

of incomplete tetanic tension, and the lesser effect on the plateau of the active state may explain the small reduction of complete tetanic tension as the decaying phase and plateau of the active state reflect incomplete and complete tetanus, respectively.

According to Edman and Kiessling (1971), the duration of the active state was prolonged without changing the rate of rise when the semitendinous muscle of the frog was stretched. If this result is applicable to cat's skeletal muscle, the peak active state may be able to reach a higher level in drug-treated preparations and this may result in relatively less reduction of tension when the muscle is elongated.

EFFECT OF DANTROLENE SODIUM ON THE INTRAFUSAL MUSCLE FIBRE

The GIa discharge during stimulation of isolated fusimotor fibres of the ventral root was recorded at various times after the drug administration to investigate the effect of dantrolene sodium on the intrafusal fibre of the muscle spindle (Fig. 4). The effect on the extrafusal muscle fibre was detected by the reduction of the tetanic tension of the same muscle.

The number of GIa discharges evoked by the contraction of the intrafusal muscle fibre decreased in parallel with the reduction of the tetanic tension of the extrafusal fibre with injection of additional drug (arrows). This indicates that the drug affects both intrafusal and extrafusal muscle fibres and the degree of the effect depends upon the dose of the drug injected.

To investigate the effect of dantrolene sodium on the dynamic response of the GIa discharge, the inter-spike interval histogram of the discharge was analysed during sinusoidal movement of the soleus with dynamic or static fusimotor stimulation (Fig. 5).

In the drug-treated preparation, the high frequency oscillation of the GIa discharge during dynamic fusimotor stimulation became irregular with a low spike frequency and the almost constant frequency of the GIa discharge during static fusimotor stimulation became oscillatory with a low spike frequency. In other words, the dynamic pattern of the GIa discharge in drug-treated preparations

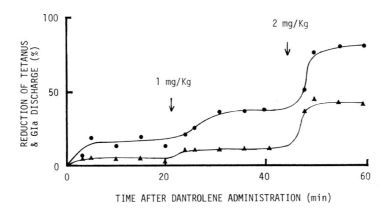

Fig. 4. Percentage reduction of GIa discharge (closed triangle) and tetanic tension (closed circle) after the injection (i.v.) of dantrolene sodium (initial dose: 1 mg/kg, i.v.). The number of GIa discharges was calculated during fusimotor stimulation (100 Hz, 0.5 msec) for 1.5 sec and the tetanic tension was measured at 1 sec after the initiation of the tetanic stimuli (100 Hz, 0.5 msec) for 1.5 sec. Note the decrease of the GIa discharge paralleled by the reduction of tetanic tension.

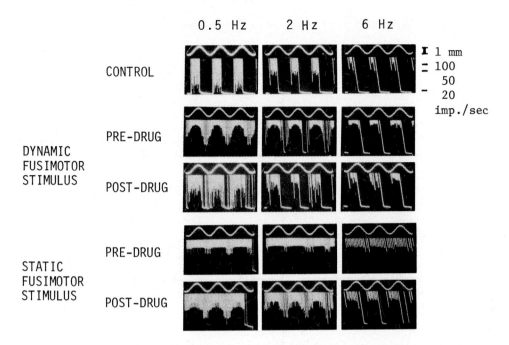

Fig. 5. Effect of dantrolene sodium (2 mg/kg, i.v.) on the dynamic response of GIa discharge during fusimotor stimulation (100 Hz, 0.5 msec). The first and second traces of each picture represent the sinusoidal stretch (2 mm peak to peak) of soleus and the inter-spike interval histogram of the GIa discharge, respectively. The pattern in the drug-treated preparation shows an intermediate type between the control response without fusimotor stimulation (uppermost picture) and the pre-drug response with each fusimotor stimulation (the 2nd and 4th pictures).

changed into the intermediate pattern between the control response without fusimotor stimulation and the pre-drug response with each fusimotor stimulation.

EFFECT OF DANTROLENE SODIUM ON THE STRETCH REFLEX

The effect of dantrolene sodium on the stretch reflex was examined during sinusoidal movement of the gastrocnemius muscle in the decerebrate cat. The sinusoidal stretch was performed by a vibrator and controlled by a velocity feedback circuit. The displacement, tension and EMG of the stretched muscle were recorded simultaneously with the GIa and GIb discharges of the same muscle from the partial dorsal root (cf. Tamai 1974).

The effect of the drug on the stretch reflex changed with the preparation. Fig. 6 shows 2 typical frequency responses of the tension, integrated EMG, maximum frequency of GIa and GIb discharges produced by 2 mm sinusoidal stretch of the gastrocnemius muscle. In one type of preparation, the integrated EMG and GIa discharges decreased after drug administration (dashed lines in the second and third pictures of the left column), while those responses in the other type of preparation

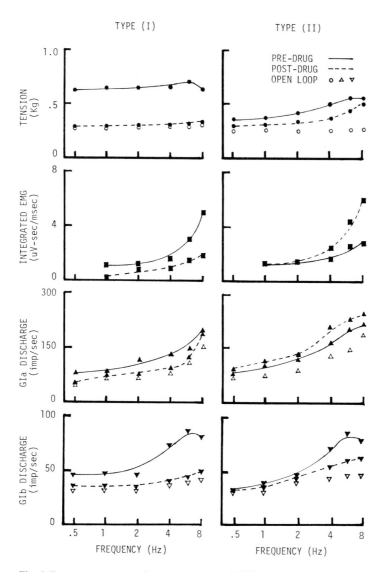

Fig. 6. Frequency response of tension, integrated EMG, GIa, and GIb responses during sinusoidal stretch of gastrocnemius (2 mm peak to peak) in 2 typical preparations. The solid and broken lines indicate the pre-drug and post-drug responses, respectively. The open symbols show the open loop responses after cutting the ventral root. See text.

(right column) increased. The reflex tension was, however, reduced in both types after the drug injection (uppermost pictures). On the other hand, the maximum frequency of the GIa discharge decreased in all drug-treated preparations (bottom pictures).

Thus, the effect of the drug on the stretch reflex is relatively complex as the effect on the extrafusal muscle fibre changes the pattern of the afferent discharges as does the effect on the intrafusal fibre (Table I). That is, the reduced tension of the

TABLE I

SUMMARY OF THE EFFECT OF DANTROLENE SODIUM ON THE MOTOR SYSTEM

The up and down arrows represent the increase and decrease of the corresponding responses, respectively.

Action site	A direct action on excitation-contraction coupling, perhaps by decreasing the amount of calcium released from the sarcoplasmic reticulum.			
Primary effect on motor system	Tension	Extrafusal muscle fibre $\downarrow\downarrow$ (pale muscle) $\quad\downarrow$ (red muscle)		Intrafusal muscle fibre $\downarrow$
Secondary effect on motor system	GIa discharge	$\uparrow$	Absence of unloading effect of extrafusal muscle fibre	$\downarrow\downarrow$ (Dynamic) $\quad\downarrow$ (Static)
	GIb discharge	$\downarrow$	Relaxation of extrafusal muscle fibre	$\downarrow$
	EMG discharge	$\uparrow$		$\downarrow$
Functional effect on motor system	Improvement of motor disability by reduced resistance in passive movement			

extrafusal fibre in the drug-treated preparation, named as the primary effect on the motor system in Table I, increases the GIa discharge by the absence of an unloading effect on the intrafusal fibre as the muscle spindle is arranged in parallel with the extrafusal fibre. On the contrary, the GIb discharge, which is an inhibitory input to the homonymous motoneurone, is decreased by the relaxation of the extrafusal fibre in the drug-treated preparation as the Golgi tendon organ has high sensitivity to the contracting muscle (Jansen and Rudjord 1964; Alnaes 1967). The reflex EMG response may, therefore, become greater in the drug-treated preparation through the increase of the GIa discharge and the decrease of the inhibitory GIb discharge. However, if the effect of the drug extends to the intrafusal fibre, the GIa discharge decreases as the sensitivity of the muscle spindle becomes low, especially in dynamic responses and the reflex EMG response may become small despite the decrease of the inhibitory GIb discharge. All of these effects in the GIa, GIb and EMG responses, here called secondary effects on the motor system, affect motor regulation as the tension of an active muscle is altered greatly by imposed movement and the degree of the alteration of tension depends upon the phase angle between the neural signal and the movement (Tamai 1974). Thus, the final effect of the drug on the movement, called here the functional effect on the motor system, may be complicated. In patients with spasticity, the functional effect of dantrolene sodium was reported as an improvement of motor disability by reduced resistance (Knutsson and Mårtensson 1976).

Finally, it is hoped that the evaluation of muscle relaxants will be performed on these 4 points: (1) the direct action site of the drug; (2) the primary effect on the motor system; (3) the secondary effects on the motor system caused by the primary effect of the drug; and (4) final functional effect on the motor system in dynamic and static conditions.

ACKNOWLEDGEMENTS

I wish to thank Dr. Richard Herman, Dr. A. Willem Monster, W. Freedman and Mrs. Barbara Cozzens for their permission to reproduce data from our collaborative studies and Dr. Takeshi Tsujimoto for his advice during the preparation of this paper.

REFERENCES

Alnaes, E. Static and dynamic properties of Golgi tendon organ in the anterior tibial and soleus muscles of the cat. Acta physiol. scand., 1967, 70: 176–187.

Edman, K.A.P. and Kiessling, A. The time course of the active state in relation to sarcomere length and movement studied in single skeletal muscle fibers of the frog. Acta physiol. scand., 1971, 81: 182–196.

Ellis, K.O. and Bryant, S.H. Excitation-contraction uncoupling in skeletal muscle by dantrolene sodium. Naunyn-Schmiedeberg's Arch. exp. Path. Pharmak., 1972, 274: 107–109.

Ellis, K.O. and Carpenter, J.F. The effect of dantrolene sodium (F-440) on skeletal muscle. Fed. Proc., 1971, 30: 670.

Ellis, K.O. and Carpenter, J.F. Studies on the mechanism of action of dantrolene sodium: a skeletal muscle relaxant. Naunyn-Schmiedeberg's Arch. exp. Path. Pharmak., 1972, 275: 83–95.

Heald, D.E. and Matsumoto, Y. Inhibition of contraction of frog skeletal muscle by dantrolene sodium. Fed. Proc., 1971, 30: 378.

Herman, R., Mayer, N. and Mecomber, S.A. Clinical pharmacophysiology of dantrolene sodium. Amer. J. phys. Med., 1972, 51: 296–311.

Honkomp, L.J., Halliday, R.P. and Wessels, F.L. Dantrolene, 1[5-(p-nitro-phenyl)furfurylidene] amino hydantoin, a unique skeletal muscle relaxant. Pharmacologist, 1970, 12: 301.

Jansen, J.K.S. and Rudjord, T. On the silent period and Golgi tendon organs of the soleus muscle of the cat. Acta physiol. scand., 1964, 62: 364–379.

Knutsson, E. and Mårtensson, A. Action of dantrolene sodium in spasticity with low dependence on fusimotor drive. J. neurol. Sci., 1976, 29: 195–212.

Kotsias, B.A. and Muchnik, S. Reversible effect of dantrolene sodium on twitch tension of rat skeletal muscle. Arch. Neurol. (Chic.), 1978, 35: 234–236.

Monster, A.W. Spasticity and the effects of dantrolene sodium. Arch. phys. Med., 1974, 55: 373–383.

Monster, A.W., Herman, R., Meek, S. and McHenry, J. Cooperative study for assessing the effect of a pharmacological agent on spasticity. Amer. J. phys. Med., 1973, 52: 163–188.

Monster, A.W., Tamai, Y. and McHenry, J. Dantrolene sodium: Its effect on extrafusal muscle fibers. Arch. phys. Med. Rehab., 1974, 55: 355–362.

Nott, M.W. and Bowman, W.C. Action of dantrolene sodium on contraction of the tibialis anterior and soleus muscles of cats under chloralose anesthesia. Clin. exp. Pharmacol. Physiol., 1974, 1: 113.

Putney, J.W. and Bianch, C.P. Site of action of dantrolene in frog sartorius muscle. J. Pharmacol. exp. Ther., 1974, 189: 202.

Snyder, H.R., Davis, C.S., Bickerton, R.K. and Halliday, R.P. 1-[(5-Arylfurfurylidene)amino]hydantoin. A new class of muscle relaxants. J. med. Chem., 1967, 10: 807–810.

Takauji, M. and Nagai, T. Effect of dantrolene sodium on the inactivation of excitation-contraction coupling in frog skeletal muscle. Jap. J. Physiol., 1977, 27: 743–754.

Tamai, Y. Mutual relationships among stretch reflex responses and applied sinusoidal movement in gastrocnemius and soleus of decerebrated cat. Wakayama med. Rep., 1974, 17: 1–18.

Tamai, Y., Monster, A.W., Herman, R. and Cozzens, B. Effect of dantrolene sodium on the gastrocnemius medialis and soleus of the cat. Wakayama med. Rep., 1973, 16: 1–10.

Tamai, Y., Herman, R. and Cozzens, B. Effect of dantrolene sodium on response of stretch reflex in the cat. Wakayama med. Rep., 1974a, 16: 37–46.

Tamai, Y., Herman, R. and Freedman, W. Reflex tension during sinusoidal movement in gastrocnemius and soleus of decerebrated cat. Jap. J. Physiol., 1974b, 24: 1–18.

Von Winkle, W.B. Calcium release from skeletal muscle sarcoplasmic reticulum: site of action of dantrolene sodium? Science, 1976, 193: 1130–1131.

Wendt, I.J. and Barclay, L.K. Effects of dantrolene on the energetics of fast- and slow-twitch muscles of the mouse. Amer. J. Physiol., 1980, 238: 56–61.

Zorychta, E., Esplin, D.W., Capek, R. and Lastrowecka, A. The actions of dantrolene on extrafusal and intrafusal muscle. Fed. Proc., 1971, 30: 669.

5. Kindling – Pharmacology and Physiology

Kyoto Symposia (EEG Suppl. No. 36)
Editors: P.A. Buser, W.A. Cobb and T. Okuma
© 1982, Elsevier Biomedical Press, Amsterdam

Mechanism of Amygdaloid Convulsive Seizure Development

JUHN A. WADA

Health Sciences Center Hospital, University of British Columbia, Vancouver, B.C. V6T 2A1 (Canada)

Convulsive generalized seizure has been shown to occur as an ultimate consequence of kindling in all the species of animals so far examined, regardless of the site of brain stimulation. This motor seizure development in amygdaloid kindling was thought initially to be due to strengthening of the limbic-limbic connection based upon the observations that simultaneous bilateral limbic stimulation facilitates, while forebrain bisection retards, amygdaloid kindling (Racine et al. 1972). In addition, stimulation of the hippocampal commissure was shown to result in one-trial kindling. The latter, however, was shown to be due to stimulation of more dorsal structures such as the cingulum or the corpus callosum (Madryga et al. 1975) rather than of the hippocampal commissure, raising the possibility of bilateral activation of the dorsal cortical areas being responsible for the development of the final stage of convulsive seizure.

Electrographically, the findings of a unique pattern of after-discharge in the midbrain reticular formation prior to the development of seizure generalization in cats and the blocking of the established kindled motor seizure by lesions of the ipsilateral midbrain reticular formation (Wada and Sato 1974, 1975) suggested the possibility that the functional linkage between the stimulated limbic site and the remote brain stem structure is important for seizure generalization. A subsequent demonstration of a positive transhemispheric transfer in rats with commissural bisection (McIntyre 1976) and of a unique ictal after-discharge pattern in the lower brain stem of Senegalese baboons, kindled from either the cortical or the amygdaloid site, supported this notion (Wada and Osawa 1976). However, lesions of the midbrain reticular formation prior to the commencement of amygdaloid stimulation failed to prevent kindling development, suggesting that an alternative route outside the lesion of the brain stem area must be available for generation of the final stage convulsive seizure.

On the other hand, an earlier study of amygdaloid kindling in rabbits indicated that the onset of motor seizure is coincident with ictal electrographic change in the cortical motor area (Tanaka 1972). The increasing complexity of neocortical after-discharge morphology was found to be associated with clinical motor seizure development of amygdaloid origin in both rats and cats. Progressive ictal electrographic participation of the anterior neocortical areas, with eventual development of interictal spike discharge, was coincident with the recruitment of ictal motor manifestations, suggesting that the anterior neocortex participates in motor seizure development (Wada et al. 1975). This is consistent with the results of amygdaloid kindling in cats with bilateral ablation of the sigmoid gyrus, in which difficulty in developing a final stage generalized convulsion was evident (Wake and Wada 1976). Among more than 200 kindled cats studied in our laboratory, the only ones that developed non-convulsive status epilepticus (stage 4 running) were the ones with bilateral ablation of the sigmoid gyri or with unilateral resection combined with bisection of the forebrain commissure. Furthermore, our observations of kindling in primates indicated that the initial motor seizure pattern in amygdaloid kindling is characterized by the involvement of the lower facial region, while prefrontal and mesial frontal cortical kindling involves the upper and lower extremities, respectively (Wada 1980). This observation is complemented by our documentation of transient post-ictal paralysis of the lower facial region in amygdaloid kindling, the upper extremity in prefrontal kindling, and the lower extremity in mesial frontal kindling during stage 3 motor seizure development. These findings suggest that ictal motor development is dependent on an initial access to a specific area of the anterior rolandic cortex from the kindling site through which motor seizure propagation is organized.

In spite of the above observations, the mechanisms underlying the ictal engagement of the rolandic cortex by stimulation of a non-motor structure such as the amygdala remain entirely uncertain. Our observations over the past years on the unique pattern of progressive change in the ictal EEG manifestations during amygdaloid kindling have provided us with a clue as to what might be the underlying mechanism. We found that the initial electrographic pattern of very conspicuous high voltage spike discharge in the amygdala becomes progressively less prominent during amygdaloid kindling. This chronological alteration of ictal EEG signatures at the kindling site suggested the possibility that the function of the amygdala in amygdaloid kindling may be primarily inhibitory and that it may be progressively altered by repeated stimulation, resulting in an activation of the neural mechanisms responsible for the motor ictal manifestations by a process of disinhibition.

In order to test this hypothesis, we examined the effect of selective destruction of amygdaloid neurones by localized infusion of kainic acid prior to the commencement of amygdaloid kindling or following its completion. Our concern about this particular experiment is the seizure-inducing property of kainic acid, particularly when it is injected into the amygdala (Ben-Ari et al. 1979a, b). Therefore, unless the kainic acid-induced seizure can be obliterated, it is theoretically possible to contaminate the data by kainic acid-induced seizures before cell destruction. In this study, kainic acid was allowed to diffuse over a period of time through an electrode cannula under deep pentobarbital anaesthesia and the electro-clinical seizures of injected animals were continuously monitored. Only animals that did not show evidence of electro-clinical seizure or neurological deficit following the injection were used for this study.

Male hooded rats of the Royal Victoria Hospital strain with an implanted cannula electrode system were used. Six μg kainic acid dissolved in 1 μl of buffered phosphate solution was infused very slowly into the amygdala through the cannula under pentobarbital anaesthesia. EEG and behaviour were monitored continuously for several days with particular attention to unusual episodic behaviour or seizure activity. Seven to 20 days elapsed before these animals were subjected to amygdaloid kindling.

With small and well localized lesions, seizure stage instability was quite apparent in spite of a rather high after-discharge threshold. Although stage 5 seizure was kindled, recapitulation of stages 1 and 2 was rather obscure. The mean after-discharge threshold was high (225 μA in contrast to 100 μA in the control group) but the number of daily stimulations required to reach stage 5 was significantly less than that of the control group. It is known that a kindled seizure can be triggered following the placement of an electrolytic lesion at the tip of the kindling electrode when a higher intensity current is applied, presumably due to activation of neurones in the periphery of the lesion (Goddard et al. 1969). Since our histological findings in this group suggested that a similar mechanism might be responsible for the development of seizures from the amygdala, animals with a much larger unilateral amygdaloid lesion were examined. The after-discharge threshold was comparable to that of the control group, yet the mean number of daily stimulations required for stage 5 seizure development was 6.3, which is significantly smaller than in the control group. It should be noted that after-discharge activity could not be detected at the amygdala during the earlier half of the induced seizure, in which recapitulation of stages 1 and 2 was absent. No significant difference was found between this group and the control group so far as stage 5 seizure manifestation was concerned. In view of the quite striking results in this group, animals with bilateral amygdaloid lesions were examined and their mean after-discharge threshold was found to be lower than that of the control group. The speed of seizure development at the secondary site as well as at the primary site was also strikingly faster than that of the control. Again, the evolution of the clinical seizure event in this group was rather rapid although stage 1 and 2 manifestations were absent. Electrographically, it was frequently impossible to be certain of the presence or absence of after-discharge in the amygdala despite the obvious display of clinical motor seizures.

Additional experiments in which the effect of post-kindling lesions of the primary site amygdala was tested showed that kindled stage 5 seizure can be triggered from the lesioned amygdala, although with a slightly higher generalized seizure triggering threshold. Deoxyglucose (DG) autograms of all the animals used in this study showed an enhancement of the glucose uptake in the interpeduncular nucleus, pars reticulata of the substantia nigra, the entopeduncular nucleus, habenula, fasciculus retroflexus of Meynert, and in the subthalamic nucleus — a finding which is identical to that in kindled amygdaloid seizure in control animals. This finding, along with the fact that we were able to establish a generalized seizure triggering threshold in these lesioned animals, suggested that the observed seizures are indeed kindled seizures.

Results of our study indicated that kainic acid lesions of the amygdala prior to amygdaloid kindling significantly facilitate the rate of convulsive seizure development. It is clear that animals can be kindled from the amygdala without neuronal components. It could be argued that the kindling in this study resulted from the stimulation of neurones in the periphery of the lesion (Goddard et al. 1969). Indeed, some elevation of the after-discharge threshold was noted with rather small and localized intra-amygdaloid lesions. However, the after-discharge thresholds in animals with much larger lesions were the same or lower than those of the control group.

The results of the prior lesion experiment suggest that the amygdaloid neurone is not necessary for amygdaloid kindling. The findings further suggest that the amygdaloid kindling accomplished in this study following kainic acid injection is most likely due to the activation of distant neurones whose axon terminals are located in the amygdala or whose axons pass through it.

The very rapid kindling following destruction of the amygdaloid neuronal mass is consistent with the assumption that the amygdaloid neurone exerts a largely inhibitory effect upon motor seizure mechanisms. It is postulated that such an inhibitory property of the amygdaloid neurone is rendered progressively less effective by repeated electrical stimulation, culminating in activation of the neuronal system responsible for motor seizures.

Animals with bilateral amygdaloid lesions showed seizure development that was strikingly more rapid with one-trial kindling than in animals with unilateral lesions. This suggests that the final motor mechanism for amygdaloid kindling receives inhibitory inputs from both amygdalae.

The amygdala is known to project to the prefrontal and motor cortices (Krettek and Price 1977; Llamas et al. 1977; Canedo et al. 1978; Macchi et al. 1978), but the extent of projection into the motor area appears rather sparse. The pattern of amygdaloid seizure development, however, indicates that a functional linkage must be made between the amygdala and the cortical motor system. Since the motor cortex is not known to project directly to the amygdala, one must look elsewhere for a possible anatomical linking mechanism to explain the present findings.

The findings of chemical kindling by cholinergic agonists (Wasterlain et al. 1981) and, by my colleague Dr. Kimura, of marked accentuation of amygdaloid kindling seizures by diisopropylfluorophosphate (DFP) pretreatment, and its elimination by atropine, a muscarinic cholinergic blocking agent, suggest that the marked change of behavioural events in amygdaloid kindled animals following DFP can be regarded in part as the result of changes in the central cholinergic system.

Recent progress in visualizing cholinergic structures in the CNS, using a choline acetyl transferase-immunohistochemical method, provides helpful information in identifying the precise localization of the cholinergic system in the mammalian CNS (Kimura et al. 1981).

In the rostral forebrain of cats, cholinergic cell bodies were found in the nucleus caudatus and putamen, the medial septal area, the nucleus of the diagonal band of Broca, the globus pallidus, the substantia innominata and the nucleus basalis of Meynert. No cholinergic neurones were found in the amygdala or the cerebral cortex, although cholinoceptive cells were unevenly distributed in these structures. It is interesting to note that the highest density of cholinoceptive cells is localized in the basal lateral nucleus of the amygdala, which is known to be the most susceptible site for kindling seizure development. Some of the pathways relating to the above structures, in which acetylcholine is believed to be used, include (a) neostriatal interneurones, (b) habenulo-interpeduncular tract, (c) septal hippocampal pathway, and (d) the substantia innominata projecting to the cerebral cortex.

To investigate the cholinergic involvement of the above pathways in amygdaloid kindling, lesions were made in rats in 5 discrete brain areas relating to the latter 3 projection systems: the diagonal band nucleus, the medial septal area, the habenular nuclei, the interpeduncular nucleus and the substantia innominata. All animals, with the exception of those with lesions of the substantia innominata, survived and responded fully to amygdaloid stimulation. Since animals with sufficient destruction of the substantia innominata failed to survive, the effect of acute lesions of this structure was examined in kindled rats. Such acute lesions resulted in a marked suppression of kindled seizures in contrast to the insignificant effect of lesions of other areas containing cholinergic neuronal populations. The finding suggests that the substantia innominata has a significant role to play in the expression of amygdaloid kindled seizure. The substantia innominata appears to receive inputs from mid and lower brain stem structures, including both dopaminergic and noradrenergic neurones (Swanson and Hartman 1975), and projects widely and diffusely to the cerebral cortex (Beccari 1943; Gorry 1963; Divac 1975; Kievit and Kuypers 1975; Jones et al., 1976; Parent et al. 1977). It is interesting to postulate that the cholinergic neurones situated in the substantia innominata also project to the cerebral cortex and the motor cortex. It is suggested that the cholinergic cell cluster located in the substantia innominata may be significantly involved in the mechanisms of generating convulsive seizures of amygdaloid origin.

REFERENCES

Beccari, N. Neurologia Comparata Anatomofunzionale dei Vertebrati compreso l'Uomo. Sansoni, Florence, 1943.

Ben-Ari, Y., Algowska, J., Tremblay, E. and Le Gal La Salle, G. A new method of status epilepticus: Intra-amygdaloid application of kainic acid elicits repetitive secondarily generalized convulsive seizures. Brain Res., 1979a, 163: 176–179.

Ben-Ari, Y., Tremblay, E., Otterson, O.P. and Naquet, R. Evidence of suggesting secondary epileptogenic lesion after kainic acid: Pretreatment with diazepam reduces distant but not local brain damage. Brain Res., 1979b, 165: 362–365.

Canedo, A., Mariotti, M., Schiettati, M. and Mancia, M. Hypothalamic and amygdaloid influences upon sensory motor cortical neurons. Brain Res., 1978, 158: 223–228.

Divac, I. Magnocellular nuclei of the basal forebrain project to neocortex, brainstem and olfactory bulb – Review of some functional correlates. Brain Res., 1975, 93: 385–398.

Goddard, G.V., McIntyre, D.C. and Leech, C.A. A permanent change in brain functions resulting from daily electrical stimulation. Exp. Neurol., 1969, 25: 295–330.

Gorry, J.D. Studies on the comparative anatomy of the ganglion basale of Meynert. Acta anat. (Basel), 1963, 55: 1–104.

Jones, E.G., Burton, H., Saper, C.B. and Swanson, L.W. Midbrain, diencephalic and cortical relationships of the basal nucleus of Meynert and associated structures in primates. J. comp. Neurol., 1976, 167: 385–420.

Kaneko, Y., Wada, J.A. and Kimura, H. Is the amygdaloid neuron necessary for amygdaloid kindling? In: J.A. Wada (Ed.), Kindling 2. Raven Press, New York, 1981: 249–264.

Kievit, J. and Kuypers, H.G.J.M. Basal forebrain and hypothalamic connections to frontal and parietal cortex in the rhesus monkey. Science, 1975, 187: 660–662.

Kimura, H., Kaneko, Y. and Wada, J.A. Catecholamine and cholinergic systems and amygdaloid kindling. In: J.A. Wada (Ed.), Kindling 2. Raven Press, New York, 1981a: 265–288.

Kimura, H., McGeer, P.L., Peng, J.H. and McGeer, E.G. Central cholinergic system: Choline acetyl transferase immunohistochemical study in the cat brain. J. comp. Neurol., 1981b, 200: 151–201.

Krettek, J.E. and Price, J.L. Projections from the amygdaloid cortex to the cerebral cortex and thalamus in the rat and cat. J. comp. Neurol., 1977, 172: 687–722.

Llamas, A., Avendano, C. and Reinoso-Suarez, F. Amygdaloid projections to prefrontal and motor cortex. Science, 1977, 195: 194–196.

Macchi, G., Bentivoglio, M., Rossini, P. and Tempesta, E. The basolateral amygdaloid projections to the neocortex in the cat. Neurosci. Newslett., 1978, 9: 347–351.

Madryga, F.J., Goddard, G.V. and Raśmussen, T.D. The kindling of motor seizures from hippocampal commissure in the rat. Physiol. Psychol., 1975, 3: 369–373.

McIntyre, D.C. Split brain rat: Transfer and interference of kindled amygdaloid convulsions. In: J.A. Wada (Ed.), Kindling. Raven Press, New York, 1976: 61–83.

Parent, A., Poirier, L.J., Boucher, R. and Butcher, L.L. Morphological characteristics of acetylcholinesterase-containing neurons in the CNS of DFP-treated monkeys. Part 2: Diencephalic and medial telencephalic structures. J. neurol. Sci., 1977, 32: 9–28.

Racine, R., Okujava, V. and Chipashivili, S. Modification of seizure activity by electrical stimulation: III. Mechanisms. Electroenceph. clin. Neurophysiol., 1972, 39: 261–271.

Swanson, L.W. and Hartman, B.K. The central adrenergic system. An immunofluorescence study of the location of cell bodies and their efferent connections in the rat using dopamine-hydroxylase as a marker. J. comp. Neurol., 1975, 163: 467–506.

Tanaka, A. Progressive changes of the behavioural and electroencephalographic responses to daily amygdaloid stimulation in rabbits. Fukuoka med. J., 1972, 63: 152–164.

Wada, J.A. Amygdaloid and frontal cortical kindling in subhuman primates. In: M. Girgis and L.G. Kiloh (Eds.), Limbic Epilepsy and the Dyscontrol Syndrome. Elsevier, Amsterdam, 1980: 133–148.

Wada, J.A. and Osawa, T. Spontaneous recurrent seizure state induced by daily electric amygdaloid stimulation in Senegalese baboons, Papio papio. Neurology (Minneap.), 1976, 26: 273–286.

Wada, J.A. and Sato, M. Generalized convulsive seizure induced by daily electrical stimulation of the amygdala in cats: correlative electrographic behavioural features. Neurology (Minneap.), 1974, 24: 565–574.

Wada, J.A. and Sato, M. Effects of unilateral lesion in the midbrain reticular formation upon kindled amygdaloid convulsion in cats. Epilepsia, 1975, 16: 693–697.

Wada, J.A., Sato, M. and McCaughran, Jr., J.A. Cortical electrographic correlates of convulsive seizure development induced by daily electrical stimulation of the amygdala in rats and cats. Folia psychiat. neurol. jap., 1975, 29: 331–339.

Wake, A. and Wada, J.A. Frontal cortical kindling in cats. In: J.A. Wada (Ed.), Kindling. Raven Press, New York, 1976: 203–214.

Wasterlain, C.G., Masulka, D. and Jonec V. Chemical kindling: A study of synaptic pharmacology. In: J.A. Wada (Ed.), Kindling 2. Raven Press, New York, 1981: 315–327.

Kyoto Symposia (EEG Suppl. No. 36)
Editors: P.A. Buser, W.A. Cobb and T. Okuma
© 1982, Elsevier Biomedical Press, Amsterdam

Amygdaloid Organization Related to the Kindling Effect

G. LE GAL LA SALLE

Laboratoire de Physiologie Nerveuse, C.N.R.S., 91190 Gif-sur-Yvette (France)

In 1967 Goddard showed that repetition of an initially subconvulsive stimulation applied in different brain areas can lead to a progressive and permanently enhanced epileptic susceptibility. He termed this phenomenon "kindling" and, 2 years later (Goddard et al. 1969), gave an extensive description of this phenomenon. Since then, the kindling effect has been intensively studied in different species by stimulating different brain areas. Of all the structures from which kindling can be induced, the amygdala is among the most sensitive, eliciting it readily. This facility explains the great number of studies dealing with amygdaloid kindling. However, in spite of the numerous data we have at present, little is yet known about the mechanisms underlying this phenomenon and many basic questions remain unsolved. For example, both hippocampus and, to a lesser extent, amygdala are well known for their high vulnerability to epileptogenic procedures or conditions. However, hippocampal kindling requires at least twice as much stimulation as does amygdaloid kindling (Goddard et al. 1969; McIntyre and Burnham 1976; Sato 1976).

In this paper, first of all, using behavioural, EEG and pharmacological data currently available, we shall give several reasons which lead us to assign a central role to the amygdala in the kindling phenomenon. Then we shall try to understand what properties of the amygdaloid complex can account for its privileged role in the elicitation of particularly rapid kindling. This reflexion on the amygdaloid organization related to kindling should allow us to specify a little further our concept of the kindling phenomenon.

WHAT EXACTLY IS THE RANK OF THE AMYGDALA IN THE HIERARCHY OF SENSITIVITY TO KINDLING?

Before trying to answer this question we would like to specify that only kindling from stimulation of the limbic system will be considered here. Cortical kindling differs on many points and does not share all the characteristics of limbic kindling (Racine 1975; Burnham 1978). In addition, because of the differences which exist between species, we shall be mainly referring to data on kindling in the rat. Stimulation of fibre tracts (Racine et al. 1972; Madryga et al. 1975; Le Gal La Salle 1979) or simultaneous stimulation of bilateral structures will also be discarded, although inducing rapid kindling.

Concerning single structures, several difficulties arise when trying to rank them according to their susceptibility for kindling. The greatest difficulty comes from the somewhat different procedural and experimental conditions used by the different authors. Amygdala (Goddard et al. 1969), pyriform cortex (Racine 1975), olfactory bulb (Cain 1977) and n. accumbens (personal result) are among the most likely candidates which can lead to the most rapid kindling. However, n. accumbens surrounds the anterior commissure from which kindling is readily obtained and this throws some doubt on its relative sensitivity. Concerning the olfactory bulb, Cain (1977) has accumulated evidence showing that kindling from the olfactory bulb may operate through the amygdala, as has already been suggested for hypothalamic kindling (Cullen and Goddard 1975). A similar possibility may also be valid for the pyriform cortex, which is very intimately associated with the amygdala. Thus, although it is difficult, if not impossible, to assign a top ranking for kindling susceptibility, the amygdala seems to stand out above all other cerebral structures in the elicitation of rapid kindling.

SIMILARITY OF THE LATE SEIZURE MANIFESTATIONS INDEPENDENTLY OF THE PRIMARY LIMBIC SITE

If the kindling rate varies widely according to the primary site of stimulation, several similarities in the gradual development of the late seizure manifestations are very striking. Whichever limbic structure is stimulated the animals always display an orderly progression from stage 1 to the final stage of kindling. The early stages differ according to their duration and the behavioural signs which are evoked; however, in all cases one can notice striking similarities in the late development of the ictal behavioural pattern among brain areas. This similarity is based on several experimental observations.

Behavioural evidence

The moment from which kindling progresses to convulsive seizure, with minor differences according to the primary site of stimulation, is mainly characterized by the appearance of oro-alimentary motor manifestations. These manifestations are somewhat different according to the species and more marked in rats and cats than in primates. In the rat they include facial motor effects, such as twitching of the eyes and movements of the vibrissae, as well as chewing and masticatory movements. This behavioural pattern is more or less related to the beginning of stage 2 in amygdaloid kindling and to stage 3 in hippocampal kindling.

It is very important to stress that such manifestations seem to involve the active participation of the amygdala. Backed up by experimental data, the existence of a close relationship has been shown between the appearance of oro-alimentary motor activity and the disorganization of the amygdaloid complex during epileptic seizures. This relationship is found in most animal species with, however, some differences in the ultimate evolution of the amygdaloid discharges*. In man, the occurrence of such early oro-alimentary signs during epileptic seizures has also been related to paroxysmal discharges that directly involve the amygdala (Munari et al. 1979).

In a previous paper (Le Gal La Salle 1981) we showed that variations in the delay of amygdaloid kindling onset was fairly well related to the time spent in the early stages (1 and 2), whereas the time spent in the late stages (3 and 4) was practically unchanged in spite of varying kindling rates. In fact, this observation seems to apply to all the limbic structures. Once the critical behavioural point has been reached, convulsive seizures develop within a very similar time span regardless of primary site location.

The preceding statement is further emphasized by data on the transfer phenomenon. After a kindled site has been established, behavioural convulsions are acquired more readily by activation of other related sites. Numerous examples of transfer exist in the literature (Racine 1972; McIntyre and Goddard 1973; McIntyre 1976; Sato 1976). From these it is possible to suggest a general rule. Independently of the primary limbic site, elicitation of a kindled seizure is always immediate, or quasi-immediate, when the secondary site of stimulation is involved with the amygdala. On the contrary, a number of additional stimulations are required to get a fully kindled seizure from secondary sites in amygdaloid kindled animals. According to all the cases reported in the literature, this number is equal to the difference between the time necessary to kindle the animal from the primary site and that necessary to kindle the animal from the amygdala. This can be verified with less than 20% error in all the examples provided up to now.

Pharmacological evidence

Pharmacological studies of anticonvulsant drugs also provide some data supporting the distinction between the early and late phases during kindling. Many substances act by suppressing the generalization without modifying the focal discharge. This is the case, for example, with amino oxyacetic acid (Le Gal La Salle 1980) and diazepam (Racine et al. 1976; Albright et al. 1980). Concerning the latter drug, a particularly interesting result is the following: we have shown that diazepam (1 mg/kg), while able to block amygdaloid kindling when given daily before stimulation, is ineffective when given only from stage 2 (unpublished result). In the latter case, kindling develops without any major modifications.

Finally, it is interesting to note that the ED_{50} calculated for the majority of anticonvulsant drugs is similar in that it suppresses the "generalized" part of the kindled seizure whatever the brain region from which the seizure is triggered. Based

---

*On this point it is particularly important to emphasize that under no circumstances can the stage 5 seizure in the rat be considered as similar to the secondarily generalized tonic-clonic seizure observed in the cat, in most primates and also in the rat after, for example, picrotoxin injection. The stage 5 seizure in the rat can more accurately be described as a bilateral complex clonic seizure or, more simply, as a full motor seizure and not as a generalized seizure.

on these results Albright et al. (1980) have suggested that "the kindled generalized convulsion is a unitary phenomenon regardless of the location of the focus." However, in contrast to the fully kindled seizure, the focal seizure induced in different brain regions is not equally suppressed by anticonvulsant drugs. Thus, all the above data add some evidence for the central role played by the amygdala and strengthen the importance of the distinction between early and late stages in kindling development.

A further source pointing out the special role of the amygdala in the development of the epileptic phenomenon comes from experiments on other models of epilepsy. In this context, of particular interest is the parallel which can be made between kindling and epilepsy induced by kainic acid. Systemic administration of low doses of kainic acid initially evokes a typical syndrome characterized by immobilization, staring and numerous episodes of "wet dog shakes" (Ben-Ari et al.1981; Lothman and Collins 1981). This syndrome is accompanied by epileptiform discharges in the hippocampal formation and septum, corresponding to an increase in deoxyglucose (DG) consumption in these two structures. In a second stage, as seen in septal kindling (Le Gal La Salle and Cavalheiro 1981), the number of wet dog shakes progressively diminishes while the first typical amygdaloid signs appear, corresponding to increased DG consumption in the amygdaloid complex and closely related areas. Thereafter, motor limbic seizures develop rapidly while the DG map then resembles that found in kindled animals (Engel et al. 1978). Thus, systemic administration of kainic acid roughly mimics hippocampal kindling. The particularly high vulnerability of the hippocampus to neurotoxic agents could explain the development of epileptic discharges from this structure. The possibility that the two models share some common neuroanatomical substrate is also illustrated by other experiments (Ben-Ari et al. 1979, 1980; Nelson et al. 1980), including the recent study of Kaijima et al. (1981) who demonstrate a strong facilitation of hippocampal kindling following microinjection of quisqualic acid (another potent glutamate analogue) into the ipsilateral amygdala in the cat.

WHAT PROPERTIES CAN CONFER A PRIVILEGED ROLE ON THE AMYGDALA DURING EARLY KINDLING DEVELOPMENT?

These few remarks confer a central role on the amygdala in the kindling effect as well as in some other experimental models of epilepsy. However, as demonstrated by lesion experiments, this role is not essential since amygdaloid lesions do not prevent the development of kindling from other structures, although they greatly lengthen the early stages (Le Gal La Salle 1979). Also, amygdaloid lesions in the rat under kainic acid do not block the development of severe limbic motor seizures, but slightly alleviate the typical amygdaloid signs (Tremblay, personal communication).

Thus, particular attention must be paid to the participation of the amygdala in the early development of kindling. Intraneuronal amygdaloid circuitry and its system of connections may be of primary importance for its particularly high capacity to kindle.

Intraneuronal amygdaloid circuits

One of the most important basic characteristics of kindling is the progressive increase in after-discharge (AD) duration. At the final stage of convulsive seizure identical AD durations are found, regardless of the stimulation site. In addition, AD duration seems to be correlated with two other basic characteristics, growth in amplitude and propagation of ADs. Concerning this last point it has been shown that ADs that cover several structures are longer than when limited to a single one (Andy and Koshino 1967). Thus, AD duration could represent a good index of the growth of amplitude and the spread of ADs.

In addition, increase in AD duration seems to be correlated with kindling development velocity (Le Gal La Salle 1981). Thus it can be postulated that some characteristics of the AD itself might be correlated with the development of kindled seizures. Since inducing AD triggers a chain reaction which, once activated, develops independently of the parameters of the initiator, the functional organization of the neuronal network which gives rise to the AD may account for its capacity to kindle.

Unfortunately the synaptic organization of the amygdala, in terms of excitation and inhibition, is still poorly known (Le Gal La Salle and Ben-Ari 1981). This is mainly due to the fact that the amygdala, unlike the hippocampus, lacks a well structured organization, and to the paucity of intracellular studies.

Racine and Zaide (1978) have recorded from amygdaloid cells in kindled animals. During epileptiform discharges a large number of units fire rhythmically and synchronously. The bursts of action potentials coincide with the epileptiform EEG "spikes." In kindled animals, burst duration and intraburst action potential frequency increase, as compared to control animals. In addition, all the responses evoked by a single stimulus pulse are followed by an inhibitory period which increases in duration as kindling progresses. This is in contrast to our results during the habituation paradigm in which the response duration progressively decreased (Ben-Ari and Le Gal La Salle 1974).

In a recent paper Fernandez de Molina et al. (1981) have shown that IPSPs are by far the most frequently observed synaptic activity and that some amygdaloid neurones are able to generate repetitive hyperpolarizing activity. On the other hand, based on recent experiments (Rayport and Kandel 1981), the possibility that ADs propagate through non-chemical synapses, which have been shown to exist in the mammalian brain, might participate in epileptogenesis and favour the spread of discharges through abnormal pathways. Nonetheless, further experiments are needed to understand the intrinsic synaptic organization of amygdaloid neurones in the elicitation of epileptiform activity.

It can be noticed when comparing amygdalar and hippocampal kindling developments that ADs, both in terms of duration and amplitude, progress much more rapidly in the amygdala. The hippocampal AD is typical because a "silent period" follows the AD in most cases. This silent period probably reflects a local inhibitory phenomenon (Racine et al. 1972) and may contribute to limiting AD duration. Thus, processes limiting AD duration seem to be an important factor capable of retarding kindling. Besides local inhibitory phenomena, tonic inhibition at the primary site or negative feedback action might account for curtailing the AD in specific structures. While explanations at the unitary level must await further experiments the organization of amygdaloid connectivity may also be a determining factor in rapid amygdaloid kindling.

Amygdaloid connections

Firstly, it is interesting to note that almost all the nuclei which compose the amygdaloid complex are strongly interconnected (Krettek and Price 1978). Thus, stimulation of a single nucleus can have strong influences on the other nuclei. From several experiments it has been shown that the more the tissue is activated, the longer are the ADs and the more rapid is the kindling. For example, this has been demonstrated by simultaneously stimulating either both amygdalae or both hippocampi (Racine et al. 1972). Equally, we have shown that amygdaloid stimulation via 2 electrodes 1 mm apart strongly increases AD duration and subsequently facilitates kindling (unpublished result).

In addition to the intra-amygdaloid connections, the amygdaloid complex has a widely distributed projecting system which connects it with many structures in different brain areas. In this respect, the pivotal position of the amygdala is again emphasized because it is a unique structure in the brain with strong links to both the extrapyramidal and limbic systems. Recently our knowledge of amygdaloid connections has greatly increased. Strong direct interconnections between the amygdala and the lower brain stem have been found that are as big as amygdalo-hypothalamic projections (Norgren 1976; Hopkins and Holstege 1978; Krettek and Price 1978). Pontine and mesencephalic projections could serve as substrate for the autonomic and somato-motor responses elicited by amygdaloid stimulation. In a previous paper (Le Gal La Salle 1981) we showed that stimulation of the central nucleus, which is preferentially linked to the lower brain stem structures, leads more rapidly to the appearance of motor signs, including masticatory movements.

Several experiments have examined the role of specific amygdaloid afferent and efferent pathways in the establishment of amygdaloid kindling. Only lesions of the stria terminalis facilitate amygdaloid kindling (Engel and Katzman 1977; Le Gal La Salle 1977). On the contrary, lesions of the ventral amygdalofugal pathway do not modify the amygdaloid kindling rate (12.5 $\pm$ 2.9 stimulations were required in sectioned animals compared with 13.1 $\pm$ 3.2 in control animals). Among other lesions, those of the medial forebrain bundle (MFB) or the anterior commissure have no effect on the kindling rate, whereas section of the ascending noradrenergic pathways facilitates amygdaloid kindling (Ehlers et al. 1980). However, all such experiments are difficult to interpret since, depending on the time between the lesion and the kindling procedure, some sprouting or more general regenerative phenomena can occur. For example, we have shown that kindled amygdaloid seizures are transitorily blocked immediately after an MFB lesion (about 5 days are sufficient to restore a full kindled seizure) whereas an MFB lesion has no effect on kindling development (unpublished result). In addition, section of a specific pathway can facilitate propagation through other pathways. It is known that the amygdala has access to numerous structures via several routes.

Finally, the problem raised by the propagation of the ADs still remains unsolved. Much evidence shows that AD alone is sufficient for kindling. Thus, a detailed analysis of AD propagation throughout kindling development should provide the most interesting information on the participation of the different structures during the gradual establishment of kindling. Unfortunately, anatomo-electrophysiological correlations are difficult to establish. A simple relationship does not seem to exist between the involvement of ADs in specific structures and behavioural manifestations. Usually ADs diffuse very early. For example, in the cat, ADs diffuse to all the recording sites within the first few days in amygdaloid kindling and by the end of stage 1 in hippocampal kindling, even when the ADs are well focussed at the stimulating site when stimulation begins (Wada and Sato 1974; Sato 1975). As first emphasized by Delgado and Sevillano (1961), 2 types of ADs should be considered: (a) propagated ADs in which the pattern corresponds with, and seems to depend on, the pattern of the primary focal seizure; (b) reactive ADs in which the pattern is triggered, but independent of the primary site ADs. The emergence of reactive discharges in the amygdala after repetition of hippocampal stimulation is related to a growth of amplitude of the ADs and corresponds to the appearance of facial twitching (Delgado and Sevillano 1961). The development of reactive discharges and their synchronization seem to be determinant factors in generalization (Ono et al. 1981). Seizure manifestations are probably dependent on both the extent of the ADs in different structures and their EEG pattern in each of these structures. In this context a more detailed analysis of AD characteristics should provide interesting information on the respective participation of different structures in the development of kindling.

Thus, while we cannot in a short paper mention all the available data, the observations reported here argue for a central role of the amygdala in early kindling development. Since differences exist depending on the species, this report has been intentionally restricted to limbic kindling in the rat, with few references to the cat and none to the monkey.

As already emphasized, these observations lead to the necessity of clearly distinguishing at least 2 phases in kindling development. The duration and the symptomatology of the first phase is strongly dependent on the structure which is stimulated. On the contrary, the second phase seems to be a unique phenomenon regardless of the primary focus location.

Although it is still needed to characterize these phases further, it is clear that the amygdala plays a special role in triggering the second phase. Oro-alimentary motor manifestations accompanied by paroxysmal activity in the amygdala appear more or less rapidly, depending on the structure stimulated, but, in all cases, these manifestations are the typical first signs of the subsequent uniform kindling development.

Probably because of the ease with which intraneuronal amygdaloid circuits are able to generate paroxysmal activity and of its unique system of projections, the amygdala may have easier access to motor circuits than other limbic structures. In this respect, the amygdala can be thought of as playing the role of interface between non-motor limbic and motor systems. However, this role is not essential, since it can be displayed by other structures, as proved by ablation experiments. In addition, this role might also be limited in time since it is probably played by other structures, such, for example, as the midbrain reticular formation, when kindling progresses.

In conclusion, these observations clearly show that kindling cannot be regarded as a global phenomenon, but rather as the succession of distinct but linked events. In this chain of events, the amygdala occupies a special position which deserves further investigation the better to estimate and understand its role in the kindling effect as well as in other models of epilepsy.

SUMMARY

Since the original observation that repetition of initially subconvulsive stimulation can lead to a progressive and permanently enhanced epileptic susceptibility, the kindling paradigm has been extensively used in epileptic research.

Because of the ease with which kindling develops following stimulation of the amygdaloid complex, this structure offers a particular interest. For example, the hippocampus, which is also known for its vulnerability to epileptogenic procedures or conditions, requires much more stimulation than the amygdala to kindle fully.

The electrical stimulation of different limbic structures evokes different electrographic and behavioural signs which are proper to each structure. When the stimulation is repeated, typical amygdaloid signs, such as oro-alimentary manifestations, appear with variable delay according to the structure. From this stage, probably involving the amygdala, the subsequent kindling development is identical, regardless of the origin of the primary focus. EEG, behavioural and pharmacological evidences are also given which support a key role for the amygdala.

The active participation of the amygdala in kindling development is discussed on the basis of our knowledge of its synaptic organization as well as of its system of interconnections. The amygdala is unique in the brain because of its strong links with both the extrapyramidal and limbic systems. The possibility that the amygdala has an easier access to the neurocircuits involved in the development of severe limbic motor seizures is suggested.

REFERENCES

Albright, P.S., McIntyre, D. and Burnham, W. Development of a new pharmacological seizure model: effects of anticonvulsants on cortical and amygdala-kindled seizures in the rat. Epilepsia, 1980, 21: 681–689.

Andy, O.J. and Koshino, K. Duration and frequency patterns of the after-discharge from septum and amygdala. Electroenceph. clin. Neurophysiol., 1967, 22: 167–173.

Ben-Ari, Y. and Le Gal La Salle, G. Lateral amygdala unit activity. II. Habituating and non-habituating neurons. Electroenceph. clin. Neurophysiol., 1974, 37: 449–461.

Ben-Ari, Y., Lagowska, J., Tremblay, E. and Le Gal La Salle, G. A new model of focal status epilepticus: intra-amygdaloid injection of kainic acid elicits repetitive secondarily generalized convulsive seizures. Brain Res., 1979, 163: 176–180.

Ben-Ari, Y., Tremblay, E. and Ottersen, O.P. Injections of kainic acid into the amygdaloid complex in the rat: an electrographic, clinical and histological study in relation to the pathology of epilepsy. Neuroscience, 1980, 5: 515–528.

Ben-Ari, Y., Tremblay, E., Riche, D., Ghilini, G. and Naquet, R. Electrographic, clinical and pathological alterations following systemic administration of kainic acid, bicuculline or pentetrazole: metabolic mapping using the deoxyglucose method with special reference to the pathology of epilepsy. Neuroscience, 1981, 6: 1361–1391.

Burnham, W.N. Cortical and limbic kindling: similarities and differences. In: K.E. Livingston and O. Hornykiewicz (Eds.), Limbic Mechanisms. Plenum Press, New York, 1978: 507–519.

Cain, D.P. Seizure development following repeated electrical stimulation of central olfactory structures. Ann. N.Y. Acad. Sci., 1977, 290: 200–216.

Cullen, N. and Goddard, G.V. Kindling in the hypothalamus and transfer to the ipsilateral amygdala. Behav. Biol., 1975, 15: 119–131.

Delgado, J.M.R. and Sevillano, M. Evolution of repeated hippocampal seizures in the cat. Electroenceph. clin. Neurophysiol., 1961, 13: 722–733.

Ehlers, C.L., Clifton, D.K. and Sawyer, C.H. Facilitation of amygdala kindling in the rat by transecting ascending noradrenergic pathways. Brain Res., 1980, 189: 274–278.

Engel, J. and Katzman, R. Facilitation of amygdaloid kindling by lesions of the stria terminalis. Brain Res., 1977, 122: 137–142.

Engel, J., Wolfson, L. and Brown, L. Anatomical correlates of electrical and behavioral events related to amygdaloid kindling. Ann. Neurol., 1978, 3: 538–544.

Fernandez de Molina, A., Yajeya, J., Colino, A. and Velasco, J. Cyclic hyperpolarizing activity in amygdaloid neurons and limbic epilepsy. In: Y. Ben-Ari (Ed.), The Amygdaloid Complex. Elsevier/North-Holland, Amsterdam, 1981: 465–474.

Goddard, G.V. Development of epileptic seizures through brain stimulation at low intensity. Nature (Lond.), 1967, 214: 1020–1021.

Goddard, G.V., McIntyre, D.C. and Leech, C.K. A permanent change in brain function resulting from daily electrical stimulation. Exp. Neurol., 1969, 25: 295–330.

Hopkins, D.A. and Holstege, G. Amygdaloid projections to the mesencephalon, pons and medulla oblongata in the cat. Exp. Brain Res., 1978, 32: 529–547.

Kaijima, M., Tanaka, T., Ohgami, S. and Yonemasu, Y. Rapid hippocampal kindling after microinjection of quisqualic acid into the ipsilateral amygdala in cats. Electroenceph. clin. Neurophysiol., 1981, 52: 3–536.

Krettek, J.E. and Price, J.L. Amygdaloid projections to subcortical structures within the basal forebrain and brain stem in the rat and cat. J. comp. Neurol., 1978, 178: 224–254.

Le Gal La Salle, G. Effets des lésions de la strie terminale sur l'effet d'embrasement chez le chat et le rat. J. Physiol. (Paris), 1977, 73: 46A.

Le Gal La Salle, G. Kindling of motor seizures from the bed nucleus of the stria terminalis. Exp. Neurol., 1979, 66: 309–318.

Le Gal La Salle, G. Inhibition of kindling induced generalized seizures by amino oxyacetic acid. Canad. J.Physiol. Pharmacol., 1980, 58: 7–11.

Le Gal La Salle, G. Amygdaloid kindling in the rat: regional differences and general properties. In: J. Wada (Ed.), Kindling 2. Raven Press, New York, 1981: 25–38.

Le Gal La Salle, G. and Ben-Ari, Y. Unit activity in the amygdaloid complex: a review. In: Y. Ben-Ari (Ed.), The Amygdaloid Complex. Elsevier/North-Holland, Amsterdam, 1981: 227–237.

Le Gal La Salle, Y. and Cavalheiro, E.A. Stimulation of septal and amygdaloid nuclei: EEG and behavioral responses during early development of kindling with special reference to wet dog shakes. Exp. Neurol., 1981, 74: 717–727.

Lothman, E.W. and Collins, R.C. Kainic acid induced limbic seizures: metabolic, behavioral, electroencephalographic and neuropathological correlates. Brain Res., 1981, 218: 299–318.

Madryga, F.J., Goddard, G.V. and Rasmusson, D.D. The kindling of motor seizures from hippocampal commissure in the rat. Physiol. Psychol., 1975, 3: 369–373.

McIntyre, D.C. and Burnham, W. Primary and "transfer" seizure development in the kindled rat. In: J.A. Wada (Ed.), Kindling. Raven Press, New York, 1976: 61–83.

McIntyre, D.C. and Goddard, G.V. Transfer, interference and spontaneous recovery of convulsions kindled from the rat amygdala. Electroenceph. clin. Neurophysiol., 1973, 35: 533–543.

Munari, C., Bancaud, J., Bonis, A., Buser, P., Talairach, J., Szikla, G. et Philippe, A. Rôle du noyau amygdalien dans la survenue de manifestations oro-alimentaires au cours des crises épileptiques chez l'homme. Rev. E.E.G. Neurophysiol., 1979, 9: 236–240.

Nelson, M.F., Zaczek, R. and Coyle, J.T. Effects of sustained seizures produced by intrahippocampal injection of kainic acid on noradrenergic neurons: evidence for local control of norepinephrine release. J. Pharmacol. exp. Ther., 1980, 214: 694–702.

Norgren, R. Taste pathways to hypothalamus and amygdala. J. comp. Neurol., 1976, 166: 17–30.

Ono, K., Baba, H. and Mori, K. A new approach to the reactive after-discharge in the development of kindling. Int. J. Neurosci., 1981, 12: 79–85.

Racine, R.J. Modification of seizure activity by electrical stimulation: cortical areas. Electroenceph. clin. Neurophysiol., 1975, 38: 1–12.

Racine, R.J., Okujava, V. and Chipashvili, S. Modification of seizure activity by electrical stimulation. III. Mechanisms. Electroenceph. clin. Neurophysiol., 1972, 32: 295–299.

Racine, R.J., Livingston, K. and Joaquin, A. Effects of procaine hydrochloride, diazepam, and diphenylhydantoin on seizure development in cortical and subcortical structures in rats. Electroenceph. clin. Neurophysiol., 1976, 38: 355–365.

Racine, R.J. and Zaide, J. A further investigation into the mechanisms underlying the kindling phenomenon. In: K.E. Livingston and O. Hornykiewicz (Eds.), Limbic Mechanisms: The Continuing Evolution of the Limbic System Concept. Plenum Press, New York, 1978: 457–493.

Rayport, S.G. and Kandel, E.R. Epileptogenic agents enhance transmission at an identified weak electrical synapse in *Aplysia*. Science, 1981, 213: 462–464.

Sato, M. Hippocampal seizure and secondary epileptogenesis in the "kindled" cat preparations. Folia psychiat. neurol. jap., 1975, 29: 239–250.

Sato, M. A study on psychomotor epilepsy with "kindled" cat preparations. Folia psychiat. neurol. jap., 1976, 30: 426–434.

Wada, J.A. and Sato, M. Generalized convulsive seizures induced by daily electrical stimulation of the amygdala in cats: correlative electrographic and behavioral features. Neurology (Minneap.), 1974, 24: 565–574.

Kyoto Symposia (EEG Suppl. No. 36)
Editors: P.A. Buser, W.A. Cobb and T. Okuma
© 1982, Elsevier Biomedical Press, Amsterdam

Mesolimbic System and Amygdaloid Kindling

M. SATO

Department of Neuropsychiatry, Okayama University Medical School, Okayama (Japan)

It has been suggested that the central catecholaminergic system may inhibit the kindling effect and its transfer to secondary brain sites. There is some evidence that pretreatment with intraventricular (Corcoran et al. 1974) or intracerebral 6-hydroxydopamine (Mason and Corcoran 1979), as well as treatment with pimozide or haloperidol (Sato et al. 1980), facilitate amygdaloid kindling, while the kindling and transference phenomena were inhibited in cats which had been sensitized to direct and indirect dopamine agonists by chronic pretreatment with methamphetamine or cocaine (Sato et al. 1980). Depletion of brain catecholamine concentration was also reported at 1 week after amygdaloid kindling in cats (Sato and Nakashima 1975). A functional role of the mesolimbic dopamine system on kindling, however, remains unexplored. The nucleus accumbens is normally regarded as a part of the mesolimbic system arising from projections of dopamine cell bodies in the A10 group of neurones in the midbrain. It receives inputs from the limbic system including entorhinal cortex, hippocampus, hypothalamus and amygdala, and it projects to the globus pallidus, substantia nigra and midbrain tegmentum (Troiano and Siegel 1978; Krayniak et al. 1981; Somogyi et al. 1981). In accord with such anatomical relationships, Troiano and Siegel (1978) described that n. accumbens may be viewed as a transitional structure between limbic and basal ganglia. In addition, several studies have implicated the mesolimbic system in psychiatric function, notably schizophrenia (Stevens 1973). In order to examine a possible mechanism underlying psychotic states in patients with temporal lobe epilepsy, it seems worth while to examine whether a limbic seizure can result in a functional alteration in n. accumbens or not. The object of the present study was 2-fold. First, to look for possible relationships between n. accumbens and limbic structures in the kindling and transference phenomena and, secondly, to examine the possible functional role of n. accumbens in the amygdaloid kindling and transference phenomena.

GENERAL METHOD

Subjects and EEG recording

Twenty adult cats weighing 2.8–3.7 kg were used. Electrodes were implanted in all cats under sodium pentobarbital anaesthesia. The electrodes were made of stainless steel and were 0.18 mm in diameter. They were insulated with teflon or glass tubing with 1 mm exposed at the tips, and were attached in pairs. Such pair of electrodes was stereotaxically implanted into n. accumbens, amygdala, hippocampus, n. caudatus and olfactory tubercle. The electrodes were fixed in position with dental cement. EEG recordings were made on a 13-channel EEG polygraph before, during and after electrical stimulation of the brain.

Procedures for kindling and transfer to secondary brain sites

The details of this procedure have been described elsewhere (Wada and Sato 1975). Briefly, the minimal stimulus intensity needed to produce localized afterdischarge (AD) was determined initially (AD threshold) and was used for daily stimulation. Stimulation was given once daily in 1 sec trains of 60 Hz sine waves, regulated by a constant current unit. Daily stimulation to the primarily kindled brain site was continued until the animal developed generalized convulsions for 5 successive days. Subsequently, the stimulus intensity was reduced daily until generalized convulsions ceased. The minimal intensity sufficient to induce generalized convulsion was designated as the final electroconvulsive threshold (FET). Two days after the final primary site stimulation, the transference session was started. A secondary site was stimulated in the same manner as the primary site, until the animal developed secondary site generalized convulsions.

Stages of amygdaloid and hippocampal seizure development

Chronological assessment of the amygdaloid and hippocampal seizure development was performed according to the methods described previously (Sato 1975; Wada and Sato 1975). Amygdaloid seizure stages were: 1, unilateral facial twitching; 2, bilateral facial twitching; 3, head nodding; 4, tonic extension of contralateral forepaw; 5, generalized clonic jerking; 6, generalized convulsion. Hippocampal seizure stages were: 1, attention response; 2, immobility; 3, autonomic manifestation; 4, bilateral facial twitching, head nodding and masticating movements; 5, tonic extension of contralateral forepaw; 6, generalized convulsion.

Histology

The brains were removed and embedded with paraffin and serially sectioned every 20 μm to confirm the electrode placement and extent of electrolytic lesion. The results described here were obtained only in cats whose electrodes were confirmed to be in the aimed sites.

EXPERIMENT 1

To look for possible relationships between n. accumbens and limbic structures, transfer from the primary site n. accumbens to secondary sites amygdala and hippocampus, and the primary site amygdala to secondary site n. accumbens were examined in the present experiment.

Method

Five cats were used for primary site n. accumbens kindling, and 6 cats were used for the primary site amygdaloid kindling. The transfer was judged positive when the number of daily stimulations required for the secondary site kindling was significantly less than that for the primary site kindling in the same brain.

Results

(1) Seizure development during n. accumbens kindling. The principal pattern of behavioural seizure development during n. accumbens kindling was divided into 6 stages: 1, searching behaviour with contraversive head turning; 2, bilateral facial twitching; 3, head nodding; 4, contraversive circling; 5, contralateral clonic hemi-convulsion; 6, generalized convulsion. All cats developed generalized convulsion after 28 (mean) daily n. accumbens stimulations. Changes in the seizure parameters are summarized in Table I. In the EEG, AD in n. accumbens, initially propagated to the ipsilateral amygdala and hippocampus, propagated bilaterally at stage 1 or 2. Increase in AD amplitude and prolongation of AD duration appeared progressively. The spiking frequency of n. accumbens AD was identical to that of amygdaloid AD in the earlier stage, and to that of hippocampal AD in the later. Interictal spike discharge, localized in n. accumbens, appeared at stage 3 or 4.

(2) EEG changes in n. accumbens during primary amygdaloid kindling. Active AD in n. accumbens which was almost isorhythmic to that of hippocampal AD appeared at stage 3 or 4 of the amygdaloid seizure development. Interictal spikes localized in n. accumbens appeared at stage 3 or 4. Both findings suggest the emergence of an electrographic epileptic focus in n. accumbens during the amygdaloid kindling.

(3) Transfer from primary site kindling to secondary sites. The data are summarized in Table I. Positive transfer was found from n. accumbens on one side to the other side, bilateral amygdala and hippocampus, and from amygdala to ipsilateral n. accumbens. Secondary site n. accumbens convulsions were longer in duration than the primary site n. accumbens convulsions.

EXPERIMENT 2

To examine a possible functional role of n. accumbens in amygdaloid kindling, the transference phenomenon and the kindled convulsion, electrolytic lesions were made in bilateral n. accumbens before and after amygdaloid kindling.

Method

Nine cats were used. Bilateral n. accumbens lesions were made before the amygdaloid kindling in 5 cats, and after kindling in 4 cats. In both cases the post-operative recovery period was more than 2 weeks. An electrolytic lesion was made by a current at 12 V for 10 min through an electrode inserted stereotaxically under anaesthesia. The electrode was made of stainless steel (2 mm in diameter), insulated with 2 mm exposed at the tip.

TABLE I

N. ACCUMBENS KINDLING AND TRANSFER TO SECONDARY SITES

	Primary n. accumbens (N=5)	Secondary n. accumbens (N=4)	Secondary amygdala (N=6)	Secondary hippocampus (N=7)	Primary amygdala (N=6)	Primary hippocampus (N=7)
Initial response						
ADT (μA)	620.0±113.4	492.5±172.4	213.3±32.6	270.0±88.9	275.0±68.9	285.7±74.8
AD duration (sec)	4.4± 9.2	11.8± 9.2	66.0±85.5	99.5±45.4***	5.4± 2.3	10.1± 4.2
Seizure stage	(I)	(0–III)	(0–VI)	(V–VI)**	(0–I)	(0–I)
Days for kindling	28.0± 9.7	9.5± 12.4*	4.7± 4.8**	1.4± 0.5***	20.2± 2.8	35.1± 4.1
Developed response						
FET (μA)	347.5±145.9	310.0±127.7	166.7±57.7	244.3±109.2	196.4±95.2	214.3±47.6
AD duration (sec)	85.0± 17.5	125.5± 47.7	127.3±62.7	122.1± 38.9	67.0±12.1	90.9± 9.0

Primary, primary site kindling; secondary, secondary site kindling after n. accumbens kindling; ADT, after-discharge threshold; FET, final electroconvulsive threshold. Seizure stages: see Method in text.

*$P < 0.05$; **$P < 0.01$; ***$P < 0.001$ vs. each primary site kindling by Student's t test.

TABLE II

EFFECTS OF N. ACCUMBENS LESION ON AMYGDALOID KINDLING AND TRANSFER TO HIPPOCAMPUS

	N. accumbens lesion			Intact control		
	Primary amygdala (N=4)	Secondary amygdala (N=4)	Secondary hippocampus (N=5)	Primary amygdala (N=6)	Secondary amygdala (N=6)	Secondary hippocampus (N=4)
Initial response						
ADT (μA)	283.3 ± 144.3	150.0 ± 57.7	180.0 ± 44.7**	275.0 ± 68.9	213.3 ± 71.2	300.0 ± 81.6
AD duration (sec)	9.3 ± 7.6	87.0 ± 59.0	117.6 ± 17.6***	5.4 ± 2.3	53.3 ± 33.5	18.8 ± 3.0**
Seizure stage	(0–I)	(0–VI)	(V–VI)**	(0–I)	(0–VI)	(I–II)
Days for kindling	21.3 ± 7.6	3.8 ± 3.4*	1.2 ± 0.4***, [a]	20.2 ± 2.8	2.7 ± 2.8***	22.0 ± 5.8*, [b]
Developed response						
FET (μA)	226.7 ± 46.2	200.0 ± 0	180.0 ± 44.7	196.4 ± 95.2	183.3 ± 40.8	225.0 ± 64.5
AD duration (sec)	88.7 ± 17.6	125.0 ± 15.4	124.0 ± 19.7*	67.0 ± 12.1	157.5 ± 23.6	133.8 ± 18.0***
All-or-none	2(+)/4	1(+)/4	5(+)/5	6(+)/6	4(+)/6	unexamined

*$P<0.005$; **$P<0.002$; ***$P<0.001$ vs. each primary site kindling by Student's t test.
[a] $P<0.01$ as compared to [b].

TABLE III

EFFECTS OF N. ACCUMBENS LESION ON AMYGDALOID KINDLED CONVULSION

	Before lesion (N = 4)	After lesion (N = 4)
Final electroconvulsive threshold (FET, μA)	131.3 ± 55.4	118.8 ± 55.4
AD duration (sec)	71.5 ± 14.3	$87.8 \pm 20.6**$
Seizure stage	VI	VI
Response to sub-FET stimulation		
AD duration (sec)	0	$3.5 \pm 0.6*$
Seizure stage	0	0–I

$*P < 0.05$; $**P < 0.02$ with one-tail Student's t test. Sub-FET was a stimulus intensity on average 37.5 μA below the final electroconvulsive threshold intensity.

Results

The data are summarized in Table II.

(1) Effects on the amygdaloid seizure development. The intensity of initial response, amygdaloid kindling rates, FET and duration of kindled convulsions were unchanged by n. accumbens lesions before starting amygdaloid kindling. Although positive transfer from the primary site amygdala to the contralateral amygdala was unchanged, transfer to the ipsilateral hippocampus was facilitated in the n. accumbens lesion group, as compared with the control group.

(2) Effects on fully developed convulsion. After amygdaloid kindling, bilateral n. accumbens lesions were made. The data are summarized in Table III. The duration of the generalized convulsion was prolonged. The all-or-none type of response with generalized convulsion to the test stimulation at FET, which is normally seen in amygdaloid and hippocampal kindled convulsions, was lost.

DISCUSSION

Interrelationships between n. accumbens and other limbic structures

The present study showed that epileptic hyperexcitability resulting from n. accumbens kindling readily transferred to the contralateral n. accumbens, bilateral amygdala and hippocampus and, in the opposite direction, the hyperexcitability due to amygdaloid kindling readily transferred to n. accumbens. In our previous reports the following positive transfers have been defined in cats: from the septal area to the hippocampus and amygdala (Sato 1976), from the hippocampus to contralateral hippocampus and bilateral amygdala (Sato 1975), from the amygdala to bilateral hippocampus, caudate nucleus and globus pallidus (Sato 1977), and from the sylvian gyrus to ipsilateral amygdala (Sato 1981) and hippocampus (Okamoto, unpublished). With these findings, it is evident that kindling in one of these structures can lead to a secondary functional alteration in the other limbic structures in cats. As the transference phenomenon has been reported to be long lasting (McIntyre and Goddard 1973), such functional alteration must be a long lasting change. This close inter-limbic relationship is consistent with the present findings that behavioural seizure manifestations appearing during n. accumbens kindling were almost identical to those of amygdaloid kindling, and that electrographic epileptic foci appeared in n. accumbens during amygdaloid kindling. As n. accumbens has been reported to form a functional link between the limbic and motor systems for the translation of motivation into action (Graybiel 1976), long lasting epileptic hyperexcitability in n. accumbens may be involved in a triggering mechanism for a psychotic state in temporal lobe epilepsy.

A possible role of n. accumbens in amygdaloid kindling

A GABAergic inhibitory projection from n. accumbens to the globus pallidus was reported recently (Pycock and Horton 1976; Jones and Mogenson 1980), while decreased GABA levels in the experimental epileptogenic focus have been reported (Van Gelder and Courtois 1972). In addition, central dopamine was reported to act inhibitorily on the progression of amygdaloid kindling in cats (Sato and Nakashima 1975; Sato 1981). The present results, however, showed that bilateral n. accumbens lesions had no effect on the amygdaloid kindling rates, whereas they lowered the final AD threshold, prolonged the duration of amygdaloid kindled convulsions, and facilitated the positive transfer from amygdala to hippocampus. These findings showed that n. accumbens has an inhibitory action on seizure initiation, seizure duration and neuronal interaction between the amygdala and hippocampus, although it has no effect on the seizure development and possible transsynaptic changes underlying the kindling.

SUMMARY

In order to study a functional change in n. accumbens resulting from the amygdaloid seizure, and to examine the role of n. accumbens in amygdaloid seizure development, 2 experiments were done: first, interaction between the n. accumbens and amygdala was studied using kindling and the transference phenomenon and, secondly, the effects of n. accumbens lesions on amygdaloid kindling and the kindled seizure were examined in cats. (1) Positive transfer from n. accumbens to amygdala and hippocampus and behavioural seizure manifestations of n. accumbens kindling identical to those of amygdaloid kindling were shown. (2) Positive transfer from amygdaloid kindling to n. accumbens, and the emergence of an EEG epileptic focus in n. accumbens during amygdaloid seizure development were found. (3) Bilateral n. accumbens lesions lowered the final after-discharge threshold, prolonged the seizure duration, and facilitated the positive transfer from amygdala to hippocampus, while it had no effect on the amygdaloid kindling rate.

Possible functional alterations in n. accumbens due to limbic seizures and a role of n. accumbens in limbic seizure development are discussed.

REFERENCES

Corcoran, M.E., Fibiger, H.C., McGeer, E.G. and Wada, J.A. Potentiation of amygdaloid kindling and metrazol-induced seizures by 6-hydroxydopamine in rat. Exp. Neurol., 1974, 45: 118–133.

Graybiel, A.M. Input-output anatomy of the basal ganglia. In: A. Barbeau (Ed.), Basal Ganglia in Health and Disease. Society for Neuroscience, Toronto, 1976.

Jones, D.L. and Mogenson, G.J. Nucleus accumbens to globus pallidus GABA projection. Brain Res., 1980, 188: 93–105.

Krayniak, P.F., Meibach, R.C. and Siegel, A. A projection from the entorhinal cortex to the nucleus accumbens in the rat. Brain Res., 1981, 209: 427–431.

Mason, S.T. and Corcoran, M.E. Catecholamine and convulsions. Brain Res., 1979, 170: 497–507.

McIntyre, D.C. and Goddard, G.V. Transfer, interference and spontaneous recovery of convulsions kindled from the rat amygdala. Electroenceph. clin. Neurophysiol., 1973, 35: 533–543.

Pycock, C. and Horton, R. Evidence for an accumbens-pallidal pathway in the rat and its possible gabaminergic control. Brain Res., 1976, 110: 629–634.

Sato, M. Hippocampal seizure and secondary epileptogenesis in the kindling cat preparations. Folia psychiat. neurol. jap., 1975, 29: 329–350.

Sato, M. A study on psychomotor epilepsy with kindled cat preparations. Folia psychiat. neurol. jap., 1976, 30: 425–435.

Sato, M. Functional changes in the caudate and accumbens nuclei during amygdaloid and hippocampal seizure development in kindled cats. Folia psychiat. neurol. jap., 1977, 31: 501–512.

Sato, M. Kindling, transference phenomenon between temporal cortex and limbic structures in cats. Adv. physiol. Sci., 1981, 17: 509–516.

Sato, M. and Nakashima, T. Kindling: secondary epileptogenesis, sleep and catecholamines. Canad. J. neurol. Sci., 1975, 30: 439–446.

Sato, M., Tomoda, T., Hikasa, N. and Otsuki, S. Inhibition of amygdaloid kindling by chronic pretreatment with cocaine or methamphetamine. Epilepsia, 1980, 21: 497–507.

Somogyi, P., Bolam, J.P., Totterdell, S. and Smith, A.D. Monosynaptic input from the nucleus accumbens-ventral striatum region to retrogradely labelled nigrostriatal neurons. Brain Res., 1981, 217: 245–263.

Stevens, J.R. An anatomy of schizophrenia. Arch. gen. Psychiat., 1973, 29: 177–189.

Troiano, R. and Siegel, A. Efferent connections of the basal forebrain in the cat: The nucleus accumbens. Exp. Neurol., 1978, 61: 185–197.

Van Gelder, N.M. and Courtois, A. Close correlation between changing content of specific amino acids in epileptogenic cortex of cats, and severity of epilepsy. Brain Res., 1972, 43: 477–484.

Wada, J.A. and Sato, M. Generalized convulsive seizure induced by daily electrical stimulation of the amygdala in cats. Neurology (Minneap.), 1975, 24: 565–574.

Kyoto Symposia (EEG Suppl. No. 36)
Editors: P.A. Buser, W.A. Cobb and T. Okuma
© 1982, Elsevier Biomedical Press, Amsterdam

Kindling in the Spinal Cord: Differential Effects on Mono- and Polysynaptic Reflexes and its Modifications by Atropine and Naloxone

A. FERNÁNDEZ-GUARDIOLA, J.M. CALVO, L.A. BARRAGÁN, R. ALVARADO and M. CONDÉS-LARA

Unidad de Investigaciones Cerebrales, Instituto Nacional de Neurología y Neurocirugía, Insurgentes Sur No. 3877, Tlalpan, Mexico 14410, D.F. and Departamento de Farmacología, Facultad de Medicina, U.N.A.M., Mexico City (Mexico)

The permanent modifications in the CNS produced by temporal lobe amygdala kindling (TLA-K), first described by Goddard (1967), have developed into a new field in the understanding of neuronal plasticity and functional organization. This technique has demonstrated the occurrence of long-term synaptic and transsynaptic modifications which culminate in epileptic seizures when adequate low intensity electrical stimulation is carried out in a specific, irreducible time sequence. The technique has also indicated the presence of the kindling effect in structures different from TLA (Goddard et al. 1969; Wada et al. 1975; Cain 1977). Long-term bioelectrical and behavioural modifications have also been observed in caudal structures, but with the absence of seizures (Stevens and Livermore 1978; Fernández-Guardiola et al. 1981a).

Regarding the general phenomenon of CNS plasticity, most of the work has been done on monosynaptic pathways, but the polysynaptic pathways have offered results of greater behavioural interest.

Several subsystems of the CNS offer the opportunity of studying both mono- and polysynaptic kindling effects, as well as antidromic phenomena. We have been able to analyse this in the visual pathway, kindling the optic chiasm and thus activating monosynaptically the lateral geniculate body, transsynaptically the visual cortex and antidromically the retina (Fernández-Guardiola et al. 1981b). We have used the evoked response to a flash as a test of the kindling effect and found an ipsilateral enhancement of these responses in all levels, including the retina.

A well known model of mono- and polysynaptic pathways is the spinal cord, where the interneuronal pathway of presynaptic inhibition has properties which correspond to complex circuitry, having two or more synapses in serial order, and such pathways have been postulated as the simplest pathways for primary afferent depolarization (PAD) in the spinal cord (Eccles et al. 1962).

Rudomín and Dutton (1969) have demonstrated in unanaesthetized spinal cats that these pathways exhibit considerable spontaneous activity which causes excitability fluctuations in the fibre terminals. Considering the above, the aim of this work consisted in kindling the spinal cord through its afferents, analysing the mono- and polysynaptic responses in spinal unanaesthetized paralysed cats. In addition, atropine was used, based upon the known cholinergic involvement in these synaptic systems (Krnjević 1969) and naloxone was tested because of its potentiating effects on the spinal polysynaptic reflex observed in non-kindled cats (Goldfarb and Hu 1976; Bell and Martin 1977). Also, this drug facilitates amygdaloid kindling (Hardy et al. 1980) and Vindrola et al. (1981) report on levels of both leu- and metenkephalin in TLA-K.

METHOD AND MATERIAL

Twelve spinal, unanaesthetized and paralysed artificially ventilated cats were used. Tracheotomy, venous dissection and spinal cord (C6-C7) section were done under ether anaesthesia. All animals were bilaterally vagotomized. The spinal cord was exposed at the low lumbar and sacral levels and the ventral roots L6, L7 and S1 were dissected and cut for recording. Electrodes were also placed over the dorsal spinal cord surface for recording the afferent volley. After placing the electrodes, the sectioned roots and the spinal cord were covered with mineral oil. The body temperature of the cats was maintained at $37-38°C$ and the ECG was continuously monitored.

Sural, peroneal, tibial and gastrocnemius nerves were dissected distally and axonotomized; bipolar silver electrodes were placed for stimulation. The nerves were covered with mineral oil and the skin was sutured.

The kindling electrical stimulation of these nerves consisted in trains of rectangular 2 msec pulses at 100 Hz, lasting for 3 sec. The current intensity varied from 200 to 400 μA. Kindling trials were preceded by a single-shock search for the reflex to be analysed, adjusting the intensity of stimulation at threshold levels. Kindling was done every 20 min and started after $4-6$ h following the spinal cord section, once the reflex response was completely stabilized. After each kindling trial, 16 single-shock responses at 0.2 Hz were averaged. The reflex recorded in two roots, the afferent volley and the stimulus artifact were recorded on tape, analysed on line and plotted. The effect of the repetitive trains was tested on the reflex responses of the same kindled nerve and, on several occasions, on the responses of the contralateral nerve also. When kindling the sural nerve, usually both the cutaneous afferent-elicited reflex response and the monosynaptic reflex from the gastrocnemius nerve were tested. Drugs used were atropine sulphate 0.5 mg/kg, and naloxone 0.4 mg/kg, dissolved in physiological saline and administered intravenously.

RESULTS

Averaging (0.2 Hz) 16 consecutive (20 min interval) mono- and polysynaptic responses revealed a great amplitude constancy of the reflexes and the afferent volley. In some experiments, a slight progressive amplitude increment was noticeable only about 4 h after the spinal cord section. In this case, the kindling procedure was delayed until 3 consecutive controls (1 h) showed the same amplitude. In 3 experiments the control test was prolonged for 7 h without detecting amplitude increment; instead no change or a small amplitude decrement was observed.

The first kindling trials (K_1–K_3) always produced a moderate amplitude enhancement of about 20% in both poly- and monosynaptic reflexes. This increase was more prominent in polysynaptic reflexes (Fig. 1) and reached its maximum in kindling trials 7–10, followed by a plateau that lasted at least for 3 h after the last kindling stimulus, usually K_{15}. Kindling also induced changes in the late components of the reflexes. In monosynaptic reflexes, elicited by peroneal nerve stimulation, a polysynaptic late component appeared that increased progressively (Fig. 2). In polysynaptic cutaneous afferent reflexes, which were not exactly time locked at the beginning of the experiment, kindling induced synchronization, elongation and faster after-discharge. This kindling induced changes propagated ipsilaterally, provoking the reflex in a previously silent ventral root adjacent to the one reflexly activated. This phenomenon was restricted to the polysynaptic components. When the contralateral homologous ventral root was recorded and the contralateral sural nerve was tested, no propagation of the kindling effect was found.

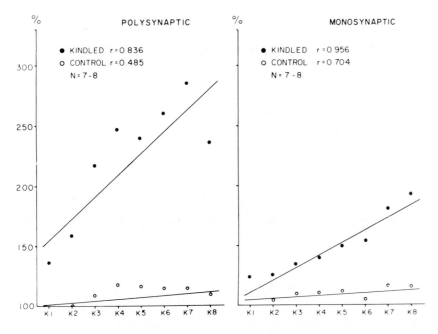

Fig. 1. Black circles: progressive increment of the polysynaptic (left) and monosynaptic (right) reflexes provoked by low intensity repetitive electrical stimulation (kindling) of the cutaneous afferent (sural) and the muscle afferent (gastrocnemius, tibial and peroneal) nerves. Each dot is the average of 128 responses from 8 cats. Ordinates: percentage amplitude values. Abscissae: kindling trials (20 min interval). White circles: average of 6–8 control reflexes elicited at the same interval in non-kindled cats.

Several experiments were carried out of kindling the sural nerve (cutaneous afferents) and testing, with 2 min delay, the gastrocnemius nerve (muscle afferents). Fig. 3 illustrates the progressive amplitude, frequency and duration increase, as mentioned, of the cutaneous polysynaptic reflex and the progressive decay of the gastrocnemius monosynaptic reflex amplitude.

Our experimental design permitted the recording of electrical stimulus intratrain responses without artifact interference despite the relatively high intensity of electrical stimulation used. The analysis of these intratrain responses showed similar changes to those described in mono- and polysynaptic single-shock test reflexes. The appearance of late polysynaptic waves, absent in the initial kindling trials, was also evident.

Atropine (0.5 mg/kg) modified the spinal cord kindling, inhibiting the progressive enhancement of amplitude, frequency and duration of the mono- and polysynaptic reflexes. Furthermore, when the maximum kindling effect was attained, a reverse effect was observed, with the greatest effect 5 min after its administration and recovery that was almost complete 30 min later.

Naloxone (0.4 mg/kg) effects were characterized by enhancement of the maximal kindling polysynaptic response, lasting up to 30 min and increasing with further kindling trials (Figs. 2 and 3). A short latency (2 min) effect was also observed. In

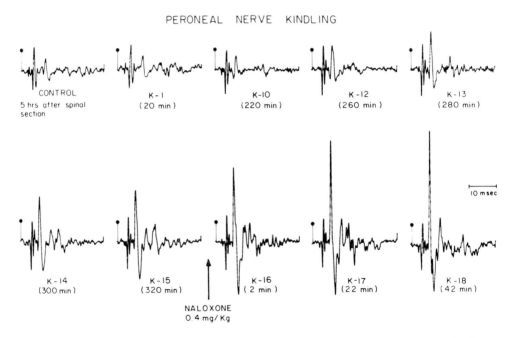

Fig. 2. Averaged mono- and polysynaptic reflexes induced by peroneal nerve single-shock stimulation in control (time 0) and after each kindling (K) trial. Each potential is the average of 16 responses analysed with a bin width of 30 μsec. Notice the slight monosynaptic increment and the more evident polysynaptic increase during kindling. After naloxone administration the polysynaptic response undergoes a further augmentation whereas the monosynaptic reflex is slightly reduced, despite the kindling trials (K-16, K-18). Dots, single-shock stimulus artifact.

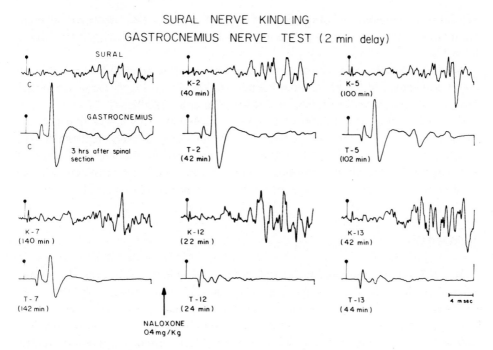

Fig. 3. Experiment showing a long latency sural nerve polysynaptic reflex progressively enhanced during kindling (upper trace). The lower trace is the averaged gastrocnemius monosynaptic reflex elicited 2 min after each sural nerve kindling trial. The monosynaptic reflex is preceded by the afferent volley. As the polysynaptic reflex increases in amplitude and in its component numbers the monosynaptic reflex progressively decreases. Both trends are noticeably accentuated by systemic naloxone, the monosynaptic reflex being almost abolished without change in the afferent volley (K-13, T-13). C, control; dots, single-shock stimulus artifacts.

contrast, diminution of the monosynaptic reflexes induced by this drug was constantly observed, even in the test-elicited reflexes of the non-kindled nerves. This was always present in the tibial and gastrocnemius monosynaptic responses.

DISCUSSION

The spinal cord reflex activity has been classically studied through experiments in which only the immediate effects were assessed. The effects of orthodromic, antidromic or direct stimulation of the spinal cord circuitry have been studied in an instantaneous manner.

Our paradigm allows observation of the middle- and long-term plastic changes that could reflect facilitation of the involved cholinergic processes, evidenced by the amplitude and frequency enhancement and the spatial propagation to the adjacent segments of the spinal cord. This is supported by the inhibitory atropine action which abolished the kindling effect, reducing the reflex responses to their control values. Moreover, the brief atropine effect (30 min) corroborates the idea that a previously augmented cholinergic activity induced by the repetitive afferent stimulation is present. This is in line with Wasterlain and Jonec's (1980) findings in TLA-K.

Another possible explanation of the progressive reflex amplitude augmentation could be changes in the enkephalin contents of the dorsal horn. These substances have been reported to be present in this area (Su et al. 1980).

Our results suggest an inhibitory role for enkephalins. This means that the cells producing the PAD could be enkephalinergic and progressively depleted by the kindling process, an idea that is indirectly corroborated by the naloxone effect of enhancement of the kindled responses. Furthermore, this is in agreement with an inhibitory enkephalinergic control of cholinergic synapses (Luján et al. 1980).

SUMMARY

We have used the kindling paradigm at the spinal cord level. In spinal, unanaesthetized, paralysed (gallamine 20 mg/kg) cats, the cutaneous afferent (sural) or the muscle afferent (gastrocnemius, tibial and peroneal) nerves were electrically stimulated at 20 min intervals with a 3 sec train (100 Hz, 2 msec pulse duration, 200–400 μA). Kindling was assessed by averaging 16 mono- or polysynaptic ventral root reflex responses produced by constant intensity single shocks. Atropine sulphate (0.5 mg/kg) and naloxone (0.4 mg/kg) effects were measured in the kindled preparation.

Kindling induced a progressive increment of the amplitude, ipsilateral propagation and after-discharge frequency. This was greater in polysynaptic responses. When testing monosynaptic responses during the kindling of cutaneous afferents, a cumulative inhibitory effect was observed. In both types of kindled response, atropine had a transient inhibitory effect. Naloxone noticeably augmented the kindled polysynaptic reflexes.

ACKNOWLEDGEMENTS

This study was supported in part by Grants 03/04/80 and 03/03/80, from the Instituto Mexicano de Psiquiatría, Mexico, D.F.

We are indebted to Dr. Rodolfo Rodríguez for commissioning Dr. L.A. Barragán to this brain research unit.

REFERENCES

Bell, J.A. and Martin, W.R. The effect of the narcotic antagonist naltrexone and nalorphine on spinal cord C-fiber reflexes evoked by electrical stimulation or radiant heat. Europ. J. Pharmacol., 1977, 42: 147–154.

Cain, D.P. Seizure development following repeated electrical stimulation of central olfactory structures. Ann. N.Y. Acad. Sci., 1977, 290: 200–216.

Eccles, J.C., Kostyuk, P.G. and Schmidt, R.F. Central pathways responsible for depolarization of primary afferent fibres. J. Physiol. (Lond.), 1962, 161: 237–257.

Fernández-Guardiola, A., Jurado, J.L. and Calvo, J.M. Repetitive low intensity electrical stimulation of cat's nonlimbic brain structures: dorsal raphe nucleus kindling. In: J.A. Wada (Ed.), Kindling, 2. Raven Press, New York, 1981a: 99–111.

Fernández-Guardiola, A., Condés-Lara, M. and Calvo, J.M. Synaptic changes induced by optic chiasm low intensity repetitive electrical stimulation: The kindling effect. In: R. Tapia and C.W. Cotman (Eds.), Regulatory Mechanisms of Synaptic Transmission. Plenum Press, New York, 1981b: 331–343.

Goddard, G.V. Development of epileptic seizures through brain stimulation at low intensity. Nature (Lond.), 1967, 214: 1020–1021.

Goddard, G.V., McIntyre, D.C. and Leech, C.K. A permanent change in brain function resulting from daily electrical stimulation. Exp. Neurol., 1969, 25: 295–330.

Goldfarb, J. and Hu, J.W. Enhancement of reflexes by naloxone in spinal cats. Neuropharmacology, 1976, 15: 785–792.

Hardy, C., Panksepp, J., Rossi, III, J. and Zolovick, A.J. Naloxone facilitates amygdaloid kindling in rats. Brain Res., 1980, 194: 293–297.

Krnjević, K. Central cholinergic pathways. Fed. Proc., 1969, 28: 113–120.

Luján, M., Valencia-Flores, G. and Rodríguez, R. Electrically induced narcotic-like dependence in the isolated guinea-pig ileum. Life Sci., 1980, 27: 1687–1693.

Rudomín, P. and Dutton, H. Effects of muscle and cutaneous afferent volleys on excitability fluctuations of Ia terminals. J. Neurophysiol., 1969, 32: 158–169.

Stevens, J. and Livermore, Jr., A. Kindling of the mesolimbic dopamine system: Animal model of psychosis. Neurology (Minneap.), 1978, 28: 36–46.

Su, T.P., Gorodetzky, C.W. and Bell, J.A. Radioimmunoassay of enkephalin: distribution in the cat spinal cord and the effect of superficial peroneal nerve stimulation. Res. Commun. Chem. Pathol. Pharmacol., 1980, 29: 43–55.

Vindrola, O., Briones, R., Asai, M. and Fernández-Guardiola, A. Amygdaloid kindling enhances the enkephalin content in rat brain. Neurosci. Lett., 1981, 21: 39–43.

Wada, J.A., Osawa, T. and Mizoguchi, T. Recurrent spontaneous seizure state induced by prefrontal kindling in Senegalese baboons, *Papio papio*. Canad. J. neurol. Sci., 1975, 2: 477–492.

Wasterlain, C.G. and Jonec, V. Cholinergic kindling: transsynaptic generation of a chronic seizure focus. Life Sci., 1980, 26: 387–391.

Kyoto Symposia (EEG Suppl. No. 36)
Editors: P.A. Buser, W.A. Cobb and T. Okuma
© 1982, Elsevier Biomedical Press, Amsterdam

Kindling: a Pharmacological Approach*

C.G. WASTERLAIN, A.M. MORIN and V. JONEC

Epilepsy and Neurology Research Laboratories, Veterans Administration Medical Center, Sepulveda, Calif. 91343, and Department of Neurology and Brain Research Institute, U.C.L.A. School of Medicine, Los Angeles, Calif. (U.S.A.)

The role of electrical current in amygdala kindling may be to release neurotransmitter. If this is true, intracerebral injection of appropriate amounts of neurotransmitters should have effects similar to electrical stimulation, with agonist and antagonist exerting appropriate actions. This was recognized by Goddard (1969) who repeatedly injected into the amygdala of rats small amounts of carbamylcholine, an agonist of the excitatory transmitter acetylcholine. The initial injections produced no behavioural change, but repeated stimulation led in about one-quarter of the animals to the progressive development of seizures. These observations were confirmed and extended by Vosu and Wise (1975) using larger amounts of carbamylcholine. We reinvestigated this phenomenon, using simple pharmacological principles to determine whether it is transsynaptically mediated, whether the type of synapse involved could be identified and how these synapses might differ from those of control, unkindled rats.

METHODS

A chemode made of a Teflon guide cannula with a bipolar twisted stainless steel electrode attached to its wall was stereotaxically implanted into the left basolateral amygdala of male Holtzman rats. For injections, the mandrel was replaced by a prefilled stainless steel tube which protruded 2 mm from the tip of the guide cannula and opened within 0.5 mm of the electrode tips. This enabled accurate delivery of volumes of 0.2–1 μl of sterile isotonic sodium chloride solution containing appropriate amounts of pharmacological agents. Following implantation, each rat was handled daily for 2 weeks, then received 1 daily injection (5 days per week) between 10 and 12 a.m. Untreated controls were handled in a similar fashion but received neither surgery nor stimulation.

Animals were killed by decapitation, following a rest period of at least 1 week. The entire brain was removed and briefly chilled on dry ice. Each brain was then placed ventral side up on a multiple razor blade device and sectioned coronally (Morin and Wasterlain 1980). Amygdala (excluding overlying cortex), hippocampus, hypothalamus, motor cortex, caudate, cerebellum and brain stem were dissected

* This work was supported by the Research Service of the Veterans Administration.

from the appropriate slice, frozen, weighed and homogenized in 0.32 M sucrose (20 mg/ml). Homogenates were used for enzyme and receptor binding assays and for protein determination by the method of Lowry et al. (1951).

The muscarinic receptor assay was based on the binding of a muscarinic agonist, [^{3}H]D,L-quinuclidinyl benzilate (3 nM) to the membranes present in whole homogenates, as described by Yamamura and Snyder (1974). Choline acetyltransferase activity was determined according to the procedure of Schrier and Shuster (1967) and McCaman and Hunt (1965). Acetylcholinesterase activity was measured according to the procedure of McCaman et al. (1968).

BEHAVIOURAL EFFECTS

Ninety-one per cent of the animals showed no behavioural response to the initial injection of 2.7 nmoles of carbamylcholine. However, a few animals did develop seizures on the first day of stimulation, and in this they differed from rats electrically kindled from amygdala. Repeated stimulation induced the progressive development of kindled seizures which resembled those induced by electrical amygdaloid kindling and were classified according to Racine (1972). We defined full kindling as the occurrence of 3 consecutive stage 5 seizures. It was remarkable that during stage 2, 3, and 4 seizure activity, the animals appeared out of touch with their environment, did not blink to threat or avoid visually threatening stimuli, and did not react to their handler. When placed at the entrance of the tube used for microwave fixation, kindled rats and handled controls normally crawl into the tube and position themselves at its extremity. During carbachol kindled seizures, rats appeared unable to crawl in the tube and were never able to position their heads in the apparatus. The initial seizure lasted from 30 sec to several minutes, and after a post-ictal period was quickly followed by other seizures, often of approximately the same intensity. With repetition, rats in stages 3, 4 and 5 frequently cycled in and out of seizure activity during a 30–60 min period and occasional animals continued to have repetitive seizures for 90 min or more. This long duration of seizure activity was expected since carbamylcholine is a poor substrate for acetylcholinesterase and therefore has a long duration of action.

ELECTROGRAPHIC DESCRIPTION

A majority of animals showed mild periodic spiking from the site of injection from the first day of stimulation, but some rats, which subsequently kindled successfully, displayed no change in electrographic activity from the amygdala on the first injection. With repeated injections, spiking became more frequent and increased in amplitude as complex paroxysmal discharges developed (Fig. 1). There was little delay between the appearance of those discharges in the amygdala and their spread to the opposite amygdala and to bilateral motor cortices. After-dischar-

CARBACHOL
DAY 1

CARBACHOL
DAY 10

CARBACHOL
+ ATROPINE
DAY 10

CARBACHOL
DAY 1
MUSCARINE-
KINDLED

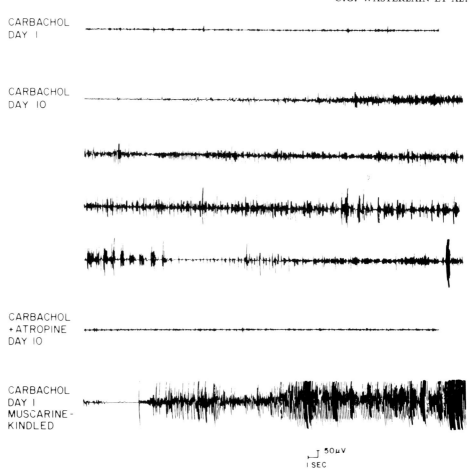

50 μV

1 SEC

Fig. 1. Electrographic record from the basolateral amygdala of male Holtzman rat following the first injection of carbachol (2.7 nmoles, 1 μl) shows minimal occasional spiking (top line). The same animal on its 10th stimulation shows prolonged seizure activity. A paired animal treated in the same way, except that each injection contained equimolar atropine (2.7 nmoles) mixed with carbachol, had a normal EEG after 10 injections. The bottom trace shows a full seizure in response to the first injection of carbachol (2.7 nmoles) in an animal previously kindled with muscarine. Compare this response to that of a similarly injected naive rat (top line).

ges were frequently delayed by 30–150 sec following injection. As they increased in complexity and duration, clinical seizures appeared and were followed by post-ictal silence. Once established, the fully kindled response of intense and complex paroxysmal activity was repeated on the majority of subsequent stimulations even after prolonged periods of rest. Considerable variability in the amplitude and duration of after-discharges was observed from day to day and bore no apparent relationship to any of the behavioural events that we measured.

DOSE DEPENDENCE AND TIME COURSE

In 6 rats, daily injections of 0.27 nmoles of carbachol produced no seizures or kindling. Injections of 1 nmole daily kindled approximately half the animals, while 2.7 nmole injections kindled the majority of rats. Progressively larger amounts of carbachol shortened kindling time, the mean time needed to reach a first stage 5 seizure being 15 ± 2.4 days after 2.7 nmoles ($N = 10$), 8.6 ± 3.5 after 5.4 nmoles ($N = 5$), 6 ± 1 after injections of 13.5 nmoles ($N = 9$), and 4.8 ± 0.6 days after injections of 27 nmoles ($N = 19$). Injections of amounts greater than 27 nmoles produced status epilepticus which was often fatal, so that kindling could not be assessed.

The duration of the interstimulus interval was critical for the rate of kindling. After 10 stimulations, rats injected 3 times a day had only reached a mean seizure stage of 0.7 ± 0.2 while animals injected once a day reached a mean seizure stage of 2 ± 0.6 and those injected twice a week had a mean seizure stage of 4.2 ± 0.8. All 3 groups had an N of 6 and eventually reached full kindling.

The change in excitability induced by repeated carbachol injection was long lasting. After 20 stimulations, 6 animals were rested for 1 week. On subsequent injection of 2.7 nmoles of carbachol they reached a mean seizure stage of 3.5 ± 1.5. After an additional 2 weeks of rest, mean seizure stage was 3 ± 1.6. After an additional 4 weeks of rest, the 3 animals whose chemodes were still usable all had a stage 5 seizure. This was repeated after an additional 8 weeks of rest.

Extensive histological studies revealed a small cavity at the tip of the chemode, a mild foreign body reaction around the cannula with occasional giant cells, but no light microscopic difference could be identified between kindled rats injected with carbachol and non-kindled controls injected with saline or with carbachol plus atropine.

MEDIATION BY MUSCARINIC SYNAPSES

Six fully kindled rats were rested for a week, then injected with 27 nmoles of carbachol mixed with 100 nmoles of D-tubocurarine, a blocker of nicotinic receptors. Mean seizure stage was 4.2 ± 0.6, showing that blockage of nicotinic receptors had no effect on the seizure intensity. At weekly intervals the experiment was repeated, replacing D-tubocurarine by varying amounts of atropine. As little as 6 pmoles of atropine significantly inhibited the seizures induced by carbachol. Equimolar mixtures of atropine and carbachol markedly reduce seizure activity, the median seizure stage on any day of carbachol plus atropine treatment being zero. In addition, use of a mixture of carbachol plus atropine injected daily into naive animals failed to produce any seizure on any day of stimulation (Table I). This suggests that blockage of nicotinic synapses had no effect on the seizures but blockage of muscarinic synapses completely prevented kindling in naive animals and significantly reduced its expression in kindled animals.

TABLE I

MEAN SEIZURE STAGE ± S.E.M. FOLLOWING INJECTION ON EACH TRIAL OF 1 μl OF STERILE ISOTONIC SOLUTION THROUGH A CHEMODE CHRONICALLY IMPLANTED IN THE LEFT BASOLATERAL AMYGDALA OF MALE HOLZMAN RATS

The solution contained NaCl only (saline group, n = 6), carbamylcholine 2.7 nmoles + NaCl (carbachol A, n = 6; B, n = 15; C, n = 6) or carbamylcholine 2.7 nmoles + atropine 2.7 nmoles + NaCl (carbachol-atropine, n = 5).

	Carbachol group A (3 trials/day)		Carbachol group B (1 trial/day)		Carbachol group C (0.3 trial/day)		Carbachol atropine (1 trial/day)		Saline group (1 trial/day)	
Trial 1	0	(6)	0.8 ± 0.3	(15)	0.5 ± 0.3	(6)	0	(5)	0	(6)
Trial 5	0.6 ± 0.4	(6)	2.3 ± 0.4	(15)	3.3 ± 0.6	(6)	0	(5)	0	(6)
Trial 10	0.9 ± 0.3	(6)	2.8 ± 0.3	(15)	3.7 ± 0.9	(6)	0	(5)	0	(6)
Last trial	3.4 ± 0.8	(6)	3.0 ± 0.5	(12)	4.5 ± 0.5	(6)	0	(5)	0	(6)
1 week rest	5	(3)	3.5 ± 1.5	(3)	3.5 ± 0.9	(5)	–		–	
2 weeks rest	5	(3)	3.0 ± 1.5	(3)	5	(5)	0.6 ± 0.3	(5)	0.7 ± 0.4	(6)
4 weeks rest	5	(1)	5	(1)	5	(1)	–		–	

The muscarinic agonist muscarine was effective in inducing kindled seizures on daily injections of 3 nmoles into the amygdala. Both seizure development and expression were very similar to those induced by carbachol. In 6 rats which were fully kindled with carbachol then rested for 1 week, injection of a subconvulsive amount of muscarine (3 nmoles) instead of producing the mild spiking and lack of behavioural change expected from the first muscarine injection, induced a generalized seizure (mean stage 3.8 ± 0.7) characteristic of kindled animals. Transfer was equally effective in the opposite direction. Six rats kindled with muscarine, upon their first carbachol injection (2.7 nmoles) had a mean seizure stage of 3.2 ± 1.5.

We injected rats with stereoisomers of the muscarinic agonist acetyl-β-methylcholine (ABM) once daily in a sterile isotonic 1 μl volume containing 3 nmoles. The (−)-isomer, which has little affinity for muscarinic receptors, produced no kindling. The (+)-isomer induced progressive seizure development which, however, remained brief and partial. Since (+)-ABM is a good substrate for cholinesterase, (+)-ABM was delivered with the cholinesterase inhibitor physostigmine. This resulted in rapid and effective kindling.

Equimolar amounts of atropine used with muscarine or carbachol completely blocked kindling. Quinuclidinyl benzilate (QNB) and scopolamine were also effective blockers of both carbachol and muscarine-induced seizures, QNB being slightly more potent and scopolamine less potent than atropine. QNB was characterized by prolonged duration of action following a single injection, which markedly decreased seizure responses to carbachol for over a week.

If kindling is mediated through a particular postsynaptic apparatus, the relative potencies of various agonists and antagonists of its transmitter should be similar in their affinities for the receptor in vitro and in their behavioural effects in vivo. Fig.

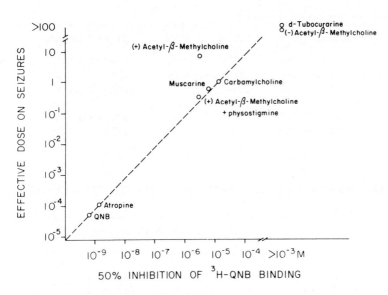

RELATIONSHIP BETWEEN KINDLING POTENCIES AND AFFINITY
FOR MUSCARINIC RECEPTORS

Fig. 2. The "effective dose" was the amount of agonist that induced at least 1 stage 5 seizure in 50% of the rats in a 20 day (1 injection/day) trial, or the amount of antagonist that prevented seizures in 50% of fully kindled animals when mixed with 2.7 nmoles of carbamylcholine in a 1 μl injection.

2 suggests that the relative potencies of muscarinic agonists and antagonists in vivo and in vitro were remarkably similar and strongly supports our interpretation that obligatory mediation through a group of muscarinic synapses reached by pharmacological agents injected into the amygdala is a feature of this type of chemical kindling.

SYNAPTIC CHEMISTRY

Assays for QNB binding sites, choline acetyltransferase and acetylcholinesterase activities revealed no difference between controls and experimentals, or between left (injected) and right (uninjected) sides in kindled animals. Other brain regions were also unaffected by the treatment (Tables II, III and IV). Concentrations of enzymes and receptors were similar to those expected in the sample regions from published values (Yamamura and Snyder 1974; Morin and Wasterlain 1980).

Since diffusion of injected pharmacological agents was relatively limited, and kindling was completely blocked by atropine or QNB, it is likely that the muscarinic receptors stimulated by the injectate were located close to the site of injection and were included in the biopsy. Since all experimental animals were fully kindled and rested for at least a week before death, these results do not exclude the possibility

TABLE II

CHOLINERGIC MUSCARINIC RECEPTORS IN BRAIN AREAS OF CARBACHOL-KINDLED RATS

[³H]QNB specifically bound (femtomoles/mg protein).

Area	Control	Carbachol-kindled	Carbachol/atropine
Left amygdala	828.6 ± 140.2 (9)	737.0 ± 126.0 (5)	820.0 ± 159.4 (3)
Right amygdala	888.4 ± 109.6 (10)	844.8 ± 141.8 (6)	913.6 ± 155.4 (4)
Cortex	1219.1 ± 85.3 (9)	1004.2 ± 167.0 (7)	1089.3 ± 172.5 (4)
Hippocampus	1116.8 ± 232.6 (9)	932.6 ± 153 (7)	1217.9 ± 262 (4)
Striatum	1347.8 ± 220.0 (10)	1212.1 ± 327 (7)	990.3 ± 146.2 (4)
Cerebellum	119.9 ± 32.9 (6)	123.4 ± 171.1 (4)	102.5 (2)

TABLE III

CHOLINE ACETYLTRANSFERASE ACTIVITY IN BRAIN AREAS OF CARBACHOL-KINDLED RATS

Area	Control	CAT activity (μmoles/g protein/h)	
		Carbachol-kindled	Carbachol/atropine
Left amygdala	51.8 ± 21.4 (n = 10)	62.8 ± 6.9 (n = 3)	53.9 (n = 1)
Right amygdala	52.8 ± 12.1 (n = 10)	65.5 ± 14.9 (n = 3)	66.3 (n = 2)
Cortex	19.4 ± 5.6 (n = 10)	17.3 ± 5.0 (n = 4)	17.8 (n = 2)
Hippocampus	25.4 ± 6.8 (n = 10)	23.4 ± 5.7 (n = 4)	24.6 (n = 2)
Striatum	67.6 ± 22.1 (n = 10)	61.0 ± 14.5 (n = 4)	44.9 (n = 2)
Cerebellum	2.7 ± 0.3 (n = 10)	2.5 ± 0.4 (n = 4)	2.8 (n = 2)

TABLE IV

CHOLINESTERASE ACTIVITY IN BRAIN AREAS OF CARBACHOL-KINDLED RATS

Area	Control (n = 10)	Cat activity (μmoles/mg protein/h)	
		Carbachol-kindled (n = 4)	Carbachol/atropine (n = 2)
Left amygdala	6.6 ± 2.4	5.1 ± 1.7	5.9
Right amygdala	7.0 ± 1.3	5.1 ± 1.9	4.8
Striatum	15.3 ± 2.3	16.3 ± 3.8	11.9
Cortex	2.1 ± 1.5	2.3 ± 0.8	1.6
Hippocampus	3.8 ± 1.9	3.9 ± 0.3	2.8
Hypothalamus	3.0 ± 0.3	2.2 ± 0.9	2.4
Brain stem	2.9 ± 0.5	2.5 ± 1.0	2.3
Cerebellum	1.3 ± 0.1	2.6 ± 1.6	2.4

that transient changes in QNB binding sites similar to those described in electrical kindling of the amygdala (McNamara 1978) might have taken place at earlier times in chemical kindling. However, since kindling persists for at least 8 weeks without stimulation (see above) and changes in QNB binding sites were not found after 1 week without stimulation, these changes would be unlikely to represent the substrate of the long lasting change in excitability which characterizes the phenomenon.

Preliminary studies (Wasterlain and Farber 1982) suggest that in vitro phosphorylation of synaptic plasma membrane proteins from the kindled hippocampus is markedly reduced compared to controls. The most striking change was seen in a protein of approximately 50,000 dalton separated by SDS-polyacrylamide gel electrophoresis. It persisted in kindled animals killed after 2 weeks without stimulation, and therefore does not appear to be a result of the seizures. Further studies will be needed to assess the significance of this finding.

CONCLUSION

The evidence summarized above suggests that the establishment of the engram of muscarinic kindling is mediated through the excitation of muscarinic receptors reached by the injected solution. In this model, the change of activity of a population of muscarinic synapses in or around the amygdala appears sufficient and necessary to cause a long lasting change in excitability resulting in an epileptic focus able to generate spontaneous seizures in some animals. The complete block of the phenomenon by 3 different muscarinic blockers, the complete failure of other receptor blockers (e.g. nicotinic) and the lack of histological changes rule out, as a source of seizures, scar formation, change in extracellular space, or glial proliferation, none of which would be altered by the addition of atropine or QNB to a solution of carbachol. It appears that this model provides the strongest evidence to date that epilepsy can be a disease of cell to cell communication and can be acquired as a result of abnormal transsynaptic activity. The induction of this phenomenon by multiple agonists, the easy and full transfer from one agonist to another, its blockage by multiple antagonists, the linearity of in vivo and in vitro potencies, and the demonstration of stereospecificity on the behaviour strongly support the view that in this model, the genesis of the epileptic focus is best explained by the aggregate hypothesis. In other words, abnormal synaptic communication is both necessary and sufficient for the genesis of an epileptic focus.

The long duration of the change in excitability induced by repeated carbachol injections raises interesting questions. A new and very abnormal behaviour was acquired by carbachol-injected rats as a result of the periodic excitation of a group of muscarinic synapses. It is intriguing that this change in excitability could persist for at least 8 weeks in the absence of further stimulation. Some of our experiments would seem to rule out the hypothesis of a constantly firing synaptic circuit required for the persistence of the new engram, since the injection of atropine did not erase the change in excitability in kindled animals, but fully abolished the seizures in many animals. As soon as the atropine was eliminated, these animals again responded to subconvulsive carbachol injections with full seizures. Reverberating circuits would presumably have been interrupted by blockage of a key component and would not have been able to return to a kindled state. Perhaps the retardation of kindling by inhibitors of protein synthesis (Jonec and Wasterlain 1979) is a clue to its nature.

The increase in response following repetitive stimulation observed in kindling is relatively characteristic of the brain, and the opposite of the adaptation, desensitization or general decrease in response on repeated stimulation observed in most organs. The complexity of cerebral circuitry and the multiplicity of feedback mechanisms in the central nervous system are such that the mediation of these changes by mechanisms such as denervation supersensitivity is not excluded. In fact, the dependence of the kindling phenomenon upon the rate of stimulation and the interstimulus interval might suggest a role for denervation supersensitivity. Feedback circuits may have to be set in motion for a certain period of time to induce either desensitization of inhibitory synapses or supersensitivity of excitatory synapses. However, the simple chemical changes of modification in the number or affinity of muscarinic receptors which one might expect in such a phenomenon were not observed. It should be noted that this evidence does not rule out involvement of muscarinic receptors in chemical kindling. QNB binding assays may measure only the antagonist form of the receptor and bear an uncertain relationship to its physiological response. Changes in presynaptic physiology or in postsynaptic biochemistry occurring beyond the receptor represent equally plausible alternatives.

The transsynaptic acquisition of an abnormal behaviour and its retention without further stimulation in adults imply that under certain circumstances transient stimulation of some receptors may be sufficient to generate long lasting abnormal behaviour, even in the adult. It might serve as a conceptual model for the acquisition of persistent abnormal behaviour which appears for the first time in the fully developed brain, such as some types of post-traumatic epilepsy, or abnormal behaviour associated with acquired psychiatric illness.

SUMMARY

Injection of a few nanomoles of the muscarinic agonists carbamylcholine, muscarine or (+)-acetyl-β-methylcholine once a day into the rat amygdala was initially subconvulsive, but on repetition led to the progressive development of kindled epileptic seizures. This behaviour was stereospecific, was potentiated by the cholinesterase inhibitor physostigmine, and was blocked by the muscarinic antagonists atropine, QNB and scopolamine. The kindling potencies of cholinergic muscarinic agonists and antagonists paralleled their relative affinities for muscarinic receptors in vitro. No changes in muscarinic receptors, in cholinesterase or in choline acetyltransferase were observed in kindled brains after a stimulation-free period of at least 1 week. These data support the aggregate hypothesis of epileptogenesis and suggest that abnormal activity through a particular group of muscarinic synapses can be sufficient to generate an epileptic focus.

ACKNOWLEDGEMENTS

We are indebted to S. Weems and I. Tanaka for technical help, and to P. Oblander and P. Shamblin for secretarial help.

REFERENCES

Goddard, G.V. Analysis of avoidance conditioning following cholinergic stimulation of amygdala. J. comp. physiol. Monogr., 1962, 2: 1–18.

Jonec, V. and Wasterlain, C.G. Effect of inhibitors of protein synthesis on the development of kindled seizures in rats. Exp. Neurol., 1979, 66: 524–532.

Lowry, O.H., Rosebrough, N.H., Farr, A.L. and Randall, R.J. Protein determination with the Folin reagent. J. biol. Chem., 1951, 193: 269–275.

McCaman, R.E. and Hunt, J.M. Microdetermination of choline acetylase in nervous tissue. J. Neurochem., 1965, 12: 253–259.

McCaman, R.E., Tomey, L.R. and McCaman, R.E. Radiometric assay of acetylcholinesterase activity in submicrogram amounts of tissue. Life Sci., 1968, 7: 233–244.

McNamara, J.P. Muscarine cholinergic receptors participate in the kindling model of epilepsy. Brain Res., 1978, 154: 415–420.

Morin, A.M. and Wasterlain, C.G. Aging and rat brain muscarinic receptors as measured by quinuclidylbensilate binding. Neurochem. Res., 1980, 5: 301–308.

Morrell, F. and Tsuru, N. Kindling in the frog: development of spontaneous epileptiform activity. Electroenceph. clin. Neurophysiol., 1976, 40: 1–11.

Racine, R.J. Modification of seizure activity by electrical stimulation. II. Motor seizure. Electroenceph. clin. Neurophysiol., 1972, 32: 281–294.

Schrier, B.K. and Shuster, L. A simplified radiochemical assay for choline acetyltransferase. J. Neurochem., 1967, 14: 977–985.

Vosu, H. and Wise, R.A. Cholinergic seizure kindling in the rat: comparison of caudate, amygdala and hippocampus. Behav. Biol., 1975, 13: 491–495.

Wasterlain, C.G. and Farber, D. A lasting change in protein phosphorylation associated with septal kindling. Brain Res., 1982, 247: 191–194.

Yamamura, H.T. and Snyder, S.H. Muscarinic cholinergic binding in rat brain. Proc. nat. Acad. Sci. (Wash.), 1974, 71: 1725–1729.

Kyoto Symposia (EEG Suppl. No. 36)
Editors: P.A. Buser, W.A. Cobb and T. Okuma
© 1982, Elsevier Biomedical Press, Amsterdam

Common Aspects of the Development of a Kindling Epileptogenic Focus in the Prepyriform Cortex of the Dog and in the Hippocampus of the Rat: Spontaneous Interictal Transients with Changing Polarities

F.H. LOPES DA SILVA[1], W.J. WADMAN[1], L.S. LEUNG[2] and K. VAN HULTEN[3]

[1]*Department of Animal Physiology, University of Amsterdam, Kruislaan 320, 1098 SM Amsterdam (The Netherlands),* [2]*Department of Psychology, University of Western Ontario, London, Ontario N6A 5C2 (Canada), and* [3]*Department of Clinical Neurophysiology, University Hospital Utrecht, Nic. Beetsstraat 24, 3511 HG Utrecht (The Netherlands)*

The "kindling" experimental model of epilepsy which was originally described by Goddard (1967) offers the attractive property that the experimental focus develops gradually and depends in a characteristic way on the pattern of electrical stimulation and probably also on the brain area and animal species. It consists essentially of periodic (usually daily) mild electrical stimulation of a brain area with a short train of pulses (e.g. 1 sec) which leads to the development of electro-behavioural epileptic seizures after a certain number of stimuli. The kindling model has been most commonly studied in rats (Goddard et al. 1969; Racine 1972a,b; McIntyre and Goddard 1973; Pinel et al. 1974, 1975), in rabbits (Tanaka 1972), in cats (Sato and Nakashima 1972; Wada and Sato 1974; Lange et al. 1977), in dogs (Van Hulten et al. 1977; Wauquier et al. 1979), in monkeys (Goddard et al. 1969; Wada and Osawa 1976), and in a modified way in frogs (Morrell and Tsuru 1976). Gaito (1974) has also suggested that the same process may occur in humans undergoing extensive electroshock treatment. The brain areas most commonly used for kindling are the amygdala and rather ill-defined areas of the temporal or frontal lobes.

Our aim in this research was to investigate the main electrophysiological phenomena characteristic of the formation of a slowly developing epileptogenic focus induced by kindling. At first we chose as preparation the prepyriform cortex (PPC) of the dog (beagle) for the following reasons: (a) it is the primary olfactory cortex with a well known set of inputs and outputs and (b) it has a rather simple 3-layered structure with a characteristic pattern of interconnections.

In the course of this study we found the intriguing phenomenon that during kindling the development of the epileptogenic focus is accompanied by the appearance of spontaneous interictal transients (SITs), or EEG spikes, with different polarities depending upon the phase of the evolution of the kindling process. This prompted us to study this phenomenon in more detail in another preparation in order to determine whether the occurrence of SITs of different polarities could be generalized to another kindling model. Therefore we studied in the second place the electrophysiology of SITs during the development of a kindled focus in the hippocampus of rat. This is a structure of choice for such an electrophysiological analysis given its well organized laminar structure (Lopes da Silva and Arnolds 1978).

Both in the PPC of dog and in the hippocampus of rat we investigated also the evoked potentials (EPs) obtained by stimulation of specific input pathways. This was of importance to help understanding the changes in SITs.

MATERIAL AND METHODS

(1) Experiments in dog

Electrodes and their placement

Three dogs (beagles) were prepared with about 40 chronically indwelling stainless steel electrodes with tip diameters of 100 μm and uninsulated up to 300 or 500 μm of the tip. The wires were twisted to form bundles of 2–5 electrodes with distances between electrode tips of 500 μm. These electrodes were stereotaxically implanted in several structures: olfactory bulb (OB), lateral olfactory tract (LOT), PPC (bilaterally), amygdala (Amy), hippocampus (Hip), reticular pontine nucleus (NRPO) and thalamic nucleus, namely the nucleus centre median (THCM). In addition, electrodes were placed subdurally or in the skull overlying the temporal lobes. The stereotaxic coordinates were based on the atlas of the beagles' brain of Dua-Sharma et al. (1970). Post-mortem histological examination was carried out and showed that the target structures were reached, namely the PPC electrodes were placed in such a way that they straddled the pyramidal cell layer.

Recording

The EEGs of the dogs were recorded with the animals in a standard behavioural situation; they were strapped into a classical treadmill provided with a displacement transducer in which they could walk actively in circles of 2.60 m diameter. This arrangement allowed the dogs' displacement to be easily converted into an electrical signal which was written on the EEG paper. The behaviour of the dogs was also monitored by means of a closed circuit TV system and, when of interest, it was recorded on video tape. EEG derivations were to a common reference electrode, a stainless steel pin placed in the frontal bone at the level of the frontal sinus. Sixteen EEG signals were transmitted by means of a 16-channel radiotelemetry system (Storm van Leeuwen and Kamp 1969). The signals were further amplified by the amplifiers of a 16-channel EEG machine (Elema-Schönander), filtered (time constant, 0.3 sec; low pass filter, 70 Hz) and written on paper together with a digital time code, the output of the displacement transducer and the pulses used for stimulation.

Stimulation

Two types of stimulation were used, for kindling (abbreviation K) and for EP investigations. Both were applied through cable connections using sliding contacts so that there was no interference with the dog's movements in the treadmill. As a generator, a Neurolog device controlled by a Digitimer (Devices) and with an isolation unit was used to provide constant current pulses. The kindling stimulus (K stimulus) consisted of 1 sec long trains of biphasic pulses (60/sec, 1 msec duration, 100 μA) applied daily through 2 electrodes placed in the PPC; these 2 electrodes were part of a bundle placed vertically in the PPC so that the last electrode of the bundle was at the level of the superficial pyramidal cell layer. One electrode used for K lay immediately above the tip of the bundle and another about 1–1.5 mm above it. The EPs were elicited by single pulses applied to the LOT. The stimuli were monophasic pulses with a duration of 200 μsec and a variable amplitude depending upon the purpose of the experiment, as described below; they were usually given at the rate of 1/sec.

Both K and EP stimuli were administered in the same behavioural condition while the dog was standing still, alert and waiting for the click of the food dispenser which signalled the food reward.

(2) Experiments in rat

Electrodes and their placement

Twelve Wistar rats were implanted with a number of stainless steel electrode bundles of 100 μm diameter with sharp cut tips in both dorsal hippocampi region CA1. Three electrodes used for stimulation were lowered to the level of the stratum radiatum in order to stimulate the Schaffer collaterals. On the basis of electrophysiological criteria (Leung 1979) a pair of electrodes (interelectrode distance 700 μm) was positioned in such a way that they straddled the CA1 pyramidal cell layer. A reference electrode was placed on the frontal bone. All electrodes were cemented in place and soldered to a connector plug.

Recording

Hippocampal EEG signals were recorded by way of 4 field-effect transistors (FETs) which were mounted on the connector plug. This was connected via a cable and a commutator to standard amplifiers. In this way the rat was allowed relative freedom of movement in its cage during recording and stimulation.

Stimulation

Although the rats were provided with recording electrodes in both dorsal hippocampi, the stimulating electrodes were placed only on the left side. The kindling stimulus and the single pulses used for the study of EPs were applied to the left dorsal hippocampus. The kindling stimulus consisted of a 1 sec long train of biphasic pulses (50/sec, 1 msec duration); it was applied daily. The EPs were elicited by single pulses (duration 100 μsec, variable amplitude, rate 1/5 sec) applied to the Schaffer collaterals.

ANALYSIS

The EPs were averaged on a CAT-400C (Mnemotron) special purpose computer and plotted on paper using an X-Y plotter. In some cases these averaged EPs were digitized by using a Tektronix type Digitizer or a common AD converter (sampling rate 2000/sec) and stored on the disk of a PDP 11/40 computer. Some samples of EEG signals were also digitized by the ADC of a Motorola Exorset microcomputer which was programmed to average a chosen number of EPs and to compute the standard deviation at each sample point. In some experiments SITs were automatically detected on the basis of an amplitude threshold criterion. After visual control to exclude artefacts these SITs could be averaged too.

HISTOLOGY

At the end of the experiments the animals were killed, perfused with saline and formalin with added potassium ferrocyanide; histological sections of the brain were made and the electrode positions were verified by the Prussian blue reaction.

RESULTS

(1) Experiments in dog

(1.1) Types of seizure: kindling (K) and spontaneous

The ultimate aim of these experiments was, of course, to find out how K of the PPC would lead to the development of electro-behavioural seizures in beagles. In 1 dog (Th), we fixed the strength of the K stimulus at 100 μA because this did not give rise to noticeable behavioural changes or after-discharges on the first application; in contrast, a K stimulus of 200 μA would induce a short train of after-discharges. After 34 K sessions (5 per week), a seizure developed. This was a complex seizure which started with a head movement, facial clonus, licking movements followed by wide opening of the mouth, turning the head and body to the right, lifting the front leg followed by loss of equilibrium so that the dog fell on his left side; while it lay on the floor, there was a rather long phase of opisthotonus followed by forelimb clonus and later also hind limb clonus and walking movements and the passage of urine. This seizure lasted about 1 min. At the end of the seizure, the animal rose up but it was obvious from the overt behaviour that it was disturbed in its spatial orientation. The performance of the conditioned task was also disturbed for a more or less long period (about 5–10 min); in this period, the dog did not react properly to the click of the food dispenser, did not pick up food which was made available and walked in the treadmill in erratic directions.

In a second dog (Ti), the current strength of the K stimulus was also fixed at 100 μA, which initially produced no after-discharges or behavioural changes. After 60 K stimuli according to the schedule described above, the dog developed a partial complex seizure with almost the same pattern as that described above; the only difference was that the very early stage was characterized by a repeated pendular movement of the head followed by an extreme and long lasting opening of the mouth.

In a third dog (C) the K stimulus had a current strength of 40 μA; after 100 K stimuli the dog developed a partial complex seizure with the same pattern as in the first case.

In electroencephalographic terms the K seizures can be described as a succession of periods: in a first period, lasting about 3 or 4 sec, there was a drastic decrease in EEG amplitude in the PPC and Amy derivations which was terminated by a first large peak or sharp wave in the same derivations; in a second period of about the same duration, a series of large amplitude peaks appeared in the PPC simultaneously with rhythmic large waves (about 11/sec) with sharp peaks in most other derivations, but less evident in OB and Hip; a third period, less well defined, was characterized mainly by small amplitude high frequency beta activity interspersed with peaks in some PPC derivations; in the Amy however, there were large rhythmic waves of about 22/sec; a fourth period was similar to the

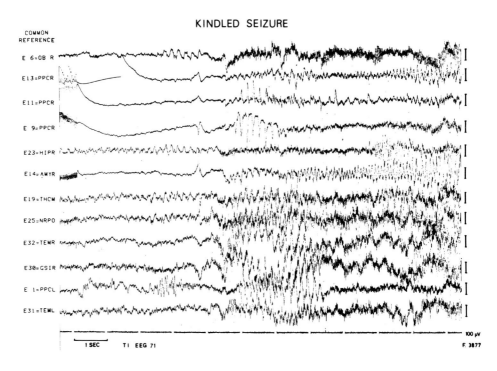

Fig. 1. (a) Samples of the EEG of a kindled seizure (dog Ti) and (b) of a spontaneous seizure. Abbreviations (for this and for other figures): OB, olfactory bulb; PPC, prepyriform cortex; Hip, hippocampus; Amy, amygdala; THCM, thalamus – centre median; NRPO, nucleus reticularis pontis oralis; TEM, temporal cortex (convexity); GSI, sigmoid gyrus; R, right side; L, left side. For description see text.

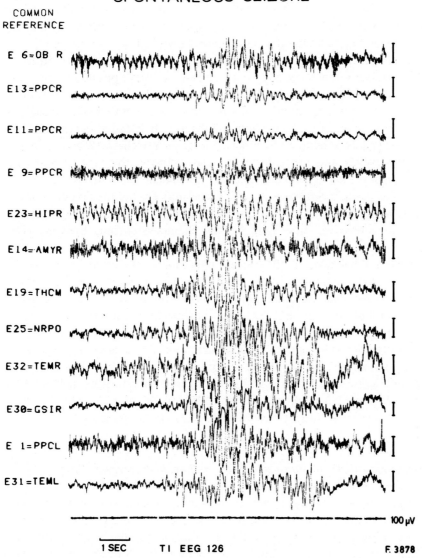

Fig. 1b.

corresponding periods of common seizures: there were large rhythmic waves of about 3–5/sec in all derivations, which increased in amplitude and gradually decreased in frequency until they terminated abruptly; this period lasted about 40–60 sec. Several variants of this type of seizure were encountered but the beginning was always almost identical.

After the first K seizure had been elicited, the continuation of the K procedure led to seizures in about 2 out of 3 times. In one of the dogs K stimuli were applied over a long time (5 weeks after the first seizure) until it was noticed that the dog suffered from repeated spontaneous seizures (without electrical stimulus) which, however, had a different character from those elicited by K, both as regards the EEG and the behaviour. Examples of the EEGs of a K-triggered seizure and one occurring spontaneously (3–4 sec) in the same animal are shown in Fig. 1.

The EEG of spontaneous seizures differed very much from the pattern described above. These seizures were initially characterized by brief episodes of rhythmic peaky waves of increasing and then decreasing amplitude, often in the form of a spindle; the main frequency within the spindle was 4–5/sec but there were important higher harmonic components. The whole spindle usually lasted about 6 sec. These EEG episodes were accompanied by a behavioural seizure characterized mainly by clonus of the eyelids and other facial muscles, namely, the nostrils and ears, sometimes accompanied by licking and jaw movements and lifting of the left foreleg; in a few cases, a certain unsteadiness was noticed, but the dog did not lose equilibrium. These episodes lasted as long as the EEG seizure pattern and thus were often difficult to observe; they could be well characterized only by using video recordings.

These EEGs and behavioural differences imply that the underlying processes for the K and the "spontaneous" seizures may differ. The question arose as to where within the brain the "spontaneous" seizures began or, in more precise terms, at which derivations did the first EEG changes characteristic of a seizure appear.

This was studied by making histograms of the number of times each EEG derivation was scored as being the first at which those EEG changes appeared. The results are summarized in Fig. 2. It can be seen that the beginning of a "spontaneous" seizure was encountered in the right temporal cortex in 46% of the cases followed by the left temporal cortex in 25% of the cases; in contrast, the K seizures always appeared to start (according to EEG visual inspection) in the PPC-amygdala area.

(1.2) Spontaneous interictal transients (SITs) and evoked potentials (EPs)

In the EEG recorded after the cessation of the after-discharges SITs were observed which presented a characteristic evolution. The most common types of SITs are shown in Fig. 3; we classified them into 2 main types: type A SITs which are mono- or biphasic sharp waves in the PPC and amygdala; type C, which are more complex waves such as very large spikes followed or not by slow waves. These type C phenomena are also accompanied by minor transient changes in other derivations such as the contralateral PPC, temporal cortex, thalamic nuclei and pontine areas. The morphology of these SITs recorded from the PPC merits special attention; whereas the SITs of type A had an initial negative-going peak at the surface of the PPC (E9) and initial positivity in deep layers (E11 and E13), the opposite was the case for type C SITs.

This is of interest for two reasons: (a) it shows that the A complexes, on the one hand, and C, on the other, depend upon different neurophysiological mechanisms, and (b) it permits a comparison with the wave forms of the EPs obtained by LOT stimulation and recorded from the same sites. It is thus of special interest to examine

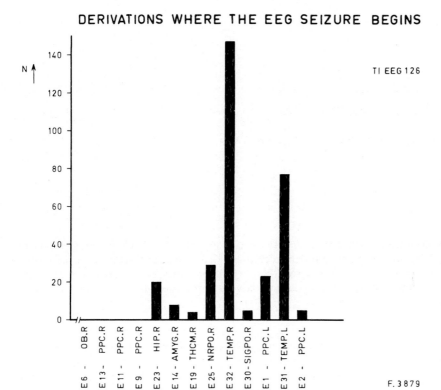

Fig. 2. Histogram showing the number of times different EEG derivations were scored as being the first where changes characteristic of a spontaneous seizure were seen. Note that the largest number was encountered in the right temporal cortex (Temp. R) followed by the left temporal cortex (Temp. L). In the hippocampus (Hip), amygdala (Amyg), thalamus centre median (ThCM), reticular pontine nucleus (NRPO), sigmoid gyrus (SIGPO), PPC (prepyriform cortex) and olfactory bulb (OB), very few (or no) events were scored.

the depth profiles of the SITs as shown in Fig. 3 in comparison with the EPs to LOT stimulation recorded at the same electrode positions; the most remarkable aspect is the polarity of the first deflection. In the EP this first wave is of negative polarity in the superficial cortical layers (E9; Fig. 3) and positive in deep layers. This is also the case for the main deflection of the type A SITs. However, it is the opposite of what was encountered for the large deflection of type C SITs. The interpretation of these results is discussed below.

In the course of K a remarkable evolution of the most common type SITs was noticed. At the beginning of K (during the first 40 sessions; dog Ti), type A SITs were the more common; at a late stage (after 53 sessions), those of type C became the more numerous. This suggests that there is a gradual transformation of the type of paroxysmal complexes, reflecting not only an increased degree of synchrony of

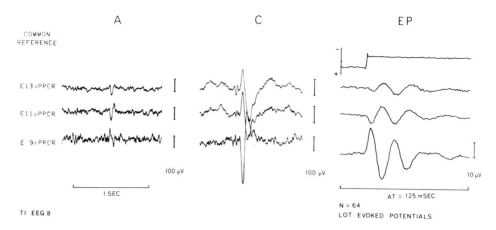

Fig. 3. Depth profile in the PPC of types of SITs along with EPs to LOT stimulation recorded from the same electrode sites. Note that the main initial deflection of type A in E9 (PPC surface) is in the negative direction, while that of E11 and E13 (depth of PPC) is in the positive direction. The same occurs for the EPs, but type C present opposite polarities. Note, however, that between E13 and E9, there is always a polarity reversal (negativity upwards).

the neuronal populations involved but also changes in the underlying neuronal processes.

(2) Experiments in rat

(2.1) Kindled seizures

At the beginning of the experiments EPs were investigated by applying 0.1 msec current pulses to the Schaffer collaterals, to set the current strength of the K stimulus; the peak current of the pulses used as K stimulus was 1.5 times the threshold for EPs. At the first applications the K stimulus did not in general evoke after-discharges, but even in the first week these might occur; after about 15–25 applications of the K stimulus behavioural seizures occurred. In some rats K was continued until stage 4 of Racine's scheme was reached, i.e., the rats presented generalized seizures with a focal onset.

(2.2) Spontaneous interictal transients (SITs) and evoked potentials (EPs)

During the first week of kindling we observed in the hippocampal EEG immediately after the cessation of after-discharges and even many hours afterwards, SITs with the following characteristics: peak amplitudes of 250 μV up to 1 mV, duration of about 80 msec, as shown in Fig. 4B; moreover they had the same polarity as the EPs elicited by stimulation of Schaffer collaterals (Fig. 4A) and they did not appear to be followed by an after-potential. These SITs were sometimes difficult to distinguish in the primary EEG record, but they could readily be recognized by using an averaging procedure. We called these rat SITs type I. Usually around the second week of kindling another type of SITs was found: type II. These

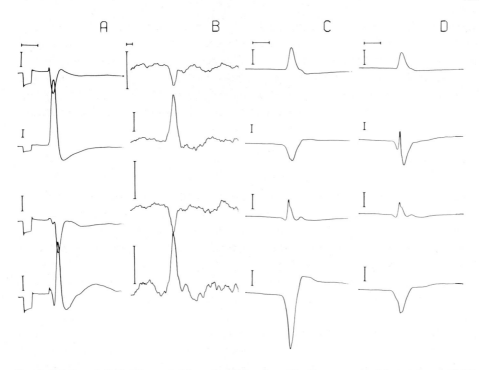

Fig. 4. SITs (panels B, C, D) recorded from the CA1 region of the hippocampus of the rat along with EPs (panel A) to stimulation of the Schaffer collaterals. The 2 traces above are from the left hippocampus which was stimulated; the 2 below are from the contralateral hippocampus. Within each hippocampus the first trace is from an electrode placed at about or above the pyramidal cell layer and the second trace is from an electrode placed at the level of the apical dendrites. Note the polarity reversal of the EPs. Type I SITs (panel B) show the same polarity as EPs but are of longer duration. Type II SITs (panel C) present the opposite polarity; note that the large initial deflection is followed by a rather slow wave of opposite polarity. Type II SITs could also present a population spike (panel D) and then the late slow wave changed in polarity. All signals are the average of 16 events. Horizontal lines: time calibration 20 msec. Vertical lines: amplitude calibration 500 μV. Negativity upwards.

had larger amplitudes (2–3 mV); the main deflection had a short duration, about 20 msec, and it was followed by a late wave of opposite polarity. SITs type II were also consistent in wave shape as illustrated by the averages of Fig. 4C. At a still later stage the SITs type II could present a clear-cut population spike in the leading edge; this population spike, when recorded at an electrode close to the cell body layer, or just below it, consisted of a sharp negative-going deflection, as shown in Fig. 4D. A similar population spike might also be seen in Schaffer collateral EPs, particularly if recorded some hours (2–3 h) after the K stimulus. In all cases, however, the slopes of the SITs were less steep than those of the corresponding EPs. It should be noted that in the same experiments in which different types of SITs were encountered the EPs presented always the same polarity; any changes in EPs were only seen at much later stages of kindling.

In all rats in which the electrodes were almost symmetrically placed the EPs elicited by one-sided stimulation of the Schaffer collaterals were isomorphic in both hippocampi; the contralateral EP lagged by 5 ± 1 msec. At the same electrodes and from both hippocampi SITs with largely similar characteristics were recorded. However, no detectable time delay between bilaterally occurring SITs could be put in evidence. This was unexpected; it may suggest that both hippocampi are affected in the same way by the kindling procedure and that most SITs are probably triggered by random inputs originating from a source which is common to both hippocampi.

DISCUSSION

As regards the dog experiments, it should be stressed that K of the PPC in the dog is possible. A particular observation, however, was that we did not find in this preparation a clear build-up of motor seizures in terms of the 5-class scheme devised by Racine (1972a, b); in contrast, it appeared that the motor seizures occurred in an all-or-none fashion. Another finding was that long-term K of the PPC in the dog can lead to the occurrence of spontaneous seizures, as has also been demonstrated for amygdaloid K in the rat (Pinel and Rovner 1978). It should be stressed that these spontaneous seizures do not appear to start at the same place as the K seizures and have quite different behavioural manifestations. Pinel and Rovner (1978) also described some spontaneously occurring seizure patterns which were different from those produced by brain stimulation. Although they did not record the EEG many times during these spontaneous seizures, they suggested that in these cases the epileptogenic foci were not restricted to the site of stimulation. Our findings support this suggestion and present clear proof that the spontaneous electro-clinical seizures differ from the kindled seizures not only in time course but also in area of origin. A question remaining is how and why does the kindled focus lead to the so-called "spontaneous focus." It should still be noted that the spontaneous seizures appeared in a dog which had been kindled bilaterally, although kindled seizures were elicited from only one side.

The electrophysiological changes occurring in the course of long-term K of the PPC have been analysed in detail. One interesting aspect is the gradual build-up of spontaneous inter-ictal transients from rather simple forms, up to polyspike complexes which are most probably due to massive neuronal depolarizations and firing of cells. Similar aspects of the SITs were also encountered in the kindled hippocampus of the rat.

A most remarkable finding was that in both the dog's PPC and rat's hippocampus there appeared SITs with different polarities, depending upon the stage of the kindling process. In the dog's PPC the SITs occurring mainly in the early stage had the same depth profile as the initial deflection of the EP elicited by LOT stimulation. It may therefore be concluded that these SITs correspond to a dipole field which in both the initial deflection of the EP and the SITs may be caused primarily by excitation of the dendrites of superficial pyramidal neurones. In contrast, the so-called type C SITs had an inverted depth profile in comparison to the initial deflection of the EP, although with a polarity reversal along the main axis of the pyramidal neurones. This leads to the conclusion that the neurophysiological process underlying type C SITs is of a different nature from that underlying type A SITs. This observation was amply confirmed in the experiments on the rat. The main finding in these experiments was the occurrence of 2 types of SITs, showing reversed polarity and appearing also at different stages in the course of kindling. The following explanation may be advanced.

It is well established that the Schaffer collateral EPs cause an extracellular negative wave below the pyramidal cell layer which corresponds to a depolarization caused by EPSPs at the apical dendrites; in this way an equivalent dipole layer is formed with a negative pole in the stratum radiatum and a positive pole lying dorsal to the pyramidal cell bodies. The simplest hypothesis, therefore, is that the SITs type I of the rat are similarly caused by a depolarization at the level of the synapses of the Schaffer collaterals, i.e., SITs type I could be a sort of large EPSP generated at the same synapses which receive the kindling stimulus. In this case the electrodes lying below the pyramidal cell layer would record a field potential corresponding to an active sink while the more dorsally lying electrode would record from a passive source.

This would be compatible with the observations of Ebersole and Levine (1975) on the evolution of a penicillin epileptogenetic focus; they showed that at low concentrations of penicillin there was an "enhancement of the physiological response" of the cells. An alternative explanation would be that SITs type I are caused by hyperpolarization at the level of the cell body, since this may cause a similar field potential profile. Although this alternative cannot be excluded in face of the present data, it appears to be less likely since hyperpolarizations (IPSPs) in the hippocampal pyramidal cells are usually of much longer duration and if they were caused by recurrent collaterals they should be preceded by an initial excitatory process revealed extracellularly as a field potential of opposite polarity. This was, however, never found. As regards the SITs type II it is clear from our findings that they represent depolarization processes involving the pyramidal cell bodies since a population spike can be encountered. In this case an electrode lying below the pyramidal cell layer would record a field potential corresponding to a passive source while the more dorsally lying electrode would record from the active sink; the fact that the negative-going population spike can be recorded even below the cell body layer indicates that, besides a large degree of synchrony, the action potential appears to invade to some extent the apical dendrites. This large depolarization may correspond to the classic paroxysmal depolarization shift (PDS).

In conclusion, the establishment of a kindling epileptogenic focus can be traced electrophysiologically as a sequence of changes in the excitability of the local neuronal population. It appears that at the onset of kindling large depolarizations are restricted to the level of the synapses to which the kindling stimulus is applied; at a later stage, when convulsions are likely to occur, the large depolarizations (PDS) migrate to the cell body.

SUMMARY

Long-term records of field potentials during kindling were analysed in 2 preparations: the prepyriform cortex (PPC) in dog and the CA1 subarea of the hippocampus in rat. Besides the occurrence of after-discharges directly following the kindling stimulus, short transients were found to occur spontaneously between seizures: spontaneous inter-ictal transients or SITs. In both the PPC and the hippocampus 2 different types of SITs were encountered. Both types corresponded to a dipole layer centred around the main local pyramidal neurones (PPC or hippocampus). One type occurred early in the course of kindling and had the same polarity as the local evoked potential (EP) produced by stimulation of the lateral olfactory tract in PPC or of the Schaffer collaterals in the hippocampus. The other type occurred at later stages and had a reversed polarity to the EP. These findings were interpreted as indicating that at the onset of kindling spontaneously occurring depolarizations corresponding to the early type of SITs are restricted to the level of the synapses to which the kindling stimulus is applied; at a later stage, when convulsions are likely to occur, large spontaneous depolarizations corresponding to the late type of SITs are generated at the level of the cell bodies.

ACKNOWLEDGEMENT

This work was partially subsidized by a grant from the Commissie Landelijk Epilepsie Onderzoek (CLEO-TNO).

REFERENCES

Dua-Sharma, S., Sharma, K.N. and Jacobs, H.L. The Canine Brain in Stereotaxic Coordinates. MIT Press, Cambridge, Mass., 1970.

Ebersole, J.S. and Levine, R.A. Abnormal neuronal response during evolution of a penicillin focus in cat visual cortex. J. Neurophysiol., 1975, 38: 250–266.

Gaito, J. The kindling effect. Physiol. Psychol., 1974, 2: 45–50.

Goddard, G.V. Development of epileptic seizures through brain stimulation at low intensity. Nature (Lond.), 1967, 214: 1020–1021.

Goddard, G.V., McIntyre, D.C. and Leech, C.K. A permanent change in brain function resulting from daily electrical stimulation. Exp. Neurol., 1969, 25: 295–330.

Lange, H., Tanaka, T. and Naquet, R. Temporo-spatial pattern of subcortical spike activity in kindling epilepsy. A statistical approach. Electroenceph. clin. Neurophysiol., 1977, 42: 564–574.

Leung, L.S. Orthodromic activation of hippocampal CA1 region of the rat. Brain Res., 1979, 176: 49–63.

Lopes da Silva, F.H. and Arnolds, D.E.A.T. Physiology of the hippocampus and related structures. Ann. Rev. Physiol., 1978, 40: 185–216.

McIntyre, D.C. and Goddard, G.V. Transfer, interference and spontaneous recovery of convulsions kindled from the rat amygdala. Electroenceph. clin. Neurophysiol., 1973, 35: 533–543.

Morrell, F. and Tsuru, N. Kindling in the frog: Development of spontaneous epileptiform activity. Electroenceph. clin. Neurophysiol., 1976, 40: 1–11.

Pinel, J.P.J. and Rovner, L.I. Experimental epileptogenesis: kindling-induced epilepsy in rats. Exp. Neurol., 1978, 58: 190–202.

Pinel, J.P.J., Phillips, A.G. and Deol, G. Effects of current intensity on kindled motor seizure activity in rats. Behav. Biol., 1974, 11: 59–68.

Pinel, J.P.J., Mucha, R.F. and Phillips, A.G. Spontaneous seizures generated in rats by kindling. A preliminary report. Physiol. Psychol., 1975, 3: 127–129.

Racine, R.J. Modification of seizure activity by electrical stimulation. I. Afterdischarge threshold. Electroenceph. clin. Neurophysiol., 1972a, 32: 269–279.

Racine, R.J. Modification of seizure activity by electrical stimulation. II. Motor seizure. Electroenceph. clin. Neurophysiol., 1972b, 32: 281–294.

Sato, M. and Nakashima, T. Kindling: Secondary epileptogenesis, sleep and catecholamines. Canad. J. neurol. Sci., 1972, 2: 439–446.

Storm van Leeuwen, W. and Kamp, A. Radiotelemetry of EEG and other biological variables in man and dog. Proc. roy. Soc. Med., 1969, 62: 401–403.

Tanaka, A. Progressive changes of behavioral and electroencephalographic responses to daily amygdaloid stimulations in rabbits. Fukuoka Acta med., 1972, 63: 152–164.

Van Hulten, K., Lopes da Silva, F.H., Lommen, J.G. and Tichelaar, M. Kindling in the prepyriform cortex in dog; analysis of local and interregional changes using evoked potentials and EEG quantification. Electroenceph. clin. Neurophysiol., 1977, 43: 567.

Wada, J.A. and Osawa, T. Spontaneous recurrent seizure state induced by daily electric amygdaloid stimulation in Senegalese baboons (*Papio papio*). Neurology (Minneap.), 1976, 26: 273–286.

Wada, J.A. and Sato, M. Generalized convulsive seizure induced by daily electrical stimulation of the amygdala in cats. Correlative electrographic and behavioral features. Neurology (Minneap.), 1974, 24: 565–574.

Wauquier, A., Ashton, D. and Mellis, W. Behavioral analysis of amygdaloid kindling in beagle dogs and the effects of clonazepam, diazepam, phenobarbital, diphenylhydantoin, and flunarizine on seizure manifestation. Exp. Neurol., 1979, 64: 579–586.

Kyoto Symposia (EEG Suppl. No. 36)
Editors: P.A. Buser, W.A. Cobb and T. Okuma
© 1982, Elsevier Biomedical Press, Amsterdam

288

Separate Analysis of Lasting Alteration in Excitatory Synapses, Inhibitory Synapses and Cellular Excitability in Association with Kindling

GRAHAM V. GODDARD

Department of Psychology, University of Otago, Dunedin (New Zealand)

Kindling is a process by which repeated stimulation of an area of the brain leads to a progressively changing response, eventually including epileptiform convulsions (Goddard et al. 1969; Racine 1978). The stimulated tissue does not appear to be altered structurally (Goddard and McIntyre 1972; Racine et al. 1975; Goddard and Douglas 1976) except after a very large number of kindled convulsions and spontaneous seizures (Scheibel 1981), but the response to stimulation is permanently changed, even when the stimulation is withheld for many months (Goddard et al. 1969; Wada et al. 1974; Wada and Osawa 1976).

Electrophysiological studies in the hippocampus and elsewhere have shown durable increases in the strength of excitatory synapses that accompany kindling (Racine et al. 1972; Douglas and Goddard 1975; Goddard and Douglas 1976; Bliss 1979). This increased excitation is very long lasting, although we do not know if it lasts as long as the kindling does (Douglas and Goddard 1975; Barnes 1979). The long-term potentiation of synapses can be caused by stimulation without seizure activity, but one of the most effective patterns for causing it (synchronous bursts at very high frequency; Douglas 1977) resembles the cellular activity that occurs during seizures and during interictal spiking (Matsumoto and Ajmone Marsan 1964; Ajmone Marsan 1969; Prince 1969; Ward 1969; Calvin 1974; Racine et al. 1975).

Another lasting change that has been observed in some of these studies is an increased excitability of the postsynaptic neurones (Bliss et al. 1982). After kindling they discharge in response to a weaker postsynaptic excitatory potential. This increase in cellular excitability is long lasting, but it does decay over several weeks (Douglas and Goddard 1975) at a rate faster than the expected loss of kindling. The excitability changes can be caused by stimulation too weak to cause long-term potentiation of the synapses, or kindling; but again, a very effective form of stimulation resembles the neural activity generated during seizures or interictal spikes (Bliss et al. 1982).

It has long been thought that some forms of epilepsy may be a consequence of reduced inhibition. Pharmacological evidence clearly shows that seizures occur when inhibition is blocked (Meldrum 1975). Here, I ask whether kindling in the hippocampus is accompanied by a lasting reduction of inhibition. A subsidiary question is whether altered inhibition might explain the long lasting increase in cellular excitability.

A model system well suited for kindling and the study of long-term changes in excitability, excitation and inhibition is the interaction of the field potentials of the perforant path input and the commissural input to the granule cells of fascia dentata. The perforant path is the major projection from the entorhinal cortex to the dentate gyrus of the hippocampal formation. The perforant path fibres terminate in the outer two-thirds of the dentate molecular layer (Hjorth-Simonsen 1972; Hjorth-Simonsen and Jeune 1972) where they make excitatory synapses on the distal two-thirds of the granule cell dendrites (Lomo 1971). The commissural afferents to the dentate gyrus arise from the contralateral hippocampal field CA4 (Laurberg 1970; Hjorth-Simonsen and Laurberg 1977) and they terminate within the inner third of the molecular layer (Blackstad 1956; Gottlieb and Cowan 1973; Deadwyler et al. 1975). These commissural and perforant path terminal fields do not overlap. Activation of the commissural afferents by stimulation of the contralateral hilus produces a strong inhibition of the granule cells so that an immediately following perforant path activation does not produce its usual response (Buzsaki et al. 1982; Czeh and Buzsaki 1982; Douglas et al. 1982). This inhibition is probably not monosynaptic, but results from commissural activation of local inhibitory interneurones (Douglas et al. 1982).

The data to be reported here are preliminary. They are taken from 14 rats with chronically implanted electrodes tested before and 2 weeks after having been kindled to various stages of behavioural convulsion. The bilaterally symmetrical electrode arrangement is shown in Fig. 1A. Procedures of surgery, stimulation, recording, computer sampling and analysis were similar to those described elsewhere (Douglas and Goddard 1975; Goddard and Douglas 1976; Douglas et al. 1982). At least 1 month was allowed for recovery from surgery and all testing was done on awake freely moving animals with their head plugs connected to the apparatus by a 1.5 m low noise shielded cable. The averaged field potentials were taken first from one hemisphere, then the connections were rearranged to take average field potentials from the other hemisphere. Kindling was by stimulation to the hilus of one hemisphere only, once or twice per day with 2 sec, 100 Hz, 150 μA, 0.5 msec diphasic pulses. The evoked potentials in both hemispheres were remeasured 2 weeks after the last kindling stimulus.

The evoked potentials were measured according to the following procedures. Pulses of diphasic constant current of predetermined duration were delivered once every 10 sec. The first pulse in a series was to the perforant path. It evoked a large field potential with 2 main components (Fig. 1B): a population EPSP due to depolarization of the granule cell dendrites (Lømo 1971), and a population spike formed from the almost synchronous discharge of many granule cells (Andersen et al. 1971). The second pulse in a series was to the contralateral hilus. It evoked a smaller field potential (Fig. 1B) that resembled an EPSP originating in the inner third of the molecular layer (Deadwyler et al. 1975; Douglas et al. 1982). The third event in a series was a pulse to the contralateral hilus followed, after a short delay, by a pulse to the perforant path. This combined stimulus evoked a compound potential which lacked, in varying degree, the population spike that normally

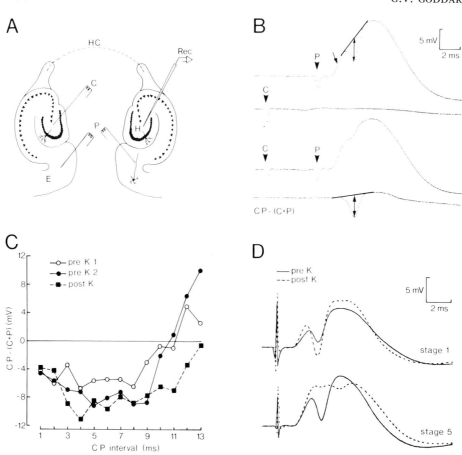

Fig. 1. A: schematic horizontal section through the hippocampi of both hemispheres showing location of electrodes. Rec, recording electrode that was also used for stimulation during kindling and when testing the contralateral hemisphere; C, stimulation electrode in contralateral hilus that was also used for recording when testing the contralateral hemisphere; P, stimulation electrodes in the perforant path of each hemisphere; E, entorhinal cortex; H, hilus; HC, hippocampal commissure. B: the upper 3 traces are examples of the potentials recorded from the hilus following a test pulse to the ipsilateral perforant path (P), a pulse to the contralateral hilus (C) and a pulse to C followed at 5 msec by a pulse to P. The population EPSP amplitude was measured at a fixed latency (arrow) and the population spike was measured vertically from the peak of the negative going deflection to a line tangent to the shoulders on either side (double headed arrow). The lower trace was computer generated from the upper 3 traces by the formula CP − (C + P) and the difference in population spike height was measured vertically from the peak difference to a line tangent to the shoulders on either side (double arrow). C: example from 1 rat showing differences in population spike heights, measured as in lower trace of B, plotted against intervals between the pulses to contralateral hilus and perforant path (CP interval). pre K1, measured before kindling; pre K2, measured after brief high frequency stimulation of perforant path that caused long-term potentiation but no seizure activity; post K, measured 2 weeks after the last of 24 after-discharges with stage 3 seizure. Note that pre K1 and pre K2 cross the zero line at about 11 msec whereas post K does not cross before 13 msec. D: wave forms from 2 rats comparing an average of 70 potentials evoked by standard test pulses to the perforant path before kindling (pre K) and 2 weeks after kindling (post K). One rat was kindled only to stage 1 with 5 after-discharges, the other was kindled to stage 5 with 20 after-discharges. Both showed an increase in the population EPSP. The stage 1 rat showed an increase in the population spike whereas the stage 5 rat showed a decrease in the population spike.

followed the stimulus to the perforant path (Fig. 1B). The diminution of this population spike was measured as in Fig. 1B and taken as an index of inhibition. It was measured in each hemisphere, before and after kindling, in 2 different series of stimulus pulses.

In the first series, the strength and duration of both the perforant path and contralateral pulses were held constant. At 10 sec intervals, pulses were delivered first to one pathway, then the other, then both, in continuously recycling triplets. The delay between the contralateral pulse and the perforant path pulse in the compound stimulus was varied in an up-down-up-down series in steps of 1 msec from 1 to 13 msec in some animals and to 20 msec in others. The 4 measures of population spike reduction at each delay were averaged and plotted as in Fig. 1C. The delay at which the measure of inhibition crossed the zero line was taken as the maximum duration of inhibition.

In the second series, pulses were again delivered at 10 sec intervals, first to one pathway then the other and then to both, in recycling triplets. But this time the interval between the contralateral pulse and the perforant path pulse was held constant in the compound stimulus, at 5 msec. With the amplitude and duration of the perforant path pulse held constant, the duration of the contralateral pulse was varied in 7 steps from 30 to 150 μsec. The measure of inhibition was repeated 10 times at each value and averaged. By inspection of these averages, the stimulus threshold for inhibition was obtained for each animal before and after kindling.

The third type of measure from these animals before and after kindling was of the amplitudes of the 2 main components (EPSP and spike) of the potential evoked by a standard test pulse to the perforant path (Fig. 1D) and the amplitude of the main component of the potential evoked by a standard test pulse to the contralateral hilus.

RESULTS

The average duration of inhibition for 6 control animals tested before and after several weeks without stimulation rose from 9.5 to 10.4 msec, a difference that was not statistically significant. Between the test before kindling and the test 2 weeks after the last kindling stimulus, the average duration of inhibition for 7 kindled animals was from 10.6 to 14.4 on the non-kindled side and from 10.1 to 13.1 on the kindled side. The apparently greater increase in the duration of inhibition in kindled animals was not statistically significant. Without further experimentation we are not at liberty to conclude that kindling causes an increase in the duration of inhibition, but it is reasonable to say that it is very unlikely that kindling causes a decrease.

The thresholds of inhibition were not measured in a matched set of control animals. They were measured before and 2 weeks after stimulation in 10 rats kindled to various stages of behavioural convulsion. Three out of 5 rats kindled to stages 1–3 showed a small increase in threshold, the other two showed no change. Three out of 5 rats kindled to at least 1 stage 5 convulsion showed an increase in threshold, the other two showed no change. On average, therefore, the thresholds tended to increase, but clearly, this increase was not a necessary condition for kindling.

The amplitudes of the potentials evoked by a standard test pulse to the contralateral hilus varied from animal to animal, both before and after kindling. Changes as a result of kindling were inconsistent, most of them showed a decrease, but some increased and some did not change.

The amplitude of the EPSP component of the potentials evoked by the standard test pulse to the perforant path was found to be larger following kindling in all 10 animals. This result is similar to a previous report (Douglas and Goddard 1975) in which kindling from an electrode in the perforant path resulted in larger population EPSPs. Here the increase, which is usually interpreted as an increase in the strength of the excitatory synapses between perforant path and granule cells, was caused by kindling stimulation of the hilus.

Contrary to expectation, the amplitude of the population spikes evoked by the standard test pulse to the perforant path did not always increase along with the EPSP increase. In fact, some animals showed decreases in the population spike even though the EPSP had increased (Fig. 1D). Population spike increases tended to be seen most often following stages 1–3 kindling whereas population spike decreases were more often seen following stage 5 kindling. A change in the relation between EPSP size and population spike size (input-output relation) is usually interpreted as a change in cellular excitability. If in fact the later stages of kindling result in decreased cellular excitability, it would be consistent with the possibility of stronger inhibition.

It is not known whether these effects last longer than the 2 week interval used here. The two main findings, while both preliminary and uncertain, imply that kindling results in a strengthening of inhibition. A larger scale study would be required to make a satisfactory test of this possibility. The present results, however, seem adequate to rule out the possibility that kindling in the hippocampus is due to lasting destruction of the local inhibitory connections.

ACKNOWLEDGEMENT

This work was supported by the Natural Sciences and Engineering Research Council Canada Grant No. A0365 to G.V. Goddard.

REFERENCES

Ajmone Marsan, C. Acute effects of topical epileptogenic agents. In: H.H. Jasper, A.A. Ward, Jr. and A. Pope (Eds.), Basic Mechanisms of the Epilepsies. Little, Brown and Company, Boston, Mass., 1969: 299–319.

Andersen, P., Bliss, T.V.P. and Skrede, K.K. Unit analysis of hippocampal population spikes. Exp. Brain Res., 1971, 13: 208–221.

Barnes, C.A. Memory deficits associated with senescence: a neurophysiological and behavioral study in the rat. J. comp. physiol. Psychol., 1979, 93: 74–104.

Blackstad, T.W. Commissural connections of the hippocampal region in the rat, with special reference to their mode of termination. J. comp. Neurol., 1956, 105: 417–537.

Bliss, T.V.P. Synaptic plasticity in the hippocampus. Trends Neurosci., 1979, 2: 42–45.

Bliss, T.V.P., Goddard, G.V. and Riives, M. Reduction of long-term potentiation in the hippocampus of the rat following selective depletion of monoamines. J. Physiol. (Lond.), 1982, under review.

Buzsaki, G., Czeh, G., Grastyán, E., Kellényi, L. and Czopf, G. Commissural and perforant path interaction in the rat hippocampus: field potentials. Exp. Brain Res., 1982, in press.

Calvin, W.H., Three modes of repetitive firing and the role of threshold time course between spikes. Brain Res., 1974, 69: 341–346.

Czeh, G. and Buzsaki, G. Unitary responses evoked by the commissural and perforant path vollies in the dentate area of the rat hippocampus. Exp. Brain Res., 1982, in press.

Deadwyler, S.A., West, J.R., Cotman, C.W. and Lynch, G.S. A neurophysiological analysis of commissural projection to the dentate gyrus of the rat. J. Neurophysiol., 1975, 38: 167–184.

Douglas, R.M. Long-lasting synaptic potentiation in the rat dentate gyrus following brief high-frequency stimulation. Brain Res., 1977, 126: 361–365.

Douglas, R.M. and Goddard, G.V., Long-term potentiation of the perforant path-granule cell synapse in the rat hippocampus. Brain Res., 1975, 86: 205–215.

Douglas, R.M., McNaughton, B.L. and Goddard, G.V. Commissural inhibition and facilitation of granule cell discharge in fascia dentata. J. comp. Neurol., 1982, in press.

Goddard, G.V. and Douglas, R.M. Does the engram of kindling model the engram of normal long term memory? In: J.A. Wada (Ed.), Kindling. Raven Press, New York, 1976: 1–18.

Goddard, G.V. and McIntyre, D.C. Some properties of a lasting epileptogenic trace kindled by repeated electrical stimulation of the amygdala in mammals. In: L.V. Laitinen and K.E. Livingston (Eds.), Surgical Approaches in Psychiatry. University Park Press, Baltimore, Md., 1972: 109–115.

Goddard, G.V., McIntyre, D.C. and Leech, C.K. A permanent change in brain function resulting from daily electrical stimulation. Exp. Neurol., 1969, 25: 295–330.

Gottlieb, D.I. and Cowan, W.M. Autoradiographic studies of the commissural and ipsilateral association connections of the hippocampus and dentate gyrus of the rat. I. The commissural connections. J. comp. Neurol., 1973, 149: 393–422.

Hjorth-Simonsen, A. Projection of the lateral part of the entorhinal area to the hippocampus and fascia dentata. J. comp. Neurol., 1972, 146: 219–232.

Hjorth-Simonsen, A. and Jeune, B. Origin and termination of the hippocampal perforant path in the rat studied by silver impregnation. J. comp. Neurol., 1972, 144: 215–232.

Hjorth-Simonsen, A. and Laurberg, S. Commissural connections of the dentate area of the rat. J. comp. Neurol., 1977, 174: 591–606.

Laurberg, S. Commissural and intrinsic connections of the rat hippocampus. J. comp. Neurol., 1970, 184: 685–708.

Lømo, T. Patterns of activation in a monosynaptic cortical pathway. The perforant path input to the dentate area of the hippocampal formation. Exp. Brain Res., 1971, 12: 18–45.

Matsumoto, H. and Ajmone Marsan, C. Cortical cellular phenomena in experimental epilepsy: Ictal manifestations. Exp. Neurol., 1964, 9: 305.

McNaughton, B.L., Douglas, R.M. and Goddard, G.V. Synaptic enhancement in fascia dentata: cooperativity among coactive afferents. Brain Res., 1978, 157: 277–293.

Meldrum, B.S. Epilepsy and GABA-mediated inhibition. Int. Rev. Neurobiol., 1975, 17: 1–36.

Miller, J.J., Baimbridge, K.G. and Goddard, G.V. Biochemical correlates of kindling-induced epilepsy in the hippocampus: the role of calcium binding protein. In: Epilepsy International Congress, Kyoto, Japan, 1981 (abstract).

Prince, D.A. Electrophysiology of "epileptic" neurons: spike generation. Electroenceph. clin. Neurophysiol., 1969, 26: 476.

Racine, R. Kindling: The first decade. Neurosurgery, 1978, 3: 234–252.

Racine, R., Gartner, J. and Burnham, W. Epileptiform activity and neural plasticity in limbic structures. Brain Res., 1972, 47: 262–268.

Racine, R., Tuff, L. and Zaide, J. Kindling, unit discharge patterns and neural plasticity. Canad. J. neurol. Sci., 1975, 2: 395–405.

Scheibel, A. Dendritic spine changes in hippocampus of rats kindled to spontaneous convulsions. Reported at Winter Conference on Brain Research, Keystone, Colo., 1981.

Wada, J.A. and Osawa, T. Spontaneous recurrent seizure state induced by daily electric amygdaloid stimulation in Senegalese baboons (*Papio papio*). Neurology (Minneap.), 1976, 26: 273–286.

Wada, J.A., Sato, M. and Corcoran, M.E. Persistent seizure susceptibility and recurrent spontaneous seizures in kindled cats. Epilepsia, 1974, 15: 465–478.

Ward, Jr., A.A. The epileptic neuron: chronic foci in animals and man. In: H.H. Jasper, A.A. Ward, Jr. and A. Pope (Eds.), Basic Mechanisms of the Epilepsies. Little, Brown and Company, Boston, Mass., 1969: 263–288.

Zimmer, J. Ipsilateral afferents to the commissural zone of the fascia dentata demonstrated in decommissurated rats, by silver impregnation. J. comp. Neurol., 1971, 142: 393–416.

6. Brain Stem Evoked Potentials: Clinical Uses

Kyoto Symposia (EEG Suppl. No. 36)
Editors: P.A. Buser, W.A. Cobb and T. Okuma
© 1982, Elsevier Biomedical Press, Amsterdam

Sensory Evoked Potentials and their Changes with Respiration in Man and Cat

MUNEO SHIMAMURA and AKIO MORI

Department of Neurophysiology, Tokyo Metropolitan Institute for Neurosciences, 2–6, Musashidai, Fuchu-city, Tokyo 183 (Japan)

It has been found that several sensory functions vary with respiration. For example, two different kinds of sensation are obtained to electrical stimuli applied percutaneously to the median nerve of a human. When stimulation is applied to the nerve during the inspiratory phase, sensation is localized at the stimulated site and the pain felt is weak; when stimulation is applied during the expiratory phase, the sense of pain is greater and spreads beyond the stimulated site (Nakayama and Hori 1966).

Neural activities have also been found to vary with respiration. Indications of neural activities that parallel respiratory changes are obtained not only from the cerebral cortex, but also from the midbrain reticular formation, the subcortical nuclei and the limbic system (Kumagai et al. 1966). Slow potentials are observed in EEGs of humans and rabbits that vary in correspondence with the respiratory phase (Gibbs et al. 1940). The readiness potential also shows changes parallel with respiration (Grozinger et al. 1973). Though respiratory fluctuations might be due to impulses in respiratory neurones acting at any level of the central nervous system, they appear to originate in the brain stem reticular formation (Kumagai et al. 1966).

In the present experiments, we studied the mechanisms of respiratory fluctuation in the somatosensory evoked cortical potentials. Cutaneously evoked cortical potentials were recorded from man and cat, to attempt to find some correlations between sensory function and sensory evoked potentials.

METHODS

Experiments were divided into 2 groups: human and chloralosed cats.

In human experiments, adult males sat in a convenient chair. EEGs were recorded from Cz and right side following mechanical stimulation of a left finger. A surface electrode was placed on the scalp near Cz and an indifferent electrode on the ear lobe. Apply mechanical stimuli to the finger, a fine bamboo stick with a blunt tip was placed about 1 mm from the skin of the finger; it was moved by electrical pulses to a solenoid. Stimuli could be applied during inspiration or expiration: a resistor transducer was fixed to a band around the chest and the respiratory curve was recorded with a pen-recording system. At the maximal point of each respiratory phase a stimulus could be delivered, controlled by a wind comparator.

In cat experiments, the animals were initially anaesthetized with ether. Tracheal canulation and venous catheterization of the femoral vein were performed. Craniotomy in the frontal region was performed. The animals were then mounted in a stereotaxic head holder, intravenously anaesthetized further with α-chloralose (30 mg/kg), immobilized with gallamine triethiodide and artificially respired. The gas mixture was adjusted to 5% CO_2 with the anaesthetic apparatus. The ventilation volume was adjusted for each animal and the frequency was 29/min to obtain continuously large amplitude evoked potentials during the experiment. The potentials were recorded 2 h after cessation of ether.

A silver ball-tipped electrode was placed on the surface of the primary somatosensory area in the cerebral cortex (gyri sigmoideus posterior) and a silver plate on the temporal muscle acted as an indifferent electrode. Mechanical and electrical stimuli were applied to the skin or cutaneous nerve of the hind limb contralateral to the recording.

The same mechanical stimulator as for man was used to apply stimuli to the hind paw at various phases of respiration. A thermistor transducer was inserted between the tracheal cannula and the respirator and the respiratory curve was recorded with a pen-recording system. Eight points were stimulated, 4 during inspiration and 4 during expiration. To avoid vibration the mechanical stimulator was set on a separate stand from the animal's head holder, the hind limb was fixed and several nerve branches innervating the hind limb and the hip were transected, but the sciatic nerve was left intact.

Electrical stimulation was applied to the central cut end of the sural nerve, which was dissected from the surrounding tissue and transected. Rectangular pulses of 0.3 msec duration were applied to the nerve through a bipolar silver wire electrode.

During the experiment, body temperature was kept at about 37°C by a rubber mat with circulated warm water and by infrared lamps, and the exposed forebrain was covered with warm mineral oil.

Fifty repetitions were averaged by a computer, as potentials in individual records were small in amplitude and large in fluctuation.

RESULTS

(I) Human SEP and its changes with respiration

Mechanical stimulation was applied to a finger of the left side and 2 component potentials, early and late, were evoked in the Cz-right ear channel. Fig. 1 shows examples of averaged sensory evoked potentials in the phases of expiration and inspiration. The early and late components were different with the phase of respiration, particularly the late component, which was smaller in the inspiratory than in the expiratory phase.

(II) Evoked potentials of the somatosensory cortex following mechanical stimulation of a hind limb in cats

Mechanical stimulation was applied to the skin around the metatarsal bone of a

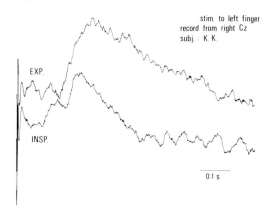

stim. to left finger
record from right Cz
subj. : K. K.

EXP.

INSP.

0.1 s

Fig. 1. SEPs of man and their respiratory fluctuations. SEPs at Cz were recorded in the expiratory phase (EXP) and the inspiratory phase (INSP). Each record was averaged 50 times.

hind limb and 3 component potentials were evoked in the somatosensory area of the cerebral cortex (Fig. 2): a surface negative spike of small amplitude and short latency (N1), a surface positive potential of large amplitude (P), and a delayed negative potential of prolonged duration (N2). In this case, several nerve branches were transected with the sciatic nerve left intact. Latencies of N1, P and N2 were 11 ± 1, 21 ± 1 and 63 ± 2.5 msec (mean ± S.D.); their amplitudes were 0.09 ± 0.01, 0.75 ± 0.05 and 0.48 ± 0.07 mV and their peak times were 18 ± 0.5, 29 ± 1 and 68–102 msec, respectively. The N2 potential varied during the respiratory phase; changes in duration were particularly marked. The peak time (t), amplitude (h) and duration (d) of the N1, P and N2 potentials were measured, and with each value at the beginning of the inspiratory phase plotted as 1.0. The peak time of N2 (N2t) was 78 msec at the beginning of the inspiratory phase; it gradually decreased and reached its shortest value of 63 msec at the shifting point from inspiration to expiration, then increased again and reached its maximum value of 102 msec at the end of the expiratory phase. The duration (N2d) was longest (310 msec) at the beginning of the inspiratory phase, then gradually decreased and reached its minimum (115 msec) at the end of this phase; it increased gradually again during the expiratory phase, and reached its maximum value at the shifting point from expiration to inspiration. The amplitude of N2 (N2h) exhibited changes with respiration, but these were small. The peak time (N1t, Pt) and the duration (N1d, Pd) of N1 and P were measured but no fluctuations corresponding with respiration were observed (N1 is not shown in Fig. 2).

Similar changes with respiration were seen after the main trunk of the sciatic nerve was transected and only the sural nerve was left intact. In this case, 3 components of the cortical potential were again obtained, but their amplitudes were slightly smaller than before the transection.

In contrast, no fluctuations in the potentials with respiration were obtained following mechanical stimulation of the hind limb, after several nerve branches, including the sural and sciatic nerves were transected, leaving intact the nerves

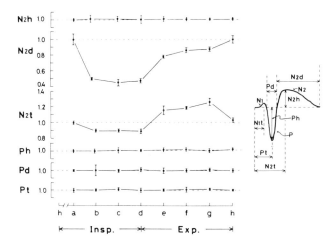

Fig. 2. Relations between the evoked potentials of the somatosensory cortex in cats and the respiratory phase. Surface negative (N1), positive (P) and prolonged negative (N2) potentials were evoked by mechanical stimulation of the hind limb. Each value of the evoked potentials was plotted against respiratory phase (a–h). Pt, Pd, Ph: peak time, duration, and amplitude of P, respectively. N2t, N2d and N2h: peak time, duration and amplitude of N2, respectively.

innervating the gastrocnemius soleus muscle. The potentials were a surface positive one of small amplitude (11 ± 1 msec latency, 32.5 ± 2 msec peak time, 87 ± 8 msec duration) and a surface negative one (103 ± 9 msec latency, 204 ± 6 msec peak time, 209 ± 9 msec duration); these wave forms were greatly different from those obtained in cats in which the sural nerve was intact.

The evoked potentials of the somatosensory cortex were obtained by electrical stimulation of the sural nerve. Three components of the potentials are N1 (8.5 ± 0.5 msec latency, 13.5 ± 1.5 msec peak time); P (18.5 ± 0.5 msec latency, 30 ± 2 msec peak time) and N2 (41.5 ± 2.5 msec latency, 48 ± 2 msec peak time). Fluctuations with respiration were seen in the electrically induced potentials but they were not very pronounced.

Evoked potentials were recorded after pentobarbital sodium administration (10 mg i.v.) under the same stimulating-recording procedures as those above. The amplitudes of all N1, P and N2 potentials were reduced; there were particularly marked reductions in the amplitude and duration of N2. The N2 potential was 60 ± 3 msec in latency, 73 ± 3 msec in peak time, 115 ± 5 msec in duration and 0.3 ± 0.04 mV in amplitude. These values were changed by respiration, but only to a small extent.

DISCUSSION

Evoked potentials from the somatosensory cortex and their respiratory fluctuation
In the present experiment, 3 component potentials, N1, P and N2 were obtained

from the somatosensory cortex in response to mechanical stimulation of a hind limb.

The peripheral sensory sources mostly originate in the skin. Mountcastle (1957) reported that 74% of the cells in the primary somatosensory cortex are activated by cutaneous nerve excitation and only 26% by nerves innervating deep tissue. In the present experiment the evoked potentials were obtained with large amplitude by mechanical stimulation of a hind limb when a cutaneous nerve remained; in contrast, potentials were small and with a different wave form following stimulation of muscle afferents in the hind limb.

Two ascending systems may be involved, lemniscal and extralemniscal reticular (Bowsher and Albe-Fessard 1965). The lemniscal system includes the ventral basal nuclei in the thalamus and the ventro-postero-lateral nucleus, which is a specific projection nucleus (Bowsher 1967). The extralemniscal reticular system includes the brain stem reticular formation, non-specific nuclei of the medial parafascicular-centro-median complex, and ventral basal nuclei (Bowsher and Albe-Fessard 1965). The thalamus connects with the somatosensory cortex through both the specific projection and the non-specific projection systems (Magoun 1952; Morison and Dempsey 1942, 1943). The non-specific projection system is also called the thalamic reticular system (Jasper 1949), and it includes the ascending reticular activating system (Magoun 1952). Jasper (1949) stated that 2 cortical potentials are evoked by stimulation of the thalamus; a short latency potential is produced by impulses travelling via the specific projection system and a long latency potential by impulses via the non-specific system, perhaps including polysynaptic pathways.

From our observations we assume that N1 and P potentials are conducted by the specific projection system, and N2 by the non-specific system. N2 potentials showed respiratory fluctuation; in the expiratory phase the latency was longer and the amplitude was larger than in the inspiratory phase. This means that N2 is more easily obtained in expiration than in inspiration. In contrast, respiratory fluctuation of N1 and P1 is not seen. We assume that the cause of the respiratory fluctuation of N2 may lie at any level of the non-specific ascending projection system, appearing to originate in the brain stem reticular formation.

In the present experiments we used chloralosed cats and it is known that anaesthesia with chloralose is associated with forms of ephaptic activity (Ascher 1965). In contrast, the spino-bulbar-spinal (SBS) reflex is unaltered by chloralose anaesthesia, although the spontaneous fluctuations of the SBS reflex are reduced (Shimamura and Yamaguchi 1967). Before starting the present experiments we tested, in awake cats, the respiratory fluctuations of the late components of the SEP from the cat's scalp following tap stimulation of the hind limb. This gave similar results to those in man, as described above. However, it was difficult to keep constancy during the experiments even though familiar cats were used.

Mechanism of respiratory fluctuation in various functions

That the late evoked potentials of the somatosensory cortex are more apt to appear in the expiratory than in the inspiratory phase suggests two possible explanations: suppression may occur during inspiration or augmentation may occur during expiration.

Similar observations of respiratory fluctuation of the SBS reflex were obtained in other experiments (Mori 1979). This reflex is related to the bulbar reticular formation (Shimamura and Livingston 1963; Shimamura et al. 1979). In the expiratory phase it has a short latency, short peak time, abrupt rising phase and large amplitude. In contrast, in the inspiratory phase, the SBS reflex has a slightly longer peak time and smaller amplitude. The fluctuation of the SBS reflex is produced by the neural activities of respiration in the bulbar reticular formation; the reflex is suppressed by impulses during inspiration, since spikes of certain reticular neurones in the medial bulbar reticular formation showed alternate firing, depending on the respiratory phase. Most of the reticular neurones showed spikes in the inspiratory phase. In contrast, reticular neurone activities underlying the SBS reflex decreased in spike frequency during inspiration.

In the present experiments, we have not analysed the reticular neurone activity underlying the SEP pathways; however, we assume that the SEP fluctuations with respiration may have similar mechanisms to those of the SBS reflex.

It is interesting to consider possible mechanisms underlying other functions which similarly show fluctuations with respiration. Nakayama and Hori (1966) and Nakayama and Suzuki (1975) reported that when electrical stimulation is percutaneously applied to the median nerve at the end of inspiration, the feeling is one of weak pain localized around the stimulation site; if stimulation is applied at the end of expiration the feeling of pain is stronger and spreads to surrounding areas. In the present experiment, somatosensory cortical potentials evoked by mechanical stimulation of a hind limb were small in the inspiratory phase but large in expiration. No direct evidence is available that pain sensations travel the same pathways as late cortical responses; however, there is some supporting observation. Fields et al. (1975, 1977) recorded the responses of spino-reticular neurones to natural peripheral stimulation, and concluded that the spino-reticular fibres play a role in the perception of pain.

SUMMARY

Cutaneously evoked cortical potentials were recorded in man and chloralosed cats, in order to analyse the neural mechanisms responsible for their fluctuation with respiration.

From the Cz region of the human scalp, 2 components of potentials, early and late, were evoked following mechanical stimulation of a finger contralateral to the recording side. These potentials varied with the phase of respiration, the late component being larger in amplitude and longer in duration when the stimulus was applied during expiration.

From the surface of the primary somatosensory cortex of the cat (gyri sigmoideus posterior), 3 components of potentials were evoked following mechanical stimulation of the skin around the contralateral hind limb. These were surface negative (N1), followed by positive (P) and delayed negative (N2) potentials. The respiratory fluctuations were mainly in the duration of N2, which was shortest at the end of the inspiratory phase, while it was longest at the shifting point from expiration to inspiration. The peak time of N2 was shortest at the end of the inspiratory phase and longest at the end of the expiratory phase. On the contrary, N1 and P potentials did not fluctuate.

The results indicate that the late components of cutaneously evoked cortical potentials vary, depending on the respiratory phase. Each response was increased during expiration and decreased during inspiration. These fluctuations may possibly originate in the brain stem reticular formation.

REFERENCES

Ascher, P. La Réaction de Sursaut du Chat Anesthésié au Chloralose. Thèse à la Faculté des Sciences de l'Université de Paris, 1965: 1–125.

Bowsher, D. The termination of secondary somatosensory neurones with the thalamus of *Macaca mulatta:* an experimental degeneration study. J. comp. Neurol., 1967, 130: 301–312.

Bowsher, D. and Albe-Fessard, D. The anatomophysiological basis of somatosensory discrimination. Int. Rev. Neurobiol., 1965, 8: 35–75.

Fields, H.L., Wagner, G.M. and Anderson, S.T. Some properties of spinal neurons projecting to the medial brain-stem reticular formation. Exp. Neurol., 1975, 47: 118–134.

Fields, H.L., Clanton, C.H. and Anderson, S.T. Somato-sensory properties of spinoreticular neurons in the cat. Brain Res., 1977, 120: 49–66.

Gibbs, F.A., Williams, D. and Gibbs, E.L. Modification of the cortical frequency spectrum by changes in CO_2, blood sugar and O_2. J. Neurophysiol., 1940, 3: 49–58.

Grozinger, B., Kronhuber, H.H. and Kriebel, J. Inter- and intrahemispheric asymmetries of brain potentials proceeding speech and phonation. Electroenceph. clin. Neurophysiol., 1973, 34: 737–783.

Jasper, H. Diffuse projection systems. The integrative action of the thalamic reticular system. Electroenceph. clin. Neurophysiol., 1949, 1: 405–420.

Kumagai, H., Sakai, F., Sakuma, A. and Hukuhara, T. Relationship between activity of respiratory center and EEG. Progr. Brain Res., 1966, 21A: 98–111.

Magoun, H.W. An ascending reticular activating in the brain stem. Arch. Neurol. Psychiat. (Chic.), 1952, 67: 145–154.

Mori, A. Evoked potentials via brain stem reticular formation and their respiratory fluctuation. Jap. J. EEG EMG, 1979, 7: 230–240.

Morison, R.S. and Dempsey, E.W. Mechanisms of thalamocortical relations. Amer. J. Physiol., 1942, 135: 281–292.

Morison, R.S. and Dempsey, E.W. Mechanism of thalamocortical augmentation and repetition. Amer. J. Physiol., 1943, 138: 297–308.

Mountcastle, V.B. Modality and topographic properties of single neurones of cat's somatic sensory cortex. J. Neurophysiol., 1957, 20: 408–434.

Nakayama, T. and Hori, T. Cortical evoked potential and subjective sensation to electric stimulation of the skin. Effects of posture and respiratory movement. Jap. J. Physiol., 1966, 16: 612–624.

Nakayama, T. and Suzuki, M. Respiratory slow potentials cortical electroencephalography. Jap. J. EEG EMG, 1975, 3: 266–270.

Shimamura, M. and Livingston, R.B. Longitudinal conduction systems serving spinal and brain stem coordination. J. Neurophysiol., 1963, 26: 258–272.

Shimamura, M. and Yamaguchi, T. Neural mechanisms of the chloralose jerk with special reference to its relationship with spino-bulbo-spinal reflex. Jap. J. Physiol., 1967, 17: 738–745.

Shimamura, M., Kogure, I. and Wada, S. Three types of reticular neurons involved in the spino-bulbo-spinal reflex of cats. Brain Res., 1979, 186: 99–113.

Kyoto Symposia (EEG Suppl. No. 36)
Editors: P.A. Buser, W.A. Cobb and T. Okuma
© 1982, Elsevier Biomedical Press, Amsterdam

Auditory Evoked Potentials Recorded Directly from the Human VIIIth Nerve and Brain Stem: Origins of their Fast and Slow Components

ISAO HASHIMOTO

Department of Neurosurgery, Tokyo Metropolitan Hospital of Fuchu, and Department of Neurophysiology, Tokyo Metropolitan Institute of Neurosciences, Fuchu, Tokyo 183 (Japan)

With recent progress in far field averaging techniques, it has become feasible to record short latency auditory and somatosensory evoked potentials from the scalp. Unique clinical contributions of brain stem auditory evoked potentials (BAEP) include diagnosis of VIIIth nerve tumours (Selters and Brackmann 1977), localization of brain stem lesions (Starr and Achor 1975; Stockard and Rossiter 1977; Hashimoto et al. 1979), early diagnosis of multiple sclerosis (Robinson and Rudge 1977), differential diagnosis of comatose patients (Starr and Achor 1975), monitoring of brain stem function during surgical manipulations in the vicinity of the brain stem (Hashimoto et al. 1980b) and evaluation of brain death (Starr 1976).

The human BAEP is characterized by slow positive (peaking at 5–6 msec) and negative waves with 5 or 7 small positive pseudorhythmic potentials superimposed. In animal studies, 5 fast components of the BAEP at the scalp were ascribed to specific intracranial sources (Lev and Sohmer 1972; Buchwald and Huang 1975) although a considerable overlap of the activities in different auditory structures was present (Jewett 1970; Huang and Buchwald 1977; Achor and Starr 1980). In contrast, the origins of the human BAEP components remain inconclusive in spite of many studies in patients in whom BAEP abnormalities were correlated with clinical and radiological findings.

Precise information on the source of each component in the human BAEP will certainly enhance the clinical utility of the BAEP. We shall present evidence from direct recording in man that the generators of the fast pseudorhythmic components and slow waves are in the VIIIth nerve, brain stem and thalamus.

METHODS

During neurosurgical procedures, records were made from surface electrodes overlying the VIIIth nerve, pons, midbrain and thalamus. Records from a depth electrode within the thalamus were taken during stereotaxic surgery for pain relief. Records were also obtained from movable electrodes within the IVth ventricle, the aqueduct of Sylvius and the IIIrd and lateral ventricles. Details of the recording electrodes were described previously (Hashimoto et al. 1981; Hashimoto 1982).

The reference electrode for intracranial recording was either an alligator clip clamped on the muscle at the edge of the craniotomy or the earlobe ipsilateral to stimulation. The scalp electrode was placed over the central region with reference to the earlobe (C3-A1 or C4-A2 montage). The input signals from the intracranial and scalp electrodes were amplified 10^4 times with a frequency response down 3 dB at 30 and 3 kHz. Usually 1000 responses were averaged except for the records from the VIIIth nerve, where the action potentials were prominent enough to be recorded in a single sweep.

An analysis time of 10 msec was employed for recording the fast components and 20 msec for the slow components. Rarefaction clicks were given to the subjects through TDH-39 transducers mounted in acoustically shielded cushions or insert earphones. The intensity of the clicks was 65 dB above threshold for each subject. The stimulus rate was 15/sec for the fast components and 5/sec for the slow components.

RESULTS

(1) VIIIth nerve

The potentials from the cochlear nerve within the internal auditory meatus (IAM) consisted of 2 or 3 positive components and 2 or 3 negative components (P1-N1-P2-N2(P3-N3)) in which the initial negative component (N1) was the largest (20–150 μV). The potentials from the more proximal portion of the VIIIth nerve were attenuated in amplitude and the initial positive (P1) and negative (N1) components had longer peak latencies than those from the IAM. The amplitude of the N1 component was quite resistant to the effect of increasing stimulus rate, which bears a close parallel to wave I over the scalp (Chiappa et al. 1979).

The onset and peak latencies of the initial positive (P1) component from the IAM were concurrent with those of wave I at the scalp and the prominent compound action potentials (N1) of the VIIIth nerve naturally occurred later than wave I (Fig. 1). Thus there is no doubt that wave I recorded from the scalp with the earlobe reference reflects the earliest potentials from the most distal part of the VIIIth nerve, which is obviously inaccessible under normal conditions.

(2) Pons

Records from the dorsal surface of the pons were characterized by 3 positive components (P2, P3 and P4) followed by a slow negative baseline shift (Fig. 2B). The P2, P3 and P4 components at the pons coincided in time with the scalp II, III and IV waves respectively.

(3) Midbrain (inferior colliculus)

In direct recording from the inferior colliculus (IC) a large slow positive wave, peaking at a similar latency to P5, was predominant and the earlier potentials were markedly attenuated. Wave V at the scalp showed close correlation with the P5

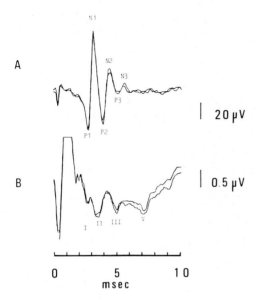

Fig. 1. Correlation of auditory evoked potentials recorded from the human VIIIth nerve and the scalp to monaural click stimulation. A and B denote records from the VIIIth nerve within the internal auditory meatus and from the scalp respectively. The onset and peak of the initial positive component (P1) from the VIIIth nerve are synchronous with those of wave I at the scalp. The peak of the compound action potential (N1) is almost concurrent with the negative peak between waves I and II and later peaks (P2, N2, P3 and N3) are in the range for waves II and III. The reference for intracranial recording is an alligator clip on the muscle at the edge of the craniotomy and for the scalp recording in this case, the external auditory meatus ipsilateral to stimulus. Positivity of the intracranial and scalp (C3) electrodes is down in this and the next figures.

although a small peak latency difference (0.3 msec) between the two was present. The potential showed a systematic change; a progressively shorter latency at increasing distance from the midbrain toward the scalp.

In the course of the present studies the author has become aware of the presence of an even larger amplitude slow negative wave following the P5. This negative wave had a longer duration, well outside the current definition of BAEPs (the responses within 8 or 10 msec). When the analysis time was extended to 20 msec, this slow negativity with an amplitude of 10–14 μV and a duration of about 10 msec was recorded from a circumscribed region of the midbrain (Hashimoto 1982). It was demonstrated in multiple intracranial records that the potentials were propagated to the scalp and the peak of the midbrain negativity coincided in time with the No component at the scalp. These components were classified conventionally as the middle latency components (MLC) (Picton et al. 1974).

(4) Thalamus

The potentials from the medial geniculate body (MGB) had 2 positive components (P5 and P6) which corresponded with waves V and VI at the scalp. The P6 was

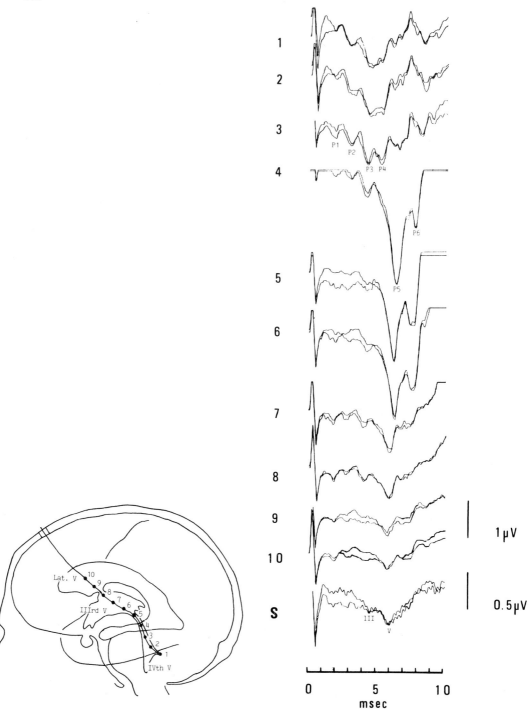

Fig. 2. A: recording electrodes located along the ventricular tube at equal intervals of 1 cm within the IVth, IIIrd and lateral ventricles and the aqueduct of Sylvius. The electrodes 1, 2 and 3 are located in the IVth ventricle (vicinity of the pons); 4 and 5 in the aqueduct of Sylvius (the midbrain); 6, 7 and 8 in the IIIrd ventricle (the thalamus) and 9 and 10 in the lateral ventricle. B: brain stem auditory evoked potentials to left monaural stimulation recorded at the various locations indicated in A. The P2, P3 and P4 components are maximal at the pontine level while P5 is largest at the midbrain level. These potentials are propagated to the scalp with amplitude reductions and minor but systematic latency shifts. S signifies scalp records from C3. The common reference for the intracranial and scalp records is the left earlobe.

maximal within the MGB and dropped off much more rapidly than the P5 with electrode displacement, suggesting that the MGB is primarily responsible for the scalp wave VI. No slow waves comparable to the midbrain potentials were recorded from the MGB except those volume conducted from the midbrain.

(5) Volume conduction of the intracranial potentials to the scalp

Identification of the intracranial source of a surface-recorded potential has been made on the basis of a concurrent maximum activity within the brain (Jewett 1970; Lev and Sohmer 1972; Achor and Starr 1980). However, intracranial and scalp potentials were not always strictly "concurrent" in peak latencies and often minor shifts were present between them, questioning the correspondence of a given intracranial activity with a scalp potential. We consider it mandatory therefore to trace the potential all the way from its intracranial maximum to the scalp. Fig. 2A and B clearly show the amplitude reductions of the potentials as a function of distance from their sources, as well as minor but systematic shifts in their latencies within the brain stem. These systematic latency shifts point to interactions of potential fields generated by multiple sources. Records from more rostral electrodes beyond the midbrain toward the scalp exhibit little or no similar shift in latencies.

DISCUSSION

It has been generally accepted that wave I at the scalp represents the summation of axonal volleys travelling along the VIIIth nerve from the cochlea to the cochlear nucleus. However, the action potentials (N1) of the VIIIth nerve recorded from an electrode within the IAM occur definitely later than the peak of wave I and the preceding small positive wave (P1), an approaching wave front, begins and ends on the same ordinate as wave I. The responses from a more proximal portion of the VIIIth nerve consist of smaller P1 and N1 components and their latencies are progressively increased at increasing distances from the cochlea. Hashimoto et al. (1980a) concluded from their experience in patients with VIIIth nerve lesions, in whom responses typically consist of a normal wave I and a complete loss of other components, that, for the generation of wave I, only the most distal structure of the VIIIth nerve needs to remain intact. Thus, wave I in humans is generated within a limited portion of the first auditory neurones; probably at or near the synaptic junction with cochlear hair cells.

The adaptation of the compound action potentials observed in the present study, which parallels that of N1 from the round window (Eggermont and Odenthal 1974) and wave I at the scalp (Chiappa et al. 1979) supports the concept that wave I represents the postsynaptic potentials of the first order neurones.

Axonal volleys from the VIIIth nerve may contribute to a later wave but much less so than do the postsynaptic potentials to wave I because the polyphasic axonal volleys generated along the VIIIth nerve tend to cancel out in the far field except for the earlier activity at the distal end of the nerve.

The conduction velocity (CV) of the human auditory nerve measured by Hashimoto et al. (1981) is approximately 13 m/sec. Engström and Rexed (1940) demonstrated that 77.1% of the auditory nerve fibres in man have diameters ranging from 2 to 5 μm.

The study by Lazorthes et al. (1961) gave similar results; the diameters were distributed from 2 to 4 μm in 80% of the total nerve fibres studied. If a conversion factor of 4.5 m/sec/μm provided by Desmedt and Cheron (1980) for human sensory fibres is applied, the CV of auditory nerve fibres is 9–23 m/sec with a mean of 16 m/sec, which fits well with the value measured directly from the human auditory nerve.

Suppose the average conduction distance between the cochlea and the cochlear nucleus was 20 mm, the mean conduction time of 20:16 = 1.25 msec would be obtained. This being the case, the earliest incoming volleys to the cochlear nucleus can be calculated, using the onset latency of the initial positive component (1.35–1.5 msec) from the IAM as 1.35 (1.5) msec + 1.25 msec = 2.60 (2.75) msec. Thus the cumulative delays from the stimulus to the earliest postsynaptic activities would be 2.60 (2.45) msec + 0.3 msec (a tentative figure for the synaptic delay at the cochlear nucleus) = 2.90 (3.05) msec. This is in the range for wave II. In fact, a large positive potential (P2), concurrent with wave II at the scalp, is recorded from the pons and undergoes a rapid change in amplitude from the pons to the midbrain. We conclude therefore that wave II represents primarily the postsynaptic potentials of the cochlear nucleus and secondarily the axonal volleys of the VIIIth nerve.

The conclusion reached in humans is consonant with animal studies that wave II is the complex resultant of potentials generated in the cochlear nucleus as well as the VIIIth nerve (Jewett 1970; Lev and Sohmer 1972; Buchwald and Huang 1975) but conflicts with the interpretation that wave II is generated solely from the intracranial portion of the VIIIth nerve on the basis of recording from the auditory nerve alone (Møller et al. 1981). One must recognize, as Arezzo et al. (1979) pointed out, that it is impossible to identify the intracranial sources of a surface-recorded potential by demonstrating a concurrent wave within a single brain site, simply because other intracranal sources may contribute to the surface-recorded potential. Thus the interpretation of intracranial records taken from single brain structures should be made with caution.

The P3 component from the pons which starts and ends in time with wave III at the scalp undergoes a rapid change in amplitude with a small displacement of the electrode within the brain stem but can be clearly traced from its maximum within the pons to the scalp. Although a brain stem auditory nucleus or tract was not specified as the generator for this component in man, the findings in the present study are certainly in general comformity with the animal studies, that the primary generator for wave III is the superior olivary complex (Jewett 1970; Lev and Sohmer 1972; Buchwald and Huang 1975; Achor and Starr 1980).

The P4 component at the level of the pons corresponding to wave IV shows the most rapid attenuation by electrode displacement and is almost merged in the following large potential (P5) at the midbrain (Fig. 2B). This is discrepant from the observations by Jewett (1970) and Lev and Sohmer (1972) in animals that IC is the most active site at this timing but is supported by Achor and Starr (1980), who demonstrated concurrent evoked activities within the various pontine nuclei but were unable to record potentials from the IC within this timing, and also by Buchwald and Huang (1975), who failed to observe any effect on wave IV of lesions of the IC. The P3 and P4 components are similarly maximal at the pontine level. However, they exhibit differential amplitude reductions by the same electrode displacement, indicating that P3 and P4 originate from different sources within the pontine auditory structures (Hashimoto et al. 1981).

While early components (P2, P3 and P4) are predominant at the pons, the P5 component corresponding to wave V is maximal at the midbrain (IC). In multiple records from the ventricular system this potential showed a progressively shorter latency at increasing distances from the midbrain to the scalp, probably due to overlap of separate potentials. Studies in patients with midbrain lesions (Stockard and Rossiter 1977; Hashimoto et al. 1979) and lesion experiments in animals (Buchwald and Huang 1975) point to the IC as the generator for wave V. Thus it is concluded that wave V is almost exclusively generated from the IC.

Following P5, a long smooth rounded wave with negative polarity is recorded from the midbrain. Its amplitude is 4–5 times larger than that of P5 and its duration is about 10 msec. The P6 component, propagated from the MGB, is superimposed on the initial rising phase of this slow negativity.

Studies of unit spikes from the IC in cats demonstrated that the latency of onset spike to clicks is distributed from 4 to 16 msec with most values falling between 6.5 and 8.5 msec (Thurlow et al. 1951; Katsuki et al. 1958; Hind et al. 1963; Huang and Buchwald 1977). These spike responses were superimposed on the slow waves, most often on the negative wave (Thurlow et al. 1951). Huang and Buchwald (1977) claimed, however, that their constant latency units in the IC contributed to the slow positive wave (V) rather than to the slow negative wave, although the IC units showed a mean latency of 8.0 ± 3.1 msec while that of the scalp wave V was 5.4 ± 0.4 msec in their records. They seem to have overlooked the following larger negative wave at the scalp, for which these IC units are actually responsible.

The slow positive and negative waves in cats resemble closely in configuration those in man. It is perhaps permissible therefore to suppose that the slow positive wave (P5) represents the incoming axonal volleys through the lateral lemniscus and the large negative slow wave, the summation of the postsynaptic potentials within the IC.

The cortical Pa wave which follows the midbrain No-Po-Na component was recorded from the primary auditory cortex in man with a peak latency of 26–34 msec (Celesia and Puletti 1971) and in cats with its peak at 12–16 msec (Kaga et al. 1980). The adaptation of the 2 (No-Po-Na and Pa) components naturally differs; while the Pa component decreases its amplitude rapidly at stimulus rates above 1/sec (Kaga et al. 1980), No-Po-Na is not affected at all by repetition rates from 8 to 33/sec (Davis and Hirsh 1979). Thus auditory evoked potentials from the brain stem include components (No, Po, Na) which are well outside the traditional category of

BAEPs. These slow brain stem potentials were neglected because their neural origins were unknown and it was difficult to rule out the myogenic responses (Bickford et al. 1964). However, with proper choice of bandpass filters (Picton et al. (1974), 10–3 kHz; Davis and Hirsh (1979), 40–3 kHz; Hashimoto et al. (1981), 30–3 kHz) and careful muscle artifact rejection, these slow potentials can be consistently recorded as well as faster BAEP components. Davis and Hirsh (1979) use this negative wave for estimating low frequency hearing loss in young children. Now that the sources of both faster BAEP components and the slow negative wave have been identified and the responses have proved to be reproducible with high repetition rates up to 33/sec, they (faster and slow components) can be of equal importance as indicators of neural mechanisms which underlie human brain stem auditory processes and as powerful means for localizing lesions within the brain stem.

SUMMARY

Brain stem auditory evoked potentials in humans are composed of fast pseudorhythmic positive waves and slow positive and negative waves. The sources of these components have been identified on the basis of the observation of amplitude increase in depth records during surgery and by tracing these potentials from their intracranial maximum to the scalp by using movable electrodes within the IVth, IIIrd and lateral ventricles.

The first wave I represents postsynaptic activities of the first auditory neurones; axonal volleys travelling along the auditory nerve do not contribute to this wave, which is obviously discrepant with the currently accepted view. Waves II and III are primarily generated within the pons, with possible contributions from the auditory nerve. Waves IV and VI originate from the pons and the medial geniculate body respectively. Both slow positive and negative waves have their origin in the inferior colliculus (IC). The slow positive waves probably represent incoming axonal volley and the negative waves, the postsynaptic potentials in the IC.

ACKNOWLEDGEMENTS

The author wishes to thank Dr. K. Yasuda, Department of Anesthesiology and Dr. H. Mizutani and other staff of the Department of Neurosurgery, Tokyo Metropolitan Hospital of Fuchu for their willing co-operation throughout recording procedures during surgery. The author is deeply indebted to Dr. M. Ebe, Mr. Y. Ishiyama, Ph.D., Department of Physiology, Dr. G. Totsuka, Department of Otolaryngology, Toranomon Hospital and Dr. M. Shimamura, Department of Neurophysiology, Tokyo Metropolitan Institute of Neurosciences, for their valuable advice and encouragement.

REFERENCES

Achor, L.J. and Starr, A. Auditory brain stem responses in the cat. I. Intracranial and extracranial recordings. Electroenceph. clin. Neurophysiol., 1980, 48: 154–173.

Arezzo, J., Legatt, A.D. and Vaughan, Jr., H.G. Topography and intracranial sources of somatosensory evoked potentials in the monkey. I. Early components. Electroenceph. clin. Neurophysiol., 1979, 46: 155–172.

Bickford, R.G., Jacobson, J.L. and Coby, D.T. Nature of average evoked potentials to sound and other stimuli in man. Ann. N.Y. Acad. Sci., 1964, 112: 204–223.

Buchwald, J.S. and Huang C.M. Far-field acoustic response: Origins in the cat. Science, 1975, 189: 382–384.

Celesia, G.G. and Puletti, F. Auditory input to the human cortex during states of drowsiness and surgical anesthesia. Electroenceph. clin. Neurophysiol., 1971, 31: 603–609.

Chiappa, K.H., Gladstone, K.J. and Young, R.R. Brain stem auditory evoked responses. Studies of waveform variations in 50 normal human subjects. Arch. Neurol. (Chic.), 1979, 36: 81–87.

Davis, H. and Hirsh, S.K. A slow brain stem response for low-frequency audiometry. Audiology, 1979, 18: 445–461.

Desmedt, J.E. and Cheron, G. Central somatosensory conduction in man: Neural generators and interpeak latencies of the far-field components recorded from neck and right or left scalp and earlobes. Electroenceph. clin. Neurophysiol., 1980, 50: 382–403.

Eggermont, J.J. and Odenthal, D.W. Electrophysiological investigation of the human cochlea. Recruitment, masking and adaptation. Audiology, 1974, 13: 1–22.

Engström, H. und Rexed, B. Über die Kaliberverhältnisse der Nervenfasern im N. stato-acusticus des Menschen. Z. mikro-anat. Forsch., 1940, 47: 448–455.

Hashimoto, I. Auditory evoked potentials from the human midbrain: slow brainstem responses. Electroenceph. clin. Neurophysiol., 1982, 53: 652–657.

Hashimoto, I. and Ishiyama, Y. Origin of brain stem auditory evoked potentials. Neurol. Med. (Tokyo), 1980, 13: 401–409.

Hashimoto, I., Ishiyama, Y. and Tozuka, G. Bilaterally recorded brainstem auditory evoked responses: their asymmetric abnormalities and lesions of the brainstem. Arch. Neurol. (Chic.), 1979, 36: 161–167.

Hashimoto, I., Ishiyama Y., Tozuka, G. and Mizutani, H. Monitoring brainstem function during posterior fossa surgery with brainstem auditory evoked potentials. In: C. Barber (Ed.), Evoked Potentials. MTP Press, Lancaster, 1980: 377–390.

Hashimoto, I., Ishiyama, Y., Yoshimoto, T. and Nemoto, S. Brainstem auditory evoked potentials recorded directly from human brainstem and thalamus. Brain, 1981, 104: 841–859.

Hind, J.E., Goldberg, J.M., Greenwood, D.D. and Rose, J.E. Some discharge characteristics of single neurons in the inferior colliculus of the cat. II. Timing of the discharges and observations on binaural stimulation. Neurophysiology, 1963, 26: 321–341.

Huang, C.M. and Buchwald, J.S. Interpretation of the vertex short-latency acoustic response: A study of single neurons in the brain stem. Brain Res., 1977, 137: 291–303.

Jewett, D.L. Volume-conducted potentials in response to auditory stimuli as detected by averaging in the cat. Electroenceph. clin. Neurophysiol., 1970, 28: 609–618.

Kaga, K., Hink, R.F., Shinoda, Y. and Suzuki, J. Evidence for a primary cortical origin of a middle latency auditory evoked potential in cats. Electroenceph. clin. Neurophysiol., 1980, 50: 254–266.

Katsuki, Y., Sumi, T., Uchiyama, H. and Watanabe, T. Electric responses of auditory neurons in cat to sound stimulation. J. Neurophysiol., 1958, 21: 569–588.

Lazorthes, G., Lacomme, Y., Gaubert, J. et Planel, H. La constitution du nerf auditif. Presse méd., 1961, 69: 1067–1068.

Lev, A. and Sohmer, H. Sources of averaged neural responses recorded in animal and human subjects during cochlear audiometry (Electrocochleogram). Arch. klin. exp. Ohr.-, Nas.-, u. Kehlk.-Heilk., 1972, 201: 79–90.

Møller, A.R., Jannetta, P., Bennett, M. and Møller, M.B. Intracranially recorded responses from the human auditory nerve: new insights into the origin of brain stem evoked potentials (BSEPs). Electroenceph. clin. Neurophysiol., 1981, 52: 18–27.

Picton, T.W., Hillyard, S.A., Krausz, H.I. and Galambos, R. Human auditory evoked potentials. I. Evaluation of components. Electroenceph. clin. Neurophysiol., 1974, 36: 176–190.

Robinson, K. and Rudge, P. Abnormalities of the auditory evoked potentials in patients with multiple sclerosis. Brain, 1977, 100: 19–40.

Selters, W.B. and Brackmann, D.E. Acoustic tumor detection with brainstem electric response audiometry. Arch. Otolaryng., 1977, 103: 181–187.

Starr, A. Auditory brain-stem responses in brain death. Brain, 1976, 99: 543–554.

Starr, A. and Achor, L.J. Auditory brain stem responses in neurological disease. Arch. Neurol. (Chic.), 1975, 32: 761–768.

Stockard, J.J. and Rossiter, V.S. Clinical and pathologic correlates of brain stem auditory response abnormalities. Neurology (Minneap.), 1977, 27: 316–325.

Thurlow, W.R., Gross, N.B., Kemp, E.H. and Lowy, K. Microelectrode studies of neural auditory activity of cat. I. Inferior colliculus. J. Neurophysiol., 1951, 14: 289–304.

Kyoto Symposia (EEG Suppl. No. 36)
Editors: P.A. Buser, W.A. Cobb and T. Okuma
© 1982, Elsevier Biomedical Press, Amsterdam

Auditory Nerve–Brain Stem Responses (ABR) in Children with Developmental Brain Disorders and in High Risk Neonates

H. SOHMER

Department of Physiology, Hebrew University-Hadassah Medical School, Jerusalem (Israel)

For many years the recording of responses of the auditory nerve and the brain stem auditory pathway (ABR) have contributed to the evaluation of auditory disorders by providing objective evidence of the presence of hearing loss and its degree (threshold) and by giving indications of the sites of lesions (Feinmesser and Sohmer 1976). ABRs have also contributed to the diagnosis of neurological disorders (Sohmer et al. 1974) of the brain stem such as tumours (Starr and Achor 1975) and multiple sclerosis (Robinson and Rudge 1977). More recently it has been shown that ABR can be helpful in the evaluation of infants and children with developmental brain disorders, here defined as dysfunctions encompassing a group of recognizable, chronic, neurologically related conditions such as psycho-motor retardation, minimal brain dysfunction, hyperkinetic behaviour, autism, learning disorders and cerebral palsy. These records in such patients are of value since they often confirm the presence of an organic brain lesion when a psychiatric condition is expected (e.g. autism). They may also give some indication of the nature and location of the lesion which can be related to the abnormal psycho-motor behaviour exhibited by these children.

The first part of this paper will report on studies of ABR in children with developmental brain disorders. The results of this phase of the study, together with the observation that many of the children studied had suffered from some congenital, perinatal or neonatal insult, led to ABR recording on very young infants who had been in the neonatal intensive care unit and then directly on those neonates who had suffered such insults. Finally, the results of the 3 parts of the study led to the hypothesis that ABR studies in high risk neonates and infants may be able to predict the later appearance of developmental brain disorders.

METHODS

The auditory nerve and brain stem evoked potentials (ABR) were elicited in response to alternating polarity click stimuli presented monaurally by an earphone at rates of 10 or 20/sec and at intensities of 70–80 dB above the threshold of the normal population (i.e. nHL). Occasionally, the electric response threshold was also obtained by determining the lowest click intensity which elicited a response. The electrical activity, recorded as the potential difference between an ipsilateral earlobe electrode and a scalp vertex electrode, was filtered (250 Hz–5kHz, 6 dB/oct), amplified and averaged (N = 585–1024). At least 2 consecutive average traces were obtained for each condition for each subject.

SUBJECTS

The patient groups included: (a) 450 infants and children referred for ABR testing by the Paediatric Department (including clinic) of the Hadassah University Hospital for evaluation of some developmental brain disorder; (b) 19 "graduates" of the neonatal intensive care unit when they were 3–4 months post full term; (c) 57 full-term neonates from the neonatal intensive and intermediate care units.

The ABR traces obtained in these patients were compared with appropriate control groups. Since several of the ABR response parameters undergo developmental changes with age (e.g. interwave latencies), 4 control groups of different ages were assembled. The control group subjects were not sedated. The first control group was made up of 34 ears from very young (1–8 h old), full term, normal neonates. These records were made using a small portable Microshev Computerized Electric Response Audiometer-C-ERA-100 (Rubinstein and Sohmer 1982). The records in the 3 additional control groups were made using a laboratory-assembled modular system. The second control group consisted of 29 ears from normal, full-term neonates of average age 7 days and the third control group included 29 ears from normal infants, 3–4 months of age (Gafni et al. 1980). The final control group was made up of 74 ears from normal 10-year-old children, boys and girls, of average intelligence (Goldman et al. 1981). Fig. 1 shows a typical response trace from each of the control groups. The figure also shows a scheme for wave identification.

Particular attention was paid to the presence or absence of typical response waves (W1, W3, W4a and b, P4) and interwave latencies (W3-W1 and P4-W1). The interwave latency P4-W1 is termed brain stem transmission time (BTT) and is relatively independent of stimulus intensity, stimulus frequency, stimulus repetition rate (for low and moderate rates – 10–20 clicks/sec) and the presence of a conductive hearing loss (Fabiani et al. 1979). Table I presents the values for the response parameters in the control groups. Abnormality was indicated by the absence of a typical response wave, although the absence or small amplitude of wave 2 or wave 5 (Jewett VI) was not considered abnormal because of their great variability in the normal population. An abnormal ABR trace was also defined as one in which a response wave latency differed from the average value of the appropriate control groups by more than 2 S.D. As often reported, it proved difficult to evaluate ABR amplitudes properly because of the large standard deviations of the average amplitudes in the control groups. Nevertheless an amplitude ratio beyond 1 S.D. of the control group average was considered as indicating possible abnormality (in spite of the low confidence of such a determination).

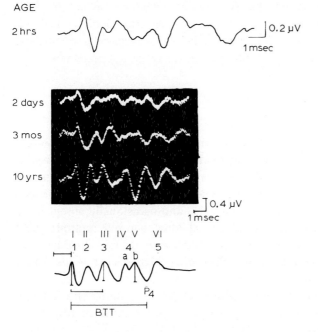

Fig. 1. ABRs in normal infants and children, showing wave identification and how latencies and amplitudes were measured. Note the decrease of BTT with age.

TABLE I

ABR PARAMETERS (AVERAGE ± S.D.) IN THE CONTROL GROUPS OF VARIOUS AGES

In the neonates A* group, a different ABR instrument was used.

Age	Latencies (msec)			Amplitudes	
	W1	W3-W1	BTT	W3/W1	W4/W1
Neonates A*	1.76 ± 0.2	2.63 ± 0.24	5.88 ± 0.31	1.17 ± 0.72	0.65 ± 0.80
Neonates B	1.65 ± 0.19	2.94 ± 0.23	5.90 ± 0.34	0.80 ± 0.23	0.87 ± 0.23
3–4 months	1.55 ± 0.19	2.63 ± 0.18	5.42 ± 0.25	0.91 ± 0.36	0.83 ± 0.30
10 years	1.37 ± 0.09	2.17 ± 0.14	4.62 ± 0.19	1.11 ± 0.40	1.28 ± 0.57

SECTION I

The first part of this study involves 450 infants and children referred for evaluation of a developmental brain disorder. In many of these infants and children (111) there was evidence of some form of congenital, perinatal or neonatal complication (e.g. neonatal hyperbilirubinaemia, perinatal asphyxia) which could have been responsible for the developmental brain disorder. ABR recording was conducted on many of the subjects under chloral hydrate, seconal or paraldehyde sedation; it has already been shown that such sedation does not affect the ABR (Sohmer et al. 1978). The ABR tests, conducted down to electric response threshold, also gave the first indication of the hearing threshold in a large number of these children in whom conventional behavioural audiometry could not be conducted.

RESULTS

A large number of the children with developmental brain disorders had abnormal ABR traces. However, in this paper we report on the 51 children in whom there were the 3 criteria of a developmental brain disorder, a congenital, perinatal or neonatal insult and an abnormal ABR. The last usually took the form of prolonged latencies (24), abnormal response wave amplitude ratios (17) and occasionally absent brain stem waves (6). The traces in several of the children showed multiple ABR abnormalities. In 18 infants and children with developmental brain disorders, the entire ABR pattern was absent even in response to the highest click levels. These children, therefore, had a profound hearing loss.

Fig. 2 shows traces from some of these children, chosen to demonstrate different types of developmental brain disorders and different types of ABR abnormalities.

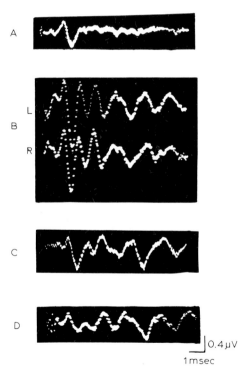

Fig. 2. ABRs in children with developmental brain disorders. The text describes the insult, the clinical state and the ABR abnormalities seen in each child. Since the ABR traces were similar for both ears in cases A, C and D, only 1 ear is shown.

Trace A is from a 1-year-old severely retarded child of consanguineous parents, born following a precipitate delivery due to foetal distress, which probably caused perinatal asphyxia. The brain stem response components are absent while the auditory nerve response (W1) is preserved. The absence of 1 or more brain stem waves does not necessarily mean structural damage to the neurones directly, since in cases of multiple sclerosis, for example, one occasionally finds absent brain stem waves with normal hearing. This is interpreted as being due to demyelination leading to loss of synchrony (Sohmer 1982). The visual cortical evoked response was also abnormal in this child. The following 2 traces are from a 3-year-old psycho-motor retarded child who was born prematurely (30–32 weeks, 1.500 kg birth weight) with episodes of apnoea. Waves 3 and 4 of the brain stem waves are much smaller in amplitude compared with the amplitude of the first wave. The response wave form therefore seems strikingly different from normal. Trace C is from a 6-year-old boy with speech disability and a history of neonatal hyperbilirubinaemia. The ABR test showed normal thresholds, demonstrating that the speech disability was not related to a hearing loss. However, the ABR BTT in this child was 5.1 msec (normal value 4.62 ± 0.19 msec). The final trace is from a 3-year-old autistic girl. BTT in this child is also prolonged (5.2 msec).

Comment

Other workers have also recorded ABRs in children with developmental disorders. For example, Sohmer and Student (1978), Skoff et al. (1980) and Rosenblum et al. (1980) found abnormal ABRs in many but not all autistic children studied and the abnormality appeared as a prolonged BTT and, in a few, as diminished amplitude of wave 3.

A similar variability of results was obtained in studies of ABRs in children diagnosed as suffering from minimal brain dysfunction (MBD) (Sohmer and Student 1978; Godby et al. 1980) since several of the MBD children had prolonged BTTs. Children with psycho-motor retardation had similar types of ABR abnormality and, in several, one or more of the brain stem responses were absent (Sohmer et al. 1979). This variability of abnormal ABR findings in the subgroups of children with developmental brain disorders seems to indicate that the subgroups studied were heterogeneous.

The ABRs have also been studied in retarded adults. Galbraith et al. (1979) and Squires et al. (1980) studied adults with Down's syndrome and adults with severe retardation of mixed, non-genetic aetiologies. They found the largest brain stem response amplitudes in the control normal group, intermediate in the mixed group and smallest in the Down's group. The BTT values in the Down's group were often shorter than those in the control group while BTT in the unknown aetiology retarded group was often greater than that in the control group. Goldman et al. (1981) also found reduced brain stem response amplitudes in a group of 10-year-old children with borderline retardation (mean IQ 81).

Sohmer and Student (1978), Student and Sohmer (1978) and Squires et al. (1980) reported that in several of their subjects with some form of developmental brain disorder, ABRs were absent even in response to the highest stimulus intensity used, indicating profound hearing loss. This too may be considered a sign of an organic (not necessarily brain) lesion in these subjects.

This study was based on the use of an evoked response technique employing auditory stimuli and eliciting responses from the auditory pathway. However, it should be pointed out that it is unlikely that the organic lesions demonstrated in these children by these techniques are limited to the auditory pathway – rather it is more likely that there is diffuse brain damage which could possibly be demonstrated by the use of additional evoked response techniques. Furthermore, even though the response studied (ABR) was generated in the brain stem, it is not likely that the abnormality was limited to it. Indeed, other types of electrical recording have also been used in the study of developmentally impaired subjects and have been shown to be abnormal. For example, the visual evoked potential from the occipital cortex was found to be abnormal in a majority of mentally retarded children studied (Shapira et al. 1973). Cortical auditory evoked responses were found to have increased amplitudes in Down's syndrome infants (Barnet and Lodge 1967). In a recent study using newer analysis techniques, the EEG in children at risk for neurological disorders and with learning disabilities has been found to have a high incidence of abnormalities (Ahn et al. 1980). Therefore this study should be complemented by using other evoked response techniques (visual and somatosensory) on homogenous subgroups of patients in order to obtain information about the functional activity of other brain regions and pathways. Following this we shall be in a position to determine whether each subgroup of children with developmental brain disorders (e.g. autism or minimal brain dysfunction) has distinct, differentiating electrophysiological abnormalities.

The findings of this study and the others reported have several interesting implications. These tests have shown that the nervous systems of many of the children in the experimental groups studied generate deviant electrophysiological responses; therefore deviant ABR traces represent electrophysiological evidence for the presence of brain damage in these children with developmental brain disorders, at least in the region of the brain stem. Thus ABR tests in such children can contribute to the diagnosis not only by providing an objective measure of their hearing acuity (which is very difficult to obtain by conventional behavioural means in such children) but also by providing objective electrophysiological evidence for an organic basis for the developmental disorder. This is especially important in the evaluation of autistic children, since a small number of workers feel that autism is due to psychogenic-emotional causes (O'Gorman 1970). On the other hand, there is much support today for the concept that autism is due to an organic brain lesion thought to involve the brain stem (Ornitz 1978), probably due to some congenital-perinatal insult (Finegan and Quarrington 1980). The ability to demonstrate deviant electrophysiological responses in such a child would constitute further evidence for an underlying organic lesion, leading to early therapeutic intervention along appropriate lines.

The final implication is that there seems to be an association between congenital, perinatal or neonatal complications, developmental brain disorders (Sechzer et al. 1973; Sohmer et al. 1979; Skoff et al. 1980; Finegan and Quarrington, 1980) and abnormal ABR. This therefore leads to the second part of this study: application of ABR recording to high risk infants.

SECTION II

In this phase, ABR recording was conducted on 19 infants, 3–4 months of age (after full term), who were hospitalized in the neonatal intensive care unit because of such factors as prematurity and respiratory distress. They had all been released to their homes and were invited back to the laboratory for the ABR test. An abnormal ABR was recorded in 9 of them. Brain stem components were absent in 2; BTT was prolonged in 3 and amplitude abnormalities were seen in 5 infants. Two of these infants with abnormal ABRs (prolonged BTT and reduced wave 3 amplitude) were showing signs of delayed development at the time of the test. The remaining 17 infants seemed to be developing normally.

Comment

The presence of an abnormal ABR in 3–4 month graduates of the intensive care unit would seem to indicate that brain damage had already occurred. As discussed above, this brain damage would probably not be limited to the brain stem and not to the auditory pathways. In addition, even though neurologically many of them appear normal, a developmental brain disorder may appear (following a clinically silent period) only when the child is expected to perform various learning, behavioural, language and motor skills. This possibility leads to the desire to follow these infants longitudinally at least until they complete the first few grades of elementary school.

Since there are already ABR signs of brain damage in many of the 3–4-month-old infants, it would also be interesting to study the ABR in neonates closer to the time of occurrence of the congenital, perinatal or neonatal insult. It had already been shown that ABRs could be recorded in neonates (Lieberman et al. 1973) and since then the ABRs have been used mainly for the auditory evaluation of neonates at risk for hearing loss. Following the demonstration that ABRs can contribute to the evaluation of adult neurological patients, several studies have been devoted to the neurological assessment of neurologically at-risk neonates. Recording in such neonates constituted the third part of this study.

SECTION III

ABR recording was conducted on a total of 57 at-risk neonates (e.g. perinatal asphyxia, hyperbilirubinaemia) when they were at full term. Twenty-six full-term neonates in the intermediate care unit because of the presence of bilirubin levels

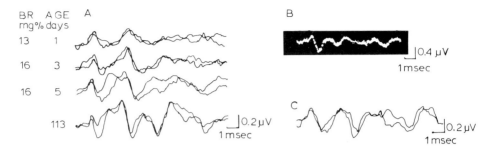

Fig. 3. ABRs in full-term neonates. Infant A had hyperbilirubinaemia and the bilirubin levels (BR) on the day of each test are shown. Infant B had neonatal meningitis and C suffered intrauterine growth retardation.

greater than 15 mg% were studied. The ABR traces were normal in 8; there were no ABRs in 2; one or more of the brain stem components were absent in 11; the BTT was prolonged in 5; the wave 3 to wave 1 interval was prolonged in 3, and there were amplitude ratio abnormalities in 11 (dominated by elevated wave 3 amplitude ratios in 6 and reduced wave 4 amplitude ratios in 2). Repeated ABR tests were conducted on 13 of these infants over periods ranging from several days to several weeks and ABR improvements were seen in 9 of them, particularly in the appearance of brain stem waves which were not apparent in earlier records (similar changes in the ABR pattern were not seen in repeated records of normal neonates). It is too soon to determine if there is a direct correlation between bilirubin levels and ABR parameters. An example in Fig. 3 shows that initially wave 4 was absent and wave 3 prolonged in latency but, with time, the latency of wave 3 shortened, its amplitude greatly increased and wave 4 appeared.

An additional group of 31 full-term neonates was studied while they were in the neonatal intensive care unit or shortly after their release. Fifteen of these infants had normal ABR traces. The example in Fig. 3B is from an infant who suffered neonatal meningitis. In this trace, obtained when he was 1 month old, the auditory nerve response is the largest and the BTT is prolonged (7.05 msec).

The ABR trace in Fig. 3C is from a full-term infant whose birth weight was 1.760 kg, with intrauterine growth retardation. The trace is abnormal since the BTT is prolonged (6.6 msec) and the amplitude of wave 3 is very large.

Comment

Several recent studies have also been devoted to the evaluation of ABRs in at-risk neonates – mainly those in whom there were periods of asphyxia (Kileny et al. 1980; Galambos and Despland 1980; Lutschg et al. 1980; Marshall et al. 1980; Salamy et al. 1980; Sanders and Amlie 1980). The types of ABR abnormality which they report are similar to those reported in this study. In addition, as in this study (hyperbilirubinaemia) several workers (Kileny et al. 1980; Sanders and Amlie 1980) also reported improvement of the ABR when the tests were repeated weeks or months later.

These findings of abnormal ABRs in neonates who have suffered a congenital, perinatal or neonatal insult demonstrate the probable vulnerability of the brain stem to such complications. Furthermore, since we assume that an abnormal ABR is functional evidence for the presence of brain damage (either biochemical or structural, focal or diffuse), these results of abnormal ABRs in at-risk neonates indicate that the brain damage has been induced close to the time of occurrence of the insult, if not concurrently with it.

In addition, as pointed out previously, the presence of an abnormal ABR does not necessarily mean that the brain damage is limited to the brain stem or to the auditory pathway. In fact, other electrophysiological studies of similar at-risk neonates have also provided evidence for damage in other brain regions. Hrbek et al. (1977) and Gambi et al. (1980) have provided evidence for abnormal visual evoked responses in asphyxiated neonates. Also the EEG in many at-risk neonates was abnormal (Despland 1980, personal communication). Evidence that perinatal insults can induce brain damage also comes from studies on experimental animals. Monkeys subjected to hypoxia at birth later developed behaviour similar to that of children with minimal brain dysfunction (Sechzer et al. 1973) or with autistic traits (Mirsky et al. 1979) and structural brain lesions have been found in the brain stem and cerebral cortex in such experimental animals (Windle, 1966; Meyers, 1967). Histological evidence of anoxic encephalopathy in the brain stem and cerebral cortex have also been found in human infants following acute asphyxial episodes (Brierley 1966; Leech and Alvord 1977).

The recovery of the ABR in older infants following periods of abnormality when these same infants were younger, as found in this study and as reported by other workers (asphyxia – Kileny et al. 1980; Sanders and Amlie 1980) does not necessarily mean complete recovery of all brain function. As suggested above, the brain damage induced by the congenital, perinatal or neonatal insult may have been widespread and while the ABR may have recovered, indicating perhaps recovery of the brain stem auditory pathway, other brain regions may still be damaged. The results of Despland (1980) seem to support this possibility; he studied the EEG of at-risk neonates with repeated EEG and clinical follow-up and found that an abnormal EEG during the initial neonatal period was correlated with an unfavourable outcome even though the EEG became normal during the later neonatal period. These considerations therefore also lead to the suggestion that at-risk neonates with initially abnormal ABRs should be studied longitudinally, even if there is later improvement of the ABR, until they conclude at least the first grade of elementary school.

GENERAL DISCUSSION

The results of this study and their implications lead to an interesting and plausible hypothesis: congenital, perinatal and neonatal insults, such as asphyxia and hyperbilirubinaemia, can induce brain damage (structural or chemical, focal or diffuse) of varying severity. Except for such conditions as inborn errors of metabolism which induce progressive, degenerative storage diseases, the perinatal insult induces the brain damage at the time of the insult. This brain damage gives rise to abnormal neuronal function and deviant electrical activity. The brain damage in some regions of the brain may be reversible with amelioration of the underlying cause (e.g. decrease in concentration of free bilirubin), while in other brain regions the effect may be irreversible. Depending upon the brain region irreversibly affected and depending upon the function of this brain region in the normal subject and the age at which this damaged region "expresses itself", a clinically silent period of varying duration may be followed by the appearance of a developmental brain disorder. Some examples of the later manifestations of such brain dysfunction include attention deficit disorders and specific learning disabilities. Therefore the recording of auditory nerve–brain stem evoked responses, perhaps complemented by other types of evoked reponse (e.g. visual (Hrbek et al. 1977) and somatosensory (Pratt et al. 1981)) and EEG, may serve as a non-invasive diagnostic tool for the early detection of brain dysfunction in at-risk neonates before the appearance of the developmental brain disorder and may predict the impending disorder.

The importance of this suggestion concerning the relationship between perinatal events, brain damage, neuronal dysfunction and the possibility that ABRs may be able to predict neuro-developmental deviations, derives from the fact that early detection of these impending behavioural deviations by electrophysiological means would lead to close and frequent observation of the infant, proper parental and educational counselling and the provision of an enriched, stimulating environment for the child to enable him to reach his full developmental potential in spite of the insult suffered at a very early age.

This hypothesis should be tested by several research groups by conducting ABR (and other) tests in a group of neonates who have suffered from congenital, perinatal or neonatal insults – making them high risks for neurological or developmental dysfunction – and in normal control neonates. These neonatal ABR records should be followed by additional ABR tests and by long-term serial follow-up of the motor, developmental, behavioural and cognitive functions of all the infants until they complete the first 2 grades of elementary school, when possible dyslexia or other forms of learning and behavioural disabilities can be assessed.

In order to appraise properly the ability of ABR recording to predict developmental disorders, we suggest that the neonates studied should be divided into at least 5 groups prior to their long-term electrophysiological and clinical follow-up: (a) normal control neonates – with normal ABRs; (b) normal control neonates with abnormal ABRs (if any); (c) high risk neonates with persistently abnormal ABRs (no recovery of ABR); (d) high risk neonates with initially abnormal ABRs which show recovery; (e) high risk neonates with persistently normal ABR.

The percentage of neonates in each of these groups in which a developmental brain disorder appears by the end of the study (at least 6 years), will provide the basis for determining the effectiveness of this hypothesis and for estimating the cost-benefit ratio of the test.

In conclusion, this hypothesis concerning the possibility that ABR recording in at-risk neonates may be able to predict the later appearance of developmental brain disorders should be studied and evaluated in several medical centres.

SUMMARY

Auditory nerve–brain stem evoked responses (ABR) have been used for many years to evaluate auditory and neurological disorders. This study is devoted to the demonstration that ABRs can also contribute to the assessment of children with developmental brain disorders, e.g. psycho-motor retardation, minimal brain dysfunction, cerebral palsy and autism. The ABR in many of these children was abnormal, providing evidence for the presence of brain damage in these children which is probably responsible for the disorder they display. Since many of these children suffered from some congenital, perinatal or neonatal insult, ABR recording was also conducted in high risk neonates and young infants. Many of these neonates and infants had abnormal ABRs and, in several, there was improvement of the ABR upon repeated testing. These findings of abnormal ABRs in children with developmental brain disorders who suffered a perinatal insult and abnormal ABRs in neonates who suffered such an insult lead to the following hypothesis: a congenital-perinatal-neonatal insult can cause, at the time of its occurrence, some form of brain damage which may be demonstrated by abnormal ABRs. The same underlying brain damage may also cause developmental brain disorders which become apparent when he is older. Therefore ABR recording during the neonatal period may contribute to the early detection of brain dysfunction in at-risk neonates and may predict the later appearance of neurological, behavioural and cognitive dysfunctions. A longitudinal experimental protocol for the testing and evaluation of this hypothesis is presented.

ACKNOWLEDGEMENTS

This study was conducted with the assistance of M. Gafni, G. Szabo, P. Fainmesser, S. Gross and R. Kinarti and the article is the results of discussions with them. Their cooperation is gratefully acknowledged.

REFERENCES

Ahn, H., Prichep, L., John, E.R., Baird, H., Trepetin, M. and Kaye, H. Developmental equations reflect brain dysfunctions. Science, 1980, 210: 1259–1262.

Barnet, A.B. and Lodge, A. Click evoked EEG responses in normal and developmentally retarded infants. Nature (Lond.), 1967, 214: 252–255.

Brierley, J.D. The influence of brain swelling, age and hypotension upon the pattern of cerebral damage in hypoxia. In: F. Luthy and A. Bischoff (Eds.), Proceedings of the Fifth International Congress of Neuropathology. Excerpta Medica, Amsterdam, 1966: 21–28.

Despland, P.A. Prognostic valve of the inactive and paroxysmal EEG in premature and full-term babies. Personal communication, 1980.

Fabiani, M., Sohmer, H., Tait, C., Gafni, M. and Kinarti, R. A functional measure of brain activity: Brainstem transmission time. Electroenceph. clin. Neurophysiol., 1979, 47: 483–491.

Feinmesser, M. and Sohmer, H. Contribution of cochlear, brainstem and cortical responses to differential diagnosis and lesion location in hearing loss. In: S.K. Hirsh, D.H. Eldredge, I.J. Hirsh and S.R. Silverman (Eds.), Essays Honoring Hallowell Davis. Washington University Press, St. Louis, Mo., 1976: 393–402.

Finegan, J.-A. and Quarrington, B. Pre-, peri-, and neonatal factors and infantile autism. In: S. Chess and A. Thomas (Eds.), Annual Progress in Child Psychiatry and Child Development. Brunner/Mazel, New York, 1980: 501–512.

Gafni, M., Sohmer, H., Gross, S., Weizman, Z. and Robinson, M.J. Analysis of auditory nerve-brainstem responses (ABR) in neonates and very young infants. Arch. Otorhinolaryngol., 1980, 229: 167–174.

Galambos, R. and Despland, P.A. The auditory brainstem response (ABR) evaluates risk factors for hearing loss in the newborn. Pediatr. Res., 1980, 14: 159–163.

Galbraith, G.C., Squires, N., Altair, D. and Giddon, J.D. Electrophysiological assessments in mentally retarded individuals: from brain stem to cortex. In: H. Begleiter (Ed.), Evoked Brain Potentials and Behavior. Plenum Press, New York, 1979: 229–248.

Gambi, D., Rossini, P.M., Albertini, G., Sollazzo, D., Torrioli, M.G. and Polidori, G.C. Follow-up of visual evoked potential in full-term and pre-term control newborns and in subjects who suffered from perinatal respiratory distress. Electroenceph. clin. Neurophysiol., 1980, 48: 509–516.

Godby, D.C., Tanguay, P.E., Oettinger, L. and Hart, A.D. Brainstem auditory evoked potentials in normal and minimally brain dysfunctioned children. Presented at Amer. Psychol. Ass., Montreal, Sept., 1980.

Goldman, Z., Sohmer, H., Godfrey, C. and Manheim, A. Auditory nerve, brainstem and cortical response correlates of learning capacity. Physiol. Behav., 1981, 26: 637–688.

Hrbek, A., Karlberg, P., Kjellmer, I., Olsson, T. and Riha, M. Clinical application of evoked electroencephalographic responses in newborn infants. I. Perinatal asphyxia. Develop. Med. Child Neurol., 1977, 19: 34–44.

Kileny, P., Connelly, C. and Robertson, C. Auditory brainstem responses in perinatal asphyxia. Int. J. Pediat. Otorhinolaryngol., 1980, 2: 147–159.

Leech, R.W. and Alvord, Jr., E.C. Anoxic-ischemic encephalopathy in the human neonatal period. Arch. Neurol. (Chic.), 1977, 34: 109–113.

Lieberman, A., Sohmer, H. and Szabo, G. Cochlear audiometry (electrocochleography) during the neonatal period. Devel. Med. Child Neurol., 1973, 15: 8–13.

Lutschg, J., Bina, M., Matsumiya, Y. and Lombroso, C.T. Brainstem auditory evoked potentials (BAEPs) in asphyxiated and neurologically abnormal newborns. Electroenceph. clin. Neurophysiol., 1980, 49: 27P.

Marshall, R.E., Reichert, T.J., Kerley, S.M. and Davis, H. Auditory function in newborn intensive-care unit patients revealed by auditory brainstem potentials. J. Pediat., 1980, 96: 731–735.

Meyers, R.E. Patterns of perinatal brain damage in the monkey. In: L.S. James, R.E. Myers and G.E. Guall (Eds.), Brain Damage in the Fetus and Newborn from Hypoxia or Asphyxia. Ross Laboratories, Columbus, Ohio, 1967: 17–21.

Mirsky, A., Orren, M., Stanton, L., Fullerton, B., Harris, S. and Myers, R. Auditory evoked potentials and auditory behavior following prenatal and perinatal asphyxia in rhesus monkeys. Develop. Psychobiol., 1979, 12: 369–379.

O'Gorman, G. The Nature of Childhood Autism. Butterworths, London, 1970.

Ornitz, E. Neurophysiologic studies. In: M. Rutter and E. Schopler (Eds.), Autism. Plenum Press, New York, 1978.

Pratt, H., Amlie, R.N. and Starr, A. Short latency mechanically evoked peripheral nerve and somatosensory potentials in newborn infants. Pediat. Res., 1981, 15: 295–298.

Robinson, K. and Rudge, P. Abnormalities of the auditory evoked potentials in patients with multiple sclerosis. Brain, 1977, 100: 19–40.

Rosenblum, S.M., Arick, J.R., Krug, D.A., Stubbs, E.G., Young, N.B. and Pelson, R.O. Auditory brainstem evoked responses in autistic children. J. Autism Develop. Disorders, 1980, 10: 215–225.

Rubinstein, A. and Sohmer, H. Latency of auditory nerve response in neonates 1–8 hours old. Ann. Otol. (St. Louis), 1982, 91: 205–208.

Salamy, A., Mendelson, T., Tooley, W.H. and Chaplin, E.R. Differential development of brainstem potentials in healthy and high-risk infants. Science, 1980, 210: 553–555.

Sanders, S.J. and Amlie, R.N. Incidence and recovery from perinatal asphyxia in newborns as measured by auditory brainstem responses (ABR). Clin. Res., 1980, 28: 126A.

Sechzer, J.A., Faro, M.D. and Windle, W.F. Studies of monkeys asphyxiated at birth: implication for minimal cerebral dysfunction. In: S. Walzer and P.H. Wolff (Eds.), Minimal Cerebral Dysfunction in Children. Grune and Stratton, New York, 1973: 13–34.

Shapira, Y., Szabo, G., Merin, S. and Auerbach, E. Electrophysiological studies of the visual system in mentally retarded children. II. Visual evoked potentials. J. pediat. Ophthal., 1973, 10: 223–225.

Skoff, B.F., Mirsky, A.F. and Turner, D. Prolonged brainstem transmission time in autism. Psychiat. Res., 1980, 2: 157–166.

Sohmer, H. Auditory evoked potentials in neurological disorders. In: E.J. Moore (Ed.), Handbook of Electrocochleography and Brainstem Electrical Responses. Grune and Stratton, New York, 1982, in press.

Sohmer, H. and Student, M. Auditory nerve and brainstem evoked responses in normal, autistic, minimal brain dysfunction and psychomotor retarded children. Electroenceph. clin. Neurophysiol., 1978, 44: 380–388.

Sohmer, H., Feinmesser, M. and Szabo, G. Sources of electrocochleographic responses as studied in patients with brain damage. Electroenceph. clin. Neurophysiol., 1974, 37: 663–669.

Sohmer, H., Gafni, M. and Chisin, R. Auditory nerve and brain stem responses: comparison in awake and unconscious subjects. Arch. Neurol. (Chic.), 1978, 35: 228–230.

Sohmer, H., Gafni, M., Tannenbaum, A., Szabo, G., Robinson, M.J. and Weitzman, Z. Auditory nerve-brain stem response abnormalities in infants with developmental disorders. In: S. Harel (Ed.), The At Risk Infant. Excerpta Medica, Amsterdam, 1979: 272–276.

Squires, N., Aine, C., Buchwald, J., Norman, R. and Galbraith, G. Auditory brainstem response abnormalities in severely and profoundly retarded adults. Electroenceph. clin. Neurophysiol., 1980, 50: 172–185.

Starr, A. and Achor, J. Auditory brainstem responses in neurological disease. Arch. Neurol. (Chic.), 1975, 32: 761–768.

Student, M. and Sohmer, H. Evidence from auditory nerve and brainstem evoked responses for an organic brain lesion in children with autistic traits. J. Autism Child. Schizo., 1978, 8: 13–20.

Windle, W.F. An experimental approach to prevention or reduction of the brain damage of birth asphyxia. Develop. Med. Child Neurol., 1966, 8: 129–140.

Kyoto Symposia (EEG Suppl. No. 36)
Editors: P.A. Buser, W.A. Cobb and T. Okuma
© 1982, Elsevier Biomedical Press, Amsterdam

328

Neural Pathways of Somatosensory Evoked Potentials: Clinical Implications

JUN KIMURA, THORU YAMADA, EZZATOLLAH SHIVAPOUR and STOKES DICKINS

Division of Clinical Electrophysiology, University Hospital and Clinics, Iowa City, Ia. 52242 (U.S.A.)

Early clinical studies suggested that all the somatosensory evoked potential (SEP) components might be dependent solely upon the integrity of the posterior column-medial lemniscal system. This view was consistent with the proposal that SEPs were mediated exclusively by the fast conducting, large myelinated sensory fibres in the peripheral nerve. However, more recent clinical and experimental studies indicate that other somatosensory pathways may provide additional, though less prominent, contributions. The possibility of a multiple, as opposed to a unitary, sensory system has important clinical implications since a prolongation of SEP interpeak intervals does not necessarily localize the lesion between the presumed sites of the respective neural generators if more than one pathway exists. The purpose of this communication is to summarize our recent observations which favour at least dual SEP pathways centrally – and possibly even peripherally.

NEURAL SOURCES OF VARIOUS PEAKS

Nomenclature

Considerable confusion exists in SEP analysis because various authors have used different systems to describe the same wave forms. For the purpose of this discussion short latency components are specified by polarity and average peak latency to the nearest millisecond, e.g., scalp recorded P9, P11, P13 and P14. Similarly, late components are designated as N19, P22, N30, P40 and N60.

Origins of short latency components

The spinal potential recorded from the cervical region after stimulation of the median nerve at the wrist is divided into 4 components, Pc9 (N9), N11, N13 and N14 (Fig. 1) (Yamada et al. 1980). The earliest component is negative relative to the ear reference electrode but positive in polarity when recorded with a non-cephalic reference; hence the name, positive cervical potential, Pc9. The scalp-recorded short latency SEP consists of 4 positive components, P9, P11, P13 and P14 using the knee reference. When referred to the ear, only P13 and P14 are identified since P9 and P11 are nearly isopotential between the scalp and ear. These 4 peaks of the cervical and scalp-recorded SEPs normally occur within the first 15 msec.

The polarity characteristics of the short latency SEPs led us to believe that a

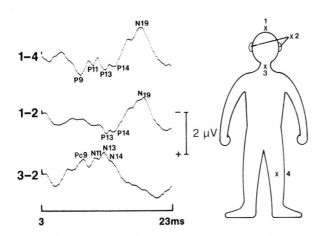

Fig. 1. Simultaneous recording from Cz (1) and low cervical (3) electrodes with ear (2) and knee (4) reference. Four positive peaks, P9, P11, P13 and P14, were recorded at Cz when using a knee reference (top trace), but P9 and P11 were absent with ear reference recording (middle trace). At the low cervical electrode, positive cervical peak Pc9 was negative in polarity relative to the "active" ear reference electrode. This was followed by 3 negative peaks, N11, N13 and N14 (bottom trace).

negative field near the generator site is responsible for the cervical potential and that the scalp-recorded peak is primarily, although perhaps not exclusively, attributable to an approaching field of positivity from the same source. Based on the polarity and mean latency, the presumed neural generators of each peak are: (1) the entry to the brachial plexus (P9 and Pc9), (2) the entry to the spinal cord (N11 and P11), (3) ascending volley of cervical cord or synaptic discharge of cuneate nucleus (N13 and P13) and (4) entry into the medial lemniscus (N14 and P14).

We do not know why the travelling impulse gives rise to SEP peaks with apparent temporal relationships to its entry to the brachial plexus (P9 and Pc9) and to the spinal cord (N11 and P11). These findings indicate, however, that the presence of a standing potential does not necessarily imply a non-propagating neural discharge such as those which occur at synapses in relay nuclei. The electrical field may alter abruptly because of change in anatomical orientation of the impulse, branching of the nerve, or alteration of the surrounding volume conductor (Kimura and Yamada 1982).

Origins of intermediate and long latency components

Following the P14, which is distributed diffusely over the entire scalp, a small but distinct negative peak, N17, occurs bilaterally in the frontal region (Fig. 2). In contrast, the first major negative peaks, N19 and N20, recorded from the central and parietal region respectively, are contralateral to the side of stimulation. The frontal negative peak, N17, is also recorded consistently from the vertex and ipsilateral central electrode, and occasionally from the contralateral central area preceding the major negative peak, N19. The topography of N17 and N19 suggests that these are 2 distinct peaks of separate neural origin. If P14 arises in the medial

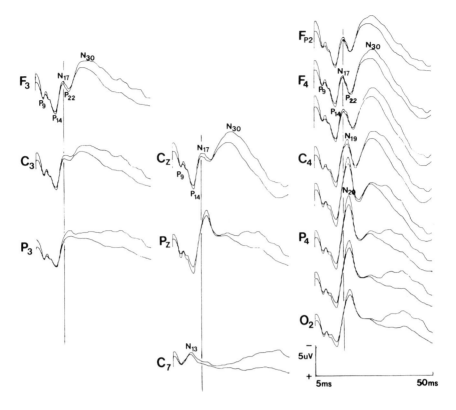

Fig. 2. Topographic display of SEPs to stimulation of the left median nerve. Electrode placement was in accordance with the 10-20 system, with a neck electrode, C7, placed just above the C7 spinous process and the reference electrode over the right shoulder. Frontal N17 (Fp2, F4) preceded central N19 (C4) and parietal N20 (P4) contralateral to the stimulus. N17 also appeared at the vertex (Cz) and frontal and central areas ipsilaterally (F3, C3).

lemniscus, then it is likely that N17 is generated subcortically, possibly reflecting a thalamic positive potential. It has generally been suggested that N19 is the first cortical potential and that the subsequent negative peak, N30, may have a separate cortical generator because of a different potential distribution. However, the origins of N17 and subsequent peaks and their field distributions remain to be elucidated.

Recent topographic studies of the short latency peaks do not support the hypothesis of a dipole relationship between parietal N20 and frontal P20. The latencies of the two are close but not the same, the P20 having a slightly later onset than the N20 (Desmedt and Cheron 1980; Kimura and Yamada 1982). Further, negative-positive peaks subsequent to P14 are shortest in latency at the frontal electrodes (N17, P20, N29) showing a progressive delay toward the central (N19, P22, N30) and parietal areas (N20, P26, N34). This finding, however, does not suggest a ''travelling wave'' since N17 can sometimes be seen as an additional separate peak preceding N19 in the central area contralateral to the stimulus. The topographic specificity for various SEP components suggests the presence of a distinct neural generator in each location.

The last negative peak, N60, appears entirely different from the preceding peaks. This component is more widely distributed over the cortex and shows greater temporal variability than the earlier peaks. It is likely that N60 is mediated through a non-specific polysynaptic pathway in contrast to the preceding peaks relayed by specific oligosynaptic routes.

PATHWAYS FOR SOMATOSENSORY POTENTIALS

Central pathways

In most early clinical studies abnormal SEPs were noted only if vibration or position sense was impaired in patients with lesions of the spinal cord (Giblin 1964; Halliday 1967), cerebral hemisphere (Williamson et al. 1970) or brain stem (Noël and Desmedt 1975). These findings suggested that all SEP components might be dependent upon the integrity of large myelinated fibres in the dorsal column-medial lemniscal system in man. However, recent experimental evidence suggests that the small myelinated fibres also contribute to the generation of cortically recorded SEPs (Andersson et al. 1972). Indeed, Katz et al. (1978) showed that stimulation with an intensity great enough to activate both large and small diameter fibres in the peroneal nerve produced SEPs even after transection of the dorsal column and spino-cervical tract in cats. More recent clinical observation described below is consistent with the experimental evidence that multiple somatosensory pathways are operant.

If N19 and N30 are mediated by 2 separate central pathways, subcortical lesions should independently affect either peak. Studying early and late SEPs in various neurological disorders, we have indeed found abnormalities of N30 and subsequent peaks in conjunction with relatively or entirely normal early components. This was noted not only in patients with cerebral lesions (Tsumoto et al. 1973; Yamada et al. 1978), but also in 11 of 50 cases with brain stem, cervical cord or peripheral nerve lesions (Yamada et al. 1982). In an additional series of 52 patients with multiple sclerosis (Yamada et al. 1982), 11 patients had single abnormalities of N30 or N60. This suggests that these late components are not solely generated by cortico-cortical activation after N19 but are mediated through the subcortical pathway. We have also encountered cases of selective involvement of the early peaks with normal late components. In 2 patients with multiple sclerosis N19 was delayed but N30 and N60 were normal. In 2 others, N30 was absent or delayed, with the preservation of a normal N60 peak. Although rare, these dissociations are difficult to explain without dual pathways for the early and late components.

Peripheral pathways

Studying the effect of ischaemia and mechanical stimulation, Shimada and Nakanishi (1979) found that a SEP was elicitable by pinprick but not by touch or tap when vibration and touch sensations were lost. Pratt et al. (1979) showed that mechanically evoked potentials were of smaller amplitude and contained fewer

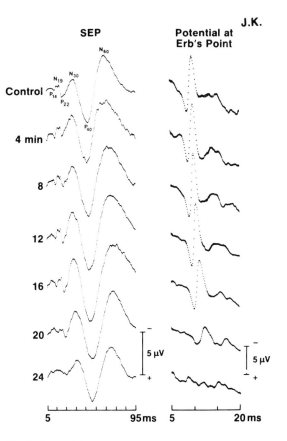

Fig. 3. Sequential changes of scalp recorded somatosensory evoked potentials (left) and Erb's potential (right) during ischaemia in a normal subject. The initial positive and negative components, P14 and N19, were affected along with Erb's potentials earlier than the later components, P22, N30, P40 and N60. The "ischaemia sensitive" peaks were no longer present after 24 min when the "ischaemia resistant" peaks were still relatively intact. (From Yamada et al. 1981.)

components than electrically evoked events, suggesting that the electrical stimulus activated more fibres synchronously than the mechanical stimulus. These findings support the contention of Tsumoto et al. (1973), that N19 may be related to the position-vibration sense, whereas N30 is attributable to the pain-temperature sense. We have also seen occasional patients with impairment of pain-temperature sense alone who showed depressed or absent N30 even if N19 was relatively preserved (Yamada et al. 1978).

Assessing the effect of limb ischaemia, induced by an inflated tourniquet, on sensory evoked potentials, we have observed a progressive increase in latency of Erb's potential as well as all the scalp-recorded SEP components (Yamada et al. 1981) (Fig. 3). The latency change of N60 was far greater than that of the earlier peaks. Similarly, the latency increased more for N30 than for N19. After 24 min of ischaemia Erb's potential could be elicited in none of the 10 subjects, and P9, P14 and N19 were recorded only in two. In contrast, P22, N30 and P40 were present in

9 subjects, and N60 in all. Thus, the selective loss of P9, P14 and N18 in the presence of the later peaks was a common, though not consistent, finding. In some subjects all the components were preserved when Erb's potential was barely appreciable, yet delay of N30 was greater than that of N19. Both the scalp-recorded SEPs and Erb's potential began to recover almost immediately after release of the cuff and returned to normal within 12–16 min.

The SEP components could be divided into groups based on their characteristic patterns of response to ischaemia induced by a pressure cuff. Those susceptible to ischaemia included Erb's potential and early SEP peaks, P9, P14 and N19. The remaining intermediate and late SEP components, P22, N30, P40 and N60, were relatively resistant to the ischaemic condition. Excluding N60, which was entirely different from the other peaks, linear regressions of latency changes were statistically analysed in the 2 groups. The two-sample test was applied for testing pair-wise regression lines for coincidence. This confirmed the presence of 2 statistically noncoincident groups; Erb's potential, P9, P14 and N19 for one, and P22, N30 and P40 as the other.

The brief effect of an inflated cuff on nerve is probably caused by ischaemia rather than mechanical compression since the largest myelinated fibres are the first to fail (Fox and Kenmore 1967). Most sensitive to ischaemia is the potential recorded from Erb's point which is subserved primarily by large myelinated fibres. Since P9, P14 and N19 are as sensitive to ischaemia as Erb's potential, these early components are probably mediated by large afferent fibres as well. In contrast, P22 and later components have different characteristics and may be mediated through independent routes, possibly involving different first-order afferent fibres, e.g., smaller myelinated fibres (Alpsan 1981).

An alternative explanation may be that central amplification compensates for peripheral conduction block. Sensory nerve potentials represent highly synchronous activity and may be sensitive to even slight desynchronization in peripheral neuropathy (Gilliatt and Sears 1958). In contrast, the cortex, operating as an integrator, may be able to generate a sizable evoked response after several synaptic relays, even if the corticopetal input is severely desynchronized (Desmedt 1971). Therefore, a few large afferent fibres which survive the effects of ischaemia may be sufficient to evoke late SEPs even when Erb's potential and early SEPs are no longer elicitable. In severe sensory neuropathy the peripheral nerve potential may be unrecordable, whereas SEP peaks are delayed but preserved.

SUMMARY

In analysing SEPs one tends to assume the presence of fixed neural generators along the sensory pathways as the primary source of successive peaks. However, the surface-positive polarity of the short latency components results presumably because the active recording electrode is located in the approaching field of the centripetal impulse. Thus, the complex wave form of the far field potential may be derived from dynamic interaction of afferent volleys, synaptic discharges and, perhaps more importantly, changes in the conduction characteristics of the surrounding tissue.

Occasional patients with brain stem or subcortical cerebral lesions show selective involvement of early components with preservation of late peaks or vice versa. These findings suggest the presence of a dual rather than unitary central pathway for SEPs since the dissociation between early and late peaks is otherwise difficult to explain. Indeed it is possible that different first-order afferent fibres are responsible for the early and late potentials. Early diminution of the Erb's potential during the course of reversible peripheral nerve dysfunction produced by a pneumatic cuff is associated with a nearly parallel diminution of the early SEP peaks, P9, P14 and N19. In contrast, the later components, P22, N30, P40 and N60, are relatively preserved initially, with some individual variability. Dissociation of the early and late components is also shown by the disproportionately greater latency increase of the latter compared to the former.

The exact mechanisms underlying dissociation between the early and late components remain to be elucidated. However, available evidence indicates that abnormalities of the early peaks may occur in association with relative preservation of late peaks in diseases of the peripheral nerve. Similarly the late components may show disproportionately greater latency increase than the early components even though the conduction abnormalities are limited to the peripheral nerve. In the clinical use of SEPs, these possibilities must always be considered before concluding that abnormalities are manifestations of a central system disease.

REFERENCES

Alpsan, D. The effect of the selective activation of different peripheral nerve fiber groups on the somatosensory evoked potentials in cat. Electroenceph. clin. Neurophysiol., 1981, 51: 589–598.

Andersson, S.A., Norrsell, K. and Norrsell, U. Spinal pathways projecting to the cerebral first somatosensory area in the monkey. J. Physiol. (Lond.), 1972, 225: 589–597.

Desmedt, J.E. Somatosensory cerebral evoked potentials in man. In: A. Rémond (Ed.), Handbook of Electroencephalography and Clinical Neurophysiology, Vol. 9. Elsevier, Amsterdam, 1971: 55–82.

Desmedt, J.E. and Cheron, G. Somatosensory evoked potentials to finger stimulation in healthy octogenarians and in young adults: wave forms, scalp topography and transit times of parietal and frontal components. Electroenceph. clin. Neurophysiol., 1980, 50: 404–425.

Fox, J.L. and Kenmore, P.I. The effect of ischemia on nerve conduction. Exp. Neurol., 1967, 17: 403–419.

Giblin, D.R. Somatosensory evoked potentials in healthy subjects and in patients with lesions of the nervous system. Ann. N.Y. Acad. Sci., 1964, 112: 93–142.

Gilliatt, R.W. and Sears, T.A. Sensory nerve action potentials in patients with peripheral nerve lesions. J. Neurol. Neurosurg. Psychiat., 1958, 21: 109–118.

Halliday, A.M. Changes in the form of cerebral evoked responses in man associated with various lesions of the nervous system. Electroenceph. clin. Neurophysiol., 1967, Suppl. 25: 178–192.

Katz, S., Martin, H.F. and Blackburn, J.G. The effects of interaction between large and small diameter fiber systems on the somatosensory evoked potential. Electroenceph. clin. Neurophysiol., 1978. 45: 45–52.

Kimura, J. and Yamada, T. Short latency somatosensory evoked potentials, following median nerve stimulation. Ann. N.Y. Acad. Sci., 1982, 388: 689–694.

Noël, P. and Desmedt, J.E. Somatosensory cerebral evoked potentials after vascular lesions of the brainstem and diencephalon. Brain, 1975, 98: 113–128.

Pratt, H., Starr, A., Amlie, R.N. and Politoske, D. Mechanically and electrically evoked somatosensory potentials in normal humans. Neurology (Minneap.), 1979, 29: 1236–1244.

Shimada, Y. and Nakanishi, T. Somatosensory evoked responses elicited by mechanical stimulations in man. Adv. neurol. Sci. (Tokyo), 1979, 23: 282–293.

Tsumoto, T., Hirose, N., Nonaka, S. and Takahashi, M. Cerebrovascular disease: changes in somatosensory evoked potentials associated with unilateral lesions. Electroenceph. clin. Neurophysiol., 1973, 35: 463–473.

Williamson, P.D., Goff, W.R. and Allison, T. Somato-sensory evoked responses in patients with unilateral cerebral lesions. Electroenceph. clin. Neurophysiol., 1970, 28: 566–575.

Yamada, T., Kimura, J., Young, S. and Powers, M. Somatosensory evoked potentials elicited by bilateral stimulation of the median nerve and its clinical application. Neurology (Minneap.), 1978, 28: 218–223.

Yamada, T., Kimura, J. and Nitz, D.M. Short latency somatosensory evoked potentials following median nerve stimulation in man. Electroenceph. clin. Neurophysiol., 1980, 48: 367–376.

Yamada, T., Muroga, T. and Kimura, J. Tourniquet induced ischemia and somatosensory evoked potentials. Neurology (Minneap.), 1981, 31: 1524–1529.

Yamada, T., Shivapour, E., Wilkinson, J.T. and Kimura, J. Short and long latency somatosensory evoked potentials in multiple sclerosis. Arch. Neurol. (Chic.), 1982, 39: 88–94.

Kyoto Symposia (EEG Suppl. No. 36)
Editors: P.A. Buser, W.A. Cobb and T. Okuma
© 1982, Elsevier Biomedical Press, Amsterdam

Origins of the Scalp-Recorded Somatosensory Far Field Potentials in Man and Cat*

T. NAKANISHI, M. TAMAKI, K. ARASAKI and N. KUDO

Department of Neurology, Institute of Clinical Medicine, and Department of Physiology, Institute of Basic Medical Sciences, University of Tsukuba, Ibaraki (Japan)

Using non-cephalic reference electrodes, short latency positive potentials preceding the cortical somatosensory evoked potentials (SEPs) have been studied in normal subjects and in patients with neurological diseases (Cracco and Cracco 1976; Anziska et al. 1978; Kritchevsky and Wiederholt 1978; Green and McLeod 1979; King and Green 1979; Anziska and Cracco 1980; Chiappa et al. 1980; Desmedt and Cheron 1980; Grisolia and Wiederholt 1980; Yamada et al. 1980; Pratt and Starr 1981). On the other hand, similar short latency positive SEPs have also been investigated in rat, cat and monkey (Wiederholt and Iragui-Madoz 1977; Iragui-Madoz and Wiederholt 1977a,b; Wiederholt 1978; Arezzo et al. 1979). Thus, it has been expected that these potentials would provide a non-invasive means of examination of the afferent somatosensory pathway in diseases of the nervous system. However, concerning the origin of each of these potentials a consensus has not been reached.

In this study, further observations on these short latency positive potentials were made in man and cat to elucidate their underlying generator sources, and a new interpretation of the origin of each of these potentials was proposed.

METHODS AND MATERIALS

Human subjects

The methods used in human subjects will be described elsewhere in detail (Nakanishi et al. 1983). Seventeen normal young volunteers (2 men, 15 women, aged 20–28 years) and 5 patients with impaired position sense due to lesions in the unilateral brain stem (3 cases) and thalamus (2 cases) were examined. They were seated comfortably in a reclining chair or rested in a supine position on a bed in a semi-darkened room with their eyes closed.

Stimulating electrodes consisting of a pair of Beckman cup electrodes were attached over the median nerve just proximal to the wrist with the cathode about 2 cm proximal to the anode. Electrical stimuli were triggered on the flat part of the ECG, with a time delay from 0.5 to 0.7 sec following each QRS complex to minimize

*This work was supported by a grant for scientific research from the Ministry of Education of Japan.

cardiac-related activity. The stimuli were 0.2 msec rectangular pulses and were adjusted to produce a small twitch of the thumb.

The inputs from 4 leads at a time were led to differential amplifiers and the output was summated by a computer. In all records, relative negativity in grid 1 resulted in an upward deflection. The frequency response of the recording apparatus was 1–2000 Hz (−3 dB). Five hundred consecutive responses were summated.

Cats

Nine adult cats weighing 2.8–3.6 kg were examined. Animals were anaesthetized intraperitoneally with sodium pentobarbital. The initial dose was 35 mg/kg, and additional doses of 5 mg/h were given intravenously in the course of the experiment to maintain absence of response to toe pinch. The animal was placed prone in a stereotactic frame with insulated ear bars to hold the head in a fixed position during recording. It was immobilized with pancuronium bromide and artificially ventilated. Rectal temperature was kept at 38–39°C with a heat lamp.

The bipolar stimulating electrode was attached to the superficial radial nerve at a proximal site on the left forelimb. Electrical stimuli were triggered from 20 to 200 msec following each QRS complex to minimize cardiac-related activity. The stimuli were 0.2 msec rectangular pulses and were adjusted to produce a maximal peripheral nerve action potential. A silver wire was placed around the forelimb rostral to the stimulating electrode and connected to ground.

Recording electrodes consisted of stainless needles inserted subcutaneously over the right sensorimotor area and in the skin of the right forepaw and earlobe contralateral to the stimulated forepaw.

Recording was performed simultaneously from the scalp with either forepaw or earlobe reference. Neuroelectric signals were amplified with differential amplifiers with a frequency response down 3 dB at 1 Hz and 3 kHz.

The computer was triggered 1 msec prior to the stimulus. The duration of the averaging epoch was 20 msec and the sampling rate was 20 μsec per point. In all experiments 500 sweeps were averaged, which were photographed from the screen of the computer oscilloscope.

Following preliminary surface recording, supracollicular transection was carried out through a posterior parietal craniotomy after ligation of both carotid arteries. A spatula was introduced rostral to the bony cerebellar tentorium in such a way that the cerebellum was not damaged. Medullo-spinal transection was performed at the medullo-cervical junction after ligation of both vertebral arteries. Finally, intrathecal anaesthesia of the cervical cord was done by injection of 1–3 ml of 1% lidocaine into the spinal canal. These transections were verified by examining the brain after experiments.

RESULTS

Human subjects

With hand reference recording, 4 positive peaks (P1, P2, P3 and P4) were

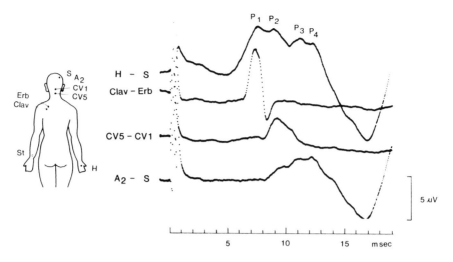

Fig. 1. Relationship between somatosensory evoked far field potentials recorded with hand reference and simultaneously recorded other responses in a normal subject. H, on the hand dorsum; S, the site 2 cm behind the C4 position; Clav, the junction where the line passing through the Erb's point and the axilla intersects with the inferior margin of the clavicle; Erb, Erb's point; CV5, over the 5th cervical spinous process; CV1, just below the base of the skull; St, stimulation. (From Nakanishi et al. (1983).)

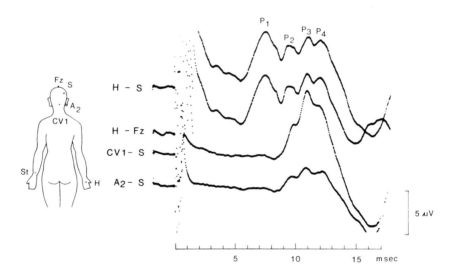

Fig. 2. Scalp-recorded potentials with hand (H), just below the base of the skull (CV1) and ear (A2) references in a normal subject. S, the site 2 cm behind the C4 position; St, stimulation. (From Nakanishi et al. (1983).)

identified in the initial portion of the scalp-recorded SEP to median nerve stimulation in normal subjects (Fig. 1, top). P1, P3 and P4 were recorded in 14 out of 17 subjects, while P2 was bilobed or poorly defined in 6 subjects. The onset and peak latencies of each of these well delineated potentials are shown in Table I. The

TABLE I

MEANS AND STANDARD DEVIATIONS OF THE ONSET AND PEAK LATENCIES OF THE SHORT LATENCY SEPs FOLLOWING MEDIAN NERVE STIMULATION AT THE WRIST IN NORMAL SUBJECTS

From Nakanishi et al. (1983).

Leads of recording	Component	Onset latency (msec)	Peak latency (msec)	Number recorded/ number tested
H-S	P1	6.4 ± 0.4	7.9 ± 0.4	14/17
	P2	8.8 ± 0.7	10.0 ± 0.5	11/17
	P3	10.7 ± 0.5	11.6 ± 0.6	14/17
	P4	12.4 ± 0.6	13.1 ± 0.7	14/17
Clav-Erb		6.6 ± 0.4	8.0 ± 0.5*	16/16
CV5-CV1	2nd comp.	8.2 ± 0.7	10.1 ± 0.7**	14/14
CV1-3A		9.1 ± 0.5	11.4 ± 0.7***	14/14
CV1-S	1st comp.	8.3 ± 0.4	10.0 ± 0.3**	13/14
	2nd comp.	10.7 ± 0.5	11.6 ± 0.4***	14/14
	3rd comp.	12.0 ± 0.5	13.0 ± 0.7****	13/14
A2-S	1st comp.	9.0 ± 0.4	10.0 ± 0.4**	15/16
	2nd comp.	10.7 ± 0.5	11.5 ± 0.6***	14/16
	3rd comp.	12.3 ± 0.7	13.0 ± 0.6****	16/16

H, on the hand dorsum; S, 2 cm behind the C_4 position; Clav, the junction where the line passing through Erb's point and the axilla intersects with the inferior margin of the clavicle; Erb, Erb's point; CV5, over the 5th cervical spinous process; CV1, just below the base of the skull; 3A, 3 cm above the base of the skull.
* Peak latency similar to that of P1.
** Peak latency similar to that of P2.
*** Peak latency similar to that of P3.
****Peak latency similar to that of P4.

peak latency of P1 was coincident with that recorded over the clavicle, and the well defined P2 was similar in peak latency to the second component recorded at CV5 (Fig. 1, Table I).

The response recorded with a high cervical reference usually consisted of 3 components (Fig. 2, 3rd). The second was identical in peak latency with P3 (Fig. 2, Table I). With earlobe reference, 3 components were also recorded (Fig. 1, bottom; Fig. 2, bottom). They were characterized by broader upward deflections, and the third component was more clearly delineated than the potential recorded with high cervical reference. The second and third components were synchronous with P3 and P4 (Figs. 1 and 2, Table I). The peak latency of the first component was similar to that of the first component recorded with high cervical reference and to that of P2. Although P2 and P3 were often equivocal when recorded with hand reference, equivalent components were better detected with the use of an ear reference.

On the other hand, in patients with impaired position sense due to a unilateral

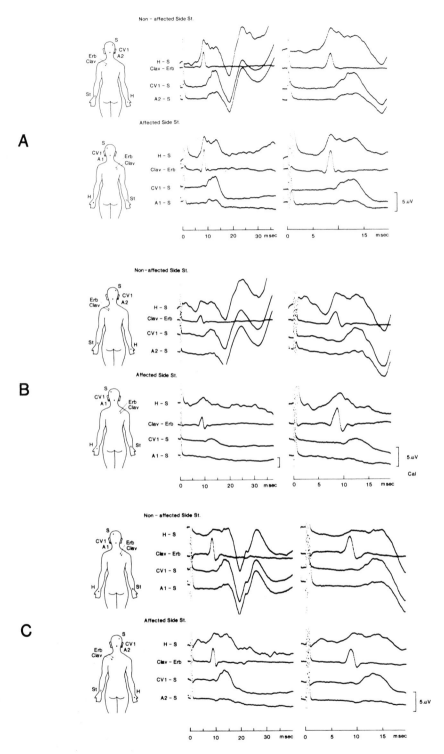

Fig. 3. SEPs obtained in patients with impaired position sense due to a unilateral lesion in the thalamus (A) and the brain stem (B, C). Short latency SEPs recorded with hand, high cervical and earlobe references were almost normal in A but abnormal in B, while in C only the short latency SEP recorded with earlobe reference was abnormal. (From Nakanishi et al. (1983).)

lesion in the thalamus, only the initial potentials were observed in hand, high cervical and earlobe reference records to stimulation of the affected side (Fig. 3A). However, 2 patients with impaired position sense due to a unilateral brain stem lesion had abnormal configurations of the initial potentials in these reference records to stimulation of the affected side (Fig. 3B). In one patient with impaired position sense due to a similar brain stem lesion only the initial positive potential recorded with earlobe reference was of abnormal configuration, while both initial potentials recorded with hand and high cervical references were not significantly altered (Fig. 3C). Stimulation of the non-affected side naturally produced normal responses in all these patients.

Cats

Following superficial radial nerve stimulation, 4 small positive potentials preceding the cortical potential (CI, CII, CIII and CIV) were recorded from the scalp electrodes over the contralateral and ipsilateral sensorimotor areas with forepaw reference in most cats (Fig. 4). Components I and IV were consistently recorded in all cats, while components II and III were often poorly defined. The onset and peak latencies of each of these well delineated potentials are shown in Table II.

With earlobe reference positive potentials preceding the cortical response were also recorded (Fig. 5, 2nd). Placing the reference on the earlobe, however, resulted in alterations of the short latency SEP wave form. It often appeared with an initial positive slope, while the positive potential corresponding to component I recorded with forepaw reference was not seen at all, and the amplitudes corresponding to components II and III were reduced.

Following supracollicular transection the cortical SEPs disappeared from both forepaw and earlobe reference records (Fig. 5, 3rd and bottom). However, both

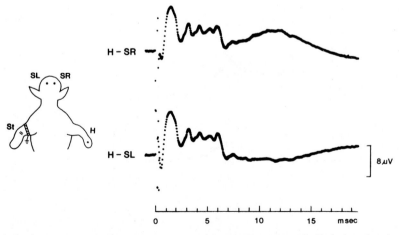

Fig. 4. SEPs recorded from the scalp electrodes contralateral and ipsilateral to the stimulated side with forepaw reference. Note similar short latency SEPs recorded from both sides of scalp.

TABLE II

MEANS AND STANDARD DEVIATIONS OF THE ONSET AND PEAK LATENCIES OF THE
SHORT LATENCY SEPs FOLLOWING SUPERFICIAL RADIAL NERVE STIMULATION AT THE
PROXIMAL SITE OF THE FOREPAW IN CATS

Leads of recording	Component	Onset latency (msec)	Peak latency (msec)
Forepaw-scalp	CI	0.7 ± 0.1	1.4 ± 0.2
	CII	2.5 ± 0.3	3.0 ± 0.4
	CIII	3.7 ± 0.6	4.0 ± 0.6
	CIV	4.7 ± 0.8	5.2 ± 0.7
Earlobe-scalp	CIa		3.0 ± 0.5
	CIIa		5.1 ± 0.6
Clavicle		1.2 ± 0.2	1.6 ± 0.2
Root at C6 level		1.4 ± 0.2	2.0 ± 0.2
Dorsal column at C1 level		2.4 ± 0.4	3.7 ± 0.4

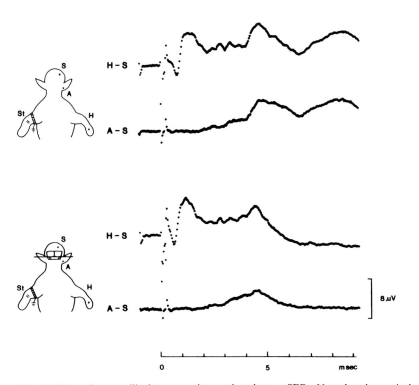

Fig. 5. Effects of supracollicular transection on short latency SEPs. Note that the cortical potentials were abolished after supracollicular transection.

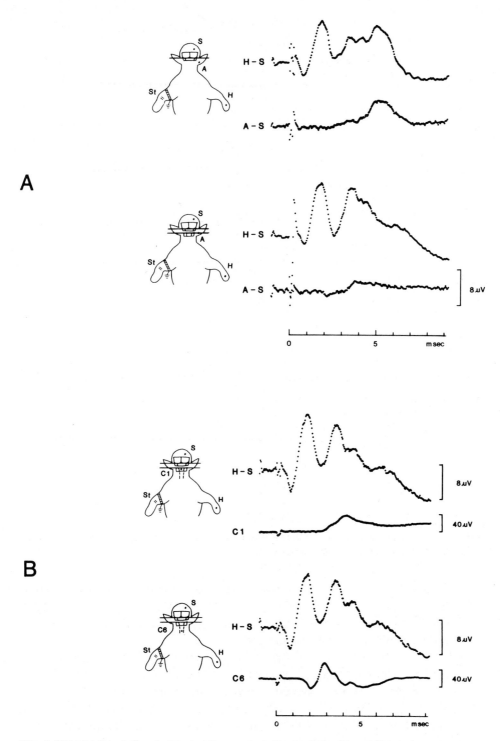

Fig. 6. Effects of medullo-spinal transection on short latency SEPs (A) and simultaneously recorded action potentials at the C1 and C6 levels (B).

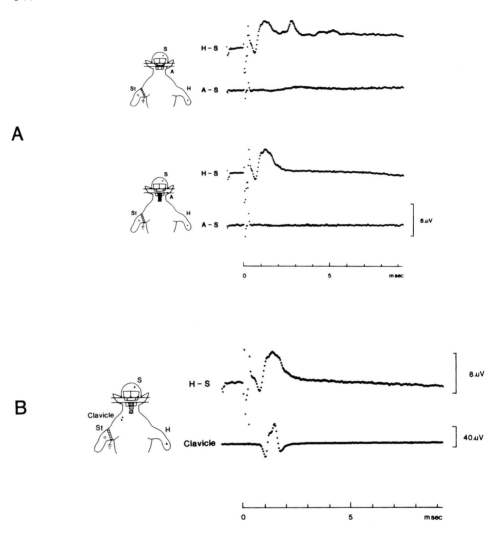

Fig. 7. Effects of intrathecal anaesthesia of the cervical cord on the short latency SEPs (A) and simultaneously recorded action potential over the clavicle (B).

components IV recorded with forepaw reference and the major positive potential recorded with earlobe reference (CIIa) persisted with slightly reduced amplitude. Components I, II and III and the initial positive potential recorded with earlobe reference (CIa) did not change significantly.

After transection at the medullo-cervical junction the amplitude of component IV was markedly reduced, while components I and III did not change significantly. In contrast, component II was remarkably increased in amplitude. On the other hand, component IIa, which corresponded to component IV, disappeared completely, while the preceding component Ia appeared clearly (Fig. 6A). The peak latency of component III was greater by 0.3 msec than that of the activity directly recorded from the dorsal column at the C1 level. Component II was longer in peak latency than the root potential directly recorded at the C6 level by 1.0 msec (Fig. 6B).

Finally, after intrathecal anaesthesia of the cervical cord with lidocaine, all components except component I recorded with forepaw reference disappeared completely. Component Ia, which remained after transection at the medullo-cervical junction, no longer existed (Fig. 7A). The peak latency of component I was coincident with that of the action potential recorded over the clavicle (Fig. 7B).

DISCUSSION

Although scalp-recorded somatosensory evoked far field potentials have been studied by many authors, who have described essentially the same findings, a consensus has not been reached concerning the neural source of each of these potentials.

Using a non-cephalic reference, 4 positive peaks preceding the cortical response were recorded in the majority of men and cats in our study. The shorter latency of these potentials in normal subjects is probably due to the shorter arm length of the subjects examined. P1 might be equivalent to the first positive potential described by Cracco and Cracco (1976), P10 of Kritchevsky and Wiederholt (1978) and P9 of Yamada et al. (1980) and Desmedt and Cheron (1980). They suggested that this potential was peripheral nerve in origin and likely to be generated in the distal portion of the brachial plexus. On the other hand, the peak latency of P1 obtained in normal subjects was coincident with that of the potential recorded over the clavicle in our study (Fig. 1, Table I). This finding is compatible with that obtained in the cat, in which component I persisted after intrathecal anaesthesia of the cervical cord. These findings suggest that P1 may be generated in the brachial plexus just beneath the clavicle. This result of the present study, however, differs from the previous report by Arezzo et al. (1979), who did not detect shorter latency peripheral nerve action potentials.

P2, with the peak latency of 10.0 ± 0.5 (S.D.) msec obtained in our study, might correspond with the second positive potential of Cracco and Cracco (1976), N11 of Jones (1977), P12 of Kritchevsky and Wiederholt (1978), N12 of Hume and Cant (1978) and P11 of Yamada et al. (1980) and Desmedt and Cheron (1980). As a possible neural source of this potential, however, several different subcortical structures have been proposed. Cracco and Cracco (1976) and Kritchevsky and Wiederholt (1978) postulated that the dorsal column nuclei and medial lemniscus may be the primary sources of this potential. Anziska et al. (1978) and Anziska and Cracco (1980) suggested that their second positive potential might arise in the cervical spinal cord or brain stem. On the other hand, Jones (1977), Hume and Cant (1978), Yamada et al. (1980) and Desmedt and Cheron (1980) proposed a generator site immediately adjacent to or just within the spinal cord. The P1-P2 latency difference obtained in our study was 2.1 msec, the same as those described by these authors. The peak latency of P2 was also similar to that of the second component recorded in CV5-CV1 leads which were located near the spinal cord (Table I).

Component II recorded in cats, furthermore, was longer in peak latency than the root potential directly recorded at the C6 level by 1.0 msec, whereas it was shorter than the cord potential at the C1 level by 0.7 msec. Moreover, component II persisted after the medullo-cervical transection. These findings suggest that P2 reflects the arrival of impulses in the low cervical cord.

P3 with the peak latency of 11.6 ± 0.6 (S.D.) msec obtained in our study may be homologous with N13 of Jones (1977), N14 of Hume and Cant (1978) and P13 of Yamada et al. (1980) and Desmedt and Cheron (1980). Cracco and Cracco (1976) and Kritchevsky and Wiederholt (1978) noted that the third positive potential was often bilobed and suggested that it might arise from the thalamus or its cortical projection fibres. As a likely generator of P3, however, many different subcortical structures such as the brain stem lemniscal pathways (Desmedt and Cheron 1980), the dorsal column nuclei (Hume and Cant 1978), the spinal grey matter or brain stem (Jones 1977) and the cervical spinal cord (Yamada et al. 1980) have been proposed. On the other hand, the peak latency of P3 obtained in our study was coincident with that of the potential recorded from the electrode just below the base of the skull. Furthermore, the potential recorded from this electrode with ear reference has been intact in patients with vascular lesions in the brain stem (Nakanishi et al. 1978). Component III recorded in cats was not significantly greater in peak latency than the action potential directly recorded from the dorsal column at the C1 level, and persisted after medullo-cervical transection (Fig. 6). These findings suggest that P3 may arise in the high cervical cord.

P4, of which the peak latency was 13.1 ± 0.7 (S.D.) msec in our study, may correspond to N14 of Jones (1977) and P14 of Yamada et al. (1980) and Desmedt and Cheron (1980). Jones (1977) thought that his N14 was generated in the brain stem or thalamus, while Yamada et al. (1980) and Desmedt and Cheron (1980) postulated that their P4 might arise in the brain stem or cerebellum. On the other hand, the peak latency of P4 was 1.5 msec greater than that of P3. P4 was also synchronous with the third component recorded in ear-scalp leads, which were almost intact in patients with lesions in the thalamus but absent or profoundly distorted in patients with vascular lesions in the brain stem (Nakanishi et al. 1978). Furthermore, component IV recorded in cats persisted with slightly reduced amplitude after supracollicular transection but was markedly reduced in amplitude by transection at the medullo-cervical junction (Fig. 6). These findings suggest that it has at least 3 generator sources; the major one lies in the brain stem or the cerebellum or both, the others in a group of cervical cord afferents that conduct at a somewhat slower velocity and in the supracollicular structures.

On the other hand, short latency positive potentials recorded with earlobe reference consisted of at least 2 components in cats; the initial positive and the later major positive one. The first component Ia was well delineated after medullo-cervical transection and similar in peak latency to component II, suggesting that it may be homologous with component I of Iragui-Madoz and Wiederholt (1977a,b) record with a nasal bone reference. It may correspond to the first positive component record with earlobe reference in man. Since the major component IIa was abolished by medullo-spinal transection but spared by a supracollicular one, it may be generated mainly in the brain stem or the cerebellum or both, and correspond to component IV recorded with forepaw reference in this study and components II and IIIA of Iragui-Madoz and Wiederholt (1977a,b). It may also correspond to the third positive component recorded with earlobe reference in man.

To the interpretation of these potentials the "dipole" concept has been applied (Cracco and Cracco 1976; Jones 1977; Desmedt and Cheron 1980; Pratt and Starr 1981). However, it was originally made on the assumption that the nerve impulse travels through an infinite, electrically homogeneous conducting medium. Since the brain and other tissues within the skull have been considered to be electrically homogeneous, each generator of electrical potential in the brain might be regarded as a "dipole". Somatosensory evoked far field potentials, especially P1 however, have been considered to originate outside the skull, as previously mentioned. The "dipole" concept, therefore, might not contribute significantly to this potential. According to our investigation of action potentials recorded by "fluid electrodes" (Nakanishi 1982), action potentials could be generated wherever the resistance of the conducting medium changed suddenly at the moment when the impulse passed through. As the impulse initiated in the median nerve travels through various regions, such as beneath the clavicle and foramen magnum, where the resistance might change suddenly, somatosensory evoked far field potentials might be recorded as if generated at such fixed sites. The earlobe electrode, moreover, may be active in contact with a relatively well conducting mass such as the auditory nerve, the internal carotid artery and the jugular vein, as Davis (1976) pointed out. Thus, short latency positive potentials mainly arising in the brain stem might be consistently recorded with an earlobe reference.

SUMMARY

Short latency somatosensory evoked potentials preceding the primary cortical potential were recorded from the scalp in man and cats. Four positive potentials (P1, P2, P3 and P4 in man, and CI, CII, CIII and CIV in cats) were observed with non-cephalic reference recording and 3 or 2 positive components (P1a, P2a and P3a in man, and CIa and CIIa in cats) were recorded with earlobe reference. (1) The latencies of these potentials and the effects of lesions on them in man and (2) the effects of (i) supracollicular and medullo-cervical transections and (ii) intrathecal anaesthesia of the cervical cord on these components in cats suggest that: (1) P1 and CI originate in the brachial plexus beneath the clavicle; (2) P2, P3 and CII, CIII are generated in the cervical cord; (3) P4 and CIV reflect activity mainly in the brain stem or the cerebellum or both; (4) P1a and CIa arise in the cervical cord; (5) P3a and CIIa reflect activity mainly in the brain stem or the cerebellum or both. As the impulse initiated in the median nerve travels through various regions where the resistance might change suddenly, these far field potentials might be recorded as if generated at fixed sites such as just beneath the clavicle and foramen magnum.

REFERENCES

Anziska, B.J. and Cracco, R.Q. Short latency somatosensory evoked potentials in brain dead patients. Arch. Neurol. (Chic.), 1980, 37: 222–225.

Anziska, B., Cracco, R.Q., Cook, A.W. and Feld, E.W. Somatosensory far field potentials: studies in normal subjects and patients with multiple sclerosis. Electroenceph. clin. Neurophysiol., 1978, 45: 602–610.

Arezzo, J., Legatt, A.D. and Vaughan, Jr., H.G. Topography and intracranial sources of somatosensory evoked potentials in the monkey. I. Early component. Electroenceph. clin. Neurophysiol., 1979, 46: 155–172.

Chiappa, K.H., Choi, S.K. and Young, R.R. Short-latency somatosensory evoked potentials following median nerve stimulation in patients with neurological lesions. In: J.E. Desmedt (Ed.), Clinical Uses of Cerebral, Brainstem and Spinal Somatosensory Evoked Potentials. Progr. clin. Neurophysiol., Vol. 7. Karger, Basel, 1980: 264–281.

Cracco, R.Q. and Cracco, J.B. Somatosensory evoked potential in man: far field potentials. Electroenceph. clin. Neurophysiol., 1976, 41: 460–466.

Davis, H. Principles of electric response audiometry. Ann. Otol. (St. Louis), 1976, Suppl. 28: 39–50.

Desmedt, J.E. and Cheron, G. Central somatosensory conduction in man: neural generators and interpeak latencies of the far field components recorded from neck and right to left scalp and earlobes. Electroenceph. clin. Neurophysiol., 1980, 50: 382–403.

Green, J.B. and McLeod, S. Short latency somatosensory evoked potentials in patients with neurological lesions. Arch. Neurol. (Chic.), 1979, 36: 846–851.

Grisolia, J.S. and Wiederholt, W.C. Short latency somatosensory evoked potentials from radial, median and ulnar nerve stimulation in man. Electroenceph. clin. Neurophysiol., 1980, 50: 375–381.

Hume, A.L. and Cant, B.R. Conduction time in central somatosensory pathways in man. Electroenceph. clin. Neurophysiol., 1978, 45: 361–375.

Iragui-Madoz, V.J. and Wiederholt, W.C. Far field somatosensory evoked potentials in the cat. Electroenceph. clin. Neurophysiol., 1977a, 43: 646–657.

Iragui-Madoz, V.J. and Wiederholt, W.C. Far-field somatosensory evoked potentials in the cat: correlation with depth recording. Electroenceph. clin. Neurophysiol., 1977b, 1: 569–574.

Jones, S.J. Short latency potentials recorded from the neck and scalp following median nerve stimulation in man. Electroenceph. clin. Neurophysiol., 1977, 43: 853–863.

King, D.W. and Green, J.B. Short latency somatosensory potentials in humans. Electroenceph. clin. Neurophysiol., 1979, 46: 702–708.

Kritchevsky, M. and Wiederholt, W.C. Short-latency somatosensory evoked potentials. Arch. Neurol. (Chic.), 1978, 35: 706–711.

Nakanishi, T. Action potentials recorded by fluid electrodes. Electroenceph. clin. Neurophysiol., 1982, 53: 343–345.

Nakanishi, T., Shimada, Y., Sakuta, M. and Toyokura, Y. The initial positive component of the scalp-recorded somatosensory evoked potential in normal subjects and in patients with neurological disorders. Electroenceph. clin. Neurophysiol., 1978, 45: 26–34.

Nakanishi, T., Tamaki, M., Ozaki, Y. and Arasaki, K. Origins of short latency somatosensory evoked potentials to median nerve stimulation. 1983, in preparation.

Pratt, H. and Starr, A. Mechanically and electrically evoked somatosensory potentials in humans: scalp and neck distributions of short latency components. Electroenceph. clin. Neurophysiol., 1981, 52: 138–147.

Wiederholt, W.C. Recovery function of short latency components of surface and depth recorded somatosensory evoked potentials in the cat. Electroenceph. clin. Neurophysiol., 1978, 45: 259–267.

Wiederholt, W.C. and Iragui-Madoz, V.J. Far field somatosensory potentials in the rat. Electroenceph. clin. Neurophysiol., 1977, 42: 456–465.

Yamada, T., Kimura, J. and Nitz, D.M. Short latency somatosensory evoked potentials following median nerve stimulation in man. Electroenceph. clin. Neurophysiol., 1980, 48: 367–376.

Kyoto Symposia (EEG Suppl. No. 36)
Editors: P.A. Buser, W.A. Cobb and T. Okuma
© 1982, Elsevier Biomedical Press, Amsterdam

Electrodiagnostic Evaluation of Radiculopathies and Plexopathies Using Somatosensory Evoked Potentials*

ANDREW EISEN and MAUREEN HOIRCH

Division of Neurology and Department of Diagnostic Neurophysiology, Vancouver General Hospital and University of British Columbia, Vancouver, B.C. V5Z 1M9 (Canada)

Conventional electrophysiology (nerve conduction studies and needle electromyography), although useful, has limited application in the assessment of radiculopathies and plexopathies. Inclusion of late waves (F wave and H reflex measurements) adds to the overall diagnostic yield of proximal lesions. They are restrictive in reflecting only motor dysfunction and S1 sensory disease respectively (Braddon and Johnson 1974; Young and Shahani 1978; Tonzola et al. 1981). Somatosensory evoked potentials (SEPs) monitor sensory information traversing roots and plexuses. Abnormalities of these might be anticipated in radiculopathies and plexopathies, especially when sensory features are predominant or occur in isolation.

The value of SEPs, evoked by segmental sensory stimulation, in diagnosing root and plexus lesions forms the basis of this report.

METHODS

Controls and patients

Normative data, details of which have been reported previously (Eisen and Elleker 1980), were derived from 102 subjects without evidence of neurological disease (Table I). Twenty-seven patients with root lesions were investigated. Their mean age was 46.2 years (range 20–66 years) and 19 were males. None had disc surgery prior to investigation and there was no evidence of neurological disease other than root involvement. Duration of symptoms to the time of study ranged from 2 weeks to 2 years (mean 11.7 months). Another group of 12 patients with plexopathies were similarly studied. Their mean age was 50.1 years (range 19–72 years) and 10 were males.

Electrophysiological methods

Stimuli of intensity 2.5 times sensory threshold (5–12.5 mA) and 0.2 msec

---

*Supported by the Multiple Sclerosis Society of Canada.

Address reprint requests to: Andrew Eisen, M.D., Diagnostic Neurophysiology (EMG), Vancouver General Hospital, 855 West 12th Avenue, Vancouver, B.C. V5Z 1M9, Canada.

TABLE I

NORMAL SOMATOSENSORY EVOKED POTENTIAL (SEP) LATENCIES

Stimulus site	Root level	Mean latency to N20 or P40 ± S.D. (msec)	Upper limit (msec) (< 3 S.D.)
Musculocutaneous	C5	17.4 ± 1.2	20.0
Thumb	C6	22.5 ± 1.1	25.0
Fingers II and III	C7	21.2 ± 1.2	25.0
Finger V	C8	22.5 ± 1.1	25.0
Saphenous	L4	33.4 ± 2.2	40.0
Superficial peroneal	L5	39.9 ± 1.8	45.0
Sural	S1	42.1 ± 1.4	45.5

duration were applied percutaneously at a rate of 5/sec to appropriate sensory nerves (Fig. 1). Thus the musculocutaneous nerve below the cubital crease, the thumb, the adjoining surfaces of the second and third digits, and the fifth digit, were considered representative of the fifth, sixth, seventh and eighth cervical dermatomes respectively and the upper, middle and lower trunks of the brachial plexus respectively. In the lower extremity the saphenous, superficial peroneal and sural nerves, reflecting L4, L5 and S1 dermatomes respectively, and the lumbar and sacral plexuses, were stimulated.

To record SEPs, scalp needle electrodes were placed at C3 or C4 (10–20 system) contralateral to the upper extremity stimulated. Cz was used as the recording site when stimulating lower extremity nerves. A cephalic referential electrode was placed at Fpz. The bandpass of the differential amplifiers was set between 200 Hz and 1.0 kHz (Eisen and Elleker 1980). Peripheral sensory nerve action potentials (SNAPs) were always simultaneously recorded (Fig. 1). A near-nerve needle recording technique was used (Buchthal et al. 1975). The time analysed was 50 and 100 msec (1024 data points) subsequent to upper and lower extremity stimulation respectively. Each set of 1024 sweeps was averaged twice to enhance time-locked events.

Latency measurements were made to N20 and P40 (Fig. 1). These peaks, labelled according to the international nomenclature (Donchin et al. 1977), reflect impulse arrival at the primary somatosensory cortex following arm and leg stimulation respectively (Allison et al. 1979; Desmedt and Cheron 1980). The latencies of the SEP and SNAP were considered abnormal if prolonged by more than 3 S.D. above their normal means (see Eisen and Elleker 1980). Amplitude measurements were considered to be too variable to be of value in absolute terms, but a side-to-side difference of 50% or more was considered abnormal. Significant dispersion with late components of the SNAP and obvious morphological desynchronization of the SEP, even when normal in latency, were also considered abnormal.

F waves were elicited by distal stimulation of appropriate upper or lower extremity mixed nerves (Kimura 1974). They were considered abnormal if (1) absent,

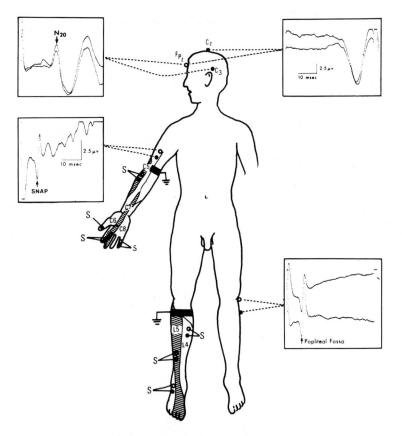

Fig. 1. Schema of stimulating and recording electrode placements for evoking SNAPs and SEPs using segmental stimulation. The potentials recorded are from a control subject.

(2) of longer latency than 32 msec when stimulating the median or ulnar nerve (Eisen et al. 1977a) or 54.5 msec when stimulating the common peroneal or tibial nerve (Eisen et al. 1977b), (3) there was a 2 msec or more side-to-side difference when employing homologous stimulating and recording sites (Fisher et al. 1978).

Physiological testing was performed with the subject comfortably reclined in a semi-darkened, air-conditioned room, maintained at an ambient temperature between 20 and 22°C.

RESULTS

Twelve (46%) and 17 (65%) respectively of the patients referred with cervical or lumbar radicular pain had an objective motor or sensory deficit. There were abnormalities of paraspinal and/or limb needle electromyography in 11 of 24 patients (46%); abnormalities of F waves in 15 of 26 patients (58%); abnormal myelograms in 7 of 17 patients (41%) and 13 of 27 (48%) patients had abnormal SEPs (Figs. 2 and 3). Correlations between these and the presence or absence of

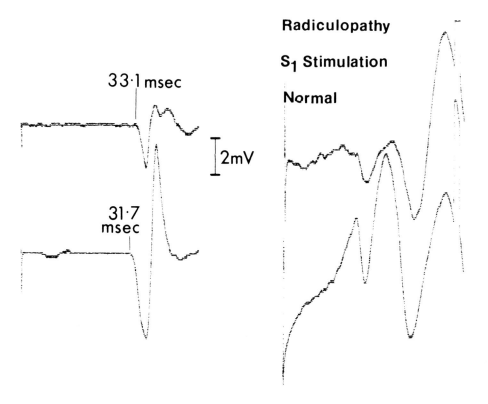

Fig. 2. H waves and SEPs recorded from a patient with a unilateral S1 radiculopathy. The top traces of each pair are the abnormal side and the potentials are prolonged in latency and reduced in amplitude compared to the bottom 2 traces, which were evoked by stimulation of the normal side.

objective clinical deficits are shown in Table II. A confirmatory SEP or F wave and EMG indicate abnormality of these tests in association with objective sensory or motor deficit respectively. Similarly, a correlation was considered confirmatory if the tests were normal in conjunction with absence of clinical deficit. A myelogram was confirmatory if abnormal in the presence of either motor or sensory signs or if normal when there was no objective deficit. A non-confirmatory test was one that was normal despite abnormal signs. Paradoxical indicates an abnormal test in the absence of objective findings.

Of the 12 patients with plexopathies, 5 had lesions of the lower trunk. SEPs evoked by stimulation of the fifth digit were absent or abnormal in 4 cases. They also had appropriately distributed EMG changes. Three patients had involvement of the entire brachial plexus. In 2, no SEPs were recordable following stimulation of cutaneous nerves representative of each trunk. The responses were prolonged in the other patient. They all had abnormal EMGs. The remaining 4 patients had respectively involvement of the middle and lower trunks, upper trunk, upper and middle trunks, and lumbar plexus (Fig. 4). In 2 the SEPs were abnormal. Overall, 9 out of 12 patients had abnormalities of SEPs evoked by stimulation of appropriate cutaneous nerves, confirming the anatomical site of the clinical lesion.

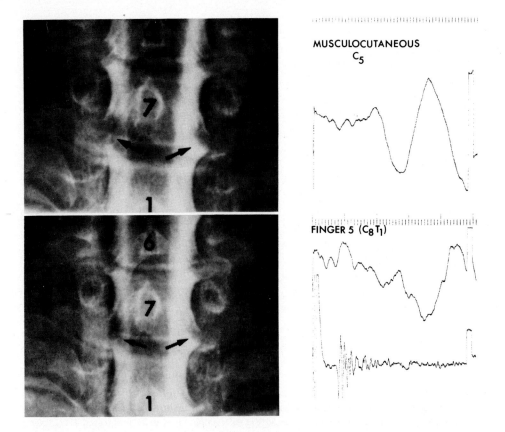

Fig. 3. The myelographic defect of the left compared to the right 8th cervical root (arrows) was associated with an appropriate motor and sensory neurological deficit. The SEP evoked by stimulation of finger 5 (C8) is dispersed and delayed. The SNAP (below) is normal. The SEP evoked by C5 stimulation (musculocutaneous) in comparison is normal.

TABLE II

COMPARATIVE YIELD OF VARIOUS ELECTROPHYSIOLOGICAL TESTS AND MYELOGRAPHY IN DIAGNOSIS OF ROOT LESIONS

	Confirmatory (%)	Non-confirmatory (%)	Paradoxical (%)
SEP	19/27 (70)	7/27 (26)	1/27 (4)
F wave	13/26 (50)	4/26 (15)	9/26 (35)
EMG	19/24 (79)	2/24 (8)	3/24 (13)
Myelogram	14/17 (82)	3/17 (18)	0

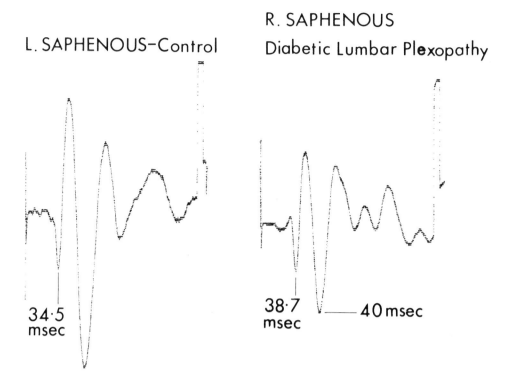

Fig. 4. Stimulation of the involved right (R) side in this patient with diabetic lumbar plexopathy produced a SEP of significantly longer latency and about 50% smaller amplitude than the uninvolved left (L) side. The conduction block was associated with a reduced recruitment of motor units on needle electromyography, but no evidence of active denervation.

DISCUSSION

In the diagnosis of central nervous system disease, the value of somatosensory evoked potentials (SEPs) is established. In comparison, the value of these tests in peripheral nervous system disease has been alluded to only rarely. For example, SEPs are recordable in the virtual absence of sensory nerve action potentials (SNAPs). Advantage can be taken of this to measure sensory conduction velocity (not otherwise possible) in some chronic or severe neuropathies (Desmedt and Noël 1973) and subsequent to nerve trauma (Assmus 1980).

Electrophysiological evaluation of proximal segments of the peripheral nervous system (roots and plexuses) can be difficult. Reliance must often be placed upon finding needle electromyographic abnormalities in appropriate myotomes. Clearly this has limited value when sensory features predominate or occur in isolation. Diagnostic use of the cervical or lumbar spinal and/or cortical SEP in the diagnosis of radiculopathies and plexopathies has been sparsely reported but holds promise (El Negamy and Sedgwick 1979; Jones 1979; Shirai et al. 1979; Ganes 1980). In these previous reports mixed nerve stimulation — usually the median nerve at the wrist — was used to elicit SEPs. This multisegmental activation, although useful in cervical spondylosis with associated myelopathy (Ganes 1980), would be unlikely to produce appreciable delay or desynchronization of the response when a single root or trunk is diseased.

In the present study there was either single root involvement or no significant root compression. This was myelographically confirmed in 63% of cases. The selective sensory stimulation used, activating one, or at most two, segmental levels, proved valuable. A positive correlation with presence (or absence) of the clinical findings occurred more frequently than that given by F wave measurements (Fisher et al. 1978), but slightly less frequently than obtained with EMG or myelogram. False positive (paradoxical) results were few, but normal SEPs were recorded in 26% of cases in which they might have been anticipated to be abnormal.

These false negatives in part reflect the limited means available at present for analysing SEPs. For example, latency prolongation may not be invariable in root compression because of the relatively short length over which conduction slowing occurs in relation to the overall length traversed by the impulses. Conduction block with resulting amplitude reduction was more useful. Side-to-side comparison was important in this regard. Morphological disruption of the response (desynchronization), although useful, was accepted as an abnormality only if obvious. Some means of quantitating this particular abnormality would be important. Because of the greater axonal length involved, delay of the SEP proved more useful in plexopathies. Using stimulation of appropriate cutaneous nerves, it was possible to determine which trunk of the plexus was predominantly involved.

No attempt was made in this study to record the cervical spinal SEP (Matthews et al. 1974). Such recording is potentially useful in root lesions and plexopathies (El Negamy and Sedgwick 1979; Jones 1979). If performed in conjunction with the cortical SEP and a nerve action potential recorded over Erb's point, it is possible to compare a pure central conduction time with one traversing the plexus and root (Eisen and Odusote 1980). Similarly, there is definite merit in using a non-cephalic referential recording montage (Cracco and Cracco 1976; Anziska et al. 1978; Cracco 1980; Desmedt and Cheron 1980). It allows for simultaneous visualization of early peaks reflecting the plexus, root, root entry zone and cuneate nucleus. Unfortunately, the cervical SEP, and more so the early components of the cortical SEP recordable with non-cephalic references, are not invariably present in normals. Using segmental sensory stimulation they are even less consistent and require averaging of several thousand responses.

SUMMARY

Segmental sensory stimulation representing cervical and lumbar dermatomes was used to elicit SEPs in 27 patients with radicular symptoms and/or signs and 12 patients with plexopathies. The test was confirmatory and aided in the anatomical localization in 19 (70%) and 9 (75%) of the respective patient groups. It is concluded that this electrophysiological test usefully complements other electrodiagnostic means of evaluating radiculopathies and plexopathies.

REFERENCES

Allison, J., Goff, W.R., Williamson, P.D. et al. On the neural origin of early components of the human somatosensory evoked response. In: J.E. Desmedt (Ed.), Clinical Uses of Cerebral Brainstem and Spinal Somatosensory EPs, Progress in Clinical Neurophysiology, Vol. 7. Karger, Basel, 1979: 51–68.

Anziska, B., Cracco, R.Q., Cook, A.W. and Feld, E.W. Somatosensory far-field potentials: Studies of normals and patients with multiple sclerosis. Electroenceph. clin. Neurophysiol., 1978, 45: 602–610.

Assmus, H. Somatosensory evoked cortical potentials in peripheral nerve lesions. In: C. Barber (Ed.), Evoked Potentials. University Park Press, Baltimore, Md., 1980: 437–442.

Braddon, R.L. and Johnson, E.W. H reflex: Review and classification with suggested clinical uses. Arch. phys. Med. Rehab., 1974, 55: 412–417.

Buchthal, F., Rosenfalck, A. and Behse, F. Sensory potentials of normal and diseased nerves. In P.J. Dyck, P.K. Thomas and E.H. Lambert (Eds.), Peripheral Neuropathy, Vol. 1. Saunders, Philadelphia, Pa., 1975: 442–464.

Cracco, R.Q. Scalp recorded potentials evoked by median nerve stimulation: subcortical potentials, travelling waves, and somatomotor potentials. In: J.E. Desmedt (Ed.), Clinical Use of Cerebral, Brainstem and Spinal Somatosensory Evoked Potentials. Prog. clin. Neurophysiol., Vol. 7. Karger, Basel, 1980: 1–14.

Cracco, R.Q. and Cracco, J.B. Somatosensory evoked potentials in man: far field potentials. Electroenceph. clin. Neurophysiol., 1976, 41: 460–466.

Desmedt, J.E. and Cheron, G. Central somatosensory conduction in man: Neural generators and interpeak latencies of the far-field components recorded from neck and right or left scalp earlobes. Electroenceph. clin. Neurophysiol., 1980, 50: 382–403.

Desmedt, J.E. and Noël, P. Average cerebral evoked potentials in the evaluation of lesions of the sensory nerves and of the central somatosensory pathway. In: J.E. Desmedt (Ed.), New Developments in Electromyography and Clinical Neurophysiology, Vol. 2. Karger, Basel, 1973: 352–371.

Donchin, E., Callaway, E., Cooper, R. et al. Publication criteria for studies of evoked potentials (EP) in man: report of a committee. In: J.E. Desmedt (Ed.), Attention, Voluntary Contraction and Event-Related Cerebral Potentials, Progress in Clinical Neurophysiology, Vol. 1. Karger, Basel, 1977: 1–11.

Eisen, A. and Elleker, G. Sensory nerve stimulation and evoked cerebral potentials. Neurology (Minneap.), 1980, 30: 1097–1105.

Eisen, A. and Odusote, K. Central and peripheral conduction times in multiple sclerosis. Electroenceph. clin. Neurophysiol., 1980, 48: 253–265.

Eisen, A., Schomer, D. and Melmed, C. The application of F-wave measurements in the differentiation of proximal and distal upper limb entrapments. Neurology (Minneap.), 1977a, 27: 662–668.

Eisen, A., Schomer, D. and Melmed, C. An electrophysiological method for examining lumbosacral root compression. Canad. J. neurol. Sci., 1977b, 4: 117–123.

El Negamy, E. and Sedgwick, E.M. Delayed cervical somatosensory potentials in cervical spondylosis. J. Neurol. Neurosurg. Psychiat., 1979, 42: 238–241.

Fisher, M.A., Shivde, A.J., Teixera, C. and Grainer, L.S. Clinical and electrophysiological appraisal of the significance of radicular injury in back pain. J. Neurol. Neurosurg. Psychiat., 1978, 41: 303–306.

Ganes, T. Somatosensory conduction times and peripheral cervical and cortical evoked potentials in patients with cervical spondylosis. J. Neurol. Neurosurg. Psychiat., 1980, 43: 683–689.

Jones, A.J. Investigation of brachial plexus traction lesions by peripheral and spinal somatosensory evoked potentials. J. Neurol. Neurosurg. Psychiat., 1979, 42: 107–116.

Kimura, J. F-wave velocity in central segment of the median and ulnar nerves. A study in normal subjects and in patients with Charcot-Marie-Tooth disease. Neurology (Minneap.), 1974, 24: 539–546.

Matthews, W.B., Beauchamp, M. and Small, D.G. Cervical somatosensory evoked responses in man. Nature (Lond.), 1974, 252: 230–232.

Shirai, Y., Ito, T. and Kota, S. A somatosensory evoked potential in patients with lumbar intervertebral disk herniations. Acta neurol. scand., 1979, 60, Suppl. 73: 80.

Tonzola, R.F., Ackil, A.A., Shahani, B.T. and Young, R.R. Usefulness of electrophysiological studies in the diagnosis of lumbosacral root disease. Ann. Neurol., 1981, 9: 305–308.

Young, R.R. and Shahani, B.T. Clinical value and limitations of F-wave determination. Muscle Nerve, 1978, 1: 248–250.

Kyoto Symposia (EEG Suppl. No. 36)
Editors: P.A. Buser, W.A. Cobb and T. Okuma
© 1982, Elsevier Biomedical Press, Amsterdam

358

Spinal Evoked Potentials

ROGER Q. CRACCO and JOAN B. CRACCO

State University of New York, Downstate Medical Center, Brooklyn, N.Y. 11203 (U.S.A.)

Evoked potentials which arise in the cauda equina and in spinal cord afferent pathways can be recorded from surface electrodes attached to the skin over the spine (Liberson et al. 1966; R.Q. Cracco 1973). Over rostral spinal cord segments these potentials are very tiny and are recorded with difficulty. The methods are the same as those used for recording potentials from the scalp, except that stimulus rates of about 7–9/sec are used, 1000–4000 responses are summated and analysis time is 20–40 msec. The frequency response of the recording apparatus is 10–3000 Hz. Simultaneous stimulation of multiple nerves, such as both peroneal nerves or both tibial nerves, increases the signal size (R.Q. Cracco et al. 1979) and this method is routinely employed in some laboratories.

Since records over the spine are often obscured by random myogenic activity, this can be minimized by recording when patients are drowsy or sleeping. Recording electrodes are attached to the skin over the spine and because of the small signal size it is important to maintain low and stable electrode impedances. Bipolar or reference records are obtained over various spinal locations. The reference electrode may be placed over the iliac crest, torso, scalp or sacrum (J.B. Cracco et al. 1975; Dimitrijevic et al. 1978; Jones and Small 1978). Reference records are often considerably noisier than bipolar records. If one is recording potentials only over the cauda equina or caudal spinal cord, far fewer responses need be summated since these potentials are much greater in amplitude than those recorded over rostral spinal cord segments. Technically satisfactory records have been obtained over this area by summating fewer than 100 responses (Dimitrijevic et al. 1978).

These potentials progressively increase in latency from lumbar to cervical recording locations (R.Q. Cracco 1973; J.B. Cracco et al. 1975, 1979) (Fig. 1). Similar potentials have been obtained from epidural leads in man (Magladery et al. 1951; Caccia et al. 1976; Ertekin 1976a,b; Shimoji et al. 1977, 1978). In bipolar surface leads over the lumbar spine, the response consists of initially positive triphasic potentials. This would be expected when recording an impulse traversing a nerve trunk in volume and is consistent with potentials arising in the roots of the cauda equina. With leads over the lower thoracic spine, which overlie caudal spinal cord segments, the response is often greater in amplitude and duration and more complex in configuration than with more rostral or more caudal leads. In adults this potential is usually initially positive and triphasic, the negative component of which has several peaks or inflections (J.B. Cracco et al. 1975). In infants and young children this response usually consists of a large positive-negative diphasic potential

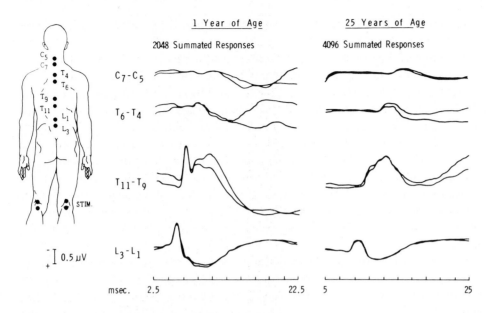

Fig. 1. Comparison of bipolar records of the spinal responses to peroneal nerve stimulation in a 1-year-old infant and an adult. Electrode placement refers to spinous process level. There is a delay of 2.5 and 5.0 msec between the stimulus and the averaging process in the infant and adult, respectively. Over the cauda equina (L3 spine) the response in both the infant and adult consists of triphasic potentials with poorly defined initial positive phases. In the infant, the response over caudal spinal cord (T11 spine) consists of a positive-negative diphasic potential followed by a broad negative-positive potential. In the adult it consists of a broad negative potential with 2 or 3 inflections. The response over rostral spinal cord in both the infant and adult consists of small, initially positive triphasic potentials with poorly defined positive phases. (From J.B. Cracco et al. 1979.)

followed by a broad negative and then, at times, by a positive potential (J.B. Cracco et al. 1975, 1979) (Fig. 1). Investigations of similar potentials recorded over caudal cord segments in cats and monkeys suggest that the initial diphasic potential arises in the intramedullary continuations of dorsal root fibres, and the subsequent potentials reflect synaptic and postsynaptic activity which is concerned with local reflex mechanisms rather than with the propagation of the response to more rostral levels (R.Q. Cracco and Evans 1978; Feldman et al. 1980).

Over rostral cord segments the response in children and adults consists of small, initially positive triphasic potentials, with poorly defined positive phases which progressively decrease in amplitude rostrally (R.Q. Cracco 1973; J.B. Cracco et al. 1975, 1979) (Fig. 1). This amplitude decrement probably reflects temporal dispersion and the greater distance between the skin recording electrodes and the spinal cord at rostral thoracic and cervical recording sites. Investigations in cats and monkeys suggest that these potentials arise in multiple, rapidly conducting afferent pathways, including the dorso-lateral columns which lie primarily ipsilateral to the stimulated peripheral nerve (Sarnowski et al. 1975; R.Q. Cracco and Evans 1978; Feldman et al. 1980). These animal studies also provide evidence which suggests that the peripheral nerve fibres which mediate these potentials recorded at all spinal levels are primarily muscle nerve rather than cutaneous nerve afferent fibres (Sarnowski et al. 1975).

The onset of the negative potential at each recording site may serve as the latency indicator and be used in determining conduction velocity, since this is thought to reflect the approximate time at which the fastest fibres contributing to a response are active under the recording electrode in reference leads and the recording electrode nearest the approaching volley in bipolar leads (Gilliatt et al. 1965). Latency differences are greater between equidistant leads placed over caudal spinal cord segments than they are between leads placed over the cauda equina or rostral spinal cord (R.Q. Cracco 1973; J.B. Cracco et al. 1979). This indicates a decrease in the speed of conduction of the response over caudal cord segments. This slowing probably reflects branching of dorsal root fibres and synaptic activity since this is the region where these fibres undergo synaptic contact in Clark's column and other nuclei.

In normal adults the mean conduction velocity of the response from lumbar to cervical recording locations is about 70 m/sec. Segmental conduction velocities are about 65 m/sec over peripheral nerve and cauda equina (point of peripheral nerve stimulation to L3 spine), 50 m/sec over caudal spinal cord (T12 to T6 spines) and 85 m/sec over rostral spinal cord (T6-C7 spines) (J.B. Cracco et al. 1979). In the newborn the segmental conduction velocities are about half those values obtained in the adult. They progressively increase with age. Peripheral conduction velocities are largely within the adult range by 3 years, whereas velocities over the spinal cord do not reach values until the fifth year (J.B. Cracco et al. 1979) (Fig. 2). This suggests that maturation of rapidly conducting spinal afferent pathways proceeds at a slower rate than maturation of rapidly conducting peripheral sensory fibres. Similar findings have been obtained in maturational studies of the scalp-recorded evoked response to median nerve stimulation. Conduction velocities in median nerve reached adult values between 12 and 18 months of age, whereas conduction velocity within central lemniscal pathways did not reach adult values until 5–7 years of age (Desmedt et al. 1973, 1976). The increase in speed of conduction in peripheral nerve and spinal cord is probably related to the increasing fibre diameter and progressive myelination which accompanies maturation. However, explanations of the differential rates of maturation of peripheral and central afferent pathways can only be speculative at this time.

In adult patients with clinically evident complete spinal cord lesions, evoked potentials recorded from surface electrodes caudal to the lesion are similar to those obtained in normal subjects. No response has been recorded in leads rostral to the lesion (R.Q. Cracco 1973) (Fig. 3). In a study of a group of infants and children with myelodysplasia from whom spinal evoked potentials and cerebral evoked potentials were recorded, there was correlation between the degree of evoked potential abnormality and the clinical status of the patients (J.B. Cracco et al. 1979, 1980a,b; J.B. Cracco and Cracco 1979). In a few of these patients it was possible to diagnose caudal displacement of the spinal cord; in these patients the large complex spinal potentials which are normally recorded over the lower thoracic spines were recorded

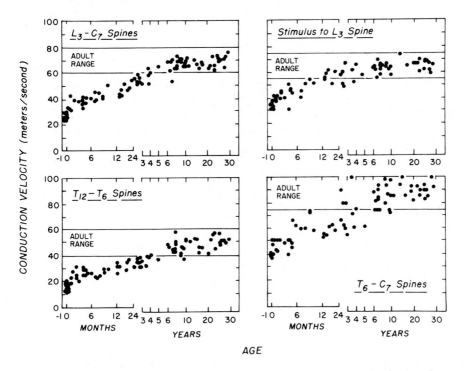

Fig. 2. Relationship between age and overall conduction velocity (L3-C7 spines) and segmental conduction velocities over peroneal nerve and cauda equina (stimulus to L3 spine), caudal spinal cord (T12-T6 spines) and rostral spinal cord (T6-C7 spines). Note the change in age scale (from months to years) on the abscissa. Infants from −1 to 0 months were premature. All conduction velocities progressively increase with age. The overall velocities are in the adult range by 5 years of age. Velocities over peroneal nerve and cauda equina increase rapidly during the first year of life and most values are in the adult range by 3 years. However, velocities over both caudal and rostral spinal cord are not in the adult range until 5–6 years of age. (From J.B. Cracco et al. 1979.)

over lumbar spinous processes. In several children with myelomeningocele a positive potential was recorded in leads immediately rostral to the lesion. This potential progressively decreased in amplitude but did not change in latency rostrally. This is a non-propagated volume-conducted potential which is consistent with physiological transection of the spinal cord. Similar positive potentials have been recorded rostral to spinal cord transections in cats and monkeys (killed end effect) (Sarnowski et al. 1975; R.Q. Cracco and Evans 1978; Feldman et al. 1980).

Spinal and scalp-recorded SEPs were studied in a group of children with degenerative diseases of the central nervous system (J.B. Cracco et al. 1980a). The conduction velocity over peroneal nerve was normal. Responses were recorded over the spinal cord in most patients but conduction velocities over the cord were slowed. Velocities over the spinal cord were slower over rostral cord segments than they were over the caudal cord. This may suggest that a "dying back" process, similar to that known to occur in some peripheral neuropathies, is operative in the spinal afferent pathways of these patients. The short latency evoked potentials to median nerve stimulation which arise within and rostral to the brain stem were absent in most of

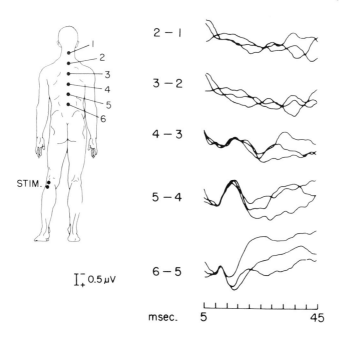

Fig. 3. Bipolar records of the spinal potential evoked by left peroneal nerve stimulation in a patient with a clinically complete spinal cord lesion at T8. Potentials caudal to the lesion (bottom 3 traces) are similar to those recorded in normal subjects. No potential is apparent in the lead in which the caudal electrode is placed over the sixth thoracic spine (trace 3-2) in relation to the lesion or in the more rostral lead (top trace). (From R.Q. Cracco 1973.)

the patients as were the longer latency potentials of cerebral cortical origin.

Spinal and peripheral nerve conduction velocities were also found to be slowed in some clinically asymptomatic juvenile diabetics (J.B. Cracco et al. 1980b). Peripheral nerve or spinal conduction velocity alone was slowed in some patients, while in others both peripheral and spinal conduction velocities were slowed. As in children with CNS degenerative disease, spinal conduction velocity over rostral spinal cord segments was chiefly affected.

Dorfman (1977) has devised a method by which conduction velocities within spinal cord afferent pathways may be indirectly estimated. He used scalp-recorded SEPs to stimulation of nerves in the lower and upper extremities as latency indicators and subtracted out the estimated peripheral conduction time by determining the F wave latencies for the stimulated peripheral nerves. He found slowing of conduction within spinal cord afferent pathways in normal elderly subjects and in some patients with diabetes and multiple sclerosis (Dorfman et al. 1978; Dorfman and Bosley 1979; Gupta and Dorfman 1980).

CONCLUSION

The recording of SEPs provides a unique opportunity to evaluate the entire neuraxis from cutaneous receptor to cerebral cortex. Information can be obtained concerning receptors, peripheral nerves, spinal cord, brain stem and cerebral cortex. When these methods are combined with those used in obtaining auditory and visual evoked potentials, it seems that it should be possible to obtain a reliable measure of the physiological integrity of the sensory systems in man.

REFERENCES

Caccia, M.R., Ubcali, E. and Andreussi, L. Spinal evoked responses recorded from the epidural space in normal and diseased humans. J. Neurol. Neurosurg. Psychiat., 1976, 39: 962–972.

Cracco, J.B. and Cracco, R.Q. Somatosensory spinal and cerebral evoked potentials in children with occult spinal dysraphism (abstr.). Neurology (Minneap.), 1979, 29: 543.

Cracco, J.B., Cracco, R.Q. and Graziani, L.J. The spinal evoked response in infants and children. Neurology (Minneap.), 1975, 25: 31–36.

Cracco, J.B., Cracco, R.Q. and Stolove, R. Spinal evoked potential in man: A maturational study. Electroenceph. clin. Neurophysiol., 1979, 46: 58–64.

Cracco, J.B., Bosch, V.V. and Cracco, R.Q. Cerebral and spinal somatosensory evoked potentials in children with CNS degenerative disease. Electroenceph. clin. Neurophysiol., 1980a, 49: 437–445.

Cracco, J.B., Castells, S. and Mark, E. Conduction velocity in peripheral nerve and spinal afferent pathways in juvenile diabetics (abstr.). Neurology (Minneap.), 1980b, 30: 370–371.

Cracco, R.Q. Spinal evoked response: Peripheral nerve stimulation in man. Electroenceph. clin. Neurophysiol., 1973, 35: 379–386.

Cracco, R.Q. and Evans, B. Spinal evoked potential in the cat. Effects of asphyxia, strychnine, cord section and compression. Electroenceph. clin. Neurophysiol., 1978, 44: 187–201.

Cracco, R.Q., Cracco, J.B. and Anziska, B.J. Somatosensory evoked potentials in man: Cerebral, subcortical, spinal and peripheral nerve potentials. Amer. J. EEG Technol., 1979, 19: 59–81.

Desmedt, J.E., Noel, P., Debecker, J. and Nameche, J. Maturation of afferent conduction velocity as studied by sensory nerve potentials and cerebral evoked potentials. In: J.E. Desmedt (Ed.), New Developments in Electromyography and Clinical Neurophysiology, Vol. 2. Karger, Basel, 1973: 52–63.

Desmedt, J.E., Brunko, E. and Debecker, J. Maturation of the somatosensory evoked potentials in normal infants and children, with special reference to the early N_1 component. Electroenceph. clin. Neurophysiol., 1976, 40: 43–58.

Dimitrijevic, M.R., Larsson, L.E., Lehmkuhl, D. and Sherwood, A.M. Evoked spinal cord and nerve root potentials in humans using a noninvasive recording technique. Electroenceph. clin. Neurophysiol., 1978, 45: 331–340.

Dorfman, L.J. Indirect estimation of spinal cord conduction velocity in man. Electroenceph. clin. Neurophysiol., 1977, 42: 26–34.

Dorfman, L.J. and Bosley, T.M. Age related changes in peripheral and central nerve conduction in man. Neurology (Minneap.), 1979, 29: 38–44.

Dorfman, L.J., Bosley, T.M. and Cummins, K.L. Electrophysiological localization of central somatosensory lesions in patients with multiple sclerosis. Electroenceph. clin. Neurophysiol., 1978, 44: 742–753.

Ertekin, C. Studies in the human evoked electrospinogram. I. The origin of the segmental evoked potentials. Acta neurol. scand., 1976a, 53: 2–30.

Ertekin, C. Studies in the human evoked electrospinogram. II. The conduction velocity along the dorsal funiculus. Acta neurol. scand., 1976b, 53: 21–38.

Feldman, M.H., Cracco, R.Q., Farmer P. and Mount, F. Spinal evoked potential in the monkey. Ann. Neurol., 1980, 7: 238–244.

Gilliatt, R.W., Melville, I.P., Velate, A.S. and Willison, R.G. A study of normal nerve action potential using an averaging technique (barrier grid storage tube). J. Neurol. Neurosurg. Psychiat., 1965, 28: 191–200.

Gupta, P.R. and Dorfman, L.J. Spinal somatosensory conduction in diabetics (abstr.). Neurology (Minneap.), 1980, 30: 414–415.

Jones, S.J. and Small, D.G. Spinal and sub-cortical evoked potentials following stimulation of the posterior tibial nerve in man. Electroenceph. clin. Neurophysiol., 1978, 44: 299–306.

Liberson, W.T., Gratzur, M., Zales, A. and Grabinski, B. Comparison of conduction velocity of motor and sensory fibers determined by different methods. Arch. phys. Med., 1966, 47: 17–23.

Magladery, J.W., Porter, W.E., Park, A.M. and Teasdall, R.D. Electrophysiological studies of nerve and reflex activity in normal man. IV. The two neuron reflex and identification of certain action potentials from spinal roots and cord. Bull. Johns Hopk. Hosp., 1951, 88: 499–519.

Sarnowski, R.J., Cracco, R.Q., Vogel, H.B. and Mount, F. Spinal evoked response in the cat. J. Neurosurg., 1975, 43: 329–336.

Shimoji, K., Matsuki, M. and Shimizu, H. Wave form characteristics and spatial distribution of evoked spinal electrogram in man. J. Neurosurg., 1977, 46: 304–310.

Shimoji, K., Shimizu, H. and Maruzama, Y. Origin of somatosensory evoked response recorded from the cervical skin surface. J. Neurosurg., 1978, 48: 980–984.

7. Functional Organization of Motor Areas in Primates and Patients with Movement Disorders

Kyoto Symposia (EEG Suppl. No. 36)
Editors: P.A. Buser, W.A. Cobb and T. Okuma
© 1982, Elsevier Biomedical Press, Amsterdam

Pathways for Short Latency Afferent Input to Motor Cortex in Monkeys

E.G. JONES

James L. O'Leary Division of Experimental Neurology and Neurological Surgery, and McDonnell Center for the Study of Higher Brain Function, Departments of Neurology and Neurological Surgery, and of Anatomy and Neurobiology, Washington University School of Medicine, St. Louis, Mo. 63110 (U.S.A.)

The idea that sensory messages emanating from working muscles serve as guides to the activities of the motor cortex is a particularly old one (Jones 1972). In recent years the principal input of this kind was thought to be mediated by the large diameter, Group I afferents that had been found to project preferentially to area 3a of the cerebral cortex, in the floor of the central sulcus (Phillips et al. 1971; Lucier et al. 1975; Heath et al. 1976; Hore et al. 1976; Jones and Porter 1980). Area 3a was then thought to complete a loop by projecting forwards to area 4 (Phillips 1969; Lucier et al. 1975) though, as reviewed below, such an anatomical connection cannot be demonstrated in primates (Jones et al. 1978; Jones and Porter 1980).

We have also been made aware that other, probably all, sensory modalities gain access to the motor cortex (Albe-Fessard and Liebeskind 1966; Welt et al. 1967; Wiesendanger 1973; Lemon and Porter 1976; Brinkman et al. 1978; Wong et al. 1978; H. Asanuma et al. 1980; Fetz et al. 1980; Tanji and Wise 1981). These inputs depend upon the integrity of the dorsal columns of the spinal cord for their section results in abolition of the peripheral receptive fields of motor cortex neurones (Brinkman et al. 1978). In this context, it seems important that lesions of the dorsal columns in man deprive the motor cortex of its capacity to compensate for peripherally imposed perturbations during performance of a repetitive movement of the finger and thumb (Marsden et al. 1977).

Because the sensory inputs to motor cortex arrive at remarkably short latency — as short as 5–8 msec in experiments involving electrical stimulation of peripheral nerves (Albe-Fessard and Liebeskind 1966; Devanandan and Heath 1975; Lucier et al. 1975; Brinkman et al. 1978; Lemon and van der Burg 1979) — some workers have suggested that these dorsal column-mediated inputs may project directly through the thalamus to the motor cortex rather than via a relay in the sensory cortex (Horne and Tracey 1979; Lemon and van der Burg 1979; H. Asanuma et al. 1980). In what follows, it will be shown that neither route is as simple as it seems.

In the monkey thalamus, short latency (ca. 5 msec) evoked potentials and unit responses to electrical stimulation of the median nerve undoubtedly extend (Horne and Tracey 1979; Lemon and van der Burg 1979; H. Asanuma et al. 1980; Tracey et al. 1980) from the traditional lemniscal relay nucleus (the VPLc nucleus of Olszewski (1952) into parts of the traditional relay to motor cortex (loosely called

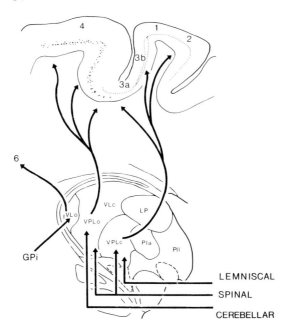

Fig. 1. Schematic representation on a sagittal section of the monkey thalamus showing segregation of lemniscal, cerebellar and pallidal inputs to thalamus and their separate projection on the cerebral cortex. From Jones and Porter (1980).

"VL" by many). Recent studies have localized these responses in the VPLo nucleus of Olszewski (1952), which is particularly easy to distinguish from VPLc in sagittal and horizontal sections. In these, it is seen to form, with its continuations, nuclei VLc, VLps and X of Olszewski, a distinctive cell-sparse zone (Jones et al. 1979; Friedman and Jones 1981; C. Asanuma et al. 1982a). Curiously, responses occurring in VPLo during perturbations of an active movement, if found at all, only appear at rather long latency (Strick 1976b; Wong et al. 1978; Macpherson et al. 1980).

The thalamic relay to area 4, as shown by anterograde and retrograde labelling, is coextensive with the cell-sparse VPLo, VLc, VLps and X complex (Strick 1976a; Jones et al. 1979; C. Asanuma et al. 1982a, b). We thus regard these as a common nuclear entity. This is further supported by the distribution of axons from the 3 deep cerebellar nuclei continuously throughout the complex (Thach and Jones 1979; Kalil 1981; C. Asanuma et al. 1982a, b) (Fig. 1). This distribution is less extensive than previously reported (Mehler and Nauta 1974; Chan-Palay 1977). There is a topography in the organization of the nuclear complex such that medial parts project laterally and lateral parts medially in area 4 while dorsal parts (VLC, VLps) project anteriorly and ventral parts (VPLo) project posteriorly (Strick 1976a; Jones et al. 1979). The distribution pattern of the cerebello-thalamic fibres from the 3 deep cerebellar nuclei implies a topographic representation of the body in each of them (Thach and Jones 1979; C. Asanuma et al. 1982b, c) (Fig. 2). Within a part of the representation in the thalamic relay to motor cortex, the terminations of fibres from the 3 deep nuclei alternate rather than overlap (C. Asanuma et al. 1982c). This may

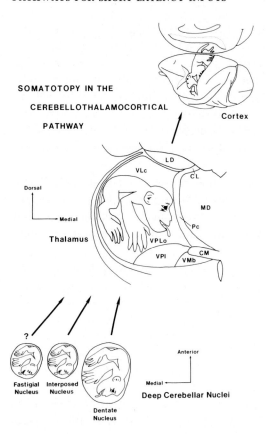

Fig. 2. Postulated somatotopy (C. Asanuma et al. 1982b) in deep cerebellar nuclei based upon distribution of fibres from different parts within known topographic representation in thalamic relay to motor cortex. Motor cortex map after Woolsey (1958). Potential multiple representations in motor cortex not figured.

imply that separate foci in motor cortex could be selectively influenced by each of the deep cerebellar nuclei. But the dendritic fields of the relay cells are so large that convergence is still possible.

The termination of axons arising in the cerebellar relay to motor cortex and those arising in the lemniscal relay to sensory cortex do not overlap in the floor of the central sulcus (Thach and Jones 1979; Friedman and Jones 1981). Area 3a receives its input, like the other 3 fields of sensory cortex (areas 3b, 1 and 2) only from the lemniscal terminal territory in VPLc and VPM (Friedman and Jones 1981) (Fig. 1).

Just as there is no convergence of the outputs of the cerebellar and lemniscal relay nuclei in the cortex, so there is no convergence of the ascending inputs to the 2 nuclei. Single labelling experiments clearly show that the cerebellar and lemniscal terminations respect the cytoarchitectonic border between the nuclei and double labelling experiments indicate no overlap (Tracey et al. 1980; C. Asanuma et al. 1982b, c; Jones and Friedman 1982). It may also be noted (Fig. 1) that the pallido-thalamic input, contrary to previous reports (Kemp and Powell 1971; Mehler and Nauta

1974), appears to be segregated (Percheron 1979; Tracey et al. 1980) from the cerebello-thalamic input, terminating only in nucleus VLo of Olszewski (1952). Also, despite some reports to the contrary (Strick 1976a) our results indicate that VLo projects to areas of cortex anterior to area 4. It is further probable that there is little encroachment of nigro-thalamic terminations on the terminal territories of pallidal and cerebellar fibres in the thalamus. Nigro-thalamic axons seem to terminate preferentially in nucleus VLm of Olszewski (Carpenter et al. 1976). The cortical target of VLm does not seem to include area 4, though this has not been extensively studied in monkeys.

The present position seems to be, therefore, that cerebellar inputs to the thalamus are much more restricted than previously reported (Kemp and Powell 1971; Mehler and Nauta 1974). The efferents of all 3 deep cerebellar nuclei terminate only in the relay to area 4 and there is no overlap with lemniscal or with pallidal or nigral inputs as previously assumed.

Because of the lack of encroachment of lemniscal terminations on the thalamic relay to motor cortex, we cannot easily account for the short latency, dorsal column-mediated inputs to the thalamus and motor cortex. The deep cerebellar nuclei are unlikely candidates for providing a short latency input since cells in them have been reported to respond only weakly, if at all, to peripheral stimulation and are said to do so at rather long latencies (20–100 msec) (Eccles et al. 1974; Allen et al. 1977; Harvey et al. 1981). The only other potential source of a short latency input is the spino-thalamic tract, whose terminations extend from the VPLc nucleus into the VPLo part of the cerebellar relay to motor cortex (Applebaum et al. 1979; Berkely 1980; Tracey et al. 1980; C. Asanuma et al. 1982b) (Fig. 1). But although many spino-thalamic axons have properties (Applebaum et al. 1975) that could account for the receptive fields of motor cortex neurones, section of the dorsal columns (Brinkman et al. 1978; H. Asanuma et al. 1980) should not interfere with the spino-thalamic tract. It is conceivable that some dorsal column pathway may exist that arises from spinal cells and, bypassing the dorsal column nuclei, terminates in VPLo but, if so, it remains to be discovered.

In view of the difficulties of obtaining conclusive anatomical support for the supposed short latency route directly through thalamus to motor cortex, it seems appropriate to re-examine the question of whether afferent influences could reach motor cortex via a relay in the sensory cortex. Such a route has not been popular on account of the repeated observations that ablation of the postcentral gyrus does not abolish peripherally evoked potentials in the motor cortex, though the potentials may be substantially diminished (Malis et al. 1953; H. Asanuma et al. 1980). It must be noted that in none of these experiments was the second somatic sensory area (SII) ablated. SII receives inputs from the lemniscal relay nucleus of the thalamus (Jones and Powell 1970) and projects via cortico-cortical fibres, to area 4 (Jones and Powell 1969; Vogt and Pandya 1977; Jones et al. 1978).

We have been able to show (Fig. 3), that areas 3a, 3b, 1 and 2 of the postcentral gyrus (Powell and Mountcastle 1959) receive inputs from different parts of the lemniscal relay nucleus of the thalamus (Jones 1972; Jones et al. 1978). These parts

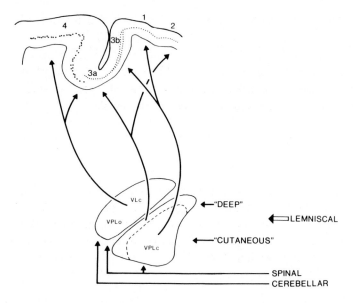

Fig. 3. Schematic figure from Friedman and Jones (1981) showing differential distribution in thalamus and separate cortical targets of deep and cutaneous components of medial lemniscus.

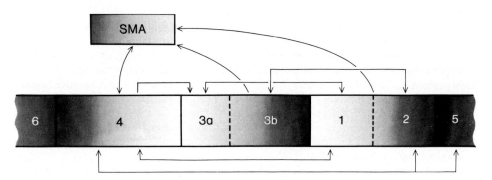

Fig. 4. Schematic figure from Jones and Porter (1980) showing pattern of cortico-cortical connectivity of pre- and postcentral cortical fields in monkeys. SMA is supplementary motor area.

can be characterized as ''deep'' or ''cutaneous'' according to the receptive field properties of their constituent neurones (Friedman and Jones 1981; Jones and Friedman 1982). Areas 3a and 2 receive inputs from the deep region which is on the antero-dorsal surface of the nucleus and areas 1 and 2 receive inputs from the cutaneous region at the centre of the nucleus (Fig. 1). These fields would then be appropriate for relaying sensory input to motor cortex, though we have no information of what sort of delay this additional step might introduce.

When we look at the cortico-cortical connectivity of the 4 post-central fields (Fig. 4), we find that it is far from simple. Of the 4 fields only area 2 projects forwards to area 4 (Vogt and Pandya 1977; Jones et al. 1978). Area 3a does not, perhaps accounting for the difficulty that most workers have experienced in demonstrating secure group I afferent inputs to area 4. Nor do areas 3b, or 1 which would be candidates for furnishing the cutaneous inputs that are particularly found in posterior parts of area 4 (Strick and Preston 1978; Tanji and Wise 1981). Therefore, if we rule out the spino-thalamic tract as the route for short latency afferent inflow to motor cortex, we are left with area 2, or conceivably with the SII area, as critical steps in any alternative cortico-cortical loop that may be responsible.

ACKNOWLEDGEMENTS

Personal work reported here was carried out in association with C. Asanuma, J.D. Coulter, S.H.C. Hendry, D.P. Friedman, R. Porter, W.T. Thach, D.J. Tracey and S.P. Wise and was supported by grants from the National Institutes of Health, United States Public Health Service and in part by grants from the National Health and Medical Research Council of Australia. E.G. Jones was for part of the time a Josiah Macy Jr. Foundation Senior Faculty Scholar.

REFERENCES

Albe-Fessard, D. et Liebeskind, J. Origines des messages somatosensitifs activant les cellules du cortex moteur chez le singe. Brain Res., 1966, 1: 127–146.

Allen, G.I., Gilbert, P.F.C., Marini, R., Schultz, W. and Yin, T.C.T. Integration of cerebral and peripheral inputs by interpositus neurons in monkey. Exp. Brain Res., 1977, 27: 81–99.

Applebaum, A.E., Beall, J.E., Foreman, R.D. and Willis, W.D. Organization and receptive fields of primate spinothalamic tract neurons. J. Neurophysiol. 1975, 38: 572–586.

Applebaum, A.E., Leonard, R.B., Kenshalo, Jr., D.R., Martin, R.F. and Willis, W.D. Nuclei in which functionally identified spinothalamic tract neurons terminate. J. comp. Neurol., 1979, 188: 575–586.

Asanuma, C., Thach, W.T. and Jones, E.G. Cytoarchitectonic delineation of the ventral lateral thalamic region in monkeys. Brain Res. Rev., 1982a, in press.

Asanuma, C., Thach, W.T. and Jones, E.G. Distribution of cerebellar terminations and their relation to other afferent terminations in the thalamic ventral lateral region. Brain Res. Rev., 1982b, in press.

Asanuma, C., Thach, W.T. and Jones, E.G. Anatomical evidence for segregated focal groupings of efferent cells and their terminal ramifications in the cerebellothalamic pathway. Brain Res. Rev., 1982c, in press.

Asanuma, H., Larsen, K.D. and Yumiya, H. Peripheral input pathways to the monkey motor cortex. Exp. Brain Res., 1980, 38: 349–355.

Berkley, K.J. Spatial relationships between the terminations of somatic sensory and motor pathways in the rostral brainstem of cats and monkeys. I. Ascending somatic sensory inputs to lateral diencephalon. J. comp. Neurol., 1980, 193: 283–317.

Brinkman, J., Bush, B.M. and Porter, R. Deficient influences of peripheral stimuli on precentral neurones in monkeys with dorsal column lesions. J. Physiol. (Lond.), 1978, 276: 27–48.

Carpenter, M.B., Nakano, K. and Kim, R. Nigrothalamic projections in the monkey demonstrated by autoradiographic technics. J. comp. Neurol., 1976, 165: 401–415.

Chan-Palay, C. Cerebellar Dentate Nucleus. Springer, Berlin, 1977.

Devanandan, M.S. and Heath, C.D. A short latency pathway from forearm nerves to area 4 of the baboon's cerebral cortex. J. Physiol. (Lond.), 1975, 248: 43–44.

Eccles, J.C., Sabah, N.H. and Táboříková, H. The pathway responsible for excitation and inhibition of fastigial neurones. Exp. Brain Res., 1974, 19: 78–99.

Fetz, E.E., Finocchio, D.V., Baker, M.A. and Soso, M.J. Sensory and motor responses of precentral cortex cells during comparable passive and active joint movements. J. Neurophysiol., 1980, 43: 1070–1089.

Friedman, D.P. and Jones, E.G. Thalamic input to areas 3a and 2 in monkeys. J. Neurophysiol., 1981, 45: 59–85.

Harvey, R.J., Porter, R. and Rawson, J.A. Discharges of intracerebellar nuclear cells in monkeys. J. Physiol. (Lond.), 1981, 297: 559–580.

Heath, C.J., Hore, J. and Phillips, C.G. Inputs from low threshold muscle and cutaneous afferents of hand and forearm to areas 3a and 3b of baboon's cerebral cortex. J. Physiol. (Lond.), 1976, 25: 199–227.

Hore, J., Preston, J.B., Durkovic, R.G. and Cheney, P.D. Responses of cortical neurons (areas 3a and 4) to ramp stretch of hindlimb muscles in the baboon. J. Neurophysiol., 1976, 39: 484–500.

Horne, M.K. and Tracey, D.J. The afferents and projections of the ventroposterolateral thalamus in the monkey. Exp. Brain Res., 1979, 36: 129–141.

Jones, E.G. The development of the "muscular sense" concept in the nineteenth century and the work of H. Charlton Bastian. J. Hist. Med., 1972, 27: 298–311.

Jones, E.G. and Friedman, D.P. Projection pattern of functional components of thalamic ventrobasal complex on monkey somatic sensory cortex. J. Neurophysiol., 1982, 48: 521–544.

Jones, E.G. and Porter, R. What is area 3a? Brain Res. Rev., 1980, 2: 1–43.

Jones, E.G. and Powell, T.P.S. Connexions of the somatic sensory cortex of the rhesus monkey. I. Ipsilateral cortical connexions. Brain, 1969, 92: 477–502.

Jones, E.G. and Powell, T.P.S. Connexions of the somatic sensory cortex of the rhesus monkey. III. Thalamic connexions. Brain, 1970, 93: 37–56.

Jones, E.G., Coulter, J.D. and Hendry, S.H.C. Intracortical connectivity of architectonic fields in the somatic sensory, motor and parietal cortex of monkeys. J. comp. Neurol., 1978, 181: 291–348.

Jones, E.G., Wise, S.P. and Coulter, J.D. Differential thalamic relationships of sensory-motor and parietal cortical fields in monkeys. J. comp. Neurol., 1979, 183: 833–882.

Kalil, K. Projections of the cerebellar and dorsal column nuclei upon the thalamus of the rhesus monkey. J. comp. Neurol., 1981, 195: 25–50.

Kemp, J.M. and Powell, T.P.S. The connexions of the striatum and globus pallidus: synthesis and speculation. Phil. Trans. B, 1971, 262: 441–457.

Kim, R., Nakano, K., Jayaraman, A. and Carpenter, M.B. Projections of the globus pallidus and adjacent structures: an autoradiographic study in the monkey. J. comp. Neurol., 1976, 169: 263–290.

Lemon, R.N. and Porter, R. Afferent input to movement-related precentral neurones in conscious monkeys. Proc. roy. Soc. B, 1976, 194: 313–339.

Lemon, R.N. and van der Burg, J. Short-latency peripheral inputs to thalamic neurones projecting to the motor cortex in the monkey. Exp. Brain Res., 1979, 36: 445–462.

Lucier, G.E., Ruegg, D.C. and Wiesendanger, M. Responses of neurones in motor cortex and in area 3a to controlled stretches of forelimb muscles in cebus monkeys. J. Physiol. (Lond.), 1975, 251: 833–853.

Macpherson, J.M., Rasmusson, D.D. and Murphy, J.T. Activities of neurons in "motor" thalamus during control of limb movement in the primate. J. Neurophysiol., 1980, 44: 11–28.

Malis, L.I., Pribram, K.H. and Kruger, L. Action potentials in motor cortex evoked by peripheral nerve stimulation. J. Neurophysiol., 1953, 16: 161–167.

Marsden, C.D., Merton, P.A., Morton, H.B. and Adam, J. The effect of posterior column lesions on servo responses from the human long thumb flexor. Brain, 1977, 100: 185–200.

Mehler, W.R. and Nauta, W.J.H. Connections of the basal ganglia and of the cerebellum. Confin. neurol. (Basel), 1974, 36: 205–222.

Olszewski, J. The Thalamus of the *Macaca mulatta*. An Atlas for Use with the Stereotaxic Instrument. Karger, Basel, 1952.

Percheron, G. The thalamic territory of cerebellar afferents and the lateral region of the thalamus of the macaque in stereotaxic ventricular coordinates. J. Hirnforsch., 1977, 18: 375–400.

Phillips, C.G. Motor apparatus of the baboon's hand. Proc. roy. Soc. B, 1969, 173: 141–174.

Phillips, C.G., Powell, T.P.S. and Wiesendanger, M. Projection from low threshold muscle afferents of hand and forearm to area 3a of baboon's cortex. J. Physiol. (Lond.), 1971, 217: 419–446.

Powell, T.P.S. and Mountcastle, V.B. Some aspects of the functional organization of the cortex of the postcentral gyrus of the monkey: a correlation of findings obtained in a single unit analysis with cytoarchitecture. Bull. Johns Hopk. Hosp., 1959, 105: 133–162.

Strick, P.L. Anatomical analysis of ventrolateral thalamic input in primate motor cortex. J. Neurophysiol., 1976a, 39: 1020–1031.

Strick, P.L. Activity of ventrolateral thalamic neurons during arm movement. J. Neurophysiol., 1976b, 39: 1032–1044.

Strick, P.L. and Preston, J.B. Multiple representation in the primate motor cortex. Brain Res., 1978, 154: 366–370.

Tanji, J. and Wise, S.P. Submodality segregation in the sensorimotor cortex of the unanesthetized monkey. J. Neurophysiol., 1981, 45: 467–481.

Thach, W.T. and Jones, E.G. The cerebellar dentatothalamic connection: terminal field, lamellae, rods and somatotopy. Brain Res., 1979, 169: 168–172.

Tracey, D.J., Asanuma, C., Jones, E.G. and Porter, R. Thalamic relay to motor cortex: afferent pathways from brain stem, cerebellum and spinal cord in monkeys. J. Neurophysiol., 1980, 44: 532–554.

Vogt, B.A. and Pandya, D.N. Cortico-cortical connections of somatic sensory cortex (areas 3, 1 and 2) in the rhesus monkey. J. comp. Neurol., 1977, 177: 179–191.

Welt, C., Aschoff, J.C., Kameda, K. and Brooks, V.B. Intra-cortical organisation of cat's motorsensory neurons. In: M.D. Yahr and D.P. Purpura (Eds.), Neurophysiological Basis of Normal and Abnormal Motor Activities. Raven Press, New York, 1967: 255–288.

Wiesendanger, M. Input from muscle and cutaneous nerves of the hand and forearm to neurones of the precentral gyrus of baboons and monkeys. J. Physiol. (Lond.), 1973, 228: 203–219.

Wong, Y.C., Kwan, H.C., MacKay, W.A. and Murphy, J.T. Spatial organization of precentral cortex in awake primates. I. Somatosensory inputs. J. Neurophysiol., 1978, 41: 1107–1120.

Woolsey, C.N. Organization of somatic sensory and motor areas of the cerebral cortex. In: H.F. Harlow and C.N. Woolsey (Eds.), The Biological and Biochemical Basis of Behavior. University of Wisconsin Press, Madison, Wis., 1958: 63–81.

Kyoto Symposia (EEG Suppl. No. 36)
Editors: P.A. Buser, W.A. Cobb and T. Okuma
© 1982, Elsevier Biomedical Press, Amsterdam

Motor Areas of the Monkey's Frontal Cerebral Cortex

COBIE BRINKMAN

Experimental Neurology Unit, John Curtin School of Medical Research, Australian National University, P.O. Box 334, Canberra 2601 (Australia)

On the basis of experiments involving stimulation and ablation of the cerebral cortex in primates it was thought for a long time that within the frontal cortex there were two distinct areas involved in the control of movement: a "motor" area largely corresponding with Brodmann's area 4, and a "premotor" area in Brodmann's area 6 on the lateral and medial surfaces of the cerebral hemisphere. Area 4 stimulation resulted in isolated movements of the contralateral extremities and body; area 6 stimulation evoked complex synergistic movements. Ablation of area 4 produced flaccid paresis while area 6 lesions caused spasticity (Fulton and Kennard 1934; Hines 1943).

This concept was questioned in more recent stimulation and ablation studies when a different organization was found: a "primary motor" area (M I) encompassing area 4 and part of area 6 on the lateral convexity of the brain, and a "supplementary motor" area (M II), located mainly in area 6 on the medial surface of the hemisphere (Woolsey et al. 1952). M I lesions were followed by flaccid paresis, while lesions of M II alone resulted in spastic paresis (Travis 1955a, b). In these studies, no evidence was found for a "premotor" area in lateral area 6 on the convexity of the brain.

The development of chronic recording techniques has made possible the examination of neuronal activity in the motor areas of the brain in conscious monkeys performing learned motor tasks. Most recordings have been made in area 4 (see Evarts, this volume) but recently, M II has also been investigated. The behaviour of neurones in the supplementary motor area (SMA) was found to differ from that of those in M I (see C. Brinkman and Porter 1979; Tanji, this volume). The results seem to point to a possible role for SMA in the programming of movements, perhaps through modulation of M I neuronal activity as, anatomically, SMA lies "upstream" of M I. Not until very recently, however, has attention been paid to the lateral parts of area 6. Like SMA, it is upstream of M I and other anatomical data also suggest that this original "premotor" area (PM) should be considered as distinct from M I.

Although few chronic recording studies have been done, so far they point to a marked influence on PM neuronal activity of visual events related to movement execution (Kubota and Hamada 1978; J. Brinkman and Porter 1979; Godschalk et al. 1981). This is not frequently seen in SMA (C. Brinkman and Porter 1979; Tanji, this volume) or M I (Godschalk et al. 1981). PM ablation studies have produced an apparent loss of control of visually guided movement (steering the hand through a hole in a perspex sheet to retrieve food; Moll and Kuijpers 1977) or an inability to perform sequences of learned movements (opening complex problem boxes) under visual guidance (Jacobsen 1934; Deuel 1977).

In contrast, SMA lesions seem to disrupt the sequencing of individual movements, a deficit looking very similar to the apraxia of some human neurological syndromes (Brinkman 1980). In addition, SMA ablations in monkeys disrupt performance of a bimanual coordination task. In the normal monkey, each hand takes a particular role, but after SMA ablation both hands tend to be used for the same part of the task. These findings are in keeping with SMA's postulated role in motor programming.

Selective lesions of neither PM nor SMA result in paresis, or gross changes of muscle tone. Paresis occurs only with M I lesions and is flaccid unless SMA is involved as well, when spasticity results (Denny-Brown and Botterell 1948; Travis 1955b; Brinkman and Kuijpers 1973). M I lesions impair the execution of movements but do not produce disturbances of visuo-motor guidance, performance of learned movements or movement sequencing.

Therefore, it seems that there are at least 3 areas in the monkey's frontal cortex related to movement control: the primary motor area, M I, the supplementary motor area, SMA, and a premotor area, PM.

REFERENCES

Brinkman, C. and Porter, R. The supplementary motor area of the monkey: activity of neurons during performance of a learned motor task. J. Neurophysiol., 1979, 42: 681–709.

Brinkman, J. Effects of supplementary motor area ablations in the monkey. Proc. Aust. physiol. pharmacol. Soc., 1980, 11: 170P.

Brinkman, J. and Kuijpers, H.G.J.M. Cerebral control of contralateral and ipsilateral arm, hand and finger movements in the split-brain rhesus monkey. Brain, 1973, 96: 653–674.

Brinkman, J. and Porter, R. "Premotor" area of the monkey's cerebral cortex: activity of neurons during performance of a learned motor task. Proc. Aust. physiol. pharmacol. Soc., 1979, 10: 198P.

Denny-Brown, D. and Botterell, E.H. The motor function of the agranular frontal cortex. Res. Publ. Ass. nerv. ment. Dis., 1948, 27: 257–346.

Devel, R.K. Loss of motor habits after cortical lesions. Neuropsychologia, 1977, 15: 205–215.

Fulton, J.F. and Kennard, M.A. A study of flaccid and spastic paralyses produced by lesions of the cerebral cortex in primates. Res. Publ. Ass. nerv. ment. Dis., 1934, 13: 158–210.

Goldschalk, M., Lemon, R.N., Nijs, H. and Kuijpers, H.G.J.M. Behaviour of neurons in monkey peri-arcuate and precentral cortex before and during visually guided arm and hand movements. Exp. Brain Res., 1981, 44: 113–116.

Hines, M. Control of movements by the cerebral cortex in primates. Biol. Rev., 1943, 18: 1–31.

Jacobsen, C.F. Influence of motor and premotor area lesions upon the retention of acquired skilled movements in monkeys and chimpanzees. Res. Publ. Ass. nerv. ment. Dis., 1934, 13: 225–247.

Kubota, K. and Hamada, I. Visual tracking and neuron activity in the peri-arcuate area in monkeys. J. Physiol. (Paris), 1978, 74: 297–313.

Moll, L. and Kuijpers, H.G.J.M. Premotor cortical ablations in monkeys: contralateral changes in visually guided reaching behaviour. Science, 1977, 198: 317–319.

Travis, A.M. Neurological deficiencies after ablation of the precentral motor area in *Macaca mulatta*. Brain, 1955a, 78: 155–173.

Travis, A.M. Neurological deficiencies following supplementary motor area lesions in *Macaca mulatta*. Brain, 1955b, 78: 174–201.

Woolsey, C.N., Settlage, P.H., Meyer, D.R., Spencer, W., Hamuy, T.P. and Travis, A.M. Patterns of localization in precentral and "supplementary" motor areas in their relation to the concept of a premotor area. Res. Publ. Ass. nerv. ment. Dis., 1952, 30: 238–264.

Kyoto Symposia (EEG Suppl. No. 36)
Editors: P.A. Buser, W.A. Cobb and T. Okuma
© 1982, Elsevier Biomedical Press, Amsterdam

Recent Studies in the Supplementary Motor Area with a Technique of Single Unit Recording from Behaving Primates

JUN TANJI and KIYOSHI KURATA

Department of Physiology, Hokkaido University, School of Medicine, Sapporo 060 (Japan)

Anatomical and physiological studies in the monkey (Penfield and Welch 1951; Woolsey et al. 1952; Wiesendanger et al. 1973) and in man (Penfield and Welch 1949; Talairach and Bancaud 1966) have provided evidence for the existence of the supplementary motor area (SMA) lying anteriorly to the precentral motor area, corresponding to the medial portion of Brodmann's area 6. Though the relevance of this area to motor control has been inferred from clinical observations and electrical stimulation or ablation studies, understanding of its functional role is still far from adequate.

Application of the single unit recording technique in awake, behaving animals recently demonstrated (Brinkman and Porter 1979) that neurones in the SMA were active in association with voluntary limb movements. Making use of this technique, further refinement of knowledge about the functional organization of this area was attempted in our laboratory. A systematic search has been made to answer the following questions concerning topographical organization of the SMA and the nature of the neuronal response. (1) How are neurones active with forelimb and hind limb movements distributed on the medial surface of the hemisphere and in the upper bank of the cingulate sulcus? (2) When an animal starts limb movements in response to a sensory cue, is the neuronal activity tightly coupled in time to the sensory stimulus or is it more associated with initiation of motor activity? What is the exact time relation between the neuronal activity and onset of the movement? (3) How different are the neuronal activities in the SMA and precentral motor cortex? (4) Apart from activities closely related to execution of movement, is there any activity in the SMA in association with some preparatory process prior to initiation of a motor task?

For this purpose macaque monkeys were trained to perform motor tasks in 3 different paradigms, which included: (1) discrete usage of forelimb and hind limb in a temporally separated manner, (2) quick wrist movements in response to 3 different cues of visual, auditory and somatosensory signals, or (3) a limb movement requiring a preparatory state of the animal to start a correct stimulus-triggered movement. With a big cylinder chronically implanted on the skull, single unit discharges were analysed in the SMA and the precentral motor cortex.

DISTRIBUTION OF NEURONES RELATED TO FORELIMB AND HIND LIMB MOVEMENTS IN SMA

In their first attempt to record discharges of single neurones in behaving animals, Brinkman and Porter (1979) noticed a general tendency that neurones active in relation to forelimb and hind limb movements were located in the rostral and caudal parts of SMA, respectively. The observation agrees with Woolsey's results but not fully with observations obtained by Penfield and Welch, who described the supplementary leg area as extending more than 10 mm anteriorly from the precentral tail area (Fig. 5 of Penfield and Welch 1951). Furthermore, other investigators failed to detect somatotopy in SMA (Wiesendanger et al. 1973; Orgogozo and Larsen 1979). These results pointed to a need for a detailed survey of neuronal activity related to forelimb and hind limb movements throughout the entire extent of SMA, including the upper bank of the cingulate sulcus. In order to study the topography by the single unit recording technique, it is essential to specify the movement as one involving muscle activity in only a limited part of the body. It is impossible to obtain precise information about topography by using animals performing unrestrained movements, since forelimb movements, for instance, are accompanied by supporting activity in axial body as well as hind limb muscles. In our studies, therefore, the following 3 procedures were taken : (1) the animal's limbs were encased in form-fitting casts and fixed at optimal joint angles for movements limited at appropriate joints, with the body weight stably sustained on a chair, (2) extensive training was done over months until the pattern of muscle activities was stabilized, and (3) the EMG was thoroughly monitored in numerous limb and axial muscles to make sure that activity was actually limited to a particular portion of the limb.

In a first series of experiments the monkey was trained to perform forelimb and hind limb movements alternately. The forelimb movements, wrist extension and flexion, and the hind limb movement, pedal pressing by plantar flexion, were triggered by visual signals and temporally separated by several seconds. Seventy-four neurones were found to be active prior to wrist extension and/or flexion. Of these 74 neurones, 38 exhibited different activities depending upon the direction of the wrist movement. None of the 74 neurones showed significant activity changes with the movement of the foot. In contrast, 86 neurones were active prior to foot movement. They did not exhibit any significant activity changes in association with the forelimb movements. Thus, no neurones exhibited positive relations to both the fore- and hind limb movements.

The depth of each extracellularly recorded neurone was recorded with respect to the cortical surface, the large-celled layers of cortex, and the subcortical white matter. Recording sites of neurones were located using the data thus obtained and by histological reconstruction of the lesion sites and electrode tracks. The recording sites were found to be located in one of three possible regions: the dorsal surface of the hemisphere, the medial face of the cortex dorsal to the cingulate sulcus and the dorsal bank of the cingulate sulcus.

Three major findings were obtained from the map showing distribution of the neurones in the SMA related to forelimb and hind limb movements: (1) neurones related to forelimb and hind limb motor tasks are distributed not only superficially but also in deeper portions of the medial face of the cortex and in the upper bank of the cingulate sulcus, (2) the location of these 2 classes of neurones are not intermingled but separated antero-posteriorly, that is, neurones related to the forelimb lie anteriorly and those related to the hind limb lie posteriorly in the SMA, and (3) neurones related to the hind limb task are located in area 6, just anterior to the hind limb and tail areas of area 4 (confirmed by positive effects of microstimulation). The third finding confirmed results obtained previously (Wise and Tanji 1981) indicating that no discrepancy exists between physiological evidence for the location of the hind limb area of SMA and the posterior boundary of area 6 determined cytoarchitectonically. Thus, the hind limb part of SMA is to be placed within area 6, not extending into area 4 as reported by Woolsey et al. (1952).

The next step of the study was to know how neurones related to distal and proximal limb movements are distributed in the forelimb area of SMA. For this purpose it was essential to establish a paradigm of motor performance in which either distal or proximal limb muscles were exclusively activated. Two monkeys were trained to sit in a chair and perform a motor task having two phases, one involving activity of digital muscles and the other calling for activation of proximal forelimb muscles. The right fore- and upper arm were fixed to an L-shaped plastic cast so that the joint angles at the elbow and wrist were 90° and 180°, respectively. The cast was attached to the chair with a pivot in such a way as to be movable by inner or outer rotation at the shoulder joint. A key was attached to the distal end of the cast which could be pressed by flexion of 4 fingers, the second to fifth digits. The monkey was required to shift the cast inwards or outwards to one of two correct holding zones of 4° which were separated by 40°. The correct holding was signalled by a green light. After the holding period of 2–4 sec, which varied unpredictably, a red light came on and instructed the monkey to press the key within 480 msec after the light onset. The monkey had to keep holding the cast in the correct zone during and even after the key press. If the cast remained in the zone 2 sec after the key press, a reward was given and the animal was asked to shift the cast to the other zone. The EMG was recorded with silver wire electrodes chronically implanted in extensors and flexors of fingers, extensors and flexors of wrist and elbow joints, as well as in muscles in the shoulder, chest, girdle and paravertebral region.

As a result of appropriate fixation of the forelimb and extensive training, temporal separation of the distal and proximal muscle activities in 2 phases of the motor task was achieved. The finger flexors, showing obvious activity increase prior to the key press, exhibited no alteration of their activity in association with shifting the cast. In contrast, triceps, supra- and infraspinatus muscles appeared to be prime movers for the outward shift and biceps and pectoralis muscles were active with inward shift movement. None of them was active in association with the key press. Paravertebral muscles and many other muscles in the girdle changed their activity with various time relations to the motor task, but their activity changes were not at all time-locked to either the shift movements or key press. Out of 562 neurones recorded in the SMA of the 2 monkeys, 225 were found to change their discharge activity before starting the forelimb movements. Sixty of them appeared to be related to the key press, 150 to the cast-shifting movement and the remaining 15 neurones to both motor acts. By mapping these neurones in the manner mentioned before, neurones related to distal forelimb movements were located more rostrally and those to proximal movements were located more caudally, though with considerable overlap. In the overlapping region, neurones related to distal movements were located more deeply.

Thus this study provided unequivocal evidence that a class of neurones in SMA are active in association with movements performed exclusively by the distal forelimb. The rostro-caudal arrangements of distal and proximal forelimb areas agree basically with the organization suggested previously (Woolsey et al. 1952; Brinkman and Porter 1979). However, the presence of neurones related to distal forelimb movements in the deeper portion of SMA, including the upper bank of the cingulate sulcus, does not agree with the motor figurine drawn by Woolsey et al. (1952).

DISCHARGE PROPERTIES OF NEURONES IN SMA AND MOTOR CORTEX

Since it was demonstrated that a large number of SMA neurones started changing their activity prior to muscular contraction, like precentral neurones (Evarts 1966), one must know how neuronal movement-related activity differs in the 2 motor representation areas. A series of experiments was designed to compare quantitatively neuronal responses in the 2 areas using animals performing forelimb movements in response to sensory signals of 3 different modalities.

Monkeys were trained to perform alternate flexion and extension at the wrist in response to visual, auditory or somatosensory triggering signals, which were given to the animal in a randomized sequence. The visual signal was a red light placed in front of the animal. The auditory signal was a tone burst of 1 kHz, 30 dB above background noise level. The tactile signal was a vibration transmitted to the monkey's hand, generated by a servo-controlled DC torque motor driven by a burst of square wave oscillation at 500 Hz. The reward was given when the correct response was initiated within 280 msec after the onset of the stimulus.

Eighty-one per cent of neurones recorded in the hand area of the precentral motor cortex were found to alter their activity in association with wrist extension and/or flexion. The neuronal response latency was calculated on the basis of the peristimulus histogram. The mean latencies of the precentral neurones to the visual, auditory and tactile signals were 157, 136 and 59 msec, respectively. These values correspond well with those obtained in previous reports (Evarts 1966, 1973). The modulation of discharge frequency was similar regardless of the modality of the sensory signal. In contrast, 38% of SMA neurones were found to be related to wrist movements. The mean latencies of SMA neurones to visual and auditory signals were 128 and 108 msec, respectively, significantly shorter than those of precentral neurones. For the tactile signal the reverse was true, though the difference was much smaller. The intensity of activity changes of SMA neurones was generally smaller. The increase or decrease of discharge frequency of individual neurones during 200 msec of the premovement period above or below background level of discharge was calculated for each movement triggered by the 3 different signals. In visually triggered movement, mean magnitudes of SMA neurones and precentral neurones were 32 and 53 impulses/sec, respectively. The difference was found to be highly significant by the Mann-Whitney U test. Similar differences were obtained for auditory and tactile triggered movements.

In 124 out of 399 movement-related SMA neurones, the magnitude of activity was different depending upon the modality of the signal to which the animal responded. For example, one of the neurones was most active in relation to visually triggered and less active with auditory triggered wrist extension. It was almost inactive when the triggering signal was tactile.

Another feature of SMA neurones different from those of the motor cortex was the presence of response time-locked to the visual or auditory stimulus. In the motor cortex, no neurones were found to be active with a close time relation to visual or auditory signals, in accordance with previous reports, although the presence of precentral neurones driven by somatosensory input is well known. Sixty-eight SMA neurones exhibited discharges time-locked to the visual and/or auditory signals.

In summary, 4 major findings emerged from this series of experiments: (1) the magnitude of movement-related activity in SMA is smaller than in precentral motor cortex; (2) the response latencies to visual and auditory signals are shorter in SMA than in motor cortex; not much difference is found in response to tactile stimuli; (3) a considerable number of movement-related neurones in SMA are found to start their activity changes time-locked to the visual or auditory stimulus; and (4) some neurones in SMA respond differently to the 3 triggering signals, which is unusual in the motor cortex. Thus it can be said that SMA neurones are more closely linked with visual and auditory inputs but less intimately connected to somatosensory input, compared to precentral neurones. Judging from the smaller magnitude of the movement-related activity, the SMA seems to play a subsidiary role in motor control, so far as a simple motor task like those performed in the present response paradigm is concerned. In this sense, the term "supplementary" appears to be appropriate.

ROLE IN HIGHER ORDER MOTOR CONTROL

In what aspects of motor performance does SMA possess more significant roles? Though we still have only a limited number of reports available, it seems that we have started on our way of approaching answers to this question. Recent studies in man and monkey suggest the role of SMA in generating a preparatory state for, or even in programming, forthcoming movements, rather than in actual execution of them.

The "readiness potential", a potential preceding initiation of movements by up to about 1 sec, is known to have its maximum at the vertex (Kornhuber and Deecke 1965). Deecke and Kornhuber (1978) found that, even in patients with bilateral parkinsonism who failed to have the readiness potential in the precentral region, the vertex maximum of the potential persisted without reduction. Judging from the location of the vertex electrode, presumably on SMA, this finding suggests a role of SMA in the process of developing a preparatory state for the impending movement. A newly developed technique of measuring regional blood flow of the cortex (presumably reflecting the level of cortical activity) provided evidence that SMA was active when subjects were simulating a motor sequence internally, without executing it (Roland et al. 1980). Furthermore, Orgogozo and Larsen (1979) found that SMA exhibited much higher blood flow during the execution of complex movement sequences than during simple muscle contractions. These observations led them to suggest a role of SMA in programming the motor sequence. These reports in man invite further studies to find what parameters of movement are programmed and in what way the preparatory process is achieved, in more precisely designed experiments.

In a subsequent study in our laboratory (Tanji et al. 1980), an attempt was made to observe how neuronal activity in the primate SMA is altered with development of a preparatory state for an impending movement. The movement required the animal to respond properly to a sudden perturbing stimulus delivered to the forearm in two different directions. An instruction as to the direction of movement (pushing or pulling the forelimb) was given several seconds before the occurrence of the stimulus. A number of SMA neurones exhibited instruction-induced changes of activity during the period intervening between the instruction and the perturbation-triggered movement. These particular neurones were not active in association with the movement per se. This finding substantiates the view that SMA plays a part in modifying sensorily triggered motor responses, known to be profoundly modified by the establishment, in advance, of a preparatory state of the animal (Evarts and Tanji 1974) or man (Hammond 1956) to initiate intended movements.

REFERENCES

Brinkman, C. and Porter, R. Supplementary motor area in the monkey: activity of neurons during performance of a learned motor task. J. Neurophysiol., 1979, 42: 681–709.

Deecke, L. and Kornhuber, H.H. An electrical sign of participation of the mesial "supplementary" motor cortex in human voluntary finger movement. Brain Res., 1978, 159: 473–476.

Evarts, E.V. Pyramidal tract activity associated with a conditioned hand movement in the monkey. J. Neurophysiol., 1966, 29: 1011–1027.

Evarts, E.V. Representation of movements and muscles by pyramidal tract neurons of the precentral motor cortex. In: M.D. Yahr and D.P. Purpura (Eds.), Neurophysiological Basis of Normal and Abnormal Motor Activities. Raven Press, New York, 1967: 215–253.

Evarts, E.V. A technique for recording activity of subcortical neurons in moving animals. Electroenceph. clin. Neurophysiol., 1968, 24: 83–86.

Evarts, E.V. Motor cortex reflexes associated with learned movement. Science, 1973, 179: 501–503.

Evarts, E.V. and Tanji, J. Gating of motor cortex reflexes by prior instruction. Brain Res., 1974, 71: 479–494.

Hammond, P.H. The influence of prior instruction to the subject on an apparently involuntary neuromuscular response. J. Physiol. (Lond.), 1956, 132: 17P–18P.

Kornhuber, H.H. and Deecke, L. Hirnpotentialänderungen bei Willkürbewegungen und passiven Bewegungen des Menschen: Bereitschaftspotential und reafferente Potentiale. Pflügers Arch. ges. Physiol., 1965, 284: 1–17.

Orgogozo, J.M. and Larsen, B. Activation of the supplementary motor area during voluntary movement in man suggests it works as a supramotor area. Science, 1979, 206: 847–850.

Penfield, W. and Welch, K. The supplementary motor area in the cerebral cortex of man. Trans. Amer. neurol. Ass., 1949, 74: 179–184.

Penfield, W. and Welch, K. The supplementary motor area of the cerebral cortex. Arch. Neurol. Psychiat. (Chic.), 1951, 66: 289–317.

Roland, P.E., Larsen, B., Lassen, N.A. and Skinhøj, E. Supplementary and other cortical areas in organization of voluntary movements in man. J. Neurophysiol., 1980, 43: 118–136.

Talairach, J. and Bancaud, J. The supplementary motor area in man. Anatomo-functional findings by stereo-electroencephalography in epilepsy. Int. J. Neurol., 1966, 5: 330–347.

Tanji, J. and Kurata, K. Neuronal activity in the cortical supplementary motor area related with distal and proximal forelimb movements. Neurosci. Lett., 1979, 12: 201–206.

Tanji, J., Taniguchi, K. and Saga, T. The supplementary motor area: Neuronal responses to motor instructions. J. Neurophysiol., 1980, 43: 60–68.

Wiesendanger, M., Seguin, J.J. and Künzle, H. The supplementary motor area – a control system for posture? In: R.B. Stein, K.C. Pearson, R.S. Smith and J.B. Redford (Eds.), Control of Posture and Locomotion. Plenum, New York, 1973: 331–346.

Wise, S.P. and Tanji, J. Supplementary and precentral motor cortex: Contrast in responsiveness to peripheral input in the hindlimb area of the unanesthetized monkey. J. comp. Neurol., 1981, 195: 433–451.

Woolsey, C.N., Settlage, P.H., Meyer, D.R., Spencer, W., Hamuy, T.P. and Travis, A.M. Patterns of localization in precentral and "supplementary" motor areas and their relation to the concept of a premotor area. Res. Publ. Ass. nerv. ment. Dis., 1952, 30: 238–264.

Kyoto Symposia (EEG Suppl. No. 36)
Editors: P.A. Buser, W.A. Cobb and T. Okuma
© 1982, Elsevier Biomedical Press, Amsterdam

Control of Voluntary Movement by the Brain: Contrasting Roles of Sensorimotor Cortex, Basal Ganglia and Cerebellum

EDWARD V. EVARTS

Laboratory of Neurophysiology, National Institute of Mental Health, Bethesda, Md. 20205 (U.S.A.)

SENSORIMOTOR CORTEX

Since the time of Herophilus (about 300 B.C.) scientists have distinguished between motor and sensory nerves and Galen argued that there were separate motor and sensory parts of the nervous system. It was not until 1822, however, that there was experimental proof for these ideas. In that year Magendie showed that surgical interruption of the nerves entering the dorsal surface of the spinal cord caused experimental animals to become insensible to even the most intense stimuli (e.g., pricks and pressures) although movement was still possible. In contrast, interruption of the nerves emerging from the ventral regions of the spinal cord paralysed movement without eliminating sensibility (see Clarke and O'Malley 1968).

Subsequent studies revealed the existence of motor and sensory areas within the cerebral cortex, but these sensory and motor areas were not as "pure" as those of the spinal cord: Woolsey (1958) showed that stimulation of the postcentral sensory area had motor effects and that the precentral motor area received sensory inputs. He introduced the term MsI for the primary motorsensory cortex located in the precentral gyrus and SmI for the primary sensorimotor cortex located in the postcentral gyrus. Quite recently Soso and Fetz (1980) have shown that neurones in SmI (like those in MsI) can discharge prior to voluntary movement, but in their studies information was not available as to whether the early discharging SmI elements were output neurones. To provide further knowledge of the functional differentiation between MsI and SmI, the activity of MsI and SmI output neurones was compared during volitional movements in the monkey (*Macaca mulatta*) (Evarts and Fromm 1981; Fromm and Evarts 1982). Unlike spinal cord output neurones to muscle, which originate entirely in the motor part of the cord, cerebral cortex output neurones to spinal cord are located in both MsI and SmI. The axons of these output neurones descend via the pyramidal tract and are called pyramidal tract neurones (PTNs). Our experimental paradigm involved the use of microelectrodes to record impulses of MsI and SmI PTNs identified by their antidromic responses to electrical stimulation of the pyramidal tract, and we compared these MsI and SmI PTNs with respect to (i) temporal relations to onset of movement, (ii) discharge frequencies as a function of strength of muscular contraction, and (iii) responsiveness to afferent stimuli.

A necessary property of neurones that initiate movement is discharge prior to muscular contraction, and while such prior discharge has been amply demonstrated for MsI PTNs, there have been no previous reports on timing of identified SmI PTNs in relation to movement onset. Onset of activity with respect to movement was determined for 208 PTNs in MsI and 72 PTNs in SmI in a paradigm in which a monkey was rewarded for (i) holding a handle in one of three different angular positions (15° supinated, 0° vertical and 15° pronated position) on the basis of a visual display and (ii) positioning the handle between these three zones by pronation or supination movements whenever a shift of the visual display indicated when and where to move. The electromyogram (EMG) of muscles involved in this task was recorded so as to relate the timing of EMG changes to the timing of changes of PTN activity.

Unlike the cytoarchitectonically homogeneous MsI (area 4), SmI contains several subdivisions: from anterior to posterior within SmI are areas 3a, 3b, 1 and 2. Immediately behind area 2 is area 5, a somatosensory association zone, and PTNs are located here as well as in the 4 subdivisions of SmI (Murray and Coulter 1981). In view of the known differences between these areas, results for PTNs were subdivided according to the cortical areas in which they were located. It was found that for area 3a of SmI, all PTNs, but none of the non-PTNs, discharged before the earliest EMG changes of the arm muscles. Discharge before the earliest EMG onset occurred less frequently in other SmI areas, with such prior discharge occurring in 55% of PTNs recorded in an area 2/5 junctional region and in 20% of the PTN population in areas 2 and 1. There were no significant timing differences between PTNs and non-PTNs in these SmI regions. For MsI (area 4), 80% of the PTNs discharged in advance of EMG onset. The total PTN population of MsI lagged that of area 3a PTNs by an average of 23 msec ($P<0.025$); this timing difference became greater (48 msec) and highly significant ($P<0.001$) if we compared mean onset time of area 3a PTNs with that of a subgroup of 33 PTNs in area 4 which were located in the rostral bank of the central sulcus adjacent to area 3a.

Previous studies have shown that activity of MsI PTNs varies as a function of strength of muscular contraction (Evarts 1968, 1969) and in the present study we compared load-related activity of 132 MsI PTNs, 39 PTNs in areas 2 and the area 2/5 junction, and 7 PTNs in area 3a. The monkey was required to maintain a given position against different static loads (including a zero load) generated by a torque motor. PTNs in each of these different areas exhibited changes in activity with load changes. A gradation of frequency with load was found in 6 of 7 PTNs in area 3a, in approximately half of the PTNs in MsI and the area 2/5 junction but in only 28% of PTNs in area 2. The mean increment in firing rate per increment in load as measured over the linear range was greatest for PTNs in area 3a, intermediate for MsI and junctional area 2/5 and least for area 2.

The data that have now been presented show that motor and sensory cortex PTNs have two features in common: discharge prior to muscular contraction and changes in discharge frequency as a function of strength of muscular contraction. The third feature according to which MsI and SmI PTNs were compared was responsiveness to afferent input evoked by passive ramp displacements. The latencies of these responses were shortest in non-PTNs of area 3a (mean: 12 msec) and were significantly longer in area 3a PTNs (mean: 20 msec). There were no clear latency differences between different SmI PTN populations, but the group mean of 22 msec for their afferent responses was significantly shorter than the mean of 26 msec in MsI PTNs. Across all cortical subdivisions there was a significant tendency for larger rapidly conducting PTNs to show dynamic ramp responses, while dynamic-static and purely static responses prevailed in slow, smaller PTNs.

Previous studies of motor cortex PTNs during voluntary movement have shown that these neurones exhibit centrally programmed discharge prior to movement onset and that, in addition, they show reflex responses to peripheral stimuli. These PTN reflex responses (called long-loop reflexes to contrast them with the analogous short-loop spinal cord reflexes) provide for automatic servocontrol of centrally programmed PTN output during voluntary movement (Evarts and Fromm 1978). The present results show that long-loop reflexes and centrally programmed discharge prior to movement are also present in many sensory cortex PTNs and that these PTNs can act on their target neurones in advance of movement. The results on PTNs in area 3a, the subdivision of SmI that receives inputs from muscle afferents (Phillips et al. 1971) were of particular interest, for within this area the PTNs discharged prior to movement onset but the non-PTNs failed to do so. While lagging PTNs in onset of activity with voluntary movement, area 3a non-PTNs were earlier than PTNs in responsiveness to peripheral stimuli. Unfortunately, we do not have information as to the laminar location of 3a non-PTNs, but it is tempting to propose that they are close to the input of the cortical column. This proposal fits with the finding of Oscarsson et al. (1966) showing stronger and shorter latency effects of muscle afferent inputs on the more superficial non-PTNs than on the deeper PTNs in cat cerebral cortex. Though delayed by an average of 8 msec with respect to non-PTNs, the reflex responses of PTNs in area 3a (and in the other SmI areas) were nevertheless earlier than the reflex responses of motor cortex PTNs. The existence of these SmI PTN reflex outputs to brain stem and spinal cord means that quite aside from further cortico-cortical processing of SmI activity leading to perception, conscious awareness and decision-making, there are immediate SmI reflex outputs that must play a part in continuous regulation of the excitability of lower centres during movement.

In conclusion, then, data on identified somatosensory cortex output neurones suggest that they contribute to the generation and control of movement, thus supporting the proposal of Woolsey (1958) that somatosensory cortex should be thought of as a sensorimotor rather than as a purely sensory area.

BASAL GANGLIA AND CEREBELLUM

Much of our current thinking concerning the way in which the basal ganglia interact with other CNS motor control areas dates from the work of Kemp and Powell (1971) showing that while the striatum receives inputs from all parts of the cerebral cortex, the output of the striatum (projected via globus pallidus to ventral thalamus and thence to cortex) returns primarily to the motor areas of the frontal lobe. Kemp and Powell noted a parallel between the widespread source of afferent input to the striatum and the widespread source of projections from cerebral cortex to brain stem relays that transmit cortical information to the cerebellum. The existence of this widespread projection from cerebral cortex to cerebellum and the relatively restricted return from the dentate nucleus via ventral thalamus to motor cortex had also been noted in the review of Evarts and Thach (1969). With more recent studies, however, it has been shown that the projection from cerebral cortex to cerebellum (via brain stem relays) arises from a more restricted cortical zone than the projection from cerebral cortex to striatum. Thus, the differences in the zones of cerebral cortex sending signals to striatum and cerebellum have in some ways become more striking than their similarities.

The patterns of projection from cerebral cortex to cerebellum via pontine nuclei have been described by Brodal (1978) and by Dhanarajan et al. (1977). In discussing the functional implications of results of studies on the projection from primate motor and somatosensory areas to the pons, Dhanarajan et al. pointed out that two hypotheses as to the role of the corticopontine projections have been extensively considered. One hypothesis (Eccles 1969; Allen and Tsukuhara 1974) held that projections from motor cortex to cerebellum and the return signals to motor cortex would provide an internal feedback loop allowing correction of motor cortex output. A second hypothesis on the cerebro-cerebellar projection focusses on its role in relation to initiation of movement. According to this hypothesis, impulses leaving association areas of parietal and frontal lobes would convey visuo-spatial information to the cerebellum for translation into impulse patterns appropriate for control of movement. For example, visuo-spatial information concerning the location, direction, and velocity of a target would be transferred from regions of the visual or parietal cortex to the cerebellum, whence computations concerning the pattern of muscle activity necessary to acquire the target would be generated and sent to motor cortex via the ventro-lateral nucleus of the thalamus.

As Dhanarajan et al. (1977) point out, the two hypotheses are not mutually exclusive, and the two sorts of cerebellar functions probably go on concurrently. Nevertheless, the results of anatomical studies carried out in the last 5 years show that the input to the pontine nuclei is considerably stronger from sensorimotor cortex than from association areas, and comparisons of projections from cerebral cortex to cerebellum via the pons and from cerebral cortex to striatum reveal some striking differences between the densities of the two projections. Thus, there are only weak projections from temporal lobe and prefrontal association cortex to the pons and thence to cerebellum (Brodal 1978), whereas both of these areas have strong projections to caudate nucleus. It is only those regions of cerebral cortex projecting densely to the putamen (areas 4, 3, 1, 2 and 5) that also have extensive projections to the pontine nuclei. In contrast, those cortical regions which project most densely to the caudate nucleus have relatively sparse projections to the pontine nuclei. These results favour a major role for the cerebro-cerebellar projection in relation to providing the cerebellum with efference copy and sensory feedback from sensorimotor cortex. As movement occurs, the efference copy signals to cerebellum would be compared to sensory feedback signals reaching the cerebellum, and error signals would be returned to motor cortex via dentate nucleus and ventro-lateral thalamus.

In addition to differing with respect to the cerebral cortical origins of their inputs, cerebellum and basal ganglia differ with respect to the thalamic and thence the cortical areas to which they in turn project: the cerebellar nuclear projection to thalamus is directed to zones that in turn project to primary motor cortex whereas the basal ganglia (via pallidum) project to more anterior thalamic nuclei that in turn project to pre-motor cortex (Kievit and Kuypers 1977; Jones et al. 1979; Thach and Jones 1979; Tracey et al. 1980).

An understanding of the functional significance of these anatomical findings has been advanced by Nauta (1981) in a recent paper presenting ideas that simplify the scheme according to which one thinks of the relationships between cerebral cortex and basal ganglia. Nauta's scheme is based on features of internal histology, neurotransmitter type and input-output patterns rather than on conventional geographical divisions determined largely by location of fibre bundles. It is proposed that "...almost the entire telencephalon can be subdivided into three concentric tiers. The outermost tier (tier I) encompasses the structures derived embryologically from the pallium, the neocortex and the allocortex. The second tier (tier II) includes the caudate nucleus, the putamen, the nucleus accumbens septi and parts of the olfactory tubercle. The third tier (tier III) is composed of the external pallidal segment, the internal pallidal segment, the non-dopaminergic part of the substantia nigra, and perhaps also parts of the substantia innominata." Nauta's formulation points to the functional unity between the globus pallidus and the non-dopaminergic substantia nigra pars reticulata (SNpr).

Results of single unit recording in behaving monkeys are consistent with Nauta's formulation. DeLong and Georgopoulos (1978) compared activity of neurones in SNpr with activity of neurones in the dopaminergic substantia nigra pars compacta (SNpc). It was found that "SNpc units had low spontaneous discharge rates and did not show clear modulation with active movements or passive manipulations. SNpr units had high spontaneous activity resembling that of internal pallidal units. Many SNpr cells were modulated by chewing, licking or swallowing movements...." DeLong and Georgopoulos concluded "that the pars reticulata of the substantia nigra and the internal segment of the globus pallidus (GPi) together form a functional entity which has been divided by the internal capsule. This is suggested by: (a) the striking similarities in the morphology of their neurones, neuropil and ultrastructure, as well as in their afferent and efferent connections, (b) the nearly identical patterns of spontaneous activity (high tonic discharge), and (c) the apparent continuation of the GPi body representation and the SNpr, with units related to licking and chewing movements located in the medial portion of GPi."

In contrast to the intense modulation of SNpr cells with active oro-facial movement, the cells of SNpc have low frequency discharge even during movements which involve intense modulation of cells in the putamen or the globus pallidus. This low frequency discharge of SNpc neurones fits with the hypothesis that the major "informational signals" to the striatum come from the cerebral cortex, with the dopaminergic nigro-striatal pathway functioning to maintain the correct operating point of the striatal neurones such that they can effectively integrate, process and transmit signals from the cerebral cortex.

The different discharge properties of neurones in SNpc as compared to those in SNpr find a certain counterpart in the cerebellum, where Purkinje cells exhibit two very different patterns of discharge depending on whether the excitation underlying the discharge originates in the parallel fibre synapses on the Purkinje cell or, alternatively, from the climbing fibres reaching the Purkinje cell from the inferior olive. The inputs to the Purkinje cell from the inferior olive generate infrequent impulses, usually occurring at a frequency of about 1 Hz. In contrast, Purkinje cell discharge resulting from parallel fibre inputs often reaches several hundred Hz. These two strikingly different discharge patterns are consistent with important differences in the functional role of inputs to the Purkinje cell from these two different sources. In commenting on this point Ekerot and Oscarsson (1981) note that "the very low discharge rate of the climbing fibres, about 1 Hz, makes it unlikely that the information carried out by these fibres is directly transferred to the frequency code of the Purkinje cells which have a background activity of 30–60 "single spikes" per second."

Indeed, rather than functioning to transfer information via immediate changes in Purkinje cell discharge, climbing fibres are thought (Marr 1969; Ito 1974) to provide for long-term changes in cerebellar cortical synapses. Ekerot and Oscarsson observed that "impulses in the climbing fibres evoke not only the classical complex spikes which can be recorded from the soma of the Purkinje cells but also prolonged depolarizing plateaus in the distal dendrites. These plateaus often last for several hundred msec and have particularly long durations in the most distal parts of the dendrites, where the parallel fibre synapses are situated." It was suggested that "the depolarizing plateaus presumably produce marked ionic and metabolic alterations in the distal dendrites. These alterations might possibly induce plastic changes in the parallel fibre synapses as required by recent hypotheses regarding the cerebellum as a site for motor learning" (Marr 1969; Ito 1978).

CONCLUDING REMARKS

Current knowledge of the ways in which the sensorimotor cortex, basal ganglia and cerebellum interact in controlling movement and motor learning has been derived from interdisciplinary studies in which electrophysiological, anatomical and behavioural techniques are combined, and it seems certain that within the next decade many additional new techniques will be combined with those already in use to work out the many unsolved riddles of motor control. The use of deoxyglucose to map brain metabolic activity, the use of receptor binding techniques to identify neurotransmitter localization in relation to neuronal activity, the use of pharmacological tools to affect certain classes of neurones selectively – all of these approaches will be used in concert to provide a more complete picture of brain mechanisms in voluntary movement.

REFERENCES

Allen, G.I. and Tsukuhara, N. Cerebrocerebellar communication systems. Physiol. Rev., 1974, 54: 957–1006.

Brodal, P. The corticopontine projection in the rhesus monkey. Brain, 1978, 101: 251–283.

Clarke, E. and O'Malley, C.D. The Human Brain and Spinal Cord. University of California Press, Berkeley, Calif., 1968.

DeLong, M.R. and Georgopoulos, A.P. The subthalamic nucleus and the substantia nigra of the monkey. Neuronal activity in relation to movement. Soc. Neurosci. Abstr., 1978, 4: 42.

Dhaharajan, P., Ruegg, D.G. and Wiesendanger, M. An anatomical investigation of the corticopontine projection in the primate (*Saimiri sciureus*). The projection from motor and somatosensory areas. Neuroscience, 1977, 2: 913–922.

Eccles, J.C. The dynamic loop hypothesis of movement control. In: K.N. Leibovic (Ed.), Information Processing in the Nervous System, Springer, New York, 1969: 245–269.

Ekerot, C.F. and Oscarsson, O. Climbing fibre elicited prolonged depolarizations in Purkinje cell dendrites. In: J. Szentágothai, J. Hamori and M. Palkovits (Eds.), Adv. Physiol. Sci., Vol. 2, Regulatory Functions of the CNS. Subsystems. 1981: 133–136.

Evarts, E.V. Relation of pyramidal tract activity to force exerted during voluntary movement. J. Neurophysiol., 1968, 31: 14–27.

Evarts, E.V. Activity of pyramidal tract neurones during postural fixation. J. Neurophysiol., 1969, 32: 375–385.

Evarts, E.V. and Fromm, C. The pyramidal tract neuron as summing point in a closed-loop control system in the monkey. In: J.E. Desmedt (Ed.), Cerebral Motor Control in Man: Long Loop Mechanisms, Progress in Clinical Neurophysiology, Vol. 4. Karger, Basel, 1978: 153–166.

Evarts, E.V. and Fromm, C. Transcortical reflexes and servo control of movement. Canad. J. Physiol. Pharmacol., 1981, 59: 757–775.

Evarts, E.V. and Thach, W.T. Motor mechanisms of the CNS: Cerebrocerebellar interrelations. Ann. Rev. Physiol., 1969, 31: 451–498.

Fromm, C. and Evarts, E.V. Pyramidal tract neurons in somatosensory cortex: central and peripheral inputs during voluntary movement. Brain Res., 1982, 238: 186–191.

Ito, M. The control mechanisms of cerebellar motor systems. In: F.O. Schmitt and F.G. Worden (Eds.), The Neurosciences, Third Study Program. MIT Press, Boston, Mass., 1974: 293–303.

Ito, M. Recent advances in cerebellar physiology and pathology. In: R.A.K. Kark, R.N. Rosenberg and L.J. Schut (Eds.), Advances in Neurology, Vol. 21. Raven Press, New York, 1978: 59–84.

Jones, E.G., Wise, S.P. and Coulter, J.D. Differential thalamic relationships of sensory-motor and parietal cortical fields in monkeys. J. comp. Neurol., 1979, 183: 833–882.

Kemp, J.M. and Powell, T.P.S. The connexions of the striatum and globus pallidus: synthesis and speculation. Phil. Trans. B, 1971, 262: 441–457.

Kievit, J. and Kuypers, H.G.J.M. Oganization of the thalamo-cortical connexions to the frontal lobe in the rhesus monkey. Exp. Brain Res., 1977, 29: 299–322.

Marr, D. A theory of cerebellar cortex. J. Physiol. (Lond.), 1969, 202: 437–470.

Murray, E.A. and Coulter, J.D. Organization of corticospinal neurons in the monkey. J. comp. Neurol., 1981, 195: 339–365.

Nauta, H.J.W. A proposed conceptual reorganization of the basal ganglia and telencephalon. Neuroscience, 1981, 4: 1875–1881.

Oscarsson, O., Rosen, I. and Sulg, I. Organization of neurones in the cat cerebral cortex that are influenced from group I muscle afferents. J. Physiol. (Lond.), 1966, 183: 189–210.

Phillips, C.G., Powell, T.P.S. and Wiesendanger, M. Projection from low-threshold muscle afferents of hand and forearm to area 3a of baboon's cortex. J. Physiol. (Lond.), 1971, 217: 419–446.

Soso, M.J. and Fetz, E.E. Responses of identified cells in postcentral cortex of awake monkeys during comparable active and passive joint movements. J. Neurophysiol., 1980, 43: 1090–1110.

Thach, W.T. and Jones, E.G. The cerebellar dentatothalamic connection: terminal field, lamellae, rods and somatotopy. Brain Res., 1979, 169: 168–172.

Tracey, D.J., Asanuma, C., Jones, E.G. and Porter, R. Thalamic relay to motor cortex: afferent pathways from brain stem, cerebellum, and spinal cord in monkeys. J. Neurophysiol., 1980, 44: 532–554.

Woolsey, C.N. Organization of somatic sensory and motor areas of the cerebral cortex. In: H.F. Harlow and C.N. Woolsey (Eds.), Biological and Biochemical Bases of Behavior. University of Wisconsin Press, Madison, Wis., 1958: 63–81.

Kyoto Symposia (EEG Suppl. No. 36)
Editors: P.A. Buser, W.A. Cobb and T. Okuma
© 1982, Elsevier Biomedical Press, Amsterdam

Separate Cell Systems in the Motor Cortex of the Monkey for the Control of Joint Movement and of Joint Stiffness

DONALD R. HUMPHREY

Laboratory of Neurophysiology, Emory University School of Medicine, Atlanta, Ga. 30322 (U.S.A.)

Even comparatively simple activities of the arm and hand appear to be governed by 2 fundamentally different control signals from central motor structures. The first of these signals evokes *reciprocal* activity in antagonist muscles, allowing a joint to be moved rapidly and smoothly from one angular position to another. In contrast, the second signal evokes a *co-activation* of antagonist muscles, so that a joint is mechanically "stiffened" and its posture is stabilized or its motion is damped. In many movements these 2 forms of muscle activity are used cooperatively, the first for movements about a particular joint, the second for postural supporting actions at adjacent joints. For example, with the arm unsupported, movements of an object by the hand are accompanied by a postural stabilization of the upper arm. Conversely, when writing on a chalkboard the fingers, wrist and elbow are stabilized by antagonist co-activation, while modulated, reciprocal activity occurs in muscles acting about the shoulder. In still other cases, antagonist muscles may be co-activated in order to increase the resistance of a joint to displacement by external forces.

Following Sherrington's early emphasis upon the concept of reciprocal innervation, the reciprocal form of antagonist muscle activity has been the subject of extensive investigation (Sherrington 1906, 1909). Much attention has been focussed recently, for example, on the central control of reciprocal movements about the wrist and elbow in both human and subhuman primates (Evarts 1966; Stark 1968; Humphrey et al. 1970; Thach 1970; Conrad and Brooks 1974; Lee and Tatton 1975; Crago et al. 1976; Polit and Bizzi 1979; Fetz and Cheney 1980). But in contrast, surprisingly little attention has been paid to the central mechanisms which produce antagonist muscle co-activation (see Smith 1981 for a recent review), despite its clear importance in a wide range of normal and perhaps also pathological motor activities (Tilney and Pike 1925; Levine and Kabat 1952; Patton and Mortensen 1971; Feldman 1980a,b).

Because of this relative paucity of information on co-activation phenomena, we have chosen to present at this symposium some new observations on the central origins of the two major control signals discussed above. Our interest in the control of antagonist co-activation began with the observation that monkeys who are trained to control the position of the wrist in the presence of perturbing forces will do so in

---

Send correspondence to: Dr. Donald Humphrey, Department of Physiology, School of Medicine, Emory University, Atlanta, Ga. 30322, U.S.A.

one or a combination of two major ways. With slow perturbations, wrist position is maintained by smoothly graded activity in the particular set of muscles whose action opposes the applied torque; when the torque alternates in direction, it is opposed by reciprocal activity in the appropriate antagonists. With rapid perturbations, however, a co-contraction effort is added, so that the wrist is stiffened tonically. Thus, by simply changing the frequency of the applied perturbation, we have been able to vary the dominance of the 2 control signals described above in the monkey's control of his wrist. Simultaneously, we have observed the behaviour of the major flexor and extensor muscles of the wrist, and of task-related neurones in the contralateral motor cortex. Our results suggest an important new hypothesis concerning the functional organization of the wrist control area of the primate motor cortex: namely, that separate cell populations may exist for (a) the separate or reciprocal control of antagonist muscles, and hence joint movement; and (b) for co-activation of these muscles, thus providing for a separate control of static joint stiffness. These same findings have recently been reported elsewhere (Humphrey and Reed 1981, 1982).

METHODS AND RESULTS

The behavioural task

The major features of our behavioural task are shown in Fig. 1. Briefly, the monkey is required to grip a small handle in a uniform way by compressing a microswitch within it, and to control its position about the axis of wrist flexion-extension in the presence of perturbing torques that are imposed about this same axis. To accomplish this task, the animal must generate a net flexor-extensor torque that is at all times approximately equal in magnitude and opposite in direction to that applied. Alternatively, he may increase the mechanical stiffness of his wrist by tonic flexor and extensor co-contraction, so that the joint is moved only slightly by the imposed torque. The torque perturbations are delivered by an electrically controlled motor, whose central shaft is connected to the handle assembly. Appropriate transducers allow measurements of angular wrist displacement from the (constant) central target position, and of the net torque exerted *by the animal* about the axis of wrist flexion and extension. Examples of the motor performance variables recorded during execution of this task are shown in Fig. 2.

Separation of neurally generated and passive mechanical contributions to task performance

In the motor task described here, we ask the animal to control his flexor and extensor muscles in such a way that the wrist appears to have a very high mechanical *stiffness*. That is, we require the animal to minimize the angular displacements of his wrist ($\Delta\theta$) in the presence of applied torques which vary sinusoidally or with triangular wave form between equal valued peaks in the flexor and extensor directions, and over a total range ΔT (typically ± 1000 g-cm, which is equivalent to a 200 g force applied to the palm of the animal's hand). The higher the apparent stiffness

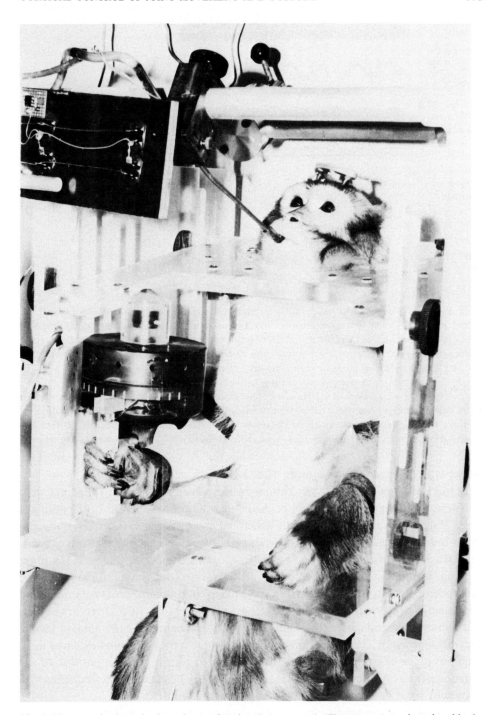

Fig. 1. Photograph of a trained monkey performing the motor task. The torque motor is enclosed in the cylindrical black housing, and a potentiometer for measurement of wrist displacement in the transparent housing immediately above; strain gauges for measurement of net wrist torque are attached to the handle assembly near the motor's lower shaft. The animal's gaze is fixed upon a small light display, which informs him of the desired position of his wrist.

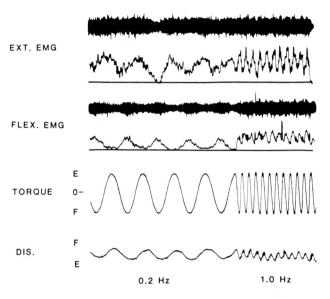

EXT. EMG

FLEX. EMG

TORQUE

DIS.

0.2 Hz   1.0 Hz

Fig. 2. Examples of motor performance variables recorded during task performance. In this example, the animal tracks a sinusoidal torque perturbation, which varies from 1000 g-cm opposing extension to 1000 g-cm opposing flexion. Each double row of EMG traces at the top shows first the unprocessed record from the major wrist extensor or flexor muscles, and immediately below this an electrically rectified then low pass filtered version of the same record (critically damped filter, 50 msec time constant). Net wrist torque is shown next, with extensor torque being upward. Wrist displacement is shown in the bottom row, with peak-to-peak values at 0.2 Hz being approximately ±3°. Note the sudden co-activation of flexor and extensor muscles, indicated by the increasing height of the processed EMG traces above the reference baseline, when the perturbation frequency is suddenly increased from 0.2 to 1.0 Hz. This co-activation produces in turn an increase in wrist stiffness, as shown by the decreased displacement at 1.0 Hz.

of the wrist, $S = \Delta T/\Delta\theta$, the more accurate is task performance.

In this task, however, there are 3 major factors which contribute to apparent wrist stiffness. The first factor is the set of passive mechanical properties of the animal's wrist. Even in the absence of neurally generated muscle activity, the mass of the animal's hand and the viscoelastic properties of his wrist and its muscular attachments may generate a torque which opposes wrist movement by external forces. In order to gauge accurately the contribution of the central nervous system to the control of joint position, the torque arising from these passive mechanical properties must first be known. The second and third factors that contribute to wrist stiffness are neurally generated. As indicated above, movement of the handle by the applied torque may be opposed by graded, reciprocal activity in the wrist flexor and extensor muscles; this mode of operation provides for a *dynamic* control of wrist position or apparent stiffness. Alternatively, the *static* stiffness may be increased, as indicated also above, by tonic co-activation of flexor and extensor muscles.

To assess first the relative contributions of neurally generated and passive mechanical factors to the control of wrist position, we performed the following set of experiments (2 monkeys, 4 replications). First, the alert monkey was required to track with wrist displacements of less than ± 4° an applied torque which varied sinusoidally between 1250 g-cm opposing flexion and 1250 g-cm opposing extension. The torque frequency was varied systematically from 0.1 to 2.0 Hz, the major range of frequencies in controlled, voluntary movements (Stark 1968). The small angular wrist movements produced by this torque were measured at each of several frequencies, and the formula given above was used to compute net wrist stiffness as a function of applied perturbation frequency. The phase angle between the applied torque and wrist movement was also measured. These data yielded plots of total wrist stiffness and tracking phase lag as a function of perturbation frequency for the actively tracking animal. The monkey was then tranquilized (7–10 mg/kg ketamine hydrochloride) and his hand was taped to the handle in a grip position similar to that used voluntarily in the alert, active state. The handle was then perturbed with a sinusoidal torque of a constant amplitude (approximately ± 200 g-cm) that was just sufficient to produce wrist movements similar to those seen during active tracking. EMG records were obtained from both flexor and extensor muscles during this procedure, to insure the absence of muscular activity. These procedures yielded plots of wrist stiffness and displacement phase lag as a function of perturbation frequency for the *passive* joint.

Plots of these 2 sets of data are shown for 2 separate experiments in Fig. 3. The results indicate clearly that the component of wrist stiffness arising from the passive mechanical properties of the joint is constant over the frequency range studied, ac-

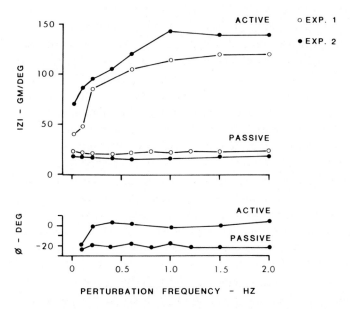

Fig. 3. Frequency dependence of apparent wrist stiffness in the actively tracking and in the tranquilized animal. Measurements of wrist stiffness as a function of applied perturbation frequency are shown for the actively tracking monkey (active curves) and for the tranquilized monkey (passive curves) for 2 separate experiments (upper panel). The phase angle between applied torque and wrist displacement are shown for one of these experiments in the lower panel. A negative phase angle indicates that displacement lags the applied torque. See the text for additional details.

counting for only 15–20% of the total stiffness seen in the alert animal at perturbation frequencies greater than 0.6 Hz. In the passive joint, wrist displacement lags the applied torque by a constant phase angle of 15–24°, due largely to a non-linear, plastic compliance. In the actively tracking animal, however, this phase lag is reduced to zero for perturbation frequencies greater than 0.4–0.6 Hz, indicating a more linear joint compliance and a better synchronization between the applied torque and the animal's opposition to it. In addition, the apparent stiffness of the wrist increased by some threefold over the frequency range studied, indicating a progressive increase in the neural drive on the flexor and extensor muscles as the perturbation frequency was raised.

Contributions of reciprocal and co-activation modes to control of wrist position and apparent stiffness

We turned next to EMG recording from the wrist flexor and extensor muscles during task performance, in order to determine how each of the modes of antagonist muscle control discussed previously contributed to the observed, frequency-dependent increase in joint stiffness. Gross intramuscular EMGs were recorded with flexible bipolar leads (1 cm tip separation), and records were obtained also from 33 sets of 3–4 distinguishable single motor units (N = 128) in the flexor and extensor carpi radialis muscles of 3 monkeys. Our major findings may be summarized briefly as follows.

At low perturbation frequencies of 0.1–0.2 Hz, wrist position is controlled principally by a graded, reciprocal activation of the flexor and extensor muscles; i.e., joint position and apparent stiffness are controlled dynamically. An example of such reciprocal muscle activity is shown by the rectified and low pass filtered EMG records from the major wrist flexor and extensor muscles in Fig. 4 (0.2 Hz column). Over the range of perturbation frequencies from 0.2 to 0.6 Hz, this reciprocal mode of control continues (Fig. 4, 0.6 Hz column). However, the muscular activity becomes better phase-locked with the applied torque; as a result, displacement phase lag decreases and the imposed torque is more rapidly and effectively opposed. Over the frequency band from 0.6 to 1.5 Hz this form of voluntary, graded tracking of the perturbation apparently becomes more difficult. Consequently, the animal now maintains his wrist position and further increases the apparent stiffness of the joint by adding a *tonic co-activation* effort to the existing reciprocal drive on the flexor and extensor muscles. The addition of this signal is shown by the rising level of the processed EMG records from the 2 muscles above the reference baseline in Fig. 4 (1.0 and 1.5 Hz columns).

The addition of these 2 muscle control signals at higher perturbation frequencies – one tonic and occurring in both flexors and extensors, the second modulated with the torque cycle and occurring reciprocally in the 2 muscle sets – was evident also at the single motor unit level, though a non-linear addition was evident due to variations in unit recruitment threshold and peak firing level. The important point to note here, however, is that *these 2 motor control signals were found to co-exist*. That is, they did not appear to be produced by one central system which changed its mode

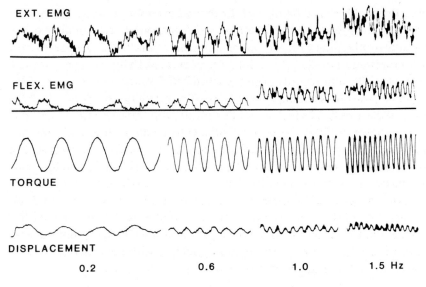

EXT. EMG

FLEX. EMG

TORQUE

DISPLACEMENT

0.2   0.6   1.0   1.5 Hz

Fig. 4. Levels of reciprocal activation and of co-activation of wrist flexor and extensor muscles as a function of applied perturbation frequency. The records are from an actively tracking monkey, whose wrist displacements were kept below ±4°. Rows 1 and 2: rectified and filtered EMG records obtained with intramuscular leads in the extensor and the flexor carpi radialis muscles. Row 3: net wrist torque. The animal's torque varies sinusoidally from 1000 g-cm in the extensor direction (upward deflection) to 1000 g-cm in the flexor direction. Row 4: angular displacements of the wrist. Displacement in the flexor direction is upward, and peak-to-peak values are approximately ±3.5° at 0.2 Hz. Perturbation frequencies are indicated at the bottom of each column. Note the reciprocal modulation in flexor and extensor EMG activity at all frequencies, and the addition of a tonic co-activation effort, signalled by the rising level of the EMG traces, at frequencies of 1.0 and 1.5 Hz.

of operation from one form of control to another. Rather, they appeared to be generated *by separate central systems,* whose outputs converged at the level of the motorneurone pool or at some more central location in the pathway leading to the spinal cord.

Separation of reciprocal and co-activation control signals at the level of the motor cortex

We set out next to determine if both of these general control signals are transmitted to the spinal cord at least in part by way of the precentral motor cortex. And, if so, we wished to determine if they were carried by a single set of cells, or by separate neuronal populations.

As a first step, we used the technique of intracortical microstimulation (ICMS; cf. Asanuma and Sakata 1967; Asanuma and Rosen 1972) to delineate the wrist control zone of the precentral motor cortex. Rather than observing evoked movements, however, we recorded the rectified and filtered EMG responses evoked in several major muscle groups of the arm by brief stimulus trains (10 current pulses, 250–300 pulse/sec, 3–40 μA intensity). In agreement with recent mapping studies (Kwan et al. 1978), the precentral wrist zone was found to contain 2–3 foci of low to intermediate threshold for activating wrist flexor and extensor muscles. These zones spanned collectively a relatively large rostro-caudal portion of area 4 and posterior area 6; partially overlapping with and surrounding this central wrist-finger area were intermediate threshold (10–25 μA) regions for evoking activity in upper arm and shoulder muscles. The unit records to be described below were all obtained from the lowest threshold focus for evoking activity in wrist flexors and extensors, which lies in caudal to middle area 4. The location of this region with respect to the arcuate and central sulci is shown in Fig. 5, where it is outlined by stimulus threshold contours.

The inner contour lines in Fig. 5 enclose regions from which activity was evoked in wrist flexor (dashed lines) or extensor carpi radialis muscles (solid lines) by a train of current pulses of 3–10 μA intensity. The outer contours enclose regions from which activity was evoked in these muscles with current pulses of 10–25 μA intensity. Panels A–C show the averaged EMG responses evoked in the indicated muscles of the arm by a train of stimuli delivered at various points within the wrist control zone (inset). The onset of stimulation coincides with the onset of the time calibration shown below each column of traces.

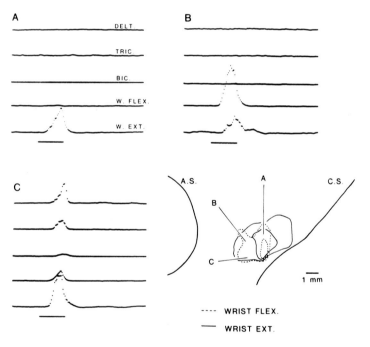

Fig. 5. Location of the stimulation-defined wrist area of the precentral motor cortex examined in the present study. The 3–10 μA and 10–20 μA zones for evoking activity in the extensor and flexor radialis muscles are indicated on a drawing of the precentral area for 1 of the 2 monkeys, as indicated in the text. A.S., arcuate sulcus; C.S., central sulcus. Examples of the averaged (N = 20 trials each), rectified and filtered EMG responses evoked in various muscle groups in the arm by stimulation at the indicated sites in the inset are shown in columns A–C. Stimulation intensities: 10 μA in A, 20 μA in B and C. Abbreviations: DELT., deltoid; TRIC., triceps; BIC., biceps; W. EXT., wrist extensor; W. FLEX., wrist flexor muscles. Time calibration (horizontal bar) in A–C = 50 msec, with the calibration beginning at the time of onset of the stimulus train. See the text for additional details.

Stimulation at an intensity of 5–10 μA within the overlapping central wrist extensor and flexor zones evoked activity only in the extensor muscle (panel A), or predominantly in the flexor muscles. In contrast, stimulation at threshold values of 12–20 μA in the *anterior* part of the surrounding zone evoked a co-activation of flexor and extensor muscles (panel B), or of several muscle groups in the arm (panel C). It is important to note that these muscle co-activation responses did not appear to be due to a simple spread of current to the lower threshold, central foci. The outer threshold contours for the 2 sets of muscles were of different shape; moreover, co-activation responses occurred with a similar threshold for two or more muscles, and the EMG responses tended to co-vary in amplitude when the stimulating current was near threshold. These results suggested that the low threshold, flexor-extensor zones were embedded within a higher threshold, more complex output system, which tended to co-activate muscles at one or more joints, as would be required for stabilization of joint positions. Interestingly, many of these co-activation responses tended to occur without significant joint movements. In the discussion below, we shall refer to the low threshold central zones and the anterior co-activation areas, respectively, as the *flexor-extensor (F-E) focus* and the *co-activation zone*.

The task-related neurones in these 2 zones behaved in significantly different ways. The first difference to be noted is in their receptive field properties. Fig. 6 shows, for

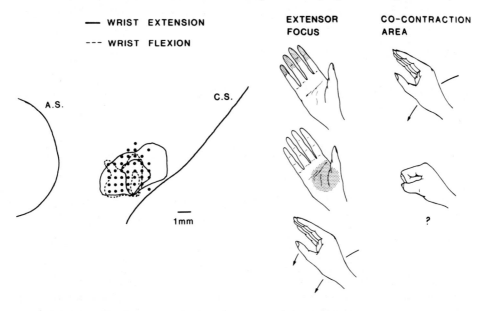

Fig. 6. Summary of receptive field properties of units in the central extensor (or F-E) zone and in the adjacent co-contraction zone of the precentral wrist area. Shown to the left is a drawing of the precentral wrist area, the location of the stimulation-defined wrist zones, and the locations within it of microelectrode penetrations (dots) for 1 of the 2 monkeys from which cortical unit records were obtained. The 2 columns to the right show the most frequently observed receptive field properties of units within the F-E focus and the co-activation area as indicated in the text. Units in the co-activation area fire only weakly in response to rapid, passive movements of the wrist, but fire briskly during the animal's voluntary gripping actions on the handle, when wrist flexor and extensor muscles are co-activated strongly.

example, the sites of electrode penetrations within the F-E focus and the co-activation zone where records were obtained from task-related units in 1 monkey (N = 210 total, N = 108 in this animal), some 40% of which were tested also for somatosensory receptive field properties. Neurones in the F-E focus were highly responsive to tactile or pressure stimuli delivered to the fingertip or the palm, or to passive flexion or extension of the wrist (Fig. 6, left-hand column). In general, neurones with cutaneous fields were localized more caudally than those responding to joint movement, as noted by previous investigators (Lemon and Porter 1976; Strick and Preston 1978; Tanji and Wise 1981). In contrast, neurones in the co-activation zone were relatively unresponsive to passive somatosensory stimuli, with only a minority firing weakly in response to rapid flexion-extension movements of the wrist. A similar declining sensitivity to somatosensory stimuli for neurones at more rostral precentral zones has been noted also by previous investigators (Lemon and Porter 1976). Yet, neurones in the co-activation zone discharged rapidly when the animal gripped a

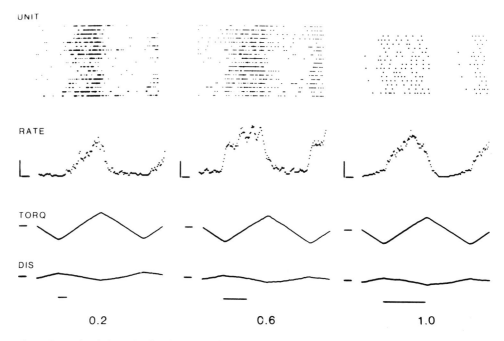

Fig. 7. Example of the task-related pattern of neuronal discharge observed most frequently in the wrist flexor-extensor focus. Each column shows for a different frequency of perturbation (0.2, 0.6, 1.0 Hz, triangular wave form) the following variables: (1) a raster display of the unit's discharge pattern during each of 15–18 consecutive perturbations; (2) the unit's average firing rate during these perturbations; (3) the average torque (TORQ) generated by the animal, with net extensor torque upwards (± 1000 g-cm total excursion); and (4) the average displacement (DIS) of the animal's wrist during each cycle, with flexion being upward (peak-to-peak displacement is approximately ± 3°). All traces in each column are aligned with respect to time. The time base is expanded for 0.6 and 1.0 Hz, to allow a comparison of phase relations (horizontal bar at the bottom of each column = 0.5 sec). The vertical bar in the firing rate averages represents 10 spikes/sec, with the horizontal bar in this and other traces indicating the zero value for that variable. Note that the unit fires in a modulated fashion in relation to wrist extensor torque. (PT cell, conduction velocity = 14 m/sec.)

rapidly perturbed handle and stabilized his wrist by flexor-extensor co-activation (Fig. 6, right-hand column).

The task-related discharge of neurones in the 2 zones also differed significantly, though some overlap in the spatial distributions of the various unit types was clearly evident (see below). Units in the F-E focus tended to fire in a graded, torque-related fashion, with discharge frequencies modulated in relation to extensor or flexor muscle activity, *but rarely in relation to both*. Moreover, the tonic background firing rates of these cells were unrelated to the rising levels of flexor-extensor co-activation seen with increasing perturbation frequencies. An example of the discharge patterns of one of these neurones is shown in Fig. 7.

In sharp contrast with the modulated firing patterns exhibited by neurones in the F-E focus were the firing patterns of task-related neurones in the co-activation zone. In this area, task-related neurones discharged at a steady or tonic rate, whose level was correlated with the degree of tonic co-activation of the wrist flexor and extensor muscles. An example of the discharge pattern of one of these units is shown in Fig. 8.

A total of 210 task-related units classifiable into these 2 general discharge pattern categories were observed in 2 monkeys. For technical reasons, we were unable to test for antidromic responses to pyramidal tract (PT) or red nucleus stimulation in one

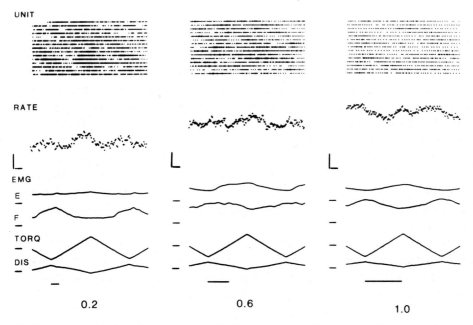

Fig. 8. Example of the pattern of task-related discharge seen most frequently in the co-activation zone. The format is similar to that in Fig. 7, except that the averaged rectified and filtered EMG records from the wrist extensor (E) and flexor (F) muscles are also shown. Note that the background level of EMG activity increases in both muscles, as evidenced by the rising level of the traces (co-activation). The unit firing rate, modulated little in relation to the torque cycle, parallels this increase in tonic co-activation level. (Cortico-rubral neurone, conduction velocity = 14 m/sec.)

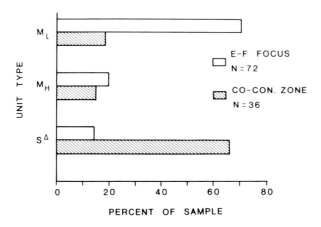

Fig. 9. Percentages of each unit type observed in the F-E focus and in the co-activation zone. M_L units discharged with a modulated rate in relation to flexor or extensor muscle torque at all frequencies of perturbation; M_H units were similar, but showed increases in the depth of firing rate modulation as the perturbation frequency rose. Both unit types were basically similar in discharge pattern to the example shown in Fig. 7. S^Δ units showed a steady (unmodulated) discharge rate, which increased (N = 26) or decreased (N = 10) in relation to the level of flexor and extensor co-activation. The example shown in Fig. 8 illustrates this type of discharge pattern. This difference in spatial distribution of the 3 unit types is highly significant statistically ($\chi^2 = 66.4$, $df = 2$, $P \ll 0.001$).

of these animals. In the second animal, however, 55% of 108 task-related neurones were PT cells, 11% were cortico-rubral neurones, and 34% could not be identified at the low stimulation currents that we were forced to use in order to escape impairment of the animal's task performance. PT neurones were encountered 4 times as frequently in the F-E focus as in the co-activation zone, whereas unidentified cells were encountered with greater relative frequency in the co-activation area; cortico-rubral neurones were found with equal frequency in both areas, though in small numbers. A classification of the 108 neurones in this animal according to discharge pattern and location yielded the frequency distributions for the 2 wrist subregions that are shown in Fig. 9. It is quite clear from these plots, and highly significant statistically, that task-related units that discharged in a modulated fashion, in relation to either wrist flexor or wrist extensor muscle activity, were seen most frequently in the F-E focus; in contrast, units firing in relation to the level of flexor-extensor co-activation, though fewer in number, were encountered most frequently in the co-activation zone. Thus, the 2 major unit types are partially intermingled spatially, but tend to cluster in separate cortical zones.

DISCUSSION

The results summarized here are in some ways preliminary. A larger sample of cortical neurones is needed, for example, with more extensive identification of their

axonal targets, before we can have strong confidence in a causal relationship between our putative "co-activation" cells and the actual co-activation of the antagonist muscles whose activity their discharge parallels. Experiments aimed at obtaining
such evidence are currently under way in our laboratory. But we have chosen to present these new data at this symposium because they suggest an important and partially new concept concerning the organization of the outputs from the precentral
motor cortex, and the parameters of motor performance which these outputs
control.

   This new concept, which is at present our working hypothesis, is shown in the
form of a flow diagram in Fig. 10. Our results suggest that there are 2 major
functional classes of output neurones in the precentral wrist area, and perhaps also
in the cortical zones which control muscles acting at other joints. The *first* class of
cells contains at least 2 subsets, with each controlling one or more synergists in a
larger set of antagonist muscles. In the example considered here, one subset of cells
controls wrist flexor motorneurones, and the second subset wrist extensor motorneurones. These neurones are controlled by 2 major sources of afferent input: an
input from central, premotor structures (central drive), and a somatotopically
precise somatosensory input from receptors in the wrist and hand. In the motor task
considered here, these neurones are activated in a modulated, reciprocal manner by
torque disturbances delivered to the wrist, which set up activity in muscle, joint and
cutaneous receptors in the hand, wrist and forearm. This modulated peripheral drive
is matched by a modulated central drive, perhaps the most important source of

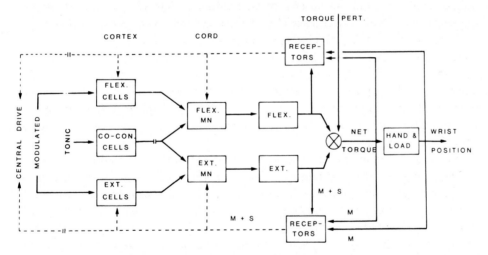

Fig. 10. Summary hypothesis concerning the major classes of output from the precentral wrist control
area. Only general directions of information flow are shown, with relay nuclei being omitted. Solid lines
indicate motor output, dashed lines somatosensory feedback. Interrupted lines indicate an uncertainty
concerning the identity of the pathways involved. The letters M or M + S are used to indicate whether
somatosensory inputs during the torque perturbation cycle used here would be modulated (M) or steady
(S). Note that no purely tonic feedback signal appears to exist, lending further support to the notion that
the co-activation neurones, unresponsive to passive somatosensory inputs, are driven principally by a
steady (non-modulated) central signal. See the text for additional details.

afferent input to these cells at low perturbation frequencies, when velocity sensitive receptors in wrist and hand would be stimulated only minimally by the applied perturbation. It is our hypothesis that these 2 subsets of cortical cells function under more natural conditions to produce precise, voluntary *movements* of the wrist under somatosensory feedback control.

The *second* class of cells performs a different function. By way of partially unknown pathways, these neurones evoke a co-activation of antagonist muscles, and thus provide for the control of the tonic impedance or stiffness of the joint. Some of these cells are PT neurones, but the majority are as yet unidentified; pathways through extrapyramidal and even cerebellar structures remain as strong possibilities. It is clear, however, that the outputs of these cells are not relayed to the spinal cord by members of the first class of neurones, for these latter cells show little in their discharge patterns that is related to tonic patterns of co-activation in the wrist muscles. The co-activation cells are relatively unaffected by somatosensory inputs, and appear to be principally under central control, as shown in Fig. 10. Note that this is precisely the arrangement needed for a system which can control joint position in the presence of unpredictable and rapid external forces, any of which might produce large variations in somatosensory input.

In summary, then, the cortical wrist zone is viewed as containing 2 major outputs: one which activates antagonist muscles singly or reciprocally, thus providing for rapid and smooth joint movement; and another which co-activates antagonist muscles at the same and perhaps adjacent joints, thus providing for postural stabilization. Note that this latter proposed output is consistent with recent studies showing a considerable divergence of cortico-spinal and rubro-spinal axon branches over several segments of the cord, providing for a dispersion of outputs to several motor nuclei (Shinoda et al. 1977, 1979; Fetz and Cheney 1980). It is consistent also with the previously advanced hypothesis that the motor cortex generates both movement and the postural adjustments that are necessary for body stability and support of that movement (Massion 1979). Finally, the co-activation system provides also for the control of joint position in the presence of rapid or unpredictable forces.

In concluding, it should be noted that this latter ''buffering'' action need not be confined only to control of joint position in the presence of external disturbances. We have all experienced a co-activation of muscles, for example, during the first executions of an unfamiliar but precise motor task. As the task is learned, the cocontraction effort subsides, to be replaced by a more economical form of distributed activity in only those muscles that are actually necessary for task performance. It is likely that the co-activation system was used during the initial phases of task performance to ''buffer'' joint movements in the presence of erroneous central signals, thus reducing movements errors. Thus, the general co-activation system envisioned here may well be used also as a means of joint position control during the early stages of motor learning. Clearly, additional studies of this important mode of motor control are needed, if we are to understand all of the roles played by the precentral motor cortex in the control of joint posture and movement.

SUMMARY

A series of new observations is described from experiments with alert monkeys, who have been trained to control the position of the wrist in the presence of perturbing forces. The results suggest that the wrist control area of the precentral motor cortex contains separate neuronal populations for the control of 2 major forms of motor output. The first activates particular groups of synergists independently, or the members of a set of antagonist muscles reciprocally; this form of activation provides, under natural conditions, for smooth movement of the joint from one position to another. The second population of cells evokes co-activation of antagonist muscles, at one or more joints in the arm. This population provides for the cortical control of the postural supporting reactions which must occur in the arm when one or more of its joints are moved. In addition, it appears to provide for a separate control of joint stiffness, thus allowing for a control of joint position in the presence of very rapid or unpredictable external force perturbations. A possible role for this system as a means of joint position control during the early phases of motor learning is also discussed.

ACKNOWLEDGEMENTS

It is a pleasure to acknowledge the important contributions of Drs. Dwain Reed and Richard Gold, and of Mr. Phillip Pellitteri to the experiments summarized here.

This research was supported by Grant No. NS 10183 from the National Institutes of Health.

REFERENCES

Asanuma, H. and Rosen, I. Topographical organization of cortical efferent zones projecting to distal forelimb muscles in the monkey. Exp. Brain Res., 1972, 14: 243–256.

Asanuma, H. and Sakata, H. Functional organization of a cortical efferent system examined with focal depth stimulation in cats. J. Neurophysiol., 1967, 30: 35–54.

Conrad, B. and Brooks, V.B. Effects of dentate cooling on rapidly alternating arm movements. J. Neurophysiol., 1974, 37: 792–804.

Crago, P.E., Houk, J.C. and Hasan, Z. Regulatory actions of the human stretch reflex. J. Neurophysiol., 1976, 39: 925–935.

Evarts, E.V. Pyramidal tract activity associated with a conditional hand movement in the monkey. J. Neurophysiol., 1966, 29: 1011–1027.

Feldman, A.G. Superposition of motor programs. I. Rhythmic forearm movements in man. Neuroscience, 1980a, 5: 81–90.

Feldman, A.G. Superposition of motor programs. II. Rapid forearm flexion in man. Neuroscience, 1980b, 5: 91–95.

Fetz, E.E. and Cheney, P.D. Postspike facilitation of forelimb muscle activity by primate corticomotoneuronal cells. J. Neurophysiol., 1980, 44: 751–772.

Humphrey, D.R. and Reed, D.J. Separate cortical systems for the control of joint movement and of joint stiffness. Neurosci. Abstr., 1981, 7: 740.

Humphrey, D.R. and Reed, D.J. Reciprocal and co-activation of antagonist muscles. New evidence for separate cortical systems in the control of joint movement and of joint stiffness. In: J. Desmedt (Ed.), Motor Control in Health and Disease. Raven Press, New York, 1983, in press.

Humphrey, D.R., Schmidt, E.M. and Thompson, W.D. Predicting measures of motor performance from multiple cortical spike trains. Science, 1970, 170: 758–762.

Kwan, H.C., MacKay, W.A., Murphy, J.T. and Wong, Y.C. Spatial organization of precentral cortex in awake primates. II. Motor outputs. J. Neurophysiol., 1978, 41: 1120–1131.

Lee, R.G. and Tatton, W.G. Motor responses to sudden limb displacements in primates with specific CNS lesions and in human patients with motor system disorders. Canad. J. neurol. Sci., 1975, 2: 285–293.

Lemon, R.N. and Porter, R. Afferent input to movement-related precentral neurones in conscious monkeys. Proc. roy. Soc. B, 1976, 194: 313–339.

Levine, M.G. and Kabat, H. Cocontraction and reciprocal innervation in voluntary movement in man. Science, 1952, 116: 115–118.

Massion, J. Role of motor cortex in postural adjustments associated with movement. In: H. Asanuma and V.J. Wilson (Eds.), Integration in the Nervous System. Igaku-Shoin, Tokyo, 1979: 239–260.

Patton, N.J. and Mortensen, O.A. An electromyographic study of reciprocal activity of muscles. Anat. Rec., 1971, 170: 255–268.

Polit, A. and Bizzi, E. Characteristics of motor programs underlying arm movements in monkeys. J. Neurophysiol., 1979, 42: 183–194.

Sherrington, C.S. The Integrative Action of the Nervous System, 2nd edn. Yale University Press, New Haven, Conn., 1906.

Sherrington, C.S. Reciprocal innervation of antagonistic muscles. Fourteenth note. On double reciprocal innervation. Proc. roy. Soc. B, 1909, 91: 249–268.

Shinoda, Y., Ghez, C. and Arnold, A. Spinal branching of rubrospinal axons in the cat. Exp. Brain Res., 1977, 30: 203–218.

Shinoda, Y., Zarzecki, P. and Asanuma, H. Spinal branching of pyramidal tract neurons in the monkey. Exp. Brain Res., 1979, 34: 59–72.

Smith, A.M. The coactivation of antagonist muscles. Canad. J. Physiol. Pharmacol., 1981, 7: 733–747.

Stark, L.S. Neurological Control Systems. Plenum Press, New York, 1968: 302–337.

Strick, P.L. and Preston, J.B. Sorting of somatosensory afferent information in primate motor cortex. Brain Res., 1978, 156: 364–368.

Tanji, J. and Wise, S.P. Submodality distribution in sensorimotor cortex of the unanesthetized monkey. J. Neurophysiol., 1981, 45: 467–481.

Thach, W.T. Discharge of cerebellar neurons related to two maintained postures and two prompt movements. I. Nuclear cell output. J. Neurophysiol., 1970, 33: 527–536.

Tilney, F. and Pike, F.H. Muscular coordination experimentally studied in its relation to the cerebellum. Arch. Neurol. Psychiat. (Chic.), 1925, 13: 289–334.

Kyoto Symposia (EEG Suppl. No. 36)
Editors: P.A. Buser, W.A. Cobb and T. Okuma
© 1982, Elsevier Biomedical Press, Amsterdam

Role of the Motor Cortex in the Initiation of Voluntary Motor Responses in the Cat

C. GHEZ, D. VICARIO, J.H. MARTIN and H. YUMIYA

Center for Neurobiology and Behavior, Columbia University, College of Physician and Surgeons, New York, N.Y. 10032 (U.S.A.)

We have previously shown that cats can be trained to make rapid and accurate tracking responses with their forelimbs in relation to a target which is suddenly displaced (Ghez and Vicario 1978a,b; Ghez 1979). Behavioural studies revealed that in the cat such motor responses are typically made with the extraordinarily short latency of 50–70 msec. Since these latencies are not affected by conditions of behavioural choice (Ghez and Vicario 1978a; Ghez 1979) we have hypothesized that neural presetting mechanisms enabled prior to the stimulus might play an important role in the sensorimotor transformation required in this tracking task. In the present study we have recorded the activity of neurones in the motor cortex of the behaving cat to determine their role in rapid reaction time responses. The questions we wished to address were: first, can the motor cortex contribute to the initiation of responses with such short reaction times? Second, do the patterns of activity of task-related neurones provide some insight into the nature of presetting mechanisms occurring prior to response initiation? Third, what relation exists between task-related neural activity and the receptive fields of neurones in the motor cortex? Abstracts of these results have been published (Vicario et al. 1980; Martin et al. 1981).

METHODS

The activity of single neurones in the motor cortex was recorded in cats trained to apply force with the forearm on a stationary lever so as to match a criterion target level. The animals were provided with a display of their force error consisting of a feeding device which was moved to the right or the left of their midline by means of a servo-controlled torque motor. Flexor or extensor adjustments in force applied to the lever by the animals were elicited by stepping the criterion target level in one or another direction after a random interval of initial alignment. This produced a shift to the right or the left in the position of the display to which the animals had to respond by making an appropriate compensatory change in the force applied to the lever. Movement of the display could be detected visually by the animals or through mechanical deflection of their vibrissae.

In a first series of experiments, animals were trained to make extensor responses to changes in target level shifting the display to the right and to make flexor responses to display shifts to the left. In a second series of experiments, a more complex paradigm was utilized. To dissociate the coding of direction and magnitude of display movement (i.e. stimulus) from that of response variables in task-related unit activity, animals were trained to respond appropriately when the polarity of displayed error was inverted, or its gain altered. Thus, a response of a given magnitude and direction could be elicited by display movements in either direction and of various sizes. Additionally, the effects of display shifts not eliciting responses were examined. In this last condition reward was withheld and unitary activity was examined following behavioural extinction (extinction trials). Peripheral receptive fields of single units and the effects of intracortical microstimulation (ICMS) from the recording sites were routinely checked. Stimuli consisted of 45 msec trains of biphasic pulses (0.02 msec per phase) at 300 Hz. Projection neurones were identified antidromically from electrodes chronically implanted in the cerebral peduncles in sites where stimulation elicited contraction of contralateral forelimb muscles at low threshold.

RESULTS

(1) Area sampled: regional differences in receptive fields and in timing of task-related activity

Penetrations were made in the lateral portions of the anterior and posterior sigmoid gyri. ICMS was applied at 500 μm intervals to ascertain the position of the electrode tip within the overall somatotopic representation in the motor cortex. Single neurones were sampled in areas where ICMS produced contraction of forelimb muscles with a threshold of 20 μA or less. Approximately 450 neurones examined showed clear temporal relations between their changes in activity and behavioural events associated with task performance. Most neurones could also be driven by peripheral stimuli applied to different body parts while the animal was at rest and not performing the tracking task.

Regional differences in receptive field characteristics and in the timing of unit activity were observed. Throughout the arm area of the motor cortex (defined by ICMS) neurones were found with clear and discrete receptive fields (simple fields) of the type described by previous authors (Welt et al. 1967; Asanuma 1975). In addition, neurones were observed with more complex receptive field characteristics (complex fields). The response of some of these neurones to peripheral stimuli was temporally labile, being brisk at times and diminishing or disappearing entirely within seconds or minutes, only to reappear a short time later (cf. also Welt et al. 1967). Other complex field cells could only be driven by moving cutaneous stimuli in a single direction while still others showed excitatory or inhibitory regions within their receptive fields, or discontinuous excitatory foci suggesting complex patterns of convergence. Taken as a group, neurones with these complex properties were preferentially located in rostral regions of area 4γ, anterior to the cruciate sulcus. While task-related neuronal activity was observed in both caudal and rostral sites, it was only in rostral regions that units were found which, on average, modulated their activity in advance of the animals' force response (lead cells). Although lead cells constituted only about 10% of the task-related units, they were subjected to more extensive evaluation because only this population could have contributed to response initiation.

Approximately 80% of lead cells had receptive fields of the complex type suggesting that lead cells receive complex convergent patterns of peripheral input. 90% of lead cells showed reciprocal response patterns characterized by increased activity with forces developed in either the flexor or extensor direction and decreased or no modulation with force developed in the opposite direction. The modulation in unit activity of these lead cells could be characterized as either phasic (14%), tonic (22%) or, in the majority of cases (64%) as mixed. In 80% of neurones the degree of modulation varied with either the rate of change of force, the steady force developed or the integrated electromyographic activity (EMG) in the agonist muscle. In neurones whose activity was modulated following the onset of force production, the change could generally be attributed to stimulation of the neurones' receptive fields which accompanied the behavioural response. For example, neurones which could be passively driven by cutaneous stimuli applied to the hair on the dorsal surface of the forearm were typically phasically active with flexor responses of the forearm.

(2) Timing of lead cell activity: stimulus synchronization

A surprising observation was that the onset of changes in unit activity of lead cells was better related in time to the occurrence of the stimulus (i.e., the display shift consequent on the target step) than to the onset of the response (operationally defined as the first change in dF/dt). This observation is illustrated in Fig. 1, which shows rasters of unit activity synchronized with the onset of force production (time zero on abscissa) sorted in order of progressively increasing reaction time. The shortest reaction times are at the top of the rasters and the longest at the bottom. The small plus signs mark the time of occurrence of the stimulus eliciting the response. Part A represents unit activity associated with a series of extensor responses elicited by display movement to the right. Part B shows activity with flexor responses following display movement to the left. Inspection of these rasters clearly shows that both increases (A) and decreases (B) in density of unit activity have a slope that parallels the stimulus mark rather than remaining aligned with the onset of the response (time zero). Fig. 1C and D illustrate the relationship between the amount of lead of increases (C) and decreases (D) in unit activity expressed as a function of reaction time. Units such as this, whose timing was better related to the occurrence of the stimulus than to that of the response, showed significant correlation coefficients and positive slopes of the lead time-reaction time regression line. Units bearing a constant lead over the onset of motor responses would be expected to exhibit a slope of zero. No units with this property were observed in our sample of lead cells. Neurones discharging after the onset of the response (lag cells) showed lead-reaction time regression slopes which were close to zero or correlation coefficients which were not

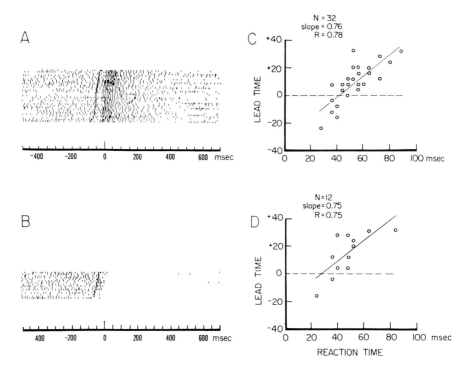

Fig. 1. Raster displays of spike activity associated with extension (A) and flexion (B). Trials are sorted and displayed from top to bottom in order of progressively increasing reaction time (RT). + signs indicate time of occurrence of shift in display position. C and D: scatter plots for lead time (time from change in unit activity to change in force exerted) as a function of reaction time (time from shift in display to onset of force change) for rasters on left.

significant. In these cases the lag was of approximately constant duration, an observation which is compatible with these cells being driven by activation of their receptive fields in the course of the behavioural response.

(3) Behavioural contingencies determining lead cell activity

The activity of lead cells was contingent on the occurrence of behavioural responses. When reinforcement was withheld and behavioural responses extinguished, changes in unit activity no longer followed shifts in the display. Additionally, peri-response time histograms of unit activity in trials where the responses were spontaneously aborted (or undershot) showed intermediate amounts of modulation. These observations suggest that target-related sensory information is conveyed to neurones in the rostral portion of the arm area of motor cortex in a contingent fashion. Two possible mechanisms may be envisaged. First, the behavioural set associated with task performance uncovered a latent receptive field in a fixed location which escaped observation when the animal was examined under passive conditions. Alternatively, the stimulus site producing excitation or inhibition in a given neurone could vary according to the direction of response required by the stimulus.

To distinguish between these possibilities we recorded the patterns of activity of lead cells in rostral motor cortex in animals trained to respond appropriately when the polarity of displayed error was inverted. With this paradigm it was possible to examine neuronal activity associated with flexor and extensor responses elicited by movements of the display to both the right and the left. Two classes of lead cells, with approximately equal numbers, were observed in rostral motor cortex. The first class showed reciprocal changes in activity (i.e. increases or decreases) contingent on the direction of force production and independent of the direction of display movement. The timing of the onset of changes of activity was, however, more consistently related to the onset of target shift than to the onset of force production. These observations suggest that display-related afferent input reaching neurones in rostral motor cortex can be selected according to behavioural set, possibly by gating mechanisms acting on neurones presynaptic to them.

In the second class of lead cells, activity was contingent on a single direction of display movement and the pattern of activity did not vary with the direction of force production by forelimb muscles. Modulation in activity of these cells while timed to the stimulus was contingent on the occurrence of the motor response. This class of cells could be important in the processing of stimulus information, leading to the development of a motor command. Alternatively, such cells might control one or more independent behavioural responses which we have observed in our behavioural paradigm. Such responses included attempts at head rotation and eye movement towards the moving display, the direction of which was independent of the polarity of displayed error and of the direction of force produced by forelimb muscles.

CONCLUSIONS

(1) The present findings suggest that the arm area of the cat motor cortex includes 2 functionally distinct regions: one rostral, the other caudal to the cruciate sulcus. For convenience, these 2 regions may be denoted as MCr and MCc. Our findings complement the earlier experiments of Pappas and Strick (1979) using micro-stimulation. Parallel anatomical studies using retrograde and anterograde transport of HRP and/or radiolabelled amino acids (Yumiya and Ghez 1981) have revealed differential cortico-cortical and thalamo-cortical projections to these 2 regions. Since the modulation of unit activity in MCc invariably lagged the onset of behavioural responses, this region cannot be considered to play a role in response initiation. Only in MCr were neurones encountered whose activity, on average, was modulated in advance of overt behaviour. While neurones in MCr could play a role in the initiation of behavioural responses, the small number of cells with this property emphasizes the importance of subcortical and other parallel pathways in mediating behaviour.

(2) A surprising observation was that the onset of lead activity was better correlated in time with the target stimulus than with the motor response. Since neuronal activity was dependent on the occurrence of the motor behaviour, the results suggest that target information may be relayed to neurones in MCr in a contingent fashion.

These observations support the notion that gating mechanisms acting presynaptically to neurones in MCr enable the efficient transfer of target information leading to motor commands. These findings suggest that similar conclusions drawn by Evarts and Tanji (1974) in relation to proprioceptive inputs may have more general implications. Thus, in the context of a task requiring spatially accurate responses to stimuli moving in one or another direction, gating mechanisms implement, within the motor cortex, a preset map that relates target and response dimensions. While aggregate lead activity in MCr could represent a command that determines both response configuration and its time of onset, it cannot be excluded that its action is also in the nature of a gating signal applied to a lower order station. Since lead activity in MCr is better timed to the occurrence of the target stimulus than to that of the response, the variance in reaction time must be strongly influenced by other mechanisms. Thus, reaction time variance may represent an emergent property resulting from the activity of multiple descending and afferent pathways acting on intercalated interneurones and motor neurones.

(3) Since both lead and lag cells often showed peripheral receptive fields in the responding limb and since sensory inputs reaching these neurones may be subject to gating mechanisms, it cannot be excluded that somatosensory inputs contribute to observed parametric relations between unit activity and force exerted.

(4) The present results suggest that the classical dichotomies drawn between sensory and motor mechanisms and between activity within the central nervous system which leads or lags behaviour may not be as useful as once thought. Consideration of the nature of information processing required in a particular task may provide a more fruitful point of departure in elucidating the neural translation between sensory events and motor responses.

REFERENCES

Asanuma, H. Recent developments in the study of the columnar arrangement of neurons within the motor cortex. Physiol. Rev., 1975, 55: 143–156.

Evarts, E.V. and Tanji, J. Gating of motor cortex reflexes by prior instruction. Brain Res., 1974, 71: 479–494.

Ghez, C. Contributions of central programs to rapid limb movement in the cat. In: H. Asanuma and V.J. Wilson (Eds.), Integration in the Nervous System. Igaku-Shoin, Tokyo, 1979: 305–320.

Ghez, C. and Vicario, D. The control of rapid limb movement in the cat. I. Response latency. Exp. Brain Res., 1978a, 33: 173–190.

Ghez, C. and Vicario, D. The control of rapid limb movement in the cat. II. Scaling of isometric force adjustments. Exp. Brain Res., 1978b, 33: 191–203.

Martin, J., Yumiya, H. and Ghez, C. Coding of target and response variables in cat motor cortex. Neurosci. Abstr., 1981, 7: 562.

Pappas, C.L. and Strick, P.L. Double representation of the distal forelimb in cat motor cortex. Brain Res., 1979, 167: 412–416.

Vicario, D., Martin, J. and Ghez, C. Discharge of neurons in cat motor cortex during voluntary muscle contraction. Neurosci. Abstr., 1980, 6: 125.

Welt, C., Aschoff, J.C., Kameda, K. and Brooks, V.B. Intracortical organization of cat's motorsensory neurons. In: M.D. Yahr and D.P. Purpura (Eds.), Neurophysiological Basis of Normal and Abnormal Motor Activities. Raven Press, New York, 1967: 255–293.

Yumiya, H. and Ghez, C. Topography of differential projections to rostral and caudal cat motor cortex. Soc. Neurosci. Abstr., 1981, 7: 562.

Kyoto Symposia (EEG Suppl. No. 36)
Editors: P.A. Buser, W.A. Cobb and T. Okuma
© 1982, Elsevier Biomedical Press, Amsterdam

Motor Deficit Following Interruption of Sensory Inputs to the Motor Cortex of the Monkey

H. ASANUMA and K. ARISSIAN

The Rockefeller University, New York, N.Y. 10021 (U.S.A.)

The importance of sensory inputs for voluntary movement has been known for a long time. In 1858 Claude Bernard reported that section of the dorsal roots produced impairment of movement in the frog and the puppy. This experiment has been repeated by many investigators and the results were confirmed in various species (Mott and Sherrington 1895; Knapp et al. 1963; Denny-Brown 1966). The role of sensory inputs to the motor cortex, however, has not been studied until recently. This is partly due to the fact that the sensory input pathway to the motor cortex was not known and it was generally thought that the input to the motor cortex comes through the sensory cortex. It has been shown recently that the motor cortex receives peripheral inputs directly from the n. ventralis postero-lateralis pars oralis (VPL_o) of the thalamus (Asanuma et al. 1979; Horne and Tracey 1979; Lemon and van der Burg 1979) and that these direct inputs are transferred primarily through the dorsal column in the monkey (Brinkman et al. 1978; Asanuma et al. 1980). These results made it possible to eliminate the sensory input to the motor cortex and study the functional deficit during movement. It will be shown that elimination of the sensory input impairs the control of fine movements as well as orientation of the hand in space.

MATERIALS AND METHODS

Three adult cynomolgus monkeys (*Macaca fascicularis*) of either sex, weighing around 3 kg, were used. They were trained to sit on a primate chair and to pick up a peanut or a raisin from a hole in a food board. Three different sizes of hole were drilled in the board and the board was turned around at various speeds while the monkey was picking up the food (Fig. 1). The animals accustomed to this situation within a week or two and became eager to sit on the chair for each day's practice. Then, operations were carried out under inhalation anaesthesia composed of a mixture of oxygen (50%) and nitrous oxide (50%) supplemented with 1.5% halothane. In 2 monkeys the postcentral gyrus of one side was exposed and removed by suction. The dura was sutured back and the skin was closed. After examination of the motor deficits, which lasted 5 and 4 weeks, the animals were re-operated and the dorsal column was sectioned bilaterally at the level of C-3 to examine the motor deficit produced by the combined lesions. In the third monkey, the sequence was reversed so

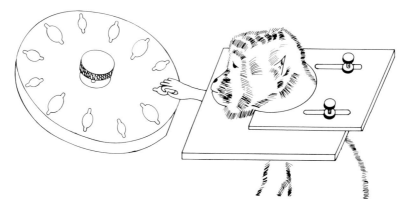

Fig. 1. The experimental paradigm for feeding the monkey. The monkey sits in front of a food board with only the neck restrained. Three sizes of hole are drilled in the board and the board rotates at various speeds. The monkey is trained to pick up a peanut or a raisin from the rotating board. When necessary, one hand is restrained so that the monkey can use only the hand of the experimental side.

that the dorsal column was sectioned first. After completion of the experiments the animals were deeply anaesthetized with nembutal (40 mg/kg) and perfused with saline followed by 10% formalin. The brain and the cervical cord were removed and frozen sections were cut and stained to examine the extents of the lesions.

RESULTS

(1) Sensory cortex ablation

In 2 of the monkeys, the sensory cortex was removed before the dorsal column section. The later histological examination revealed that in both monkeys the ablation extended to areas 1, 2, 3b, 5 and caudal part of area 3a, but not to areas 4 and 7. The medio-lateral extent was from the neck to the hind limb areas, as judged by the distribution of evoked potentials in the same species (Asanuma et al. 1980). It has been shown that lesions of the postcentral cortex produce very little motor deficit (Travis and Woolsey 1956; Denny-Brown 1966; Tatton et al. 1975). Our observation was similar to those made by the previous investigators.

Immediately after recovery from the anaesthesia, the monkeys looked curiously at the hand contralateral to the ablated cortex and, when given a peanut, used the ipsilateral hand. However, both monkeys quickly adapted to the new situation and after a few hours started using the contralateral hand in much the same manner as the ipsilateral hand. The tactile placing reaction was lost during the entire period of observation after the operation. Although the behaviour of the monkeys in the cage looked nearly normal from 2 or 3 h after the operation, further examination of the hand skill, using the turning food board, revealed some clumsiness in using the contralateral hand. Fig. 2 (upper graph) shows the results. The skill of picking up the food from the hole was severely impaired on the day after operation, but returned nearly to normal within a week and stayed at that level for the rest of the

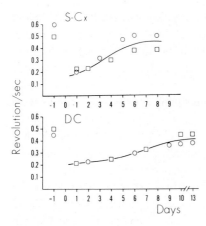

Fig. 2. Recovery of hand skill after operative procedure. The ordinates show the speed of rotation and the abscissae show the days after surgery. In all the trials shown, only the medium size holes were used, and the maximum speed at which the monkey could pick up the peanuts in 50% of the trials is plotted. The speed of 0.5 c/sec is the speed at which the experimenter starts experiencing difficulty in putting the food in the correct hole. Results from 2 different monkeys are shown in each graph (□ or ○). Upper graph: recovery of skill after contralateral sensory cortex ablation. Lower graph: recovery after bilateral dorsal column section.

period (4 and 5 weeks). During the initial stage, the monkeys could bring the hand to the hole without any trouble, but could not use the proper fingers (thumb and index) to pick up the peanut. Instead, both monkeys tried to use all of the fingers, giving the impression that the lack of tactile sensation impaired the ability to select the proper fingers. This clumsiness recovered rapidly and they started to use the proper fingers within a few days, although the usage was a little clumsier than normal. The course of the recovery gave the impression that visual guidance substituted for the function previously served by tactile sensation.

(2) Dorsal column section

In 1 monkey, the dorsal column was sectioned first, but in the other 2 the section was made after the cortical ablation. Later histological examination revealed that in all 3 cases, the dorsal columns of both sides were cut completely and in 1 case, the incision reached to a part of the grey matter, but not to the lateral column.

The monkey with only dorsal column section behaved normally even immediately after the operation. She could stand and walk normally and could climb the cage. However, further examination of hand skill with the food board showed some deficit in motor function. Although she could bring the hand to a stationary hole, she could not bring the hand to a rotating hole. When she tried to pick up a peanut from a stationary hole, she could not coordinate the thumb and the index finger and used all fingers in concert. The loss of orientation and coordination recovered gradually and after 2 weeks the ability of picking up the peanut came back nearly to normal, although there was still some clumsiness. Fig. 2 (lower graph) shows the recovery process. The loss of the tactile placing reaction was difficult to judge.

Gilman and Denny-Brown (1966) reported that the reaction was permanently lost in the forelimb, but not in the hind limb. Brinkman et al. (1978) reported that minimal disturbance of contact placing was noticed only when the dorsal surface of the hand or fingers was touched. Our observation agrees with that of the previous investigators in that the tactile placing reaction was not lost in the hind limb. However, in the forelimb, it was difficult to determine whether the stimuli were purely tactile or partly proprioceptive. A light touch to the hair of the dorsal hand, which in intact monkeys elicits a prompt reaction, did not produce the reaction, but touch to the skin of the same area sometimes elicited a slowly executed reaction. This weakness of response persisted during the entire period of observation.

The effect of dorsal column section was observed in 2 other monkeys using the hand contralateral to the intact cortex and the results were essentially similar. There was a loss of orientation in the hand movement and coordination of fingers which recovered gradually within 2 weeks.

(3) Sensory cortex ablation plus dorsal column section

In 2 monkeys, the sensory cortex was removed first and in 1 monkey, the dorsal column was sectioned first. The extent of cortical ablation in 3 monkeys and the re-

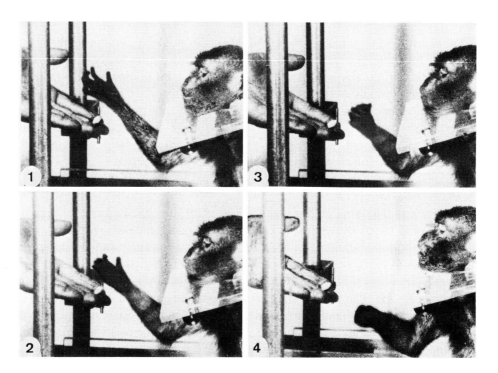

Fig. 3. Motor deficit produced by contralateral sensory cortex ablation plus bilateral dorsal column section. The monkey lost the ability to orient the hand in space as well as fine manipulation of the fingers. The illustration shows frames of a motion picture. The numbers indicate the sequence of the movement. The monkey tried to pick up a peanut from the experimenter's hand, but could not reach it. Further details are given in the text.

sults obtained in both procedures were similar. After recovery from the second operation, the monkeys could stand in the cage cautiously, but tended to fall when they tried to walk. The hand contralateral to the cortical lesion was paralysed and they did not try to use it at all. Several days after the operation, they tried to use this hand occasionally, but the movements were disoriented and could not reach the target. The ability to manipulate individual fingers was lost in spite of intact visual guidance. When seated in the chair in front of the food board, they could pick up the food occasionally from the largest hole, using all fingers in concert only when the board was not moving, but could not pick up the food from the board moving at very slow speed (0.01 c/sec). When a peanut was brought in front of the monkey, he (or she) tried hard to pick it up, using all fingers, but in many trials the hand could not reach the target. Fig. 3 shows an example. Occasional success encouraged her and kept her trying. When she picked up the peanut, she looked at the hand and brought the food cautiously to the mouth, but still tended to drop the food when she tried to eat. The results from the other monkeys were similar. This severe disturbance of motor function did not recover during the period of observation which lasted 4–5 weeks after the second operation.

It has been reported that ablation of the sensory cortex does not impair the motor function of the adjoining precentral cortex examined by the intracortical microstimulation method (Asanuma et al. 1979). The possible effect of dorsal column section on the function of the motor cortex was examined in 2 monkeys by intracortical microstimulation at the termination of the experiments. The threshold current for eliciting movements and the size of cortical efferent zones within the motor cortex were not different from those of normal monkeys.

DISCUSSION

To examine the possible functional role of peripheral inputs to the motor cortex we have destroyed the sensory cortex and sectioned the dorsal columns, which are the two major sources of peripheral inputs to the motor cortex. The motor deficit produced by elimination of both inputs was far more severe than that produced by one alone. In the case of sensory cortex ablation, the motor cortex still receives a sensory input directly from the thalamus (Asanuma et al. 1979) which may explain the remarkably small motor deficit. The impairment in movement was more severe when the dorsal column was cut than when the sensory cortex was removed. This may be attributed to the elimination of the direct input to the motor cortex as well as a part of the input to the sensory cortex which comes through the dorsal column. However, the deficit recovered rapidly and after 2 weeks, the motor skill returned nearly to normal. Several mechanisms may account for this recovery but a likely interpretation is that the peripheral information coming through the spino-thalamic tract to the sensory cortex which was transferred to the motor cortex compensated for the function of the direct input to the motor cortex. Persistent severe motor deficit after removal of both inputs to the motor cortex may support this interpretation.

The results suggest that both the direct and the transcortical inputs to the motor cortex are important in the regulation of voluntary movements but each input can compensate for the function of the other. It should be emphasized, however, that the peripheral information is not an indispensable factor for the control of voluntary movements. It has been shown (Knapp et al. 1963) that section of the dorsal roots paralyses the monkey, but the motor function recovers after careful training. The recovery, however, is not perfect and it seems clear that the peripheral input plays an important role in the smooth pursuit of voluntary movements.

How, then, do peripheral inputs to the motor cortex participate in the smooth execution of movements? It has been shown that the basic module of the motor cortex is the cortical efferent zone which projects most heavily to a particular muscle. It has also been shown that each efferent zone receives a peripheral input related to the contraction of the target muscle (Asanuma 1975). It has been proposed that this input serves as modulator of the efferent zones by changing their excitabilities rather than by initiating the movement (Asanuma 1981). This may work in the following way: when a monkey sitting in front of a turning food board wants to pick up a peanut, she or he waits until the food approaches. During this time, the muscles that would be activated are already in a preparatory stage and their tone is already increased. During this time, afferent impulses from the receptors associated with the would-be activated muscle are increased, resulting in the increased circulation of impulses between the cortical efferent zones and the target muscles. This results in increase of the excitability of related efferent zones and relay nuclei involved in the circuits and, at the same time, inhibits the other efferent zones by surround inhibition. When a command signal from other areas of the central nervous system arrives and the movement is executed, the peripheral signals are reinforced and continuously send information back to the cortical efferent zones about the actual state of the limb and automatically change the excitability of the zones to produce smooth accurate movements. When the movement is completed, the circulation of impulses is shifted to other loop circuits to produce other types of movement. The above hypothesis is yet to be proved, but the impairment of smooth movement after dorsal column section observed in this experiment supports this interpretation. The function of this corticoperipheral circuit, however, seems to be compensated for by the input from the sensory cortex, the neuronal mechanisms of which are yet to be elucidated.

SUMMARY

The possible functional role of sensory inputs in voluntary movements was examined by severing the sensory input pathways to the motor cortex. The somatic sensory cortex and the dorsal column, which are known to be the two major sources of the peripheral inputs to the motor cortex, were ablated or sectioned. The deficit produced by sensory cortex ablation or dorsal column section was not prominent and the function recovered within a week or two as long as the other input was intact, but elimination of both inputs produced severe impairment in movements such as loss of orientation in space and of manipulation of individual fingers. The possible role of the afferent input is discussed and it is proposed that it participates in the smooth pursuit of movement by continuously changing the excitability of cortical efferent zones.

ACKNOWLEDGEMENTS

The authors would like to express their thanks to Drs. E.M. Kosar and A.D. Miller for their valuable comments on the manuscript and to Ms. M.E. Genther for typing it.

This research was supported by the NIH Grant NS-10705.

REFERENCES

Asanuma, H. Recent development in the study of the columnar arrangement within the motor cortex. Physiol. Rev., 1975, 55: 143–156.

Asanuma, H. Functional role of sensory inputs to the motor cortex. Progr. Neurobiol., 1981, 16: 241–262.

Asanuma, H., Larsen, K.D. and Yumiya, H. Direct sensory pathways to the motor cortex in the monkey. In: H. Asanuma and V.J. Wilson (Eds.), A Basis of Cortical Reflexes. Igaku-shoin, Tokyo, 1979: 223–238.

Asanuma, H., Larsen, K.D. and Yumiya, H. Peripheral input pathways to the monkey motor cortex. Exp. Brain Res., 1980, 38: 349–355.

Bernard, C. Leons sur la Physiologie et la Pathologie de Système Nerveux. J.B. Baillière, Paris, 1858: 246–266.

Brinkman, J., Bush, B.M. and Porter, R. Deficient influences of peripheral stimuli on precentral neurones in monkeys with dorsal column lesions. J. Physiol. (Lond.), 1978, 276: 27–48.

Denny-Brown, D. The Cerebral Control of Movement. Thomas, Springfield, Ill., 1966.

Gilman, S. and Denny-Brown, D. Disorders of movement and behavior following dorsal column lesions. Brain, 1966, 89/3: 397–418.

Horne, M.K. and Tracey, D.J. The afferents and projections of the ventroposterolateral thalamus in the monkey. Exp. Brain Res., 1979, 36: 129–141.

Knapp, H.D., Taub, E. and Berman, A.J. Movements in monkeys with deafferented forelimbs. Exp. Neurol., 1963, 7: 305–315.

Lemon, R.N. and van der Burg, J. Short-latency peripheral inputs to thalamic neurones projecting to the motor cortex in the monkey. Exp. Brain Res., 1979, 36: 445–462.

Mott, F.W. and Sherrington, C.S. Experiments upon the influence of sensory nerves upon movement and nutrition of the limb. Proc. roy. Soc., 1895, 57: 481–488.

Tatton, W.G., Forner, S.D., Gerstein, G.L., Chambers, W.W. and Liu, C.M. The effect of postcentral cortical lesions on motor responses to sudden upper limb displacements in monkeys. Brain Res., 1975, 96: 108–113.

Travis, A.M. and Woolsey, C.N. Motor performance of monkeys after bilateral partial and total cerebral decortications. Amer. J. phys. Med., 1956, 35: 273–289.

Kyoto Symposia (EEG Suppl. No. 36)
Editors: P.A. Buser, W.A. Cobb and T. Okuma

Interaction between Sensory Input and Motor Output during Rapid Learned Movements in Man

ROBERT G. LEE and GREGORY E. LUCIER

Department of Clinical Neurosciences and Neuroscience Research Group, University of Calgary, Calgary, Alberta (Canada)

The question which we wish to address in this short review concerns the mechanisms which serve to compensate for unexpected load conditions during voluntary movements, particularly the very fast so-called "ballistic" type of movement. We shall focus on two specific aspects of this question. First, is motor output modified by sensory feedback during rapid "pre-programmed" voluntary movements, and secondly, if this is the case, are the changes mediated by short latency spinal reflexes or by long latency supraspinal or long loop reflexes?

We cannot discuss ballistic movements without reference to the hypothesis proposed a number of years ago by Kornhuber (1971). Although there are certain flaws in this hypothesis, it has served as the basis for a number of experimental studies. Kornhuber proposed that voluntary movements could be separated into two major categories – ballistic movements and ramp movements. Undoubtedly this idea arose at least partially from studies on the eye movement control system where there seems to be a clear separation between saccadic movements and pursuit movements. According to Kornhuber ballistic movements are very rapid movements which take place too quickly to allow any regulation by sensory feedback. The pattern or program for activation of the various participating muscles is transmitted in its entirety to spinal motor centres and the full sequence of the movement is acted out without any opportunity for modification by sensory feedback. Kornhuber suggested that this type of movement was pre-programmed by the cerebellum. Ramp movements are slower movements which are continuously controlled by sensory input from the moving parts, and Kornhuber proposed that these were programmed in the basal ganglia.

There are some obvious problems when we attempt to fit various types of movements into these two categories. First, there is not any universal agreement as to what constitutes a ballistic movement. Shooting a rifle at a target is obviously ballistic – in fact this is where the terminology originated. Throwing a ball or hitting a golf shot is probably similar – certainly once the ball is released no amount of "body english" is going to change its course during that particular trial. However, there is some doubt as to whether a quick movement to a specified endpoint, often indicated by a visual target on an oscilloscope, is ballistic in the true sense. This is the type of movement which has been studied in both experimental animals and human subjects, and visual and proprioceptive feedback would seem to be involved to at least some extent. The other problem is that highly trained subjects performing skilled movements such as gymnastics or playing a piano appear capable of modifying their motor programs in response to changing external conditions even during very rapid movements. It may be that there is a continuous spectrum of movements ranging from very slow to very fast rather than two distinct categories with separate central control systems.

Several investigators have designed experiments on human subjects to test the Kornhuber hypothesis for ballistic movements. Desmedt and Godaux (1978) applied sudden unexpected increases in load while subjects were performing voluntary abduction movements of the index finger. When these perturbations occurred during ballistic movements there was no evidence of any reflex compensation. The earliest increase in EMG activity did not occur until 132 msec or longer after the perturbation. During a slower ramp movement the load increase resulted in an EMG response after 52 msec, a latency which corresponds to that of an M2 or long loop response (Lee and Tatton 1975). However, if the load increase was applied very early during a ballistic task, prior to actual onset of movement, the increase in EMG output did occur at the expected time of an M2 response. It was concluded that reflex activity corresponding in time to a long loop M2 response is used to compensate for load changes during ramp movements. Similar compensation occurs during ballistic movements if the perturbation occurs sufficiently early during the evolving pattern of movement.

In a similar study Dufresne et al. (1978) demonstrated a compensatory increase in biceps EMG when torque perturbations were applied to oppose rapid voluntary flexion movements of the elbow. They studied movements at various velocities and concluded that motor output was modified by these perturbations irrespective of the speed of movement.

Hallett and Marsden (1979) have examined the effects of perturbations applied at various times during a ballistic flexion movement of the human thumb. These perturbations were arranged to either release the pre-existing load or to increase it in a manner which would either halt the movement or reverse it so that the muscle was suddenly stretched. During both the stretch and halt conditions there was a definite accentuation of the second burst of EMG activity from the agonist muscle which is part of the normal triphasic EMG pattern associated with ballistic movements. When the perturbation resulted in stretch of the muscle there was also a small reflex EMG response occurring between the first and second agonist bursts. This began approximately 45 msec after the perturbation.

From these studies and others it is clear that load changes during ballistic movements do result in some type of reflex activity. Whether this is mediated by spinal reflexes or long loop mechanisms, or a combination of the two, is not entirely certain.

Recent experiments in our laboratory have been designed to look at a slightly different aspect of this problem. The question which we have asked is as follows: if after repeated practice a subject has learned to perform a rapid movement for a specified distance against a standard load, what happens if the load unexpectedly becomes larger or smaller than what the subject has programmed for? In the previous studies summarized above sudden load perturbations were applied during the course of a voluntary movement. Our method differed in that the load change occurred prior to the onset of any EMG activity or movement.

We studied rapid flexion movements of the wrist over an angle of approximately 40°. EMG activity was recorded with surface electrodes over the wrist flexors and extensors. A potentiometer in the apparatus recorded position or angle of the wrist joint. A torque motor was used to apply varying amounts of load and a torque transducer coupled to the shaft of the motor provided a signal indicating the forces occurring between subject's arm and the apparatus. Each trial started with the handle resting against a mechanical stop. This insured that the subjects did not sense any change in load until muscle contraction or movement actually commenced. A microswitch in the stop was released as the movement started and provided a reference point for averaging of responses.

The subjects were provided with a visual display consisting of an open square controlled by the computer program and a solid square representing the position of the wrist joint. At random times the open square suddenly jumped a distance representing 40° of the wrist movement and the subject was required to make a rapid wrist flexion movement to place the solid square within the open square. To insure that the movements were rapid we set a time limit of 100 msec for movement over this distance. This resulted in movements with a minimum velocity of 400°/sec. Trials which were not completed within this time limit were discarded and not included in further analysis.

After several minutes of practice the subjects learned to move the handle this distance against a small standard load so that almost all trials were completed within 100 msec. The movement became almost automatic and we could say that the subject had developed a "motor program" for this simple movement to produce the required degree of activation of agonist and antagonist muscles. Once the pattern for this movement had been learned the load on the handle was unexpectedly increased to a value several times greater than the control load on a small percentage of random trials. The EMG activity, handle position, and torque for these trials were selectively averaged and responses were compared to those obtained during movements against the standard expected load. Ten responses were averaged for each load condition.

A representative recording from one normal subject is shown in Fig. 1. The solid traces represent averaged position and EMG recordings for the movements occurring against the small standard load which the subject expected. The superimposed dotted traces are the responses for the movements against an unexpected large load – about 8 times greater than the standard load in this example. Ballistic movements were associated with a characteristic triphasic EMG pattern. There was an initial burst from the agonist (flexor) muscle followed by a burst from the antagonist muscle and then a second less well defined agonist burst. In the example shown in Fig. 1 there is some initial tonic activity in the extensor muscles which is suppressed at the time of the first agonist burst.

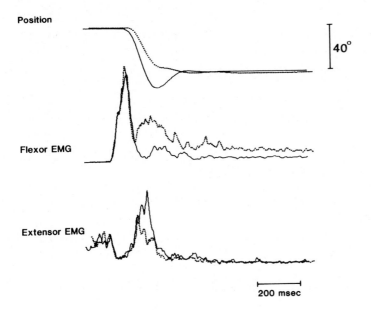

Fig. 1. Rapid flexion movements of the wrist against a small standard load (solid traces) and against an unexpected large load (dotted traces). The load increase occurred prior to the onset of movement and was maintained throughout the task. Each trace represents an average of 10 movements. EMG activity was rectified prior to averaging. The compensatory changes in EMG output are indicated by the points at which the dotted traces and solid traces diverge.

Examination of the position traces reveals that, when the load is larger than what the subject predicted, movement occurs at a slower velocity and there is less over-shoot of the target than during the standard task. Interestingly, the time required to complete the trial and stabilize the handle in the new target location is about the same in each case. Inspection of the flexor EMG recordings reveals that the initial agonist burst is almost identical in each case. However, when the load was larger than what was anticipated there was a sudden increase in EMG activity from the agonist muscle which represents the compensation for the increased load. This is indicated by the point at which the dotted and solid EMG traces diverge. At the same time there is a compensatory decrease of EMG output from the antagonist (extensor) muscle.

Two important questions arise from these observations. First, what is the latency of the compensatory changes in EMG output and, secondly, what receptors and pathways are responsible for this apparent change in the motor program? Since we are not dealing here with a perturbation or precise stimulus, latency is not a simple determination. It depends on what we choose as a reference point. The time at which movement commences can be readily determined from the position traces, and the changes in EMG output begin very soon following this, 20–30 msec in the group of normal subjects we have studied. However, it is probable that afferent activity signalling the increase or decrease in load occurs before there is any actual movement. The muscle begins to contract and force is applied to the handle for at least

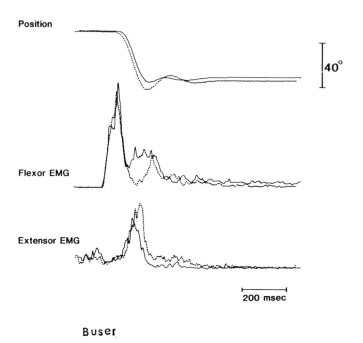

Position

40°

Flexor EMG

Extensor EMG

200 msec

Buser

Fig. 2. Rapid flexion movements of the wrist against a moderately large standard load (solid traces) and against an unexpected smaller load (dotted traces).

a short period before movement occurs. Inspection of the torque recordings (not shown in Figs. 1 and 2) revealed that the change in EMG output begin 30–40 msec following the earliest change in torque. The point at which torque begins to change would seem to represent the earliest time at which any afferent activity could begin to provide information concerning changes in load conditions.

These are very short latencies. They are considerably less than the latency of the M2 or long loop response for these muscles which normally occurs at 55–60 msec following application of a load perturbation. This short latency suggests that load compensation in this particular type of task is mediated, at least in part, by spinal reflex mechanisms.

What are the mechanisms responsible for this short latency change in EMG output? This is not a stretch reflex in the true sense because the change in EMG response occurs at a time when the muscle is still shortening, when we might expect that the spindles are at least partially unloaded. Could Golgi tendon organs be involved? We know that they become active during voluntary contraction and are sensitive to small changes in tension or force. However, most of the available evidence suggests that they inhibit motoneurones for their muscle of origin so it seems unlikely that excitation of Golgi receptors would result in increased EMG output.

Spindle primary endings and Ia afferent pathways appear to be the most logical candidates to mediate these changes, despite the fact that the muscle is being shortened rather than stretched. During a normal ballistic movement against a standard load there is co-activation of alpha and gamma motoneurones to prevent unloading of the spindle as the extrafusal fibres shorten. When movement occurs against an unexpected large load, alpha and gamma motoneurones initially receive the same central command as they did previously. The intrafusal fibres shorten by an amount which would be appropriate for the movement against a standard load.

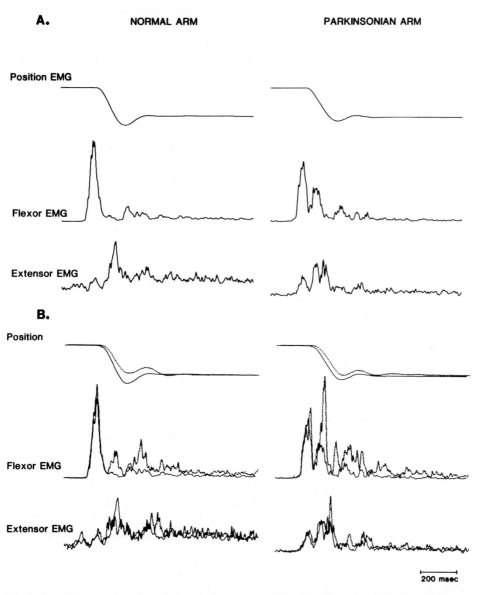

Fig. 3. Rapid flexion movements of the wrist in a patient with mild unilateral parkinsonism. Responses at the top (A) were obtained with the subject working against a small expected load. In B, responses for movements against an unexpected large load (dotted traces) are superimposed upon the responses for the standard load.

However, because of the increased load the velocity of movement is reduced. At any point in time there is relatively less shortening of extrafusal fibres. Rather than being unloaded, the spindle at this point could be considered to be inappropriately loaded. The resulting alpha-gamma mismatch could cause increased firing over Ia pathways and a short latency increase in EMG output.

With further refinement, this type of approach could provide information concerning errors in motor programming in patients with neurologic disorders affecting motor function. Fig. 3 illustrates recordings obtained from a patient with early unilateral Parkinson's disease. The top half of the figure compares responses from the normal arm and the parkinsonian arm for ballistic movements against a small load which the subject expected. The clinically normal arm shows the usual type of triphasic EMG pattern, although there is perhaps more tonic activation of the extensor muscles than in most normal subjects. In the parkinsonian arm movement occurs at a slower rate. Two abnormalities are apparent in the EMG pattern on this side. First there is co-activation of the antagonist muscle at the same time as the initial burst from the agonist. In normal subjects there is usually inhibition of the antagonist at this time (see Fig. 1). In the parkinsonian arm there is also a second burst of activity from the agonist muscle which occurs much earlier than the usual second agonist burst for this type of movement. In fact, this occurs at approximately the same time as the compensatory EMG burst in normal subjects working against unexpectedly large loads.

The bottom half of Fig. 3 is arranged in a manner similar to Fig. 1. The dotted traces represent responses associated with movements against an unexpected large load and are superimposed on the responses for movement against the small standard load. The compensatory increase in agonist EMG from the normal arm is similar to what is seen in normal subjects. In the parkinsonian arm there is a marked accentuation of this compensatory EMG output. It is tempting to speculate that this may be related in some manner to the abnormally large M2 responses which have been demonstrated in parkinsonism (Lee and Tatton 1975), although, as has already been noted, the latency of this response is considerably shorter than that of the M2 response in either normals or parkinsonians.

To summarize, these results provide evidence that there is reflex compensation for unexpected changes in external loads even during very fast learned or pre-programmed movements occurring at velocities greater than 400°/sec. These compensatory changes occur at relatively short latencies and are probably mediated by spinal reflexes rather than by long-loop mechanisms. Although ballistic movements may be pre-programmed, mechanisms appear to exist at the spinal level to modify motor programs if load conditions are other than what was expected.

ACKNOWLEDGEMENT

This work was supported by the Medical Research Council of Canada.

REFERENCES

Desmedt, J.E. and Godaux, E. Ballistic skilled movements: load compensation and patterning of the motor commands. In: J.E. Desmedt (Ed.), Cerebral Motor Control in Man: Long Loop Mechanisms, Progr. Clin. Neurophysiol., Vol. 4. Karger, Basel, 1978, 21–55.

Dufresne, J.R., Gurfinkel, V.S., Soechting, J.F. and Terzuolo, L.A. Response to transient disturbances during intentional forearm flexion in man. Brain Res., 1978, 150: 103–115.

Hallett, M. and Marsden, C.D. Ballistic flexion movements of the human thumb. J. Physiol. (Lond.), 1979, 294: 33–50.

Kornhuber, H.H. Motor functions of cerebellum and basal ganglia: the cerebello-cortical saccadic (ballistic) clock, the cerebellonuclear hold regulator and the basal ganglia ramp (voluntary speed smooth movements) generator. Kybernetik, 1971, 8: 157–162.

Lee, R.G. and Tatton, W.G. Motor responses to sudden limb displacements in primates with specific CNS lesions and in human patients with motor system disorders. Canad. J. neurol. Sci., 1975, 2: 285–293.

Kyoto Symposia (EEG Suppl. No. 36)
Editors: P.A. Buser, W.A. Cobb and T. Okuma
© 1982, Elsevier Biomedical Press, Amsterdam

430

Studies on the Normal and Disordered Human Motor Cortex

C.D. MARSDEN

University Department of Neurology, Institute of Psychiatry, de Crespigny Park, London SE5 8AF (England)

In this report I shall discuss two issues: (1) what sort of movements does the human motor cortex command?; (2) what sort of disorders occur when the human motor cortex is damaged? The studies to be described were conducted in collaboration with Dr. P.A. Merton and Mr. H.B. Morton for the physiological investigations, and with Drs. J.C. Rothwell and J. Obeso for the observations on patients with motor cortical diseases.

NORMAL MOTOR CORTEX FUNCTION

Stimulation of the normal human motor cortex

It has been difficult to study the human motor cortex other than during surgical operations, when by definition the subject is not normal, and conditions for recording or experimental observation are less than ideal. Recently, however, Merton and Morton (1980) have developed a new technique for doing so without even breaking the skin. The procedure developed out of experiments with Hill in which Merton and he were attempting to find a means of fully activating human muscle by direct stimulation. They found that the problem of pain could be overcome by using very high voltage pulses of extremely short duration (Hill et al. 1980). The same technique was then applied to the brain. Initially, a special stimulator delivering 1000 V from a condenser with a time constant of about 10 μsec was used; now however, we employ voltages of 350–500 V with a time constant of about 100 μsec. Such stimuli are delivered through surface silver-silver chloride electrodes or saline-dampened pad electrodes. They cause a sharp jolt which some find painless, while others experience discomfort.

Anodal shocks applied over the surface markings of the hand area of the motor cortex, with the cathode a few centimetres in front, easily elicited contraction of hand and forearm muscles in all of the 20 subjects we have studied. The first point to emphasize is the topography of the response.

Site of response to motor cortical stimulation

At first it was expected that great care in positioning the electrodes would be required to stimulate different muscles, but it was soon found that "cortical stimulation is unique; you simply decide what muscles you want to excite and it excites them'' (Marsden et al. 1982). The point was that while large voltages were required to excite a relaxed muscle, a slight voluntary contraction considerably reduced the threshold for stimulating that active muscle or group of muscles. Thus, by voluntary contraction it proved possible to excite proximal and distal muscles of both the arm and the leg. The latency of the onset of the EMG response in forearm muscles was about 16 msec, in hand muscles about 23 msec (Fig. 1) and in foot muscles about 34 msec in a moderately tall subject. These latencies imply fast conduction, probably in direct cortico-motoneurone pathways.

Sensation of the response

The subject does not feel that he is moving the limb; there is no sensation of effort, nor is there any discernible sensation referred to the moving limb. The impression is that the limb is moved by some external agent.

Character of the response

The effect of a single anodal motor cortex shock, or a train of such shocks, is to generate a fairly synchronous muscle action potential, followed by a silent period, which sometimes terminates in a rebound burst of activity (Fig. 1). The resulting muscle response is always a simple muscle twitch. Reciprocal inhibition, simple synergies and complex motor programs are never produced. The movement that occurs depends upon the muscles that are contracting at the time of the cortical shock.

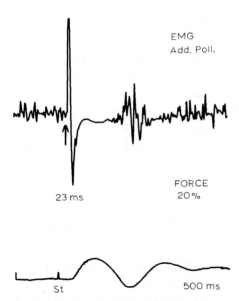

Fig. 1. Electromyogram (EMG) above and force record below from left adductor pollicis following motor cortical stimulation by a single anodal shock applied to the right scalp at the surface marking of the hand area. The subject (PAM) was exerting a background contraction of adductor pollicis to 20% of maximum. A single record is shown. The shock artefact is displayed 100 msec after the start of the sweep. A synchronous EMG action potential occurs with onset some 23 msec later.

Both the size of the action potential (and of the mechanical twitch resulting) and the duration of the subsequent silent period increase with increasing shock strength.

Cortical stimulation can command the whole muscle output

Although the EMG potential produced by a single shock to the motor cortex is synchronous, it is not as large as that which can be evoked by a supramaximal shock delivered directly to the motor nerve; presumably this is because of dispersion of the motor volley in cortico-motoneurone pathways. Marsden et al. (1981), however, were able to show that maximal twitches of adductor pollicis could be obtained by motor cortex stimulation. The mechanical twitch obtained by motor cortex stimulation was identical to that obtained by supramaximal stimulation of both ulnar and median nerves at the wrist, allowing for conduction delays.

Asterixis

The muscle twitch caused by a motor cortex shock is followed by a silent period in the EMG, associated with a lapse in muscle contraction. If the subject is maintaining a posture, say with the pronated arms outstretched, both an abrupt dorsiflexion of the wrist and fingers caused by the extensor twitch, and the subsequent brief drop of the hands are quite obvious. If the subject exerts a strong background force, or fully dorsiflexes the wrists and fingers, a motor cortex shock causes only the postural lapse, which is clinically indistinguishable from asterixis.

DISORDERED MOTOR CORTICAL FUNCTION

I will not discuss the well known effects of extensive damage to human motor cortex, which produce paralysis in a characteristic distribution, either with hypotonia or hypertonia, depending upon the extent of the lesion.

Rather, I wish to concentrate upon those clinical disorders in which there are abnormal cortical motor discharges. I believe it is possible to recognise 3 separate mechanisms by which such positive (in the sense of Hughlings Jackson) motor cortical phenomena occur.

(1) Spontaneous epilepsia partialis continua

In this situation there are repetitive, spontaneous focal muscle twitches localized to one part of the body, often the hand, which continue for days, weeks or months, often not ceasing in sleep. Many such cases have been described (see the review by Thomas et al. 1977). The output pathways from the motor cortex must be intact in such patients, otherwise there could be no cortically induced myoclonus. Damage elsewhere, perhaps in thalamus or even cerebellum or basal ganglia, causes loss of some inhibitory control of cortical function, such as to liberate a rhythmic, repetitive cortical discharge. Such cortical activity may, on occasion, spread to cause a typical Jacksonian motor seizure, or may become generalized to cause a grand mal fit.

(2) Cortical reflex myoclonus (somatosensory)

In these patients, reviewed elsewhere by Hallett et al. (1979), peripheral stimuli generate myoclonic jerks. Such patients often exhibit exaggerated giant sensory evoked potentials, indicating a loss of normal inhibition of cortical response to peripheral stimuli. The latter may be cutaneous in some patients, or muscle stretch in others, or a mixture of both. What seems to have occurred in these individuals is an exaggerated operation of normal transcortical cutaneous and stretch reflex mechanisms (Marsden et al. 1973).

The condition may be unilateral, or even confined to one limb, in some patients. Such focal cortical reflex myoclonus is often accompanied by unilateral exaggeration of the sensory evoked potentials. In others, the disorder is more widespread, but still an individual peripheral stimulus tends to evoke a local or focal myoclonic jerk in that limb. In other words, the jerking in such patients may be called multifocal rather than truly generalized.

In addition to myoclonic jerks evoked by extraneous peripheral stimuli, many such patients may exhibit myoclonus during voluntary movement ("action myoclonus"). However, this is not true spontaneous myoclonus, for voluntary movement itself generates peripheral input (quite apart from any internal "re-afference"). Thus, for example, Vallbo (1974) has shown that voluntary activation of muscle causes a burst of activity in human muscle spindle afferents, illustrating maintenance of normal alpha co-activation in these circumstances. Such a spindle volley may, itself, generate a myoclonic jerk in patients with cortical reflex myoclonus. Action myoclonus, therefore, may be provoked by mechanisms similar to those causing myoclonic jerking in response to external peripheral stimuli.

Cortical reflex myoclonus has been identified in patients with post-hypoxic myoclonus, post-traumatic myoclonus, post-encephalitic myoclonus, familial myoclonic epilepsy, spino-cerebellar degenerations of the Ramsay-Hunt variety, and in other symptomatic myoclonias.

As in epilepsia partialis continua, the output pathways from the motor cortex must be intact in this condition, but whether fast, direct cortico-motoneurone pathways are used in all cases or whether slower, indirect cortico-reticular or cortico-rubral pathways may be involved in some patients is not yet known.

(3) Cortical reflex myoclonus (auditory or visual)

Isolated photosensitive myoclonus is well recognized in some patients with epileptic myoclonus (Jeavons and Harding 1975). Isolated auditorily provoked myoclonus may underly some of the cases of excessive startle to sound that are included under the rubric of hyperreflexia but this has not been established. Many patients with diffuse progressive cerebral degenerations may exhibit myoclonus in response to sensory stimuli other than, or in addition to, somatosensory input. Thus patients with GM2 storage disease (Tay-Sach's) and its variants, or with ceroid neuronal lipofuscinosis (Batten) may exhibit myoclonic startle to a flash of light or a sudden sound, as well as to a tap on the bed. Presumably one mechanism for such photically or auditorily induced myoclonus is an exaggerated motor cortical response to cortico-cortical input from visual and auditory processing areas of the cerebral cortex. However, such detailed physiology requires further investigation.

CONCLUSION

The motor cortex may be looked upon as the "final common pathway" from cerebral cortex to spinal motoneurones. When destroyed, its loss leads to the negative phenomenon of focal paralysis. When its inhibitory inputs are damaged, or perhaps even when its internal arrangements are disturbed, it may either spontaneously discharge or it may respond excessively to a range of peripheral sensory, visual or auditory inputs to cause reflex myoclonus.

REFERENCES

Hallett, M., Chadwick, D. and Marsden, C.D. Cortical reflex myoclonus. Neurology (Minneap.), 1979, 29: 1107–1125.

Hill, D.K., McDonnell, M.J. and Merton, P.A. Direct stimulation of the adductor pollicis in man. J. Physiol. (Lond.), 1980, 300: 2–3P.

Jeavons, P.M. and Harding, G.F.A. Photosensitive epilepsy: a Review of the Literature and a Study of 460 Patients. Heinemann, London, 1975.

Marsden, C.D., Merton, P.A. and Morton, H.B. Is the human stretch reflex cortical rather than spinal? Lancet, 1973, 1: 759–761.

Marsden, C.D., Merton, P.A. and Morton, H.B. Maximal twitches from stimulation of the motor cortex in man. J. Physiol. (Lond.), 1981, 312: 5P.

Marsden, C.D., Merton, P.A. and Morton, H.B. Stimulation of the brain through the scalp in human subjects. In: J.E. Desmedt (Ed.), Motor Control Mechanisms in Man. Raven Press, New York, 1982, in press.

Merton, P.A. and Morton, H.B. Stimulation of the cerebral cortex in the intact human subject. Nature (Lond.), 1980, 285: 227 .

Thomas, J., Regan, M.J. and Klass, D.W. Epilepsia partialis continua. A review of 32 cases. Arch. Neurol. (Chic.), 1977, 34: 266–275.

Vallbo, A.B. Human muscle spindle discharge during isometric voluntary contractions. Acta physiol. scand., 1974, 90: 319–336.

8. Blood Levels of Drugs and the EEG

Kyoto Symposia (EEG Suppl. No. 36)
Editors: P.A. Buser, W.A. Cobb and T. Okuma
© 1982, Elsevier Biomedical Press, Amsterdam

437

Blood Levels of Drugs and the EEG — Introduction

H. MEINARDI (Chairman)

Instituut voor Epilepsiebestrijding "Meer en Bosch", P.O. Box 21, 2100 AA Heemstede
(The Netherlands)

During this symposium experts will discuss the tool of electroencephalography in the management of the pharmacotherapy of epilepsy.

There are two major questions.

(1) The use of drug profiles: (a) Can one subtract the drug effect from the EEG of the patient in order to obtain the true pattern of the brain function? (b) Can one classify drugs with respect to their therapeutic target on the basis of the EEG profile in healthy persons or animals? (c) Can one estimate from the EEG drug profile whether insufficient amounts of medication are given, notwithstanding adequate serum levels, or whether an abnormal reaction to medication is the basis of the therapeutic failure?

(2) What aspects have to be kept in mind when judging electroencephalograms in persons who take drugs?

I should like to mention the problem of drug withdrawal. For example, psychiatric patients have been classified as suffering from partial epilepsy with partial complex seizures because, after withdrawal of medication in order to obtain a "clean" EEG, spikes appeared in the temporal region; nicotine or, more correctly, smoking influences the EEG and even more so when the smoker is deprived of it. This phenomenon should be taken into account when studying the EEG, but particularly so when specific alterations due to drug therapy are under consideration.

Apart from the parameters studied by those who have investigated the influence of psychotropic drugs on the EEG, i.e., the power spectrum and the evoked responses, in the study of AED inter-ictal spikes are another measure which one might expect to be relevant in judging AED efficacy.

In studies on drug profiles in healthy volunteers rigid criteria have been applied with respect to the basic EEG pattern, the time of day and the amount of sleep on the day prior to the investigation.

The comparison of the drug profile in patients with the standardized drug profile in healthy persons may be complicated by the absence of standard conditions in the patient in the first place. Animal experiments may help to solve some of these problems. However, species differences may thwart these endeavours. Are, for example, reactions in less developed brains more stable, thus explaining differences in the findings of Drs. Lockhard and coworkers and of Dr. Binnie and coworkers?

Kyoto Symposia (EEG Suppl. No. 36)
Editors: P.A. Buser, W.A. Cobb and T. Okuma
© 1982, Elsevier Biomedical Press, Amsterdam

438

Therapeutic Concentration of Antiepileptic Drugs and the Severity of Epileptogenesis

MASAKAZU SEINO and NORIO KAKEGAWA

National Epilepsy Center, Shizuoka Higashi Hospital, Shizuoka 420 (Japan)

The therapeutic ranges of serum concentrations have been reported for the commonly used antiepileptic drugs; however, open studies, especially of polytherapy, are always an unsatisfactory way of examining the problem because too many factors are left uncontrolled. Lund (1974) was the first investigator to set up a prospective study on phenytoin levels. He suggested that the optimal level for each patient may have been dependent upon the severity of epilepsy. However, it was not proved.

For this reason, Schmidt and Janz (1977) carried out a prospective study on patients with grand mal seizures and reported that patients who needed high concentrations of phenytoin or phenobarbital (including primidone-derived phenobarbital) had a more severe form of epilepsy than those requiring lower concentrations. The severity of epilepsy in this study was quantified categorically by the frequency of grand mal seizures of each patient. According to their definition, the initial therapeutic concentrations were those of the patients whose grand mal seizures were completely controlled. The concentrations thus defined were unequivocally higher than the therapeutic maintenance concentrations of the patients who had a seizure-free period of several years. This finding was shown in a between-patient study rather than in a within-patient study; the possibility that the therapeutic concentrations might change during the course of epilepsy as a consequence of drug treatment was suggested.

In this context, a long-term observation was made in our clinic on epileptic patients who were eventually treated by monotherapy with either sodium valproate or carbamazepine. Emphasis was placed on a within-patient study rather than a between-patient one, and both the clinical seizures and EEG paroxysms were taken into account to evaluate the effect of antiepileptic drug treatment. On the other hand, a series of kindling experiments was carried out on cats to explore the variability of seizure threshold associated with long-standing medication and to examine whether the steady state therapeutic concentrations of antiepileptic drugs could modify the dissemination of epileptic discharges in time and space, as reflected clinically and electrographically.

Address correspondence to: Dr. M. Seino, National Epilepsy Center, Shizuoka Higashi Hospital, 886 Urushiyama, Shizuoka 420, Japan.

(1) SODIUM VALPROATE

A long-term observation was made on 176 patients who were successfully treated by chronic administration of sodium valproate as a sole drug. The mean age of the patients was 19.7 years, the mean duration of epilepsy was 9.7 years and the observation period of sodium valproate monotherapy extended from 12 to 57 months. Of the 176 patients, 127 were of primary generalized and 44 were of secondary generalized epilepsy. The seizure type was mostly generalized, either convulsive or non-convulsive. Blood specimens were taken as a rule 2.5 h after the first morning dose and the levels were determined either by gas liquid chromatography or the enzyme immunoassay technique (EMIT).

Fig. 1 illustrates a schematized course of drug treatment by polypharmacy toward monopharmacy. The clinical seizures were not sufficiently controlled during the polypharmacy regimen. When the more appropriate drug, sodium valproate in this series, was chosen and added to the previous medication a marked decrease of clinical seizures resulted. The co-medication was totally switched to monopharmacy and the patient's clinical seizures became completely suppressed thereafter, although inter-ictal epileptic discharges remained. In the course of treatment, two different steady state concentrations of the drug in question were distinguished. First, when the clinical seizures were completely suppressed by the introduction or increase of sodium valproate, the resultant level of dipropyl acetate was defined as an effect-developing concentration. On the other hand, when the long-standing suppression of clinical seizures was sustained, in spite of decreasing the dose or changing other

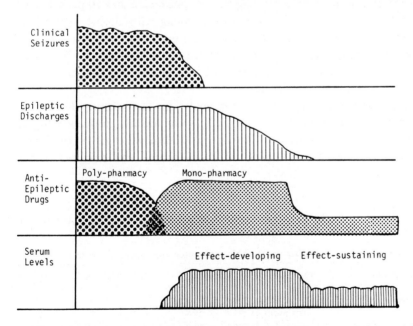

Fig. 1. Schematic presentation of the effect developing and sustaining concentrations in the long-term treatment course from polypharmacy toward monopharmacy.

drugs to sodium valproate as the sole drug, the resultant level was defined as an effect-sustaining concentration.

The effect-developing concentration of dipropyl acetate thus defined was significantly higher in the 176 patients who were eventually placed on sodium valproate successfully as compared with the effect-sustaining concentration, with respect to both tonic-clonic seizures; $104.8 \pm 28.3 \mu g/ml$ vs. $71.0 \pm 25.8 \mu g/ml$, and absence seizures; $120.8 \pm 30.9 \mu g/ml$ vs. $84.0 \pm 23.9 \mu g/ml$ (Table I) (Kakegawa et al. 1979). The difference between the two therapeutic concentrations was approximately related to the different doses of sodium valproate. Nonetheless, it is evident that the drug levels are a more reliable parameter than the oral doses to evaluate the therapeutic significance since there exists considerable inter- and intra-individual variability in the dose-level relationship of sodium valproate (Miyakoshi et al. 1979). These results basically agree with the finding of Schmidt and Janz (1977), who suggested that the between-patient variability of therapeutic values might reflect the different degrees of the severity of epilepsy. In this study, this possibility was reconfirmed by a within-patient observation over an extended period of time.

(2) CARBAMAZEPINE

An additional series of clinical studies was conducted on carbamazepine monotherapy. The subjects were 84 patients with partial seizures: 22 patients were totally untreated before the commencement of carbamazepine and 50 patients had generalized tonic-clonic convulsions occasionally, along with simple or complex partial seizures. The mean age was 23.5 years, the duration of epilepsy was 11.6 years and the monotherapy follow-up period ranged from 2 to 4 years. The serum carbamazepine concentrations were measured by EMIT from blood specimens taken as a rule 2.5 h after the first morning dose.

As in the previous study, two different concentrations were distinguished. The effect-developing concentration ($9.4 \pm 2.7 \mu g/ml$) was again significantly higher than the sustaining concentration ($6.1 \pm 1.6 \mu g/ml$) (Kakegawa et al. 1981b) (Table II). This finding on the carbamazepine effect on simple and complex partial

TABLE I

EFFECT-DEVELOPING AND SUSTAINING CONCENTRATIONS IN SODIUM VALPROATE MONOTHERAPY

GE, generalized epilepsy; GTC, generalized tonic-clonic convulsion; Abs, absence seizure.

AED	Diagnosis		Therapeutic levels ($\mu g/ml$)		Dose (mg/kg)	N
SV	GE	GTC	Developing	104.8 ± 28.3	18.1 ± 32.9	109
			Sustaining	71.0 ± 25.8	11.7 ± 4.2	40
SV	GE	Abs	Developing	120.8 ± 30.9	21.3 ± 7.3	48
			Sustaining	84.0 ± 23.9	15.3 ± 5.3	13

TABLE II

EFFECT-DEVELOPING AND SUSTAINING CONCENTRATIONS IN CARBAMAZEPINE MONOTHERAPY

Status	Level (µg/ml)	Dose (mg/kg)	N
Developing	9.4 ± 2.7	10.2 ± 3.8	45
Sustaining	6.1 ± 1.6	8.4 ± 3.5	16

seizures, including secondarily generalized tonic-clonic convulsions, also supports a hypothesis that the therapeutic concentrations may become lower as a consequence of drug treatment when successfully conducted during the long course of epilepsy (Seino 1980).

In the course of drug treatment it is often found that the inter-ictal epileptic paroxysms apparently remain long after the complete suppression of clinical seizures. Fig. 2 illustrates the decay of focal spike occurrence (mean number of spikes in the anterior temporal region per 5 min during light sleep) in relation to the steady state concentration of carbamazepine. The patient was a female, 23 years of age, with partial complex seizures occasionally evolving to generalized tonic-clonic convulsions. She had been untreated for 3 years prior to the commencement of carbamazepine. Within 1 week after the introduction of carbamazepine, both partial complex seizures and generalized convulsions were successfully suppressed. Nevertheless, the focal spike discharges persisted for 5 months while the serum levels were constantly maintained above 7 µg/ml. It is obvious that there is no direct temporal relation between the carbamazepine levels and EEG paroxysmal discharges.

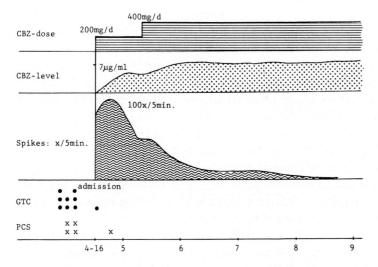

Fig. 2. A female patient with partial complex seizures (PCS) often evolving to generalized tonic-clonic convulsion (GTC) since age 10, untreated for the previous 3 years.

TABLE III

DURATION OF CLINICAL AND EEG SEIZURE MANIFESTATIONS PERSISTING AFTER THE COMMENCEMENT OF MONOTHERAPY

SV, sodium valproate; CBZ, carbamazepine.

Epilepsy	AED	Clinical seizure		N	EEG seizure		N
		Month	Max-min		Month	Max-min	
Primary generalized	SV	0.2	(0–7)	91	16.7	(1–61)	52
Secondary generalized	SV	1.1	(0–7)	37	20.0	(1–56)	25
Partial	CBZ	1.6	(0–8)	51	15.8	(1–33)	9

The duration of both the clinical and EEG seizure manifestations that persisted following the commencement of monotherapy, using either sodium valproate or carbamazepine, with respect to the type of epilepsy is shown in Table III. The seizures of primary generalized epilepsy, regardless of whether convulsive or non-convulsive, were controlled by sodium valproate in most cases within a week. Those of secondary generalized epilepsy controlled also by sodium valproate, and those of partial epilepsy controlled by carbamazepine, required more than 1 month. In contrast, the EEG seizure discharges persisted more than 1.5 year, irrespective of the type of epilepsy, following complete freedom from clinical seizures. Thus, there is a delayed onset of the therapeutic effect which works to suppress clinical seizures; the length of the delay depends on the aetiology of the epilepsy, whether idiopathic or symptomatic.

(3) AN EXPERIMENTAL STUDY

Since antiepileptic drugs in clinical practice are given for extended periods of time, it is essential that they be evaluated in experimental models during long-term treatment. A series of long-range experiments was carried out to evaluate conventional and potential new drugs, using kindled cats whose final stage of generalized convulsions was already established, as opposed to kindling animals whose clinical stages were still developing.

Fig. 3 illustrates the time course of a cat (No. 63) that was exposed to consecutive amygdaloid kindling stimulation for more than 6 months. The details of the experimental methods followed those of Wada and Sato (1974). Four drug sessions were introduced, with each session lasting for 2–3 weeks followed by a 2 week post-drug intermission. Stimulation was given 6 days a week, and the drugs were all given by mouth once a day, 7 days a week (Fig. 3).

The first drug tried was AD 810. This is a newly developed antiepileptic compound, 3-sulfamoylmethyl-1,2-benzisoxazole, which is at present undergoing phase 1 trials. The elimination half-life was about 60 h in humans and 20 h in cats (Ito et al. 1981). In the first drug session, a 50 mg dose of AD 810 orally given for

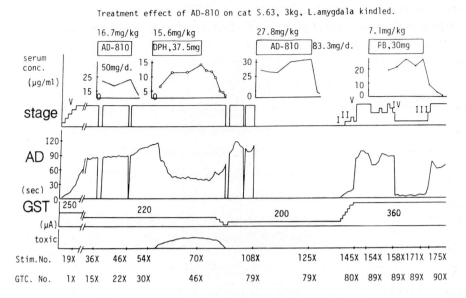

Fig 3. Treatment effect of chronic oral medication of AD 810 and diphenylhydantoin (DPH) examined in amygdaloid-kindled preparation of a cat. AD, after-discharge; GST, generalized seizure triggering threshold.

13 days failed to suppress the established generalized seizures. The serum levels of the compound were at about 20 μg/ml. On the contrary, in the third session, the generalized seizures were totally abolished by giving an increased dose of the compound not only during the medication period, with the steady state concentrations above 25 μg/ml, but also for 2 weeks following the discontinuation of the drug even though the serum level was zero. In other words, the therapeutic effect was definitely carried over in the post-drug period, as was demonstrated in valproate-infused monkeys with alumina cream foci by Lockard and Levy (1976). It was noteworthy that post-drug rekindling was only successfully elicited when the generalized seizure triggering threshold was increased from 200 to 360 μA; that is, the seizure susceptibility was obviously lowered as a consequence of chronic medication accompanied by complete suppression of clinical seizures. A similar phenomenon regarding generalized seizure triggering thresholds was reconfirmed in 4 other cats.

In a second series, 37.5 mg of phenytoin were given orally for 19 days, yielding serum levels above 10 μg/ml which resulted in the appearance of toxic signs such as ataxia and drowsiness. Nevertheless, the clinical seizure stage never regressed throughout the drug session. These results agree with the findings of Wada et al. (1976) that prophylactic administration of phenytoin was totally ineffective in suppressing established convulsions in amygdaloid-kindled cats.

Fig. 4 shows the seizure discharge propagation on the 52nd day of kindling immediately before phenytoin medication. The after-discharges generalized toward both subcortical and cortical structures and terminated 79 sec after stimulation. In contrast, on the 70th day of kindling, or on the 20th day of phenytoin medication, the after-discharge propagated more rapidly to the midbrain reticular formation and the cortex as compared with the pre-drug kindling (Fig. 5). It then generalized to the entire brain as early as 14 sec after stimulation followed by exaggerated clonic

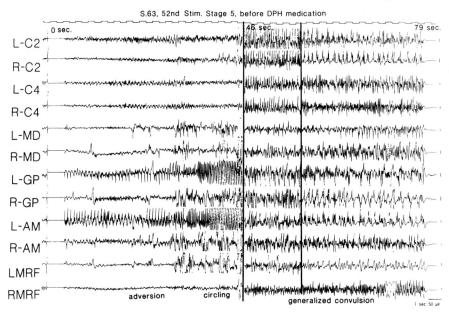

Fig. 4. Pattern of after-discharge propagation before the administration of phenytoin. C, cortex; MD, nucleus medialis dorsalis of thalamus; GP, globus pallidus; AM, amygdala (L-AM is the stimulation site); MRF, midbrain reticular formation.

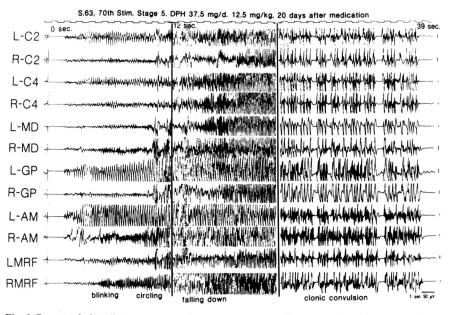

Fig. 5. Pattern of after-discharge propagation on the 20th day after phenytoin medication. Abbreviations are the same as in Fig. 4.

convulsions. The whole seizure duration was 39 sec, which was about one-half of the pre-drug kindling time (Kakegawa et al. 1981a).

SUMMARY

In sodium valproate monotherapy for generalized seizures and carbamazepine for partial seizures, it was found in a within-patient follow-up study that the effect-developing concentrations which were sufficient to suppress the clinical seizures were significantly higher than the effect-sustaining concentrations by which long-standing suppression was maintained. There was a delayed onset of therapeutic effect which worked to suppress the clinical and electrographic seizure manifestations, and the length of the delay depended on the nature of the epilepsy.

In animal experiments, the possibility that the severity of epilepsy may become milder as a consequence of successful pharmacotherapy was reconfirmed in amygdaloid-kindled cats on chronic medication in place of kindling animals on acute prophylactic medication. Only when the established generalized seizures were completely suppressed, was the generalized seizure triggering threshold evidently elevated.

Since epilepsy is a long-standing condition lasting for years to decades, short-spanned cross-sectional observations are often misleading. Whatever relationship might exist between the blood levels of antiepileptic drugs and the paroxysmal discharges in the EEG, the severity of epileptogenesis as well as the longitudinal time course must always be taken into consideration in the drug treatment of epilepsy.

ACKNOWLEDGEMENT

This work was supported in part by research grants from the Ministry of Health and Welfare for nervous diseases, 1979 and 1980.

REFERENCES

Ito, T., Sekine, M., Shimizu, M., Ishida, S. and Seino, M. Pharmacokinetic studies on AD-810, a new antiepileptic compound: phase 1 trials. Abstracts Epilepsy International Congress, 1981: 188–189.

Kakegawa, N., Miyakoshi, M. and Seino, M. Monopharmacy by sodium valproate and the blood concentration. Abstracts 11th Epilepsy International Symposium, Florence, 1979: 153.

Kakegawa, N., Higashi, T., Morikawa, T., Osawa, T. and Seino, M. Treatment effects of a new antiepileptic compound, AD-810 on kindled cats. Abstracts Epilepsy International Congress, 1981a: 189–190.

Kakegawa, N., Miyakoshi, N. and Seino, M. Carbamazepine monopharmacy for 80 patients with partial seizures. Abstracts Epilepsy International Congress, 1981b: 256.

Lockard, J.S. and Levy, R. Valproic acid: Reversibly acting drug? Epilepsia, 1976, 17: 477–479.

Lund, L. Anticonvulsant effect of diphenylhydantoin relative to plasma levels. A prospective 3-year study in ambulant patients with generalized epileptic seizures. Arch. Neurol. (Chic.), 1974, 31: 289–294.

Miyakoshi, M., Kakegawa, N., Sagisaka, M. and Seino, M. Serum concentration of sodium valproate — Age factor and an interaction with phenytoin. (In Japanese.) Brain Develop., 1979, 11: 567–576.

Schmidt, D. and Janz, D. Therapeutic plasma concentrations of phenytoin and phenobarbitone. In: C. Gardner-Thorpe (Ed.), Antiepileptic Drug Monitoring. Pitman Medical, London, 1977: 214–225.

Seino, M. Clinical implication of therapeutic serum concentration of antiepileptic drugs. Brain Develop., 1980, 2: 241.

Wada, J.A. and Sato, M. Generalized convulsive seizure induced by daily electrical stimulation of the amygdala in cats: correlative electrographic and behavioral features. Neurology (Minneap.), 1974, 24: 565–574.

Wada, J.A., Sato, M., Wake, A., Green, J.R. and Troupin, A.S. Prophylactic effects of phenytoin, phenobarbital, and carbamazepine examined in kindling cat preparations. Arch. Neurol. (Chic.), 1976, 33: 426–434.

Kyoto Symposia (EEG Suppl. No. 36)
Editors: P.A. Buser, W.A. Cobb and T. Okuma
© 1982, Elsevier Biomedical Press, Amsterdam

447

Blood Levels and the Quantitative EEG Response to CNS-Active Drugs: Retrospective Observations*

P. IRWIN and M. FINK

Department of Psychiatry and the Long Island Research Institute, Health Sciences Center, State University of New York at Stony Brook, Stony Brook, N.Y. 11794 (U.S.A.)

The principal therapies in the treatment of epileptic patients and the mentally ill are drugs which are active in the central nervous system (CNS). Evidence for CNS activity has been provided by the computer quantified electroencephalogram (EEG). In experiments designed to include EEG measurements before and after drug administration, it has been shown that psychoactive substances alter the distribution of EEG frequencies in patterns associated with their clinical effects (Fink 1969, 1978, 1980). The variable influence of psychosocial factors on the EEG, such as situational anxiety and drowsiness related to sleep time, is minimized in crossover designs using placebo controls.

Quantitative EEG data in normal volunteers can establish whether a drug is psychoactive and, therefore, of probable clinical use in the treatment of the mentally ill. Such data also permit: estimation of the time course of the drug response; classification of drugs; identification of differences between doses, drug formulations and routes of administration; and comparison of the potency of compounds of the same class.

Conclusions in these pharmaco-EEG studies are based on statistical inferences from a group of subjects given a single low dose of drug. Within these groups, however, individual responses may vary greatly. While the processes intervening between drug ingestion and the EEG response in man are complex, techniques for measuring drug concentration in the blood have been investigated. We sought 2 relationships between blood drug levels and the EEG response: the correlation within subjects over time and the correlation across subjects at a single time. We review here the results from previously reported studies and discuss a general problem in drug-response relationships. More detailed descriptions of the methods and findings are reported in Fink et al. (1976, 1977, 1979).

METHODS

In these studies, we examined single doses of substances given to normal, healthy, male volunteers, between 19 and 29 years old, and weighing between 50 and 90 kg. Written consent was obtained from each subject during a screening interview in

---

* Aided, in part, by grants from the International Association for Psychiatric Research, St. James, N.Y. 11780, U.S.A.

which procedures were demonstrated and study purposes, risks, and range of drug effects were explained. Two of the studies were placebo controlled and designed for a balanced drug order. A minimum of 1 week intervened between repeated sessions. The EEG was recorded from bipolar leads for 15 min, using subdermal electrodes. Subjects were resting with their eyes closed. Records were made before, and at fixed intervals after, drug administration. Vigilance was controlled by having subjects open their eyes for 40 sec every 5 min and by a continuous performance task (Fink 1978). The left occipital to vertex derivation was quantified by baseline crossing or power spectral density analysis, using an IBM 1800 computer analytic system. Blood sampling followed EEG recording. EEG variables which statistically discriminated drug from placebo were selected for association with blood drug levels.

OBSERVATIONS

(A) Diazepam and bromazepam (Fink et al. 1976)

Diazepam and bromazepam are benzodiazepines, recommended as sedative anxiolytics for psychiatric patients. In this study, bromazepam was an investigational drug and diazepam was used as a standard for comparison. The EEG and blood were sampled in 12 volunteers before, and at 0.5, 1, and 2 h after, oral ingestion of diazepam (10 mg), bromazepam (9 mg) or placebo.

These doses of diazepam and bromazepam elicited a characteristic behavioural and EEG fast (13–35 c/sec) response at 1 and 2 h after dosing (Fig. 1). They were equivalent in time course and in the potency of their effect on the EEG. The blood levels of bromazepam, however, were approximately half those of diazepam. The

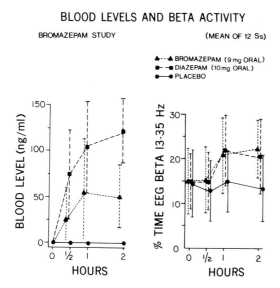

Fig. 1. Blood drug concentrations and EEG beta activity (means and standard deviations of 12 subjects). Both EEG and blood drug levels show peak values at 1 and 2 h post-drug. Taken from Fink et al. 1976.

sensitivity of the assay for bromazepam was 10 ng/ml, as compared to 1 ng/ml for diazepam.

Within 11 of the subjects, there were good temporal relationships between drug minus placebo differences in EEG fast activity and the blood drug concentration. But there were large individual differences in response sensitivity and in drug levels. EEG change and blood drug levels were not correlated across subjects at any single time of sampling for either drug.

(B) Mianserin (Fink et al. 1977)

Mianserin (GB-94) is a tetracyclic antidepressant substance. Early in the course of investigation of this compound, 4 volunteers received 15 mg on 2 occasions at least 10 days apart. This dose of mianserin was selected to ensure measurable levels of free base in the plasma, although EEG changes were demonstrable at one-third this dose. Twenty minutes of EEG were recorded before dosing and at 0.25, 0.5, 1, 2, 3, 5, 7 and 24 h afterwards. Each recording was followed by a blood and urine sample and measurement of the critical flicker-fusion frequency. During the EEG recording, a count was kept of buzzer button releases and, at 5 min intervals, subjects were asked to rate their alertness.

Data were averaged over the 4 subjects in each session separately. Among EEG variables, delta (0.5–4.5 c/sec) activity showed the greatest change from baseline. For comparison of the time courses of the various measures, the means for each measure were transformed to a percentage of the maximum mean change from the pre-drug level (Fig. 2). The changes in plasma drug levels corresponded well with the changes in each response measure and were similar in the two sessions. There was a latency of less than 1 h between the peak drug concentration and the peaks of the other measures. After 24 h, the EEG alone among the response measures reflected the continued activity of mianserin. Other response measures showed a return to baseline. Mianserin levels in the blood and urine were still measurable at this time.

This study demonstrated that within-subject relationships between plasma drug levels and response measures were highly replicable. Of the measures of response, the EEG showed the most consistent time relationship to drug concentration.

(C) Phenytoin (Fink et al. 1979)

A series of studies was undertaken with the anticonvulsant phenytoin (diphenylhydantoin, DPH). In pilot experiments, we explored dosing strategies and determined the minimum doses and times of sampling at which effects on the EEG were measurable. In 2 subjects, blood samples were drawn at times of EEG recording up to 8 h after dosing. An increase in the EEG average frequency corresponded to a rise in the plasma concentration of phenytoin after a divided dose of 1 g (Fig. 3). In 1 subject (P.B.) plasma levels and EEG average frequency showed a rise to a peak in the 4th hour after initial dosing. In the 2nd subject (F.H.), a rise to the peak occurred for both measures in the 6th hour.

Based on these and other EEG data, we designed a phenytoin-placebo study in which the EEG and blood were sampled in 12 volunteers before, and at multiple

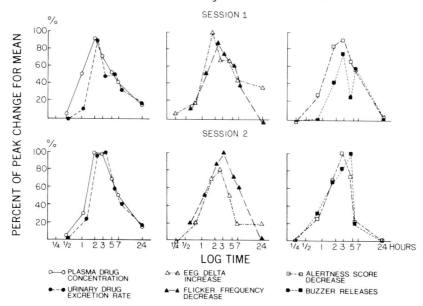

Fig. 2. Mean differences (post-drug minus baseline) of 4 subjects, expressed as percentages of the maximum mean difference in either session. The similarity in time course between EEG and plasma drug levels is seen to replicate. See Fink et al. 1977.

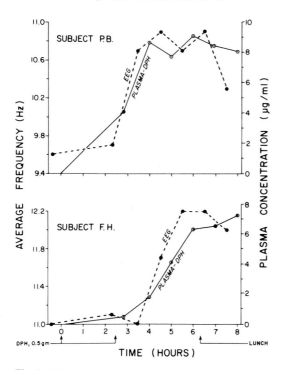

Fig. 3. EEG average frequency and plasma drug levels before and after administration of a divided dose of 1 g of phenytoin (DPH) to 2 subjects. EEG and plasma drug levels show parallel latencies to peak. Taken from Fink et al. 1979.

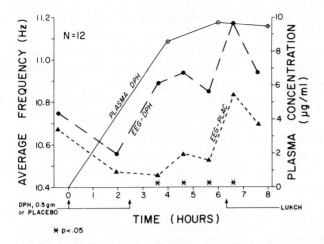

Fig. 4. EEG average frequency and plasma drug levels before and after administration of a divided dose of 1 g phenytoin (DPH) and EEG average frequency before and after placebo administration (means of 12 subjects). Asterisks indicate main effect of drug in analysis of covariance. Taken from Fink et al. 1979.

times after a divided dose of either 1 g of phenytoin or placebo. Half of the dose was administered at time 0 and the other half after 2.5 h, with EEG sampling at 2, 3.5, 4.5, 5.5, 6.5 and 7.5 h, and blood sampling at 4, 6 and 8 h.

In this study, the average phenytoin plasma level in the 12 subjects rose to a peak by the 6th hour, and remained on a plateau for the duration of the session (Fig. 4). The latency to response after dosing varied among individuals with the rate of rise in the plasma drug levels. Again, we failed to find a significant correlation across subjects between EEG responses and plasma levels of drug.

DISCUSSION

These studies show a relationship, with varying latency, between plasma concentrations and the quantified EEG response to drugs in analyses within subjects over time, but not in group data at a single time. Inferences from these studies are limited by the small samples and the single doses used.

A few authors have investigated the relationship between EEG and blood drug levels in patients, using larger samples and "steady state" drug concentrations. Rosadini and Sannita (1979) computer-analysed EEG records from 29 adult patients treated for generalized epilepsy. At the time of referral, the patients had been free from seizures for many months and were on differing daily doses of phenobarbital. The authors found a correlation ($r = 0.34$; $P = 0.01$) between EEG average frequency and the plasma concentration of phenobarbital at drug levels below 40 μg/ml; but the extent to which the within-subject correlations contributed to this relationship is unclear, since they showed 59 data points from 29 patients.

An additional complication arises from the fact that, unlike blood drug level measurements, the value of an EEG measure at baseline is not zero, and is not uniform among subjects. Consequently, it is unclear what measure of EEG has ordinal biological meaning across individuals. We have sought a correlation between EEG data and blood drug levels using post-drug EEG values, post-drug EEG differences from baseline and post-drug EEG differences from post-placebo at corresponding times. The latter approach improved the within-subject correlation in some cases, but no approach yielded a significant correlation across subjects. We are presently exploring a normalizing transform which relates the change in an EEG measure to the mean and variability of baseline and post-placebo data for each subject separately. In other studies, we have succesfully used this transform to identify a direct dose relationship to EEG response (Fink and Irwin 1981). We have also found a new measure, the spectral difference index, to be useful in assessing the global effects of substances on EEG (Irwin 1982). This index is an average per Hz of the absolute difference between post-drug and baseline 1−30 Hz relative power spectra. We believe that, across subjects, plasma drug levels may better correlate with these measures than with the activity in individual frequency bands, the mean frequency, or the mean amplitude, but the issue requires additional study.

SUMMARY

Quantitative EEG measures provide reliable, non-invasive indices of CNS effects of drugs in man. In pharmaco-EEG studies of CNS-active substances, we found that EEG changes correlated with blood drug levels within individuals over time, and showed the correlation to be replicable. Across individuals at single times, however, correlations were not evident. In seeking relationships across subjects, techniques which adjust for EEG baseline differences between subjects are under investigation.

REFERENCES

Fink, M. EEG and human psychopharmacology. Ann. Rev. Pharmacol., 1969, 9: 241−258.

Fink, M. EEG and psychopharmacology. Electroenceph. clin. Neurophysiol., 1978, 45: 41−56.

Fink, M. An objective classification of psychoactive drugs. Prog. Neuropsychopharmacol., 1980, 4: 495−502.

Fink, M. and Irwin, P. Pharmaco-electroencephalographic study of brotizolam, a novel hypnotic: comparison with flurazepam. Clin. Pharmacol. Ther., 1981, 30: 336−342.

Fink, M., Irwin, P., Weinfeld, R.E., Schwartz, M.A. and Conney, A.H. Blood levels and electroencephalographic effects of diazepam and bromazepam. Clin. Pharmacol. Ther., 1976, 20: 184−191.

Fink, M., Irwin, P., Gastpar, M. and de Ridder, J.J. EEG, blood level, and behavioral effects of the antidepressant mianserin (ORG GB-94). Psychopharmacologia (Berl.), 1977, 54: 249−254.

Fink, M., Irwin, P., Sannita, W., Papakostas, Y. and Green, M.A. Phenytoin: EEG effects and plasma levels in volunteers. Ther. Drug Monitor., 1979, 1: 93−103.

Irwin, P. Spectral difference index: a single EEG measure of drug effect. Electroenceph. clin. Neurophysiol., 1982, 54: 342−346.

Rosadini, G. and Sannita, W.G. Quantitative EEG in relation to plasma concentration during treatment with antiepileptic drugs. In: B. Saletu, P. Barner and L. Hollister (Eds.), Neuropsychopharmacology. Pergamon Press, Oxford, 1979: 417−425.

Kyoto Symposia (EEG Suppl. No. 36)
Editors: P.A. Buser, W.A. Cobb and T. Okuma
© 1982, Elsevier Biomedical Press, Amsterdam

The Influence of Antiepileptic Drugs on the Electroencephalogram: a Review of Controlled Clinical Studies*

DIETER SCHMIDT

Abteilung für Neurologie, Klinikum Charlottenburg, Freie Universität Berlin, Spandauer Damm 130, 1000 Berlin 19 (F.R.G.)

Our knowledge of the effects of antiepileptic drugs (AED) on the EEG in humans has improved in recent years through a number of methodological refinements. These include the quantitative determination of AED in plasma and the introduction of controls in EEG trials. Ideally, serial EEG observations are performed in the same patient at different plasma concentrations — preferably during one drug treatment. Furthermore, intensive monitoring of EEG for 24 h or longer and additional sophisticated quantitative analytical techniques such as computerized analysis and the use of evoked potentials have been made feasible by recent technological developments (Wolpaw and Penry 1978; Lopes da Silva et al. 1979; Saito 1979). A number of reviews covered the relationship of EEG and antiepileptic drugs at a time when therapeutic drug monitoring was less available (Müller and Müller 1972; Ketz 1974; Bente 1975; Gastaut and Tassinari 1975; Longo 1977). It is therefore the aim of this review to include primarily controlled clinical studies with measurements of plasma concentrations of antiepileptic drugs and adequate controls.

BENZODIAZEPINES

The EEG effects of benzodiazepines and more specifically of clonazepam and diazepam were recently reviewed by Browne (1976), Browne and Penry (1973), Pinder et al. (1976) and Schmidt (1982). A number of studies support a good correlation of serial EEG changes and the plasma concentration of diazepam and clonazepam (Table I). Booker and Celesia (1973) demonstrated that suppression of spontaneous paroxysmal discharges and protection against flickering light stimulation in photosensitive subjects were correlated with the serum concentration of diazepam. Fink et al. (1976) correlated blood levels with EEG effects of diazepam in volunteers; diazepam caused an increase in beta activity (above 13 c/sec) and a decrease in alpha activity (9–11 c/sec) in the EEG. There was only a weak correlation between plasma levels of diazepam and the amount of increased beta

---

* With support of the Deutsche Forschungsgemeinschaft (Schm 448-5-3).

TABLE I

CONTROLLED TRIALS ON THE EFFECT OF ANTIEPILEPTIC DRUGS ON THE HUMAN EEG

| Drug | EEG changes | Correlation of EEG changes with | | Authors |
		Plasma concentration of an antiepileptic drug	Seizure frequency	
Carbamazepine	Focal paroxysmal discharge	No	No	Monaco et al. 1980
Clonazepam	Increase in beta activity	Yes, not in all patients	n.s.	Dumermuth et al. 1976, 1977
Diazepam	Suppression of paroxysmal discharge and photosensitivity; increase in beta activity decrease in alpha activity	Yes	Yes	Booker and Celesia 1973
		Weak	n.s.	Fink et al. 1976
Phenobarbital	Focal paroxysmal discharge; increase in absolute power of fast frequencies (> 16 c/sec)	Yes	Yes	Buchthal et al. 1968; Kellaway et al. 1978; Sannita et al. 1980

n.s. = not studied.

activity. The possible use of quantitative beta assessment in patients receiving mostly clonazepam was recently studied by Dumermuth et al. (1976, 1977). In a few cases there was a good correlation with the clonazepam blood levels, but in most cases the correlation was questionable (Dumermuth et al. 1976).

Evidence for the suppression of paroxysmal discharges (Kato and Mori 1977; Kurokawa et al. 1979) and also of clinical seizures in acute treatment of status epilepticus (Bücking 1977; Congdon and Forsythe 1980; Schmidt 1981) by intravenous diazepam and clonazepam is well documented. Furthermore, long-term treatment with oral clonazepam was shown to reduce the frequency and the duration of spike-wave paroxysms in 12 h telemetered EEGs (Dreifuss et al. 1975). During chronic treatment with clonazepam the correlation between EEG changes and clinical seizure frequency was found to be poor in patients with focal epilepsy (Bielmann et al. 1978).

CARBAMAZEPINE

A double-blind study of carbamazepine and the EEG of epileptic patients revealed a significant increase in diffuse slow waves and an increase in generalized epileptic discharges without significant correlation with seizure incidence (Table I). Also, hyperventilation-induced generalized epileptic discharges were more frequent in patients with a high seizure incidence compared to patients with a low seizure incidence and patients taking phenytoin. No significant focal EEG changes were observed during carbamazepine treatment. There was no relationship between the amounts of EEG epileptiform activity and the serum levels of either carbamazepine or phenytoin. This conclusion was, however, based on single EEG observations in each patient. Unfortunately, no serial observations were performed (Wilkus et al. 1978). EEG telemetry did not reveal a statistically significant difference in the number of paroxysmal discharges between carbamazepine and primidone in a study on epileptic outpatients. Power density spectral analysis showed that the patients had significantly more beta activity while on primidone and more theta activity while on carbamazepine (Rodin et al. 1976).

In another study on the EEG, seizures and plasma level correlations in patients on chronic treatment with carbamazepine, the EEG was substantially unchanged and did not correlate with the fluctuations in dose variations and seizure frequency. The majority of patients with improved seizure control had plasma levels of 5–10 μg/ml carbamazepine, and irregular and frankly abnormal EEGs (Monaco et al. 1980). In one investigation, carbamazepine led to some increase in paroxysmal focal discharges with variable correlations with seizure frequency (Pryse-Phillips and Jeavons 1970). The authors suggested that the EEG is of limited value in the evaluation of the therapeutic efficacy of carbamazepine.

ETHOSUXIMIDE

The evidence is not yet available that the clinical control or suppression of paroxysmal discharges is directly related to plasma levels of ethosuximide in those patients who are capable of complete control by this drug (Penry et al. 1972). In a recent study, treatment with ethosuximide altered the pattern of time modulation of spike-wave activity in generalized epilepsy and eventually, when the spike-and-wave activity was reduced to a low level, the time distribution became random (Kellaway et al. 1980).

PHENOBARBITAL

The relation of EEG and seizures to phenobarbital in the serum was investigated as early as 1968 by Buchthal et al. (Table I). In serial observations of the EEG they reported on 11 patients with grand mal epilepsy that the paroxysmal activity in the EEG decreased with increasing concentrations of phenobarbital in the serum. The incidence was reduced to one-tenth of the initial value at a mean concentration of 10 μg/ml with a range of 3–22 μg/ml (Buchthal et al. 1968). In a more recent study, Kellaway et al. (1978) monitored 12 children with partial seizures and spike foci for 24 or 36 h before and following treatment with phenobarbital. The EEG spikes were counted and measured using computer-assisted visual analysis. Prior to treatment there was no correlation between the number of spikes and the manner of their occurrence and clinical seizure control. However, a direct quantitative relationship was found between the effect of phenobarbital on the spike discharges and its effect on clinical seizures. In 6 of 11 children with complete seizure control absence of spike activity was found in the post-treatment monitoring study. In the other 5 patients, a 20–30% reduction in the number of spikes occurred, but the major change was a reduction in the amplitude, duration and field area of the spike. In the former group, with increasing blood levels of phenobarbital, the spike discharges disappeared first in rapid eye movement sleep, then in the awake state, and finally in nocturnal slow wave sleep. The authors convincingly demonstrated a correlation of susceptibility of inter-ictal spikes to phenobarbital plasma concentrations.

The effect of diazepam and phenobarbital on the EEG was studied in newborns by Couto-Sales et al. (1979). Plasma levels of phenobarbital and diazepam were measured at the time of the EEG recording and ranged from 3 to 26 μg/ml phenobarbital and 0 to 2.75 μg/ml diazepam. The authors concluded that the observed EEG changes were related to the severity of the clinical condition and not due to the influence of the drugs.

In an investigation on EEG effects and plasma concentrations of phenobarbital in volunteers, a single dose of phenobarbital resulted in plasma concentrations of 2.1–7.6 μg/ml 1 h after the administration and was followed by a consistent increase in the absolute power of EEG frequencies above 16 c/sec. The EEG changes and plasma levels were substantially parallel in time course with a 5–7 h delay for the

EEG effects (Sannita et al. 1980). In a single observation Niedermeyer et al. (1977) noted the absence of drug-induced beta activity in epileptic patients with severe epilepsy. The authors wondered whether the absence of a fast drug response may be a sign of serious cerebral impairment. In a single dose experimental study in rats there was a good correlation of serum levels of phenobarbital and fast EEG changes. When serum levels were higher than 25 μg/ml, the b_1 and b_2 bands increased. Above 35 μg/ml theta waves decreased significantly (Sato 1980). The author suggests that the significant increase of fast waves resulted from the inhibition of the reticular system and the significant decrease of theta waves at higher phenobarbital levels mainly resulted from depression of the cortex.

Finally, EEG changes are also observed during the withdrawal of barbiturates in addicts (Essig and Fraser 1958). Patients with epilepsy have also been reported to show significant EEG changes during withdrawal (Spencer et al. 1981). These EEG changes include mainly the activation of focal discharges.

PHENYTOIN

Over 20 years ago, in the first paper on EEG correlations with serum levels of phenytoin, Buchthal et al. (1960) noted a reduced incidence of paroxysmal abnormalities in the EEG when the serum concentration of phenytoin was above 10 μg/ml, while it was increased with serum levels below 10 μg/ml (Table II). Several years later a quantitative study was done on the acute effects of intravenous phenytoin on the EEGs of 8 epileptic patients (Riehl and McIntyre 1968). The EEG data were automatically analysed and quantitated, using the frequency : voltage ratio as an index of EEG activity. In that study 250 mg phenytoin induced a moderate degree (20–25%) of slowing or a concomitant increase in amplitude, or both, 10–15 min after the end of the injection. No changes were observed in non-epileptic controls and in the unaffected hemisphere of patients with unilateral EEG abnormalities. This suggests that the phenytoin effect may be influenced by existing alterations in the blood-brain barrier or indicate a preferential effect of the drug for abnormal neurones. Which of these considerations is more relevant is still not known today. In a recent study, EEG effects and plasma levels were investigated in volunteers (Fink et al. 1979) following oral administration of phenytoin. The EEG showed decreases in power in the slow frequencies and increases in the fast frequencies, accompanied by an increase in mean frequency. These changes occurred at phenytoin plasma levels of more than 8 μg/ml. Furthermore, the time course and the intensity of the EEG effects were correlated. EEG changes at plasma levels of 8–12 μg/ml were not associated with behavioural toxic signs.

A number of recent reports dealt with EEG changes in patients with clinical signs of phenytoin toxicity. Nordentoft-Jensen and Grynderup (1966) found transitory increases of 5–7 c/sec slow waves correlated with increased phenytoin plasma concentrations and clinical drug toxicity. Iivanainen et al. (1978) showed a higher incidence of EEG abnormalities in mentally retarded epileptic patients as compared

TABLE II

CONTROLLED TRIALS ON THE EFFECT OF ANTIEPILEPTIC DRUGS ON THE HUMAN EEG

Drug	EEG changes	Correlation of EEG changes with		Authors
		Plasma concentration of an antiepileptic drug	Seizure frequency	
Phenytoin	Focal paroxysmal discharge; slowing of frequency, decrease in power in slow frequencies; increase in fast frequencies sharp transients	Yes	Yes	Buchthal et al. 1960; Nordentoft-Jensen and Grynderup 1966; Riehl and McIntyre 1968; Fink et al. 1979; Wilkus and Green 1974; Carrie 1976
Phenytoin and phenobarbital or primidone	Slowing of background; paroxysmal discharge	Yes	Yes	Rowan et al. 1975; Shimuzu 1979
	paroxysmal discharge	No	No	Couto-Sales et al. 1979
Primidone	Slowing of background	Yes	Clinical toxicity	Brillman et al. 1974
Sodium valproate	Generalized paroxysmal discharge	Yes	Yes, delayed	Rowan et al. 1979a, b, 1980; Adams et al. 1978; Bruni et al. 1980
	Generalized and focal paroxysmal discharge	No	No	Gram et al. 1977; Villarreal et al. 1978

to phenytoin-treated patients without intoxication. Unfortunately, serial observations were not performed.

Roseman (1961) described serial EEG observations showing a slowing in the alpha range in mild cases and marked high voltage delta activity, sometimes occurring in paroxysms, in severe cases of phenytoin intoxication. He suggested that the combination of mild clinical toxicity and slowed alpha activity may be used as a satisfactory index to judge the titrating end point of a particular dosage of phenytoin in the management of seizures. More recently, Ahmad et al. (1975) showed an increase in the dominant EEG frequency from 4–6 to 6–7 c/sec in a patient recovering from phenytoin intoxication. A generalized slowing characterized by 5–7 c/sec theta activity mixed with low voltage fast activity was also reported in patients with phenytoin intoxication by Murphy and Goldstein (1974) and Logan and Freeman (1969). Levy and Fenichel (1965) described a marked increase in slow activity with hypersynchronous 4–12 c/sec waves in a patient with phenytoin-activated seizures.

A negative study with retrospective design found no correlation between single EEG observations and the plasma concentration of phenytoin and phenobarbital (Bendarzewska-Nawrocka and Pietruszewska 1980). In recent years, however, a number of prospective studies confirmed that there is a good correlation of EEG changes and the plasma concentration of phenytoin. Wilkus and Green (1974) reported that the amount of paroxysmal discharges decreased with increased plasma levels of phenytoin in 11 of 13 patients when the waking EEG was studied. In the sleeping EEG, however, a good correlation was found in only 7 of 11 patients. In a quantitative analysis of EEG background rhythms in patients with epilepsy, the slow background activity was correlated with a number of variables. These included high serum levels of phenobarbital or phenytoin, high seizure frequencies, early onset of epilepsy and complex partial seizures (Shimuzu 1979). The degree of slow EEG background activity increased with the number of these factors involved.

Finally, in a rather complex study, the frequency of inter-ictal "sharp transients" in the EEG decreased with falling phenytoin plasma levels and increased with raised phenytoin plasma levels (Carrie 1976). The diagnostic relevance of sharp transients in relation to paroxysmal discharges is still a matter of discussion (Dodrill and Wilkus 1978).

PRIMIDONE

In a recent study on seizure activity and anticonvulsant drug concentrations, 24 h monitoring revealed a good correlation of suppression of paroxysmal discharges in the EEG and increased serum levels of phenytoin and primidone in patients receiving both drugs together (Rowan et al. 1975) (Table II). Accordingly, the withdrawal of phenytoin was associated with a recrudescence of seizures and paroxysmal discharges in the EEG (Rowan et al. 1975). In a study on the effects of primidone withdrawal in 3 patients with intractable complex partial seizures, uncontrolled by phenytoin-primidone combined treatment, a surprising clinical finding was seen. After a temporary increase in seizures the number of complex partial seizures fell below the pre-withdrawal frequency in 2 patients and was unchanged in 1 patient. The paroxysmal discharges disappeared in 1 patient who became seizure-free after withdrawal (Schmidt et al. 1978) (Fig. 1).

The EEG changes associated with primidone intoxication were described in detail by Brillman et al. (1974). In 1 patient the EEG showed a large amount of low voltage fast activity superimposed on a background of 8–10 c/sec alpha activity and generalized slow activity. At the time of recording the plasma concentration of primidone was around 100 μg/ml. At day 17 dominant alpha activity had returned

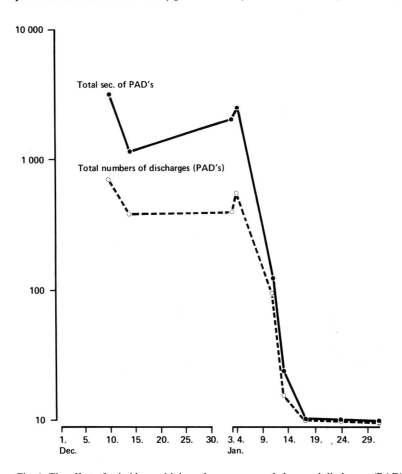

Fig. 1. The effect of primidone withdrawal on paroxysmal abnormal discharges (PAD) in a patient with complex partial seizures. The number and the total duration of paroxysmal abnormal discharges decreased at the 9th day after the withdrawal of primidone in this patient, uncontrolled by combined phenytoin and primidone treatment. At day 22 no more paroxysmal abnormal discharges were detectable in the print-out of the telemetered 8 h EEG. Following a temporary increase in seizure frequency the patient became seizure-free following the withdrawal of primidone and has been seizure-free for 2 years (Schmidt et al. 1978). The pathogenetic mechanism involved in the beneficial effect of the withdrawal of primidone in this patient is not known.

but photosensitivity was observed for the first time. On day 23 the EEG was normal and without photosensitivity.

SODIUM VALPROATE

The reported EEG effects of valproate have recently been reviewed by Bruni and Wilder (1979) (Table II). Based on serial 24 h serum level monitoring of sodium valproate, Rowan et al. (1980) have been able to show a relatively good correlation between, on the one hand, a decline in paroxysmal discharges and clinical seizures and, on the other, increasing doses of valproate. A summary of 24 h monitoring studies in 28 patients suggests that all except one of those improving as a result of sodium valproate, partly in combination with ethosuximide, had mean concentrations of 60 μg/ml or above (Rowan et al. 1980). In a recent study on clinical response, EEG changes and serum sodium valproate levels, in most cases the only EEG change observed during valproate administration was a decrease in epileptiform activity which correlated well with improvement of seizure frequency (Adams et al. 1978). In an additional report on serial monitoring of EEG and serum levels of sodium valproate, diurnal paroxysmal discharges and clinical seizures declined in association with starting valproate therapy or increasing the total daily dose of valproate. The extent and the duration of the depression of paroxysmal discharges and seizures varied in this report (Rowan et al. 1979b).

The correlation of clinical and EEG responses was excellent in 90% of all patients in one study after 1 year of treatment with sodium valproate. Only 2 out of 22 patients showed a good clinical response without a good EEG response; the lack of EEG improvement is unexplained. Furthermore, the clinical response may be prompt while the EEG response is delayed (Bruni et al. 1980).

A good correlation between a reduction of paroxysmal discharges and plasma concentration of valproate assumes that there is no delayed effect of the drug at zero plasma levels. Persistence of effects of valproate on paroxysmal discharges at a time when no valproate is detectable in plasma, has however recently been shown (Pellegrini et al. 1978). In an investigation on the effect of valproate on generalized penicillin seizures in the cat, there was a poor correlation between the degree of reduction of epileptic bursts and valproate plasma levels obtained 1 and 7 h after valproate administration. A delayed effect of valproate has also been shown for the photoconvulsive response in men. The effect appeared 3 h after attainment of peak sodium valproate concentration and lasted up to 5 days (Rowan et al. 1979a).

It is therefore not surprising that a number of reports did not find a good correlation of EEG changes or clinical improvement and sodium valproate plasma levels. In a controlled trial of sodium valproate in patients with various types of epilepsy, there was no correlation of reduced frequency of seizures or EEG ratings and the concentration of sodium valproate (Gram et al. 1977). Furthermore, there was no correlation between plasma concentrations of sodium valproate and EEG changes, but clinical improvement occurred at plasma levels exceeding 60 μg/ml (Villarreal et al. 1978).

Valproate may cause slowing of the background activity (Miribel and Marinier 1968). Computer analysis has revealed some increase in slow frequencies early, and later an increase in the beta frequencies (Sackellares et al. 1978). Others did not observe any consistent change in the EEG background when the records were analysed visually (Lagenstein et al. 1978; Bruni et al. 1980). Only 1 patient out of 22 had an increase in beta frequencies (Bruni et al. 1980). Intoxication with sodium valproate was accompanied by marked slowing of the background rhythms but no increase in beta activity (Adams et al. 1978) or generalized high voltage bisynchronous delta activity (Sackellares et al. 1979). The EEG may remain unchanged despite an acute intoxication of sodium valproate (Chadwick et al. 1979).

In a study on baboons, background EEG changes following valproate administration consisted of an increase in total spectral power with relative power changes in the 10–20 c/sec range. Furthermore, the magnitude of the EEG changes was related to the blood levels of valproate (Ehlers et al. 1980).

GENERAL COMMENTS

In a recent review of spectral EEG analysis of drug effects, Künkel et al. (1976) suggested to consider the topography, the drug effect in the EEG, and the relationship between neuroticism score and drug effect. This was shown to be of significance when the effect of diazepam on the EEG was monitored (Heinze and Künkel 1979). Another aspect of drug-induced EEG changes involved the identification of neuropsychological correlates of the EEG in anticonvulsant-treated patients with epilepsy (Dodrill and Wilkus 1978). The neuropsychological correlate of the topographic distribution and average rate of occurrence of discharges were studied (Dodrill and Wilkus 1976; Wilkus and Dodrill 1976). When the rates of occurrence of discharges were compared to the neuropsychological test scores, results were closely correlated with the EEG findings. In general, individuals with a discharge rate of more than 1/min did worse than those with fewer discharges. The preliminary results suggest that EEG paroxysmal discharges serve as an index of brain function and have a bearing upon the neuropsychological performance of patients with epilepsy (Wilkus and Dodrill 1976).

The intensive monitoring of sodium valproate treatment has led to the recognition of a delayed or carry over effect of sodium valproate in experimental animals (Lockard and Levy 1976) and in humans (Rowan et al. 1979a). Furthermore, there is preliminary clinical evidence that once or twice daily regimens of sodium valproate are just as effective as a more frequent distribution of the daily dose (Jeavons et al. 1980). This finding challenges the generally accepted principle of antiepileptic drug therapy that a stable plasma concentration is necessary for maximum therapeutic effect. These data suggest that the clinical effect of valproate may be related to the peak concentration achieved and be unrelated to the pattern of rapidly fluctuating levels of sodium valproate. It is therefore conceivable that further increase of intensive monitoring of sodium valproate will create new insights into the clinical value of achieving peak concentrations rather than of aiming at a minimal fluctuation of plasma levels.

Finally, one is struck by the paucity of data concerning an area where we need more information, namely the effect of antiepileptic drugs on the EEG in epileptic patients receiving long-term antiepileptic drug treatment. The clinical relevance of changes in the EEG background is quite unclear. Changes in background activity may be drug induced, genetic factors possibly correlated with the type of epilepsy or the intellectual development of the epileptic patient have also to be considered. The prognostic value of the background activity for the seizure prognosis and the psychosocial performance of the individual patient is a vastly unexplored area of research. Furthermore, our knowledge of the relationship of paroxysmal activity and therapeutic outcome is minimal. Consequently, the value of EEG data as a measure of therapeutic outcome is still controversial and deserves further study.

SUMMARY

The effect of antiepileptic drugs on the EEG was studied in a review of 23 controlled trials with therapeutic drug monitoring and serial EEG observations. There is a good correlation of suppression of paroxysmal discharges and an increase in the plasma concentrations of diazepam, phenobarbital, phenytoin, alone or in combination with phenobarbital or primidone. The correlation is variable during treatment with carbamazepine and in patients with focal discharge receiving sodium valproate or a delayed response to sodium valproate treatment. An increase in beta activity is correlated with a raised plasma concentration of clonazepam, phenytoin and phenobarbital, but not in all patients receiving these drugs. The degree and the localization of cerebral impairment seem to influence the drug-induced fast EEG response. Slowing of background occurs with high plasma concentrations of diazepam, phenytoin, alone or in combination with phenobarbital or primidone.

The correlation of paroxysmal discharges with clinical seizure frequency is good for phenobarbital, phenytoin, alone or in combination. The correlation is variable for carbamazepine and the delayed response to sodium valproate. A slowing of background activity is correlated with clinical drug toxicity due to carbamazepine, phenytoin, phenobarbital and primidone treatment in most patients.

REFERENCES

Adams, D.J., Luders, H. and Pippenger, Ch. Sodium valproate in the treatment of intractable seizure disorders: a clinical and electroencephalographic study. Neurology (Minneap.), 1978, 28: 152–157.

Ahmad, S., Laidlaw, J., Houghton, G.W. and Richens, A. Involuntary movements caused by phenytoin intoxication in epileptic patients. J. Neurol. Neurosurg. Psychiat., 1975, 38: 225–231.

Bendarzewska-Nawrocka, B. and Pietruszewska, E. Relationship between blood serum luminal and diphenylhydantoin level and the results of treatment and other clinical data in drug-resistant epilepsy. Neurol. Neurochir. Psychiat. pol., 1980, 14: 39–45.

Bente, D. Antikonvulsiva und Elektroenzephalogramm. Bibl. psychiat,., 1975, 151: 182–189.

Bielmann, P., Levac, T. and Gagnon, M.A. Clonazepam: Its efficacy in association with phenytoin and phenobarbital in mental patients with generalized major motor seizures. Int. J. clin. Pharmacol., 1978, 16: 268–273.

Booker, H.E. and Celesia, G.G. Serum concentrations of diazepam in subjects with epilepsy. Arch. Neurol. (Chic.), 1973, 29: 191–194.

Brillman, J., Gallagher, B.B. and Mattson, R.H. Acute primidone intoxication. Arch. Neurol. (Chic.), 1974, 30: 255–258.

Browne, T.R. Clonazepam — A review of a new anticonvulsant drug. Arch. Neurol. (Chic.), 1976, 33: 326–332.

Browne, T.R. and Penry, J.K. Benzodiazepines in the treatment of epilepsy. A review. Epilepsia, 1973, 14: 277–310.

Bruni, J. and Wilder, B.J. Valproic acid. Review of a new antiepileptic drug. Arch. Neurol. (Chic.), 1979, 36: 393–398.

Bruni, J., Wilder, B.J., Bauman, A.W. and Willmore, L.J. Clinical efficacy and long-term effects of valproic acid therapy on spike-and-wave discharges. Neurology (Minneap.), 1980, 30: 42–46.

Buchthal, F., Svensmark, O. and Schiller, P.J. Clinical and electroencephalographic correlations with serum levels of diphenylhydantoin. Arch. Neurol. (Chic.), 1960, 2: 624–630.

Buchthal, F., Svensmark, O. and Simonsen, H. Relation of EEG and seizures to phenobarbital in serum. Arch. Neurol. (Chic.), 1968, 19: 567–572.

Bücking, P.H. Elektroklinische Korrelationen während der antikonvulsiven Behandlung des Status epilepticus und chronischer Epilepsien fokaler Genese mit CLonazepam. Schweiz. Arch. Neurol. Neurochir. Psychiat., 1977, 121: 187–205.

Carrie, J.R.G. Computer-assisted EEG sharp-transient detection and quantification during overnight recordings in an epileptic patient. In: P. Kellaway and I. Petersén (Eds.), Quantitative Analytic Studies in Epilepsy. Raven Press, New York, 1976: 225–235.

Chadwick, D.W., Cumming, W.J.K., Livingstone, I. and Cartlidge, N.E.F. Acute intoxication with sodium valproate. Ann. Neurol., 1979, 6: 552–553.

Congdon, P.J. and Forsythe, W.I. Intravenous clonazepam in the treatment of status epilepticus in children. Epilepsia, 1980, 21: 97–102.

Couto-Sales, S., Rey, E., Radvanyi, M.F. et Dreyfus-Brisac, C. Essai d'évaluation des thérapeutiques (diazépam, phénobarbital) sur l'E.E.G. néonatal pendant les premières 24 h du traitement. Rev. E.E.G. Neurophysiol., 1979, 9: 26–34.

Dodrill, C.B. and Wilkus, R.J. Neuropsychological correlates of the electroencephalogram in epileptics. II. The waking posterior rhythm and its interaction with epileptiform activity. Epilepsia, 1976, 17: 101–109.

Dodrill, C.B. and Wilkus, R.J. Neuropsychological correlates of anticonvulsants and epileptiform discharges in adult epileptics. In: W.A. Cobb and H. Van Duijn (Eds.), Contemporary Clinical Neurophysiology. Elsevier, Amsterdam, 1978: 259–267.

Dreifuss, F.E., Penry, J.K., Rose, S.W., Kupferberg, H.J., Dyken, P. and Sato, S. Serum clonazepam concentrations in children with absence seizures. Neurology (Minneap.), 1975, 25: 255–258.

Dumermuth, G., Gasser, T., Hecker, A., Herdan, M. and Lange, B. Exploration of EEG components in the beta frequency range. In: P. Kellaway and I. Petersén (Eds.), Quantitative Analytic Studies in Epilepsy. Raven Press, New York, 1976: 533–558.

Dumermuth, G., Gasser, T., Germann, P., Hecker, A., Herdan, M. and Lange, B. Studies on EEG activities in the beta band. Europ. Neurol., 1977, 16: 197–202.

Ehlers, C.L., Mulbry, L.W. and Killam, E.K. EEG and anticonvulsant effects of dipropylacetic acid and dipropylacetamide in the baboon Papio papio. Electroenceph. clin. Neurophysiol., 1980, 49: 391–400.

Essig, C.F. and Fraser, H.F. Electroencephalographic changes in man during use and withdrawal of barbiturates in moderate dosage. Electroenceph. clin. Neurophysiol., 1958, 10: 649–656.

Fink, M., Irwin, P., Weinfeld, R.E., Schwartz, M.A. and Conney, A.H. Blood levels and electroencephalographic effects of diazepam and bromazepam. Clin. Pharmacol. Ther., 1976, 20: 184–191.

Fink, M., Irwin, P., Sannita, W., Papakostas, Y. and Green, M.A. Phenytoin: EEG effects and plasma levels in volunteers. Ther. Drug Monitor., 1979, 1: 93–103.

Gastaut, H. and Tassinari, C.A. (Eds.) Epilepsies. Handbook of Electroencephalography and Clinical Neurophysiology, Vol. 13A. Elsevier, Amsterdam, 1975.

Gram, L., Wulff, K., Rasmussen, K.E., Flachs, H., Würtz-Jørgensen, A., Sommerbeck, K.W. and Løhren, V. Valproate sodium: a controlled clinical trial including monitoring of drug levels. Epilepsia, 1977, 18: 141–148.

Heinze, H.-J. and Künkel, H. The significance of personality traits in EEG evaluation of drug effects. Pharmacopsychiatry, 1979, 12: 155–164.

Iivanainen, M., Viukari, M., Seppäläinen, A.-M. and Helle, E.-P. Electroencephalography and phenytoin toxicity in mentally retarded epileptic patients. J. Neurol. Neurosurg. Psychiat., 1978, 41: 272–277.

Jeavons, P.M., Covanis, A., Gupta, A.K. and Clark, J.E. Monotherapy with sodium valproate in childhood epilepsy. In: M.J. Parsonage and A.D.S. Caldwell (Eds.), The Place of Sodium Valproate in the Treatment of Epilepsy. Academic Press, London, 1980: 53–60.

Kato, H. and Mori, T. A clinical and electroencephalographic study on antiepileptic activity of clonazepam. Folia psychiat. neurol. jap., 1977, 31: 183–194.

Kellaway, P., Frost, J.D. and Hrachovy, R.A. Relationship between clinical state, ictal and interictal EEG discharges, and serum drug levels: partial seizures/phenobarbital. Ann. Neurol., 1978, 4: 197.

Kellaway, P., Frost, J.D. and Crawley, J.W. Time modulation of spike-and-wave activity in generalized epilepsy. Ann. Neurol., 1980, 8: 491–500.

Ketz, E. Wirkung von Antikonvulsiva und psychotropen Drogen auf das EEG. Z.EEG-EMG, 1974, 5: 99–106.

Künkel, H., Luba, A. and Niethardt, P. Topographic and psychosomatic aspects of spectral EEG analysis of drug effects. In: P. Kellaway and I. Petersén (Eds.), Quantitative Analytic Studies in Epilepsy. Raven Press, New York, 1976: 207–223.

Kurokawa, T., Yokota, K., Mitsudome, A., Shibata, R., Takashima, S. and Goya, N. Diagnostic and prognostic significance of electroencephalography with intravenous diazepam in epilepsy. Folia psychiat. neurol. jap., 1979, 33: 15–20.

Lagenstein, I., Sternowsky, H.J., Blaschke, E., Rothe, M. and Fehr, R. Treatment of childhood epilepsy with dipropylacetic acid (DPA). Arch. Psychiat. Nervenkr., 1978, 226: 43–55.

Levy, L.L. and Fenichel, G.M. Diphenylhydantoin activated seizures. Neurology (Minneap.), 1965, 15: 716–722.

Lockard, J.S. and Levy, R.H. Valproic acid: reversibly acting drug? Epilepsia, 1976, 17: 477–479.

Logan, W.J. and Freeman, J.M. Pseudodegenerative disease due to diphenylhydantoin intoxication. Arch. Neurol. (Chic.), 1969, 21: 631–637.

Longo, V.G. (Ed.) Effect of Drugs on the EEG. Handbook of Electroencephalography and Clinical Neurophysiology, Vol. 7C. Elsevier, Amsterdam, 1977.

Lopes da Silva, F.H., Kamp, A., Mars, N.J.I., Bultstra, G., Lommen, J.G. and Van Hulten, K. Quantitative analysis of EEGs in epileptic patients. Pharmacopsychiatry, 1979, 12: 191–199.

Miribel, J. et Marinier, R. Modifications électroencéphalographiques chez des enfants épileptiques traités par le Dépakène. Rev. neurol., 1968, 119: 313–320.

Monaco, F., Riccio, A., Morselli, P.L. and Mutani, R. EEG, seizures and plasma level correlations in patients on chronic treatment with carbamazepine. Electroenceph. clin. Neurophysiol., 1980, 48: 51P.

Müller, J. und Müller, D. Hirnelektrische Korrelate bei Überdosierung von antikonvulsiven Medikamenten. Nervenarzt, 1972, 43: 270–272.

Murphy, M.J. and Goldstein, M.N. Diphenylhydantoin-induced asterixis. A clinical study. J. Amer. med. Ass., 1974, 229: 538–540.

Niedermeyer, E., Yarworth, S. and Zobniw, A.M. Absence of drug-induced β-activity in the electroencephalogram. Europ. Neurol., 1977, 15: 77–84.

Nordentoft-Jensen, B. and Grynderup, V. Studies on the metabolism of phenytoin. Epilepsia, 1966, 7: 238–245.

Pellegrini, A., Gloor, P. and Sherwin, A.L. Effect of valproate sodium on generalized penicillin epilepsy in the cat. Epilepsia, 1978, 19: 351–360.

Penry, J.K., Porter, R.J. and Dreifuss, F.E. Ethosuximide. Relation of plasma levels to clinical control. In: D.M. Woodbury, J.K. Penry and R.P. Schmidt (Eds.), Antiepileptic Drugs. Raven Press, New York, 1972: 431–441.

Pinder, R.M., Brogden, R.N., Speight, T.M. and Avery, G.S. Clonazepam: A review of its pharmacological properties and therapeutic efficacy in epilepsy. Drugs, 1976, 12: 321–361.

Pryse-Phillips, W.E.M. and Jeavons, P.M. Effect of carbamazepine (Tegretol) on the electroencephalograph and ward behaviour of patients with chronic epilepsy. Epilepsia, 1970, 11: 263–273.

Riehl, J.-L. and McIntyre, H.B. A quantitative study of the acute effects of diphenylhydantoin on the electroencephalogram of epileptic patients. Neurology (Minneap.), 1968, 18: 1107–1112.

Rodin, E.A., Rim, C.S., Kitano, H., Lewis, R. and Rennick, P.M. A comparison of the effectiveness of primidone versus carbamazepine in epileptic outpatients. J. nerv. ment. Dis., 1976, 163: 41–46.

Roseman, E. Dilantin toxicity. A clinical and electroencephalographic study. Neurology (Minneap.), 1961, 11: 912–921.

Rowan, A.J., Pippenger, C.E., McGregor, P.A. and French, J.H. Seizure activity and anticonvulsant drug concentration. Arch. Neurol. (Chic.), 1975, 32: 281–288.

Rowan, A.J., Binnie, C.D., Warfield, C.A., Meinardi, H. and Meijer, J.W.A. The delayed effect of sodium valproate on the photoconvulsive response in man. Epilepsia, 1979a, 20: 61–68.

Rowan, A.J., Binnie, C.D., de Beer-Pawlikowski, N.K.B., Goedhart, D.M., Gutter, T., van der Geest, P., Meinardi, H. and Meijer, J.W.A. Sodium valproate: Serial monitoring of EEG and serum levels. Neurology (Minneap.), 1979b, 29: 1450–1459.

Rowan, A.J., Binnie, C.D., de Beer-Pawlikowski, N.K.B., Goedhart, D.M., Gutter, T., van der Geest, P., Meijer, J.W.A. and Meinardi, H. Serial twenty-four-hour serum level monitoring in the study of sodium valproate. In: M.J. Parsonage and A.D.S. Caldwell (Eds.), The Place of Sodium Valproate in the Treatment of Epilepsy. Academic Press, London, 1980: 115–122.

Sackellares, J.C., Sato, S., Dreifuss, F.E. and Penry, J.K. The effect of valproic acid on the EEG background. Abstract Epilepsy International Symposium, Vancouver, Canada, 1978: 27.

Sackellares, J.C., Lee, S.I. and Dreifuss, F.E. Stupor following administration of valproic acid to patients receiving other antiepileptic drugs. Epilepsia, 1979, 20: 697–703.

Saito, M. Drug-induced EEG changes studied on two-dimensional rectangular coordinates using principal component analysis. Pharmacopsychiatry, 1979, 12: 59–68.

Sannita, W.G., Rapallino, M.V., Rodriguez, G. and Rosadini, G. EEG effects and plasma concentrations of phenobarbital in volunteers. Neuropharmacology, 1980, 19: 927–930.

Sato, H. Relationship between serum levels and fast EEG activities in rats by a single administration of phenobarbital. Electroenceph. clin. Neurophysiol., 1980, 50: 509–514.

Schmidt, D. Behandlung der Epilepsien. Georg Thieme Verlag, Stuttgart, 1981.

Schmidt, D. Diazepam. In: D.M. Woodbury, J.K. Penry and C.E. Pippenger (Eds.), Antiepileptic Drugs, 2nd Ed. Raven Press, New York, 1982: 711–735.

Schmidt, D., Kupferberg, H.J., Porter, R.J. and Penry, J.K. Primidone withdrawal in patients with intractable epilepsy. Abstracts Epilepsy International Symposium, Vancouver, Canada, 1978: 26.

Shimuzu, H. Quantitative analysis of EEG basic rhythms in epileptics. Brain Nerve (Tokyo), 1979, 31: 1161–1172.

Spencer, S.S., Spencer, D.D., Williamson, P.D. and Mattson, R.H. Ictal effects of anticonvulsant medication withdrawal in epileptic patients. Epilepsia, 1981, 22: 297–307.

Villarreal, H.J., Wilder, B.J., Willmore, L.J., Bauman, A.W., Hammond, E.J. and Bruni, J. Effect of valproic acid on spike and wave discharges in patients with absence seizures. Neurology (Minneap.), 1978, 28: 886–891.

Wilkus, R.J. and Dodrill, C.B. Neuropsychological correlates of the electroencephalogram in epileptics: I. Topographic distribution and average rate of epileptiform activity. Epilepsia, 1976, 17: 89–100.

Wilkus, R.J. and Green, J.R. Electroencephalographic investigations during evaluation of the antiepileptic agent sulthiame. Epilepsia, 1974, 15: 13–25.

Wilkus, R.J., Dodrill, C.B. and Troupin, A.S. Carbamazepine and the electroencephalogram of epileptics: A double blind study in comparison to phenytoin. Epilepsia, 1978, 19: 283–291.

Wolpaw, J.R. and Penry, J.K. Acute and chronic antiepileptic drug effect on the T complex interhemispheric latency difference. Epilepsia, 1978, 19: 99–107.

Kyoto Symposia (EEG Suppl. No. 36)
Editors: P.A. Buser, W.A. Cobb and T. Okuma
© 1982, Elsevier Biomedical Press, Amsterdam

Assessment of Antiepileptic Drug Toxicity by Eye Movements

PAULO R.M. BITTENCOURT[1,*] and ALAN RICHENS[2]

[1]*The National Hospital, Queen Square, London WC1N 3BG, and* [2]*Department of Pharmacology and Materia Medica, Welsh National School of Medicine, Heath Park, Cardiff CF4 (England)*

Accurate assessment of antiepileptic drug toxicity in man poses a variety of methodological problems. Patients reaching the care of physicians with a special interest in epilepsy are usually those with long-standing severe disease, maintained on a variety of antiepileptic drug regimes. Fig. 1 is a simplification of the task faced by the researcher interested in the origin of the signs and symptoms of central nervous system dysfunction displayed by such patients. Irreversible damage in the brains of epileptic patients was reported before the availability of most of the currently used antiepileptic agents (Spielmeyer 1920). There is continuing discussion on whether the neuronal loss, particularly in the cerebellum, is due to long-term phenytoin treatment with intercurrent bouts of acute toxicity, or to the epileptic process in itself, particularly factors associated with high frequency of generalized tonic clonic seizures (Dam 1972; Salcman et al. 1978). Brain function may be temporarily impaired in patients with high serum antiepileptic drug concentrations (Hoppener et al. 1980), or during seizures of a variety of types.

Many strategies can be used in order to circumvent the problem of a number of variables producing the changes one wishes to study. Newly diagnosed patients can be followed longitudinally over a long period of time on monotherapeutic drug regimens, but the paucity of studies in the literature attests to the difficulty in carrying them out. When drug toxicity is in question studies in healthy volunteers may be helpful, as they isolate the variable to be investigated. It is clear, though, that results of such studies must be interpreted in the light of data obtained in patients. If factors such as those of Fig. 1 are taken into account, much may be learnt from patients with epilepsy of varying severity and type.

The chosen measure of brain dysfunction must be sensitive, its assessment must be objective and quantitative, and patients' co-operation needs to be decreased to a minimum. Recent studies have demonstrated that neurophysiological specificity should also be considered in the choice of a measure of drug toxicity (Bittencourt et al. 1981). Analogue rating scales, tests of psychomotor function, and standard EEG techniques represent the joint action of many neurophysiological systems, and are thus less likely to produce linearly distributed data than other measures which are

---

* Present address and address for further correspondence: Hospital e Maternidade Sao Carlos, Avenida Francisco H dos Santos 1540, Cx Postal 2433, Curitiba-Parana 80000, Brazil.

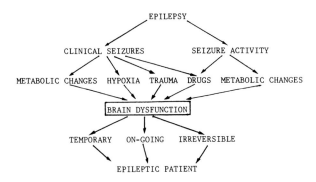

Fig. 1. Causative factors and types of brain dysfunction to be considered in patients with epilepsy.

the product of better defined neurophysiological systems, such as specific EEG measures (Fink et al. 1976) and the peak velocity of saccadic eye movements (Bittencourt et al. 1981).

We chose to look at oculomotor function in healthy and epileptic subjects. The choice of eye movements was due to their well recognized impairment by a variety of centrally acting compounds (Wilkinson 1976; Bittencourt and Richens 1981), and also the clinical observation that epileptic patients often display striking abnormalities of oculomotor function (Riker et al. 1978; Hoppener et al. 1980).

RELEVANT PHYSIOLOGY

The basic purpose of eye movements is accurate vision, a matter made complicated by the requirements of binocular vision and by the fact that our heads as well as most visual targets tend to be continually moving in a disorganized fashion. Furthermore, high quality vision is only achieved when the image of the target rests on the fovea centralis, an area occupying approximately 0.01% of the total retinal area (Steinman 1975). In order to move this minute high resolution visual field around we use movements which either maintain fixation on a given visual target or change gaze from one target to the next as quickly as possible (Collewijn 1977). Fixation and thus vision is possible during the slow phases of nystagmus, during doll's head eye movements, and during smooth pursuit (Carpenter 1977). Rapid changes in gaze direction are made either in the form of voluntary saccades or as the fast phases of the various forms of nystagmus. Vergence is the omnipresent type of eye movement, but as its control has been shown to be independent of that of version eye movements (Rashbass and Westheimer 1961), we have chosen to concentrate on version movements, that is those in which both eyes move conjugately.

A simplified classification of version eye movements is presented in Fig. 2. It is based on the 3 main oculomotor systems, which can among them generate all types of version eye movement, pathological or not. There is now evidence that the

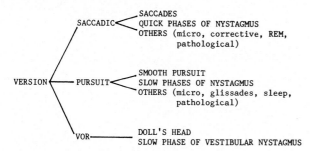

Fig. 2. Brief classification of version eye movements.

pontine circuits responsible for the generation of voluntary saccades are the same which produce the fast phases of all types of nystagmus, such as square wave jerks, micro-saccades, or the movements of REM sleep (Zee and Robinson 1979). Similarly there is evidence that smooth pursuit eye movements are generated by an independent oculomotor system (Robinson 1965), which in turn is capable of producing a variety of slow eye movements, such as micro-drift and saccades (Carpenter 1977). This system is involved in the production of the slow phases of a variety of nystagmus, to which the basic vestibulo-ocular (doll's head) reflex is also related (for further discussion see Robinson 1975; Bittencourt 1981).

It thus may be concluded that rapid and efficient assessment of oculomotor function should include one major manifestation of each of the oculomotor systems. For these reasons we have chosen to look at visually evoked smooth pursuit and saccadic eye movements and at doll's head eye movements. The latter type will not be discussed further as it has not been demonstrated to be impaired in experimental pharmacological situations, even when severe impairment of smooth pursuit and saccades was observed (Wilkinson et al. 1974; Bittencourt et al. 1980).

THE STANDARD EYE MOVEMENT TEST PROCEDURE

Silver-silver chloride electrodes were placed lateral to both outer canthi, with a similar reference electrode on the forehead. Subjects sat in semi-darkness with the head on a head rest and were asked to follow a point source of light moving horizontally across a 650 mm wide oscilloscope. In the smooth pursuit test target displacement subtended an angle of 30° in relation to the subject's nasion. The frequency of sinusoidal spot oscillation was varied so that the maximum angular velocity increased progressively from 28 to 122°/sec. Testing of saccadic eye movements was carried out by using a sequence of stimuli which induced step-like displacements of the spot on the oscilloscope, subtending angles of 15, 20, 25, 30, 35 and 40° in relation to the subject's nasion. The resulting eye movements were recorded by direct-coupled electro-oculography and stored on magnetic tape.

Smooth pursuit was analysed either visually (Bittencourt et al. 1980) or by computer (Bittencourt et al. 1982). Both procedures are based on the finding that as

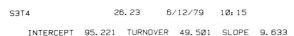

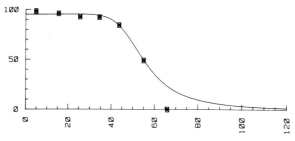

Fig. 3. Smooth pursuit velocity is calculated by plotting smooth pursuit percentage (ratio of smooth pursuit to saccadic tracking, vertical axis) against target velocity (horizontal axis), after which a curve is fitted to the data. The "turnover" of the function is the final measure of smooth pursuit velocity.

target velocity increases, saccades progressively replace smooth pursuit in the eye movement traces (Rashbass 1961). In the computer analysis, the ratio of smooth pursuit to saccadic eye movements is calculated and plotted against target velocity, after which a curve is fitted, and the measure of smooth pursuit velocity calculated (Fig. 3).

Saccades were computer-analysed according to a procedure reported in detail elsewhere (Bittencourt et al. 1981). The duration and peak velocity of a standard sequence of saccades are calculated and plotted against amplitude, after which the final measures of peak velocity and duration are extracted (Fig. 4). Both programs have built-in calibration checks, so that the analysis does not proceed unless a

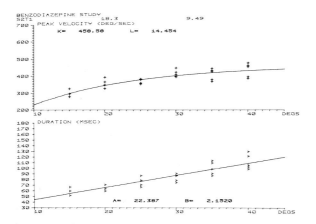

Fig. 4. The peak velocity and duration of each detected saccade (respectively above and below, horizontal axis) are plotted against amplitude, after which a convenient function is fitted to the data. K (the asymptote of the exponential) is the final measure of peak saccadic velocity, while the duration at which the line crosses 30° is the final measure of duration.

number of conditions are fulfilled. These and video monitoring of experiments involving epileptic patients were considered sufficient to decrease the influence of possible epileptic seizures on performance.

PATIENTS WITH SEVERE EPILEPSY ON POLYTHERAPY

In this preliminary study a group of patients with severe disabling epilepsy was compared with healthy subjects matched for age and sex (Bittencourt et al. 1980). The 12 patients had a mean age of 24 years, and a mean duration of epilepsy of 17 years. They were maintained on polytherapeutic drug regimens, and did not show evident signs of acute antiepileptic drug toxicity, such as non-extinguishable nystagmus, dysarthria, ataxia, involuntary movements, slowness of thought or behavioural changes (Plaa 1975; Trimble and Reynolds 1976). The patients were residents at the Chalfont Centre for Epilepsy. The 8 healthy subjects were free of drugs or evident disease, and comprised medical and para-medical staff. All were studied repeatedly over a period of 6 months.

Smooth pursuit velocity was determined according to the method of Bittencourt et al. (1980). The range of smooth pursuit velocities in patients and controls is shown in Fig. 5. It was 40% and statistically significantly smaller in the patients than in the controls.

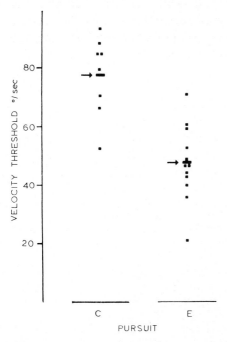

Fig. 5. Smooth pursuit velocity in 12 epileptic (E) and 8 control (C) subjects. Reproduced from Bittencourt et al. (1980).

Patients were subdivided in 2 groups, one which had "major" changes in treatment (resulting in a drop of phenytoin or phenobarbitone levels from therapeutic to non-detectable, or from toxic to therapeutic) and another whose serum concentrations remained unchanged over the 6 months. Smooth pursuit velocity improved without exception in those who had reductions in treatment, while it did not change significantly in the minor change group (Fig. 6). The latter group, though, was still significantly worse than the healthy subjects. The main conclusion of this study was that smooth pursuit velocity was shown to be impaired in treated epileptic patients, and it appeared to oscillate with changes in the drug treatment, more specifically reductions in dosage of phenytoin or barbiturates. It was not clear how much of the impairment was due to central nervous system damage associated with long-standing severe epilepsy.

PATIENTS WITH LESS SEVERE EPILEPSY ON MONOTHERAPY

Patients attending the National Hospital's epilepsy clinic (Prof. A. Richens) were referred for the eye movement test when they had been maintained on monotherapeutic drug regimens for at least 3 months previous to the study, with no episodes of acute drug toxicity or status epilepticus. There was no evidence of acute drug toxicity at the time of testing, by the above criteria.

A total of 18 patients was studied (Fig. 7). The control group was made up of 12 female and 8 male medical and para-medical staff who were free of drugs and of ocular or central nervous system disease. They were aged 24 ± 4 years. Patients and subjects underwent the standard eye movement test procedure, peak saccadic and smooth pursuit velocity being determined by computer as referred to above.

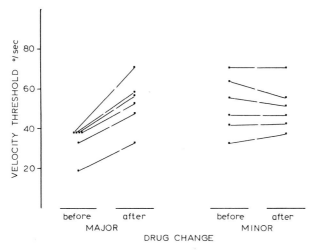

Fig. 6. Effect of major or minor changes in phenytoin or phenobarbitone serum concentration on smooth pursuit velocity. Reproduced from Bittencourt et al. (1980).

The 3 groups of patients had smooth pursuit velocities lower than the controls (Fig. 8) and not different from each other. The phenytoin group mean was 23%, and the carbamazepine and valproate means 15%, lower than the mean smooth pursuit velocity of the control group. Patients on sodium valproate had significantly

		CBZ	DPH	VAL
SEIZURE TYPE	absences	1	1	1
	CPS	2	1	3
	CPS+GM	3	2	1
	GM	–	2	1
LENGTH OF HISTORY (years)		7.3±4.8	7.3±5.2	10.3±5.3
GM FREQUENCY (past year)		0.5/month	0.7/month	0.1/month
AGE		22.3±5.4	23.6±6.1	19.1±2.3
SEX		5♀ 1♂	3♀ 3♂	4♀ 2♂
DRUG SERUM CONCENTRATIONS (umol/l)		37.7±16	77±43	403±230

Fig. 7. Summary of data on epileptic patients on monotherapy with carbamazepine (CBZ), phenytoin (DPH) and sodium valproate (VAL). Seizure types are absences, complex partial seizures (CPS) and generalized tonic clonic (GM). Values are either means or means and standard deviations.

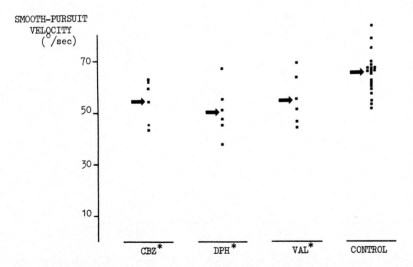

Fig. 8. Smooth pursuit velocity in 8 control subjects (64.7 ± 8, mean ± S.D.), 6 patients on carbamazepine (CBZ, 54.6 ± 8, mean ± S.D.), 6 on phenytoin (DPH, 50.5 ± 10, mean ± S.D.), and 6 on sodium valproate (VAL, 54.8 ± 10, mean ± S.D.) (* = $P < 0.05$).

lowered peak saccadic velocities when compared to the phenytoin and control groups (Fig. 9). Peak saccadic velocity in the valproate group was 17% lower than in the controls. The group on carbamazepine had peak saccadic velocities 10%, but not significantly, lower than the controls.

The results of this experiment in patients with less severe epilepsy on simpler drug regimens demonstrate that abnormal smooth pursuit is commonly found in epileptic patients, irrespective of their drug treatment. Taken in conjunction with the experiment in patients with severe epilepsy, it is suggested that the smooth pursuit abnormality is related partly to underlying CNS damage due to epilepsy and chronic drug treatment, and partly to certain antiepileptic compounds, more specifically phenytoin and barbiturates.

The peak velocity of saccadic eye movements is less commonly impaired in epileptic patients than smooth pursuit, a point emphasized by the absence of reports suggesting impairment of saccades in the literature. Although none of the patients reported here had obvious saccade slowing (Fig. 9), subdivision in groups according to their drug treatment showed that those patients on sodium valproate had saccades marginally slower than the controls. The finding that peak saccadic velocity in the

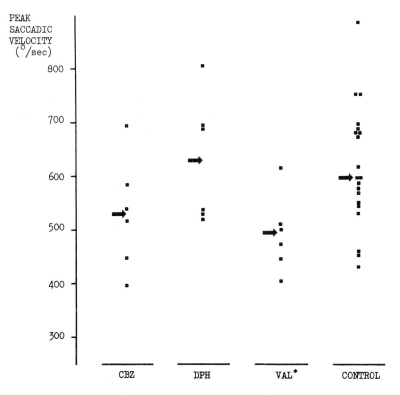

Fig. 9. Peak saccadic velocity in 20 control subjects (599.3 ± 92, mean ± S.D.), 6 patients on carbamazepine (CBZ, 530 ± 105, mean ± S.D.), 6 on phenytoin (DPH, 629 ± 118, mean ± S.D.), and 6 on sodium valproate (VAL, 492 ± 72, mean ± S.D.) (* = $P < 0.05$ compared with DPH and $P < 0.01$ compared with controls).

valproate group was lower than in patients on phenytoin, suggests that this effect is associated with the drug treatment rather than with underlying brain damage common to the 3 groups of patients. The effect of barbiturates on eye movements is well known (Bergman et al. 1952). Rashbass (1959) showed that intravenous thiopentone suppressed smooth pursuit in healthy subjects, who then used solely saccades for visual tracking. In unpublished observations (Tedeschi, Bittencourt, Smith and Richens, in preparation), both saccadic and smooth pursuit velocities were shown to be impaired after a therapeutic dose of amylobarbitone.

Phenytoin overdosage has long been recognized as inducing signs suggestive of cerebellar or brain stem dysfunction, especially when serum concentration is above 80–100 μmol/l (Richens 1976). Even at lower concentrations similar signs can be demonstrated and their magnitude does not appear to correlate in any simple manner with phenytoin concentration (Riker et al. 1978; Bittencourt et al. 1980). An interaction between drug and epilepsy-induced disease provides an adequate explanation for this lack of correlation.

EXPERIMENTS IN HEALTHY SUBJECTS

The objective of these experiments was to compare the effects on eye movements of single oral doses of centrally acting compounds. The design used was double blind and randomized. All studies were carried out in groups of 5 or 6 healthy male subjects, aged 20–40 years. They were free of drugs and disease and had standardized breakfasts on each trial day, which took place at 1–2 week intervals. The standard eye movement test procedure was performed before and at frequent intervals up to 12 h after administration of the treatments. Smooth pursuit and peak saccadic velocity were analysed by computer, as referred to above.

Blood samples were taken before each test. Phenytoin and valproic acid serum concentrations were measured by gas chromatography, while carbamazepine was measured by EMIT, in the Clinical Pharmacology Unit, Institute of Neurology. Clonazepam was measured by gas-liquid chromatography with an electron capture detector, according to the method of Toseland and Wicks (1981) in the Department of Clinical Chemistry, Guy's Hospital (Dr. P.A. Toseland).

There were no significant differences in either smooth pursuit or peak saccadic velocity between 0 and 8 h after oral administration of placebo or sodium valproate (600 mg). Valproic acid concentrations reached a peak at 1 h (439 $\pm$ 37 μmol/l, mean $\pm$ S.D.) and slowly decreased until 8 h (259 $\pm$ 41 μmol/l, mean $\pm$ S.D.). At the time of the peak the concentrations were comparable to those found in the patients on monotherapeutic drug regimens (Fig. 7) who had mildly decreased peak saccadic velocity. These results can be explained in the light of the findings of Rowan et al. (1979), who showed rather elegantly that the effect of sodium valproate on photosensitivity may take hours to be demonstrable, and may outlast peak serum levels for up to 5 days. If the results in patients can be confirmed, they suggest that peak saccadic velocity may be a convenient indicator of the pharmacological, i.e., antiepileptic, effect of sodium valproate.

Both smooth pursuit and peak saccadic velocity were significantly decreased after oral administration of clonazepam (1 mg) when compared with placebo (Fig. 10). The changes in eye movement velocities were time-locked to the oscillations in serum clonazepam concentration. These results are in disagreement with statements in a recent review of the properties of antiepileptic drugs which suggested a range of 60–220 nmol/l as therapeutic for patients on clonazepam (Morselli and Franco-Morselli 1980). Although the data presented here were acquired from healthy volunteers exposed acutely to the drug, it demonstrated an impairment of 20–30% in both measures at clonazepam concentrations of 30 nmol/l (Fig. 10), half of what

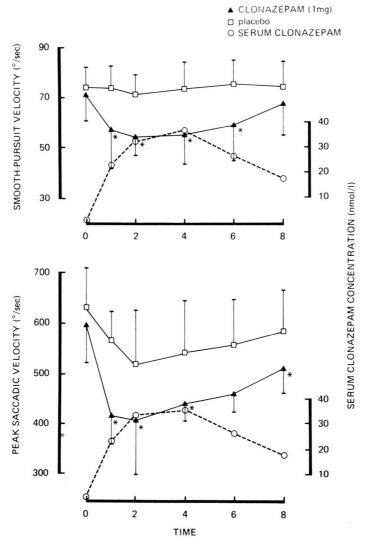

Fig. 10. Smooth pursuit and peak saccadic velocity (mean ± S.D.) and serum clonazepam concentration (mean) before and until 8 h after oral administration of 1 mg clonazepam to 5 healthy subjects, compared with placebo (* = $P<0.05$).

was suggested as the lower limit of the therapeutic range. As shown in previous studies, such impairment in peak saccadic velocity is associated with severe drowsiness and clumsiness (Bittencourt et al. 1981), and because there is a linear relationship between serum benzodiazepine concentration and effect on such measures (Bittencourt et al. 1981; Bittencourt and Dhillon 1981), the level of arousal at least can be predicted to be severely impaired at serum concentrations on the low side of this proposed therapeutic range. This range may of course be appropriate for some patients who have developed considerable tolerance to the effects of clonazepam and are thus maintained on doses of 5 mg daily or more, but not for epileptic populations as a whole.

As far as eye movements can tell there are no significant qualitative pharmacodynamic differences between benzodiazepine compounds used for a variety of clinical purposes. Fig. 11 shows the changes in peak saccadic velocity after oral administration of therapeutic doses of nitrazepam, temazepam, diazepam, flurazepam and desmethyl-diazepam. Like clonazepam (Fig. 10), all induced falls in peak saccadic velocity which reflected the oscillations in measurable serum concentrations. In other experiments (Bittencourt et al. 1982) it has been demonstrated that smooth pursuit eye movements are similarly affected. A review of the literature which claims qualitative differences between benzodiazepine compounds showed that most studies on which such views are based can be criticized seriously for their methodology, as the majority did not measure serum concentrations, did not account for quantitative differences in the pharmacological effects, and did not use reliable measures of the effect (Bittencourt and Dhillon 1981).

The effect of benzodiazepines on eye movements is typically related to the serum concentrations of those drugs, which can be accurately detected in body fluids (Bittencourt et al. 1981, 1982). It was only in the case of drugs such as flurazepam, which are extensively and rapidly metabolized into a variety of metabolites, making difficult the accurate assessment of serum concentrations, that a relationship

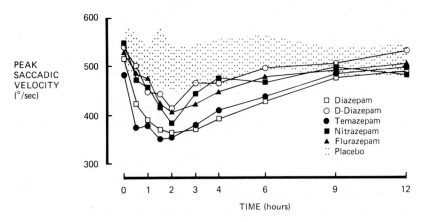

Fig. 11. Peak saccadic velocity after oral administration of the various benzodiazepines (mean) and placebo (mean ± S.D.) in 6 healthy subjects. Reproduced from Bittencourt et al. (1981).

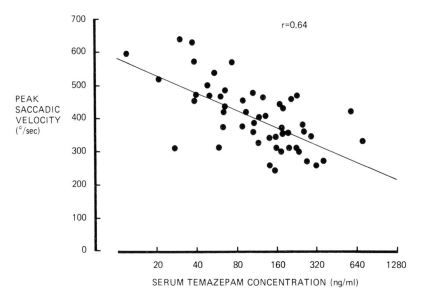

Fig. 12. Negative linear correlation between peak saccadic velocity and serum temazepam concentration ($r = -0.631$, $P<0.01$) in 6 healthy subjects, between 30 min and 12 h after oral administration of 20 mg temazepam. Reproduced from Bittencourt et al. (1981).

between serum concentration and effect could not be established. Fig. 12 shows the clear relationship between serum temazepam concentration and peak saccadic velocity in a group of 6 subjects who were studied between 0 and 12 h after oral administration of 20 mg temazepam. In other studies (Bittencourt et al. 1981, 1982) we have demonstrated similar relationships between peak saccadic velocity and the serum concentrations of diazepam and nitrazepam, and between smooth pursuit velocity and the serum concentrations of nitrazepam, temazepam and diazepam. These data are in direct disagreement with reviews of the pharmacological properties of benzodiazepines which claimed no relationship between benzodiazepine concentration and effect on the brain (Bellantuono et al. 1980; Hindmarch 1980). The methodology of the studies on which these statements were based can also be criticized (Bittencourt and Dhillon 1981). In conclusion, we would like to suggest that if benzodiazepines are to be used in epileptic patients, they should be chosen on the base of factors such as pharmacokinetic properties, and not because of alleged specific antiepileptic properties. Furthermore, a linear relationship between serum concentration and effect can be expected, if both are being accurately and specifically measured.

In a further study on health subjects (Bittencourt and Richens 1981) we have demonstrated that both smooth pursuit and peak saccadic velocity are impaired after oral administration of carbamazepine. In Fig. 13 the eye movement velocities have been plotted against serum carbamazepine, in a group of subjects who had either 400 or 1000 mg orally as a single dose. While smooth pursuit velocity was linearly related to serum carbamazepine concentration, peak saccadic velocity was

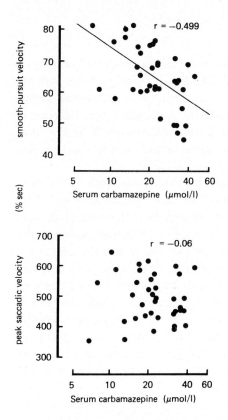

Fig. 13. Presence of linear negative correlation between smooth pursuit velocity and serum carbamazepine concentration (n = 37, $r = -0.499$, $P < 0.01$), and absence of correlation between peak saccadic velocity and serum carbamazepine concentration (n = 37, $r = -0.06$, $P > 0.05$), between 1 and 8 h after oral administration of 400 mg (5 subjects) and 1000 mg (5 subjects) carbamazepine.

clearly not. The correlation coefficients as well as the plots suggest that while the effect of carbamazepine on smooth pursuit was concentration-dependent that on peak saccadic velocity was not. These findings suggest different and at least partly independent mechanisms of action for the 2 effects of carbamazepine on the oculomotor system.

The linear correlation between serum carbamazepine and smooth pursuit velocity (Fig. 13) is of special interest, because impaired smooth pursuit is likely to be important in the production of many of the side effects of carbamazepine therapy such as diplopia, blurred vision and dizziness (Hoppener et al. 1980). These complaints are similar to those of patients with abnormalities of head-eye coordination which often can be explained by abnormalities of the vestibulo-ocular reflexes, as demonstrated in epileptic patients (Bittencourt et al. 1980). In fact, such side effects of carbamazepine appear in relation to oscillations in serum drug concentration (Hoppener et al. 1980; Morselli and Franco-Morselli 1980), and suggest involvement of structures within the posterior fossa (Baloh and Honrubia 1979). Thus, smooth pursuit may be used as a measure of some of the common side effects of carbamazepine.

CONCLUSION

The findings discussed here demonstrate that smooth pursuit velocity is commonly decreased in epileptic patients, and that this abnormality is due partly to the epileptic process in itself and partly to the drug treatment at the time of testing, in the case of phenytoin, barbiturates, carbamazepine and clonazepam. Decrease of the velocity of saccadic eye movements is less commonly observed and is more clearly associated with treatment with carbamazepine, benzodiazepines and possibly sodium valproate.

The implications of these findings are many. In terms of the mode of action of antiepileptic drugs, it is of interest that clonazepam and sodium valproate, both active against generalized seizures (Richens 1976), can be differentiated by their effects on the oculomotor system. Similarly, phenytoin and carbamazepine, active against partial seizures, had distinct effects on smooth pursuit and saccades.

Impairment of smooth pursuit implies impaired visual fixation due to defective suppression of the vestibulo-ocular reflex, and to possible impairment of optokinetic mechanisms (Baloh et al. 1980; Bittencourt et al. 1980). The results reported here indicate that epileptic patients, especially those with longer-standing and more severe epilepsy, or those on carbamazepine, benzodiazepines, phenytoin and barbiturates, have substantial abnormalities of such mechanisms, which may lead to oscillopsia and other types of blurred vision, especially during head movement.

ACKNOWLEDGEMENTS

This work was supported by grants of the Wellcome Foundation and of the Thorn Epilepsy Research Fund.

REFERENCES

Baloh, R.W. and Honrubia, V. Clinical Neurophysiology of the Vestibular System. Davis, Philadelphia, Pa., 1979.

Baloh, R.W., Yee, R.D. and Honrubia, V. Optokinetic nystagmus and parietal lobe lesions. Ann. Neurol., 1980, 7: 269–276.

Bellantuono, C., Reggi, V., Tognoni, G. and Garattini, S. Benzodiazepines: clinical pharmacology and therapeutic use. Drugs, 1980, 19: 195–219.

Bergman, P.S., Nathanson, M. and Bender, M.B. Electrical recordings of normal and abnormal eye movements modified by drugs. Arch. Neurol. (Chic.), 1952, 67: 357–374.

Bittencourt, P.R.M. The Effect of some Centrally-Acting Drugs on Smooth Pursuit and Saccadic Eye Movements in Man. Ph.D. Thesis, University of London, 1981: 9–68.

Bittencourt, P.R.M. and Dhillon, S. Benzodiazepines: clinical aspects. In: A. Richens and V. Marks (Eds.), Therapeutic Drug Monitoring. Churchill-Livingstone, Edinburgh, 1981: 275–282.

Bittencourt, P.R.M. and Richens, A. Serum drug concentrations and effects on smooth pursuit and saccadic eye movements. In: Abstracts of the 12th World Congress of Neurology, ICS 584. Excerpta Medica, Amsterdam, 1981.

481

Bittencourt, P.R.M., Gresty, M.A. and Richens, A. Quantitative assessment of smooth pursuit eye movements in healthy and epileptic subjects. J. Neurol. Neurosurg. Psychiat., 1980, 43: 1119–1125.

Bittencourt, P.R.M., Wade, P., Smith, A.T. and Richens, A. The relationship between peak velocity of saccadic eye movements and serum benzodiazepine concentration. Brit. J. clin. Pharmacol., 1981, 11: 523–533.

Bittencourt, P.R.M., Wade, P., Smith, A.T. and Richens, A. Benzodiazepines impair smooth pursuit eye movements. Clin. Pharmacol. Ther., 1982, in press.

Carpenter, R.H.S. Movements of the Eyes. Pion, London, 1977.

Collewijn, H. Gaze in freely moving subjects. In: R.G. Baker and A. Berthoz (Eds.), Control of Gaze by Brain Stem Neurons. Elsevier, Amsterdam, 1977: 13–22.

Dam, M. The density and ultrastructure of the Purkinje cells following diphenylhydantoin treatment in animals and man. Acta neurol. scand., 1972, 49 (Suppl.): 3–65.

Fink, M., Irwin, P., Weinfeld, R.E., Schwartz, M.A. and Conney, A.H. Blood levels and electroencephalographic effects of diazepam and bromazepam. Clin. Pharmacol. Ther., 1976, 20: 184–191.

Hindmarch, I. Psychomotor function and psychoactive drugs. Brit. J. clin. Pharmacol., 1980, 10: 189–210.

Hoppener, R.J., Kuyer, A., Meijer, J.W.A. and Hulsman, J. Correlation between daily fluctuations or carbamazepine serum levels and intermittent side-effects. Epilepsia, 1980, 21: 341–350.

Morselli, P.L. and Franco-Morselli, R. Clinical pharmacokinetics of antiepileptic drugs in adults. Pharmacol. Ther., 1980, 10: 65–101.

Plaa, G.L. Acute toxicity of antiepileptic drugs. Epilepsia, 1975, 16: 183–191.

Rashbass, C. Barbiturate nystagmus and the mechanisms of visual fixation. Nature (Lond.), 1959, 183: 897–898.

Rashbass, C. The relationship between saccadic and smooth tracking eye movements. J. Physiol. (Lond.), 1961, 159: 326–338.

Rashbass, C. and Westheimer, G. Disjunctive eye movements. J. Physiol. (Lond.), 1961, 159: 339–360.

Richens, A. Drug Treatment of Epilepsy. Henry Kimpton, London, 1976.

Riker, W.K., Downes, H., Olsen, G.D. and Smith, B. Conjugate lateral gaze nystagmus and free phenytoin concentrations in plasma: lack of correlation. Epilepsia, 1978, 19: 93–98.

Robinson, D.A. The mechanics of human smooth pursuit eye movement. J. Physiol. (Lond.), 1965, 180: 569–591.

Robinson, D.A. Oculomotor control signals. In: G. Lennerstrand and P. Bach-y-Rita, Basic Mechanisms of Ocular Motility and their Clinical Implications. Pergamon Press, New York, 1975: 337–374.

Rowan, A.J., Binnie, C.D., Warfield, C.A., Meinardi, H. and Meijer, J.W.A. The delayed effect of sodium valproate on the photoconvulsive response in man. Epilepsia, 1979, 20: 61–68.

Salcman, M., Defendini, R., Correll, J. and Gilman, S. Neuropathological changes in cerebellar biopsies of epileptic patients. Ann. Neurol., 1978, 3: 10–19.

Spielmeyer, W. Über einige Beziehungen zwischen Gouglien-Zellveränderungen und glosen Erscheinungen, besonders im Kleinhirn. Z. ges. Neurol. Psychiat., 1920, 54: 1–38.

Steinman, R.M. Oculomotor effects on vision. In: G. Lennerstrand and P. Bach-y-Rita (Eds.), Basic Mechanisms of Ocular Motility and their Clinical Implications. Pergamon Press, New York, 1975: 395–416.

Toseland, P.A. and Wicks, J.F.C. Principles of gas chromatography. In: A. Richens and V. Marks (Eds.), Therapeutic Drug Monitoring. Churchill-Livingstone, Edinburgh, 1981: 85–109.

Trimble, M.R. and Reynolds, E.H. Anticonvulsant drugs and mental symptoms: a review. Psychol. Med., 1976, 6: 169–178.

Wilkinson, I.M.S. The influence of drugs and alcohol upon human eye movement. Proc. roy. Soc. Med., 1976, 69: 479–480.

Wilkinson, I.M.S., Kime, R. and Purnell, M. Alcohol and human eye movement. Brain, 1974, 97: 785–792.

Zee, D.S. and Robinson, D.A. A hypothetical explanation of saccadic oscillations. Ann. Neurol., 1979, 5: 405–414.

Kyoto Symposia (EEG Suppl. No. 36)
Editors: P.A. Buser, W.A. Cobb and T. Okuma
© 1982, Elsevier Biomedical Press, Amsterdam

Should EEG Recording Be Included in Clinical Trials on New Antiepileptic Drugs?

P.L. MORSELLI[1], L. BOSSI[1] and C. MUNARI[2]

[1]*Department of Clinical Research, LERS-SYNTHELABO, 58, rue de la Glacière, 75013 Paris, and*
[2]*INSERM, Unité 97, 2 ter, rue d'Alésia, 75014 Paris (France)*

In this report we shall discuss the possible value of the EEG both as a *diagnostic variable* and an *outcome variable* during clinical trials on antiepileptic drugs (AEDs). Before coming to the point, we would like to recall the main characteristics of diagnostic variables and outcome variables in clinical trials aiming at the assessment of the effectiveness and the safety of a new drug.

Diagnostic variables should, of course, be relevant to the disorders to be treated, e.g., play a significant role in the definition of the patients' pathological syndrome, and should be expressed according to an accepted classification. In clinical trials, diagnostic variables are considered mainly in the inclusion and exclusion criteria.

Outcome variables are relevant for the assessment of the effects of the drug; therefore they have to be not only valid and reliable, and specifically related to the disorder to be treated, but also measurable on a properly defined scale (which may be quantitative, ordinal or binary), standardized and sensitive to change.

To answer the question: "Should EEG recordings be included in clinical trials on new AEDs?" we shall analyse: (1) the attitude of regulatory or public health agencies as expressed by recommended guidelines, and (2) the attitude of the clinical investigators, as expressed in published clinical trials.

The recommendations of the International League Against Epilepsy (ILAE), the Food and Drug Administration (FDA), and the European Economic Community (EEC) can be summarized as follows.

The ILAE guidelines (ILAE 1973) state that "for assessing the effectiveness of a drug during phase II trials the use of electroencephalography is desirable but not mandatory unless there is a specific indication (absences) for performing the test" and that for phase III trials "the use of electroencephalography may be indicated for a *specific drug* both pre-test and during test drug administration. These tests are mandatory if prior studies (phase I and phase II) indicate that the EEG may be affected by the drug." On the other hand, the "patients should be classified by all identifiable variables... The three most important primary variables in these patients are (1) classification by clinical and electroencephalographic pattern of seizure according to the International Classification of Epileptic Seizures (ICES), (2) age of patient, (3) presence or absence of cerebral lesion."

The FDA guidelines (FDA 1977) state that "for assessing the effectiveness of new AEDs, electroencephalography is desirable but not mandatory unless there is a specific indication for performing the test and if prior studies indicate that the EEG may be affected by the drug. Furthermore, in other than grand mal seizures (e.g. absences) newer methods of quantification (e.g. telemetry) are highly recommended." For the selection of the patients, EEG, on the contrary, is considered an essential criterion.

The proposed EEC guidelines (personal communication) recommend that "effects on EEG should be recorded systematically, at least in some studies, irrespective of whether or not they correlate with the anticonvulsant potential of the drugs; in ambulant cases and in particular in petit mal cases use of telemetry may be advisable."

It appears that, while the 3 sources agree on the need for EEG as a diagnostic variable, there is some disagreement concerning the need for EEG as an outcome variable during clinical trials; in patients other than with absence seizures, EEG recording during the trial is considered to be desirable but not mandatory according to the ILAE and FDA guidelines; on the contrary, it is formally requested during phase II and phase III clinical trials in the EEC recommendations. The reasons for such a request are not stated.

In order to verify how the EEG is taken into account in the practice of clinical trials on new AEDs, we analysed 101 papers obtained through a Medlar search for the years 1975–1980.

The results can be summarized as follows: (a) in all trials EEG was performed for diagnostic purposes and in most of them it was monitored during the trial; (b) however, in 51 reports EEG data are not mentioned at all in the discussion; (c) in 50 reports EEG data are mentioned in the discussion section; they are considered as an important factor in 25 reports only (determinant in 10). In 13 reports, EEG data are discussed but they are not considered as an important factor for the conclusions. In the remaining 12 reports, EEG data are discussed but only to underline that *they are not a relevant index*, and are frequently in contrast with data on clinical efficacy.

By grouping the papers according to the drug under study it appears that the EEG is discussed 13 times out of 14 in trials on benzodiazepines, 22 times out of 55 for valproic acid, 12 times out of 28 for carbamazepine, 2 times out of 2 for ethosuximide and 2 times out of 3 for miscellaneous drugs.

In other words, EEG data are unanimously considered very important and determinant for the interpretation of the results only in the case of ethosuximide and benzodiazepines.

In the case of valproic acid most of the papers in which EEG is discussed as an important factor deal with absence seizures. For carbamazepine all the papers but one in which EEG is discussed (12/28) agree on the fact that EEG data were not relevant for evaluating the clinical outcome and that they were often in disagreement with the clinical results.

It appears clearly from this analysis that in practice EEG recording is systematically and unanimously taken into account as an outcome variable only in absence seizures.

This is understandable since in absence seizures (a) clinical signs may be difficult to observe; (b) a good correlation has been established between spike and wave discharges and absences (Penry et al. 1975); (c) quantitation of frequency and duration of paroxysms permits an evaluation of drug effects in absences (Browne et al. 1975).

The clinical investigators therefore appear to agree with the guidelines in accepting the value of the EEG as a *diagnostic variable*, while its usefulness as an *outcome variable* is controversial.

In trying to analyse the possible reasons for this limited use of the EEG, one necessarily has to consider the methodology employed.

In most of the studies mentioned, "routine" EEG was performed. This term generally indicates short-time recording (about 20 min), during which activation is obtained through the easiest and least risky methods: hyperventilation and photic stimulation. This technique may obviously supply some useful information about the background activity, its reactivity, the photosensitivity, etc.; however, it is equally true that it seldom permits the recording of ictal events.

If we consider the great variability of inter-ictal abnormalities, both in their frequency and, quite often, in their topography, the interest of the "routine" EEG in the monitoring of epileptic patients other than with absence seizures appears indeed to be limited.

In addition, it is known that many factors such as age, interval from last fit, level of vigilance, emotional state of the patient, time of day, metabolic factors (e.g. fasting or non-fasting, etc.) and environmental conditions may influence and modify the EEG record and should be clearly defined; this is never done for "routine" EEGs, which are therefore poorly standardized and only apparently objective.

Finally, to be suitable for quantitation of a drug effect, an outcome variable has to be measurable on a properly defined scale.

In most of the available reports there is no attempt at a rational scoring of EEG data, taking into account the variables mentioned above.

On the basis of these considerations we feel that it is legitimate to say that the "routine" EEG is inadequate to be considered as an outcome variable in clinical trials on new AEDs.

However, today a possible improvement is offered by more sophisticated techniques such as prolonged EEG recording (radiotelemetry, cable telemetry and cassette recording), and simultaneous EEG and video recording, both with or without computerized analysis.

As already discussed in several papers (Porter et al. 1971, 1977; Ives et al. 1976; Rowan et al. 1978) these techniques have advantages and disadvantages.

We should remember that in fact the increased length of recording permits a reduced influence of interfering environmental factors, reduced variability and, of course, increased information. Furthermore, these techniques offer the possibility of the evaluation of relationships between the EEG and clinical aspects, AED blood concentrations and psychological or psychometric testing. The data can be stored for automatic analysis and, in the case of radiotelemetry and cassette recording, the

EEG recording takes place in a more "naturalistic" situation.

The main drawbacks are the cost of the equipment, the limited availability of these techniques, the need for specially trained personnel, and the limited number of patients which can be studied. Furthermore, in the case of cassette recording a possible malfunctioning of the system may go undetected for some time. Because of this and of previously mentioned factors, the risk of dropouts may be increased.

The major points which should be mentioned, because they are very important with respect to clinical trials, are, firstly, data reduction and secondly, but equally important, the fact that up to now the potential value of these techniques for assessing drug efficacy in controlled clinical trials has not yet been fully exploited. In fact, no sound data are available on this specific topic.

CONCLUSIONS

Going back to the initial question "Should EEG be included in clinical trials on new AEDs?" we may answer that: (a) as a diagnostic variable both "routine" EEG and prolonged recording are very valuable tools; there is, however, a need for better definition and standardization; (b) as an outcome variable, "routine" EEG should not be taken into consideration. The information which can be obtained by this technique is in fact not reliable, poorly standardized, not properly measurable.

Prolonged records are extremely useful in absence seizures. They are probably useful also in other types of seizure than grand mal, but no specific data are available up to now.

If we accept these conclusions, should EEG recording be systematically included in each phase II and phase III clinical trial on new AEDs?

As a diagnostic variable: yes.

As an outcome variable: its usefulness and value will depend on the type of seizure under study, on the drug studied and on the EEG results obtained during preclinical and early clinical testing. At the present level of information, the *systematic* use of either "routine" EEG or prolonged recording cannot be recommended and more data are needed to prove its value in the assessment of efficacy and safety in other than absence seizures.

REFERENCES

Browne, T.R., Dreifuss, F.E., Dyken, P.R., Goode, D.J., Penry, J.K., Porter, R.J., White, B.G. and White, P.T. Ethosuximide in the treatment of absence (petit mal) seizures. Neurology (Minneap.), 1975, 25: 515–524.

FDA Guidelines for the Clinical Evaluation of Anticonvulsant Drugs (adults and children).U.S. Department of Health, Education and Welfare; FDA September 1977, HEW (FDA) 77-3045. U.S. Government Printing Office, Washington, D.C., 1977.

ILAE Principles for Clinical Testing of Antiepileptic Drugs. Epilepsia, 1973, 14: 451–458.

Ives, I.R., Thompson, C.J. and Gloor, P. Seizure monitoring: a new tool in electro-encephalography. Electroenceph. clin. Neurophysiol., 1976, 41: 422–427.

Penry, J.K., Porter, R.J. and Dreifuss, F.E. Simultaneous recording of absence seizures with video tape and electro-encephalography: a study of 374 seizures in 48 patients. Brain, 1975, 98: 427–440.

Porter, R.J., Wolf, Jr., A.A and Penry, J.K. Human electro-encephalographic telemetry. Amer. J. EEG Technol., 1971, 11: 145–159.

Porter, R.J., Penry, J.K. and Lacy, J.R. Diagnostic and therapeutic reevaluation of patients with intractable epilepsy. Neurology (Minneap.), 1977, 27: 1006–1007.

Rowan, A.J., Binnie, C.P., de Beer-Pawlikowski, N.K.B., Goedhart, D.M., Guther, Th., van Parys, J.A.P., Meinardi, H. and Meyer, J.W.A. 24 hour EEG studies with very frequent serum antiepileptic drug concentration determinations in the study of sodium valproate. In: H. Meinardi and A.J. Rowan (Eds.), Advances in Epileptology 1977. Swets and Zeitlinger, Amsterdam, 1978: 255–260.

Kyoto Symposia (EEG Suppl. No. 36)
Editors: P.A. Buser, W.A. Cobb and T. Okuma
© 1982, Elsevier Biomedical Press, Amsterdam

EEG Quantification of Drug Level Effects in Monkey Model of Partial Epilepsy*

JOAN S. LOCKARD (in collaboration with RENÉ H. LEVY, LARRY L. DuCHARME and WILLIAM C. CONGDON)

Department of Neurological Surgery, University of Washington, Seattle, Wash. 98195 (U.S.A.)

EEG inter-ictal sharp activity has been utilized qualitatively in patients as a diagnostic tool of epilepsy and to facilitate the localization of epileptic foci (e.g., Ojemann 1980). The quantification of EEG spikes has rarely been employed, as have seizures, as an indicant of the degree of severity of the disease. Several studies (see review, Lockard 1980) of our monkey model of partial epilepsy have suggested that the frequency of EEG inter-ictal spikes may be clinically useful to assess therapeutic efficacy, providing more data per unit of time than seizures. Although the few clinical studies (e.g., Gibbs and Gibbs 1952; Ajmone Marsan and Ralston 1957; Buchthal et al. 1968; Wilkus and Dodrill 1976; Wilkus et al. 1978) that have correlated EEG inter-ictal paroxysms with number of seizures have not consistently found a strong relationship, serial EEG recording in the same patient under controlled conditions and therapy was rarely conducted. In contrast, such recording is the rule in our alumina-gel primate model, and correlations between the frequency of inter-ictal spikes and overt seizures have been generally high, not only with classic anticonvulsants such as phenytoin but newer drugs such as valproate and the experimental compounds cinromide and progabide.

Since the classic paper by Brodie and Reid (1969), plasma drug level confirmation of adequate dosing in patients has become routine in epilepsy centres and in the private practice of many neurologists. Also, drug levels have become useful data in animal models of drug effects. Dose-response curves of antiepileptic compounds have been complemented by documentation of their efficacious ranges of plasma concentration. However, the opportunity for frequent, non-intrusive blood sampling on a chronic basis to address pharmacological problems, such as the induction of metabolic enzymes and drug dose/time dependence, has not been generally available. Here again, the chronic monkey model is particularly suited.

Therefore, the intent of the present paper is to illustrate the scientific value and clinical utility of EEG quantification of drug level effects. The concordance, or lack thereof, among EEG, seizure and plasma drug level data will be provided for: (a) the

Correspondence should be sent to: Joan S. Lockard, Ph.D., Department of Neurological Surgery, University of Washington (RI-20), Seattle, Wash. 98195, U.S.A.

*This research was supported by NINCDS Contract Nos. N01-NS-1-2282 and N01-NS-2349, and Grant No. NS-04053. The author is an affiliate of the Child Development and Mental Retardation Center of the University of Washington.

classical anticonvulsants phenytoin, phenobarbital, primidone and ethosuximide; (b) the newer antiepileptic agents carbamazepine, valproate and clonazepam; and (c) the experimental compounds cinromide and progabide. These data represent some 10 years of studies, i.e., a total of approximately 12,000 awake or sleeping EEG recording hours and again as many hours in sleep staging and in the manual counting and collation of spikes.

Finally, an attempt will be made to integrate the findings in terms of the role EEG quantification may come to play in clinical epilepsy of partial seizures and its drug therapy. For example, if it can be shown that anticonvulsants affect EEG spikes in an analogous fashion to their effects on clinical seizures, then short-term EEG studies during the initiation of antiepileptic treatment for the first time, or when a drug regimen change is indicated clinically, may be able to forecast the likelihood of the new medication's effectiveness. If such forecasts are feasible — even if only in some patients — the savings in time, effort and cost to both physician and patient will be appreciable.

METHODS

Epileptic preparation

Rhesus monkeys (*Macaca mulatta*; adolescent males) are made experimentally epileptic in the Kopeloff et al. (1942) tradition. Approximately 0.2 ml of aluminum hydroxide is injected subpially in the left pre- and postcentral gyri, sensorimotor, hand and face areas as confirmed by electrical cortical stimulation during sterile craniotomy. The animals start to exhibit both EEG epileptiform activity and focal seizures between 6 and 10 weeks post injection. Subsequently, the monkeys gradually manifest secondarily generalized tonic-clonic seizures, reaching a relatively stable baseline of both partial and generalized seizure frequency by 4–6 months post injection.

EEG methods

Three months prior to the commencement of any study, each monkey is implanted with an EEG head plug (Lockard et al. 1980) which comprises an 8-channel, 9 skull screw electrode montage (Fig. 1). The top 4 channels are used for sleep staging (0–4, REM) and the bottom 4 for detection and quantification of inter-ictal EEG epileptiform activity. At a standard EEG polygraph speed of 30 mm/sec, the number of spikes/10 sec page, or number of spikes/min for lengthy records, is obtained. Inter-ictal spikes are defined as phase-reversed fast activity, unilateral on the epileptogenic focus side, less than 80 msec in duration, more than 100 mV in amplitude, having a velocity of the rising phase of 2 mV/msec or greater. At least 2 half-hour day EEG recordings per animal per week are used to ascertain diurnal spike frequency. One all-night recording is conducted every 2–3 weeks for each monkey for the duration of the study to quantify nocturnal inter-ictal spikes and to correlate them with the sleep stages in which they occur.

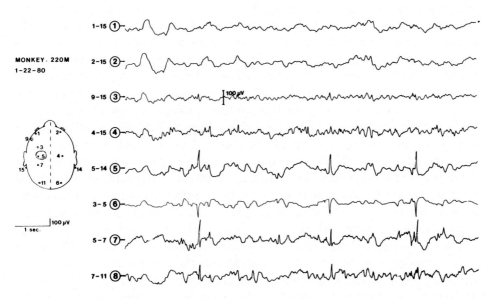

Fig. 1. EEG montage. Illustrative of night recording for staging sleep (channels 1–4) and detecting epileptiform bursts (spikes/min, channels 5–8). Electrode 9 in temporalis muscle and nos. 14 and 15 implanted in mastoid processes. Time constant 0.4 sec for channels 1 and 2; 0.05 sec for channel 3; and 0.12 sec for channels 4–8. Sensitivity of channel 3 (tonic EMG) is greater than all other channels. Electrical focus at electrode 5. (Adapted from Lockard 1980.)

Catheterization

Several months prior to the commencement of a study, each animal is trained to accept a naso-gastric tube for oral administration of drug or is equipped, depending upon alternative modes of drug administration, with 2–3 chronically tested indwelling catheters (Lockard 1980): (a) a jugular catheter for blood sampling to ascertain plasma drug concentrations, (b) a jejunal cannula for gastric administration of drug in suspension, (c) a catheter in the intraperitoneal cavity to allow periodic i.p. bolusing of drug, and (d) a femoral catheter for constant rate intravenous drug infusion.

During a drug study, 2 blood samples (maintenance samples) are taken on different days of the week, at the same time of day for each animal, to ascertain steady state concentrations of the agent(s) under investigation. In addition, 3 different series of 5–7 blood samples are obtained: one at the commencement of drug administration prior to the achievement of steady state; a second series every 2 weeks, which involves all-day sampling (1 sample every 2–3 h for 24 h); and a third period of samples at the time of drug withdrawal, during the drug elimination phase. If, for purposes of health and exercise the monkeys must be caged before, after or during a study, their cannulation tubing can be closed off in a heparin lock and sterilely tucked under the skin for the duration of the caging. The cages are instrumented for seizure recording during the interim and the catheters are usually viable for up to 3 months of such dormancy.

Seizure monitoring

During a study each monkey is maintained in a primate chair (or cage if possible) instrumented with an accelerometer for continuous polygraph read-out of all gross motor activity. Groups of 3 adjacent monkeys are monitored continuously by a closed circuit TV system with infrared vidicon and video recorder (4 systems for 12 animals). Infrared lights at night (1800–0600 h), video time/date generators and constant speed polygraph recordings allow 24 h coverage of clinical seizures. Just beneath the motor activity channel for each monkey, a single channel of slow speed EEG (0.25 mm/sec) is also written out (Lockard et al. 1980). A minicomputer programmed to detect seizure envelopes on the polygraphs automatically activates the respective videotape recorder to visually record the clinical seizures. The criteria for detection of the seizure envelopes are contiguous pen excursions simultaneously on any pair of motor and slow speed EEG channels which are of a particular minimal duration and amplitude.

The video tapes are reviewed daily for clinical verification of seizures. The motor activity envelopes of the verified seizures become the permanent data from which frequency, duration and severity (i.e., mean amplitude of the envelope), and time of occurrence are automatically saved by the computer. This methodology provides nearly 100% accuracy in seizure detection and quantification.

Behavioural and health measures

During a study, the monkeys are automatically fed, each animal having a food pellet dispenser on its primate chair, a lever for activating the dispenser, and a panel of stimulus lights to indicate the particular operant schedule of reinforcement required to achieve the pellets. Seven different combinations of time and number of lever responses (i.e., rate) are computer programmed, the particular schedule for any given study being determined to optimize the behavioural assessment of the treatment under evaluation.

Daily charts of water, food pellet and fruit consumption, and urine and faeces elimination are maintained as additional indicators of the health of the monkeys. Red and white blood cell counts, hematocrits, platelet counts, urine analyses, kidney and liver function, BUN, albumin, and fibrinogen tests are done routinely (usually once every 1–3 weeks). Also, daily collations of seizure and EEG data are made for immediate feedback regarding the state of health of the animals under study so that intervention on behalf of the monkeys may be made in a timely fashion, if it becomes necessary.

RESULTS

Standard anticonvulsants, levels and therapeutic effects

Illustrative of the correlation between frequency of spikes and seizures in the primate model are the data of a study in which the comparative efficacy of phenytoin, phenobarbital and primidone was assessed in epileptic monkeys (N = 9) for a period of 8 months (Lockard et al. 1975). Groups of 3 monkeys each received the drugs separately in a counterbalanced order for a period of 6 weeks (consisting of 3 drug steps of 2 weeks each), preceded and followed by baseline weeks of no drug. As shown in Table I, the frequency of seizures in several animals (N = 5) correlated significantly with the number of interictal spikes ($r = 0.42$ $P = 0.05$ to $r = 0.87$, $P<0.001$), and were inversely related to drug plasma levels ($r = -0.41$, $P = 0.05$ to $r = -0.76$, $P<0.001$). These effects are illustrated in Fig. 2 for 1 monkey.

Valproate levels and therapeutic effects

In a study on the efficacy of valproic acid in our monkey model (Lockard et al. 1977) the importance of frequent plasma drug levels and EEG recording became very evident. The therapeutic effects of valproic acid compared to ethosuximide were evaluated in 12 epileptic monkeys. Both drugs were known to be efficacious for absence type seizures, so the objective was to test whether valproate was a broad spectrum anticonvulsant, also effective against gross motor seizures, for which ethosuximide was not. Since both drugs are soluble in an aqueous solution, and since the half-life of valproate is very short (0.5–2 h) in monkeys, the mode of administration was by constant rate intravenous infusion. The monkeys were divided randomly into 2 drug groups of 6 animals each. The valproate animals, in 3 dosage steps for 3 weeks each, achieved mean plasma drug levels during the day of approximately 50, 100 and 150 μg/ml, respectively. The ethosuximide animals received 2 dosage steps resulting in mean plasma drug levels of 50 and 100 μg/ml. The interesting finding for our purposes here concerns the endogenous fluctuation in plasma concentration which both drugs manifested, but particularly valproic acid (Fig. 3). Even with a constant rate of intravenous infusion the mean diurnal

TABLE I

CORRELATIONS AMONG SEIZURE FREQUENCY, AVERAGE NUMBER OF SPIKES PER 10 SEC AND PLASMA DRUG LEVEL

Monkey	Number of seizures/ave number of spikes per 10 sec		Number of seizures/plasma drug level		Ave number of spikes per 10 sec/plasma drug level	
	r	P	r	P	r	P
1	0.63	<0.005	−0.41	0.05	−0.56	<0.02
2	0.55	<0.02	0.08	ns*	−0.47	<0.05
3	0.87	<0.001	0.05	ns	−0.26	ns*
4	−0.05	ns*	−0.42	0.05	0.10	ns
5	0.01	ns	−0.23	ns	−0.40	<0.10
6	−0.21	ns	−0.37	ns	−0.39	<0.10
7	0.54	<0.02	−0.16	ns	−0.22	ns
8	0.42	0.05	−0.76	<0.001	−0.32	<0.15
9	0.04	ns	0.12	ns	0.04	ns

$P < 0.05$, statistically significant; $0.15 > P > 0.05$, approaching statistical significance.
* Not approaching statistical significance.

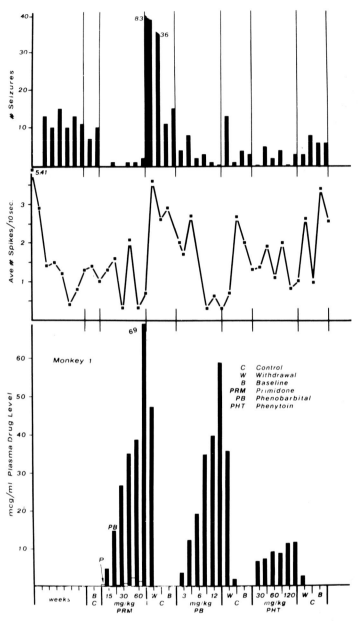

Fig. 2. Relationship of clinical seizure frequency, mean number of EEG inter-ictal spikes, and plasma drug levels, illustrated by the weekly data of 1 monkey. For concomitant time periods, a direct correlation between number of seizures and number of spikes and an inverse correlation of each with plasma drug level are indicated. (Adapted from Lockard et al. 1975.)

fluctuation in plasma valproate level was 36% and considerably more (100%) in some animals. These endogenous oscillations in plasma valproate concentration permitted correlations of therapeutic effects with drug levels on an hour by hour basis.

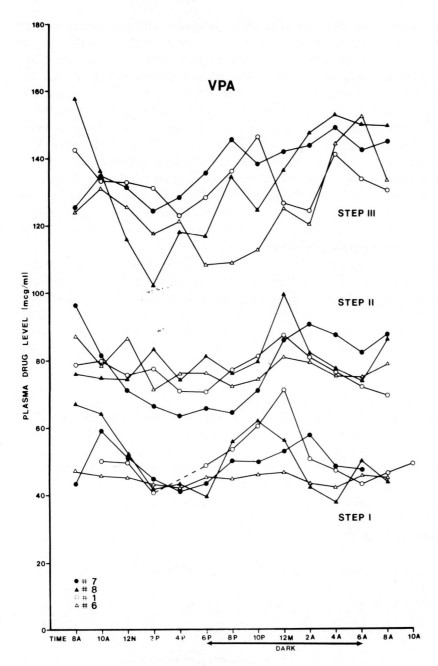

Fig. 3. Circadian oscillation in valproate plasma levels. One sample every 2 h for 24 h in 4 monkeys at drug steps I, II, and III (plasma concentrations of approximately 50, 100, and 150 μg/ml, respectively). All data gathered during steady state constant rate intravenous infusion. Mean diurnal fluctuations, 33%; much more in some monkeys. (Adapted from Lockard et al. 1977.)

Heretofore it has been generally assumed for patients on chronic medications that swings in plasma drug levels as a function of dosing regimen resulted in no noticeable changes in therapeutic effects at the moment. However, as shown in Fig. 4 for the primate model, a reasonably close relationship was found between the frequency of EEG inter-ictal spikes in all-night EEG records and plasma valproate levels sampled every 2 h. As drug concentrations increased during the early morning hours, the number of spikes decreased; in turn, with the decrease in plasma levels toward 6 a.m., the frequency of spikes increased ($r = -0.71$ to -0.99, $P < 0.10$; N $= 6$). Although these data are intimately confounded with the stage of sleep, they are in the direction opposite from that which would be predicted. More spikes would be expected in the deeper stages of sleep in the middle of the night and fewer in stage I as 6 a.m. was approached — the reverse occurred. Therefore, it seems reasonable to assume that the increasing valproate plasma concentrations were correlated with the decrease in spikes during the night.

An outcome consistent with this assumption was evident in the EEG inter-ictal spike data gathered during the waking hours, as shown in Fig. 5. Valproate decreased inter-ictal spikes ($t = 1.98$, $P < 0.10$; N $= 12$), an effect which carried over into the subsequent baseline period. A similar result was found in terms of seizure frequency (Fig. 6: $t = 2.40$, $P < 0.05$; N $= 12$). As predicted, ethosuximide did not have comparable effects in this model of partial epilepsy (see Table II: ESM).

Clonazepam levels and therapeutic effects

This study (Lockard et al. 1979a) was conducted to assess the effect of clonazepam on focal motor or partial seizures in epileptic monkeys (N $= 6$), since some ambiguity existed in the patient literature of other countries and because approval had not been given for this seizure category by the Food and Drug Administration in the U.S.A. (Browne 1976). Clonazepam was administered by constant rate intravenous infusion at a concentration to achieve plasma levels of

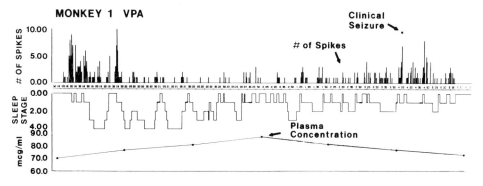

Fig. 4. Correlation of pharmacological effects and plasma valproate levels. EEG inter-ictal spikes/min (top) and drug concentration (bottom) at night; sleep stage (middle; 0–4, REM). Illustrative of an inverse relationship between plasma concentration and number of spikes in 1 monkey. (Adapted from Lockard et al. 1977.)

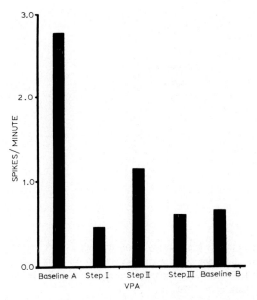

Fig. 5. EEG inter-ictal spikes (day samples); means for 12 monkeys shown for each study phase. Baseline B is post-drug phase immediately following cessation of valproic acid administered by constant rate intravenous infusion. (Adapted from Lockard et al. 1977.)

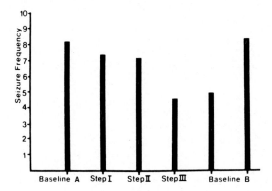

Fig. 6. Non-reversibility of valproate effects. Mean seizure frequency of monkeys (N = 12) during steady state days (last 10 days of 14 days) of each study phase. Return to former seizure frequency delayed by 2 weeks in post-drug period. Valproate plasma levels effectively zero 24 h after cessation of drug administration by constant rate intravenous infusion. (Adapted from Lockard et al. 1977.)

approximately 30 ng/ml in drug step I (3 weeks) and at least double that level in drug step II (3 weeks). The results indicated that clonazepam is effective against focal motor and secondarily generalized tonic-clonic seizures (Fig. 7), particularly when its concentration in plasma is equal to or greater than 60 ng/ml.

Consistent with the seizure data, the mean frequency of inter-ictal spikes during the day EEG samples (Fig. 8) of several monkeys decreased with clonazepam treatment but especially during the all-night EEG records on drug step II (t = 4.47, $P < 0.01$; N = 6), as illustrated in Fig. 9.

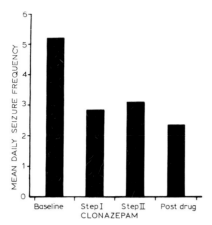

Fig. 7. Mean daily seizure frequency for the last 2 weeks (i.e., steady state) of each 3 week period (baseline, steps I and II, and post-drug periods) for clonazepam-treated monkeys (N = 6). Drug steps I and II by constant rate intravenous infusion in 35% PEG 400 gave plasma concentrations of 30 ng/ml and ≥ 60 ng/ml, respectively. (Adapted from Lockard et al. 1979a.)

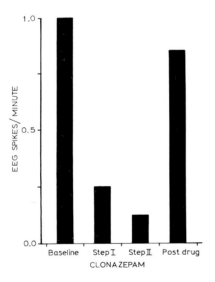

Fig. 8. Mean EEG inter-ictal spikes per minute during day samples for clonazepam-treated monkeys for the last 2 weeks (i.e., steady state) of each 3 week period (baseline period, steps I and II, and post-drug periods). Steps I and II gave plasma concentrations of 30 ng/ml and ≥ 60 ng/ml, respectively. (Adapted from Lockard et al. 1979a.)

Cinromide levels and therapeutic effects

In an evaluation of the Burroughs-Wellcome experimental anticonvulsant cinromide in the monkey model (Lockard et al. 1979b), *some* seizure efficacy was evident at plasma concentrations of 7–14 µg/ml of the drug's major metabolite. With the exception of 1 animal (N = 6), no secondarily generalized seizures were exhibited during drug administration by constant rate intravenous infusion, but

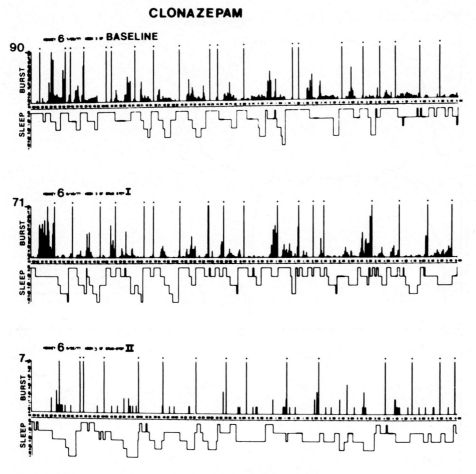

Fig. 9. EEG inter-ictal spikes per minute (bursts) and sleep stages (0–4 and REM, shown as dark horizontal line) during all-night records for monkey 6 for pre-drug baseline (top tracing). Drug step I, 30 ng/ml; drug step II, ≥ 60 ng/ml. Triangles indicate bursts terminating in clinical seizures. EEG spikes decreased during drug administration by constant rate intravenous infusion in 35% PEG 400. (Adapted from Lockard et al. 1979a.)

such seizures were evident during baseline periods. Again, EEG inter-ictal spikes decreased significantly for several animals in both the day and in the all-night records, as illustrated in Figs. 10 and 11, respectively.

Other anticonvulsants, levels and therapeutic effects

The general findings for other antiepileptic compounds tested in the monkey model are summarized in Table II; space does not allow a review of the details of each study. The effective plasma level range is indicated for each drug, with the exception of albutoin, ABT, for which there was no assay available at the time. Also indicated is whether the plasma drug range attenuated (↓), augmented (↑) or the data were ambiguous (?) or not gathered (−) with respect to partial seizures, generalized seizures and inter-ictal spikes, respectively.

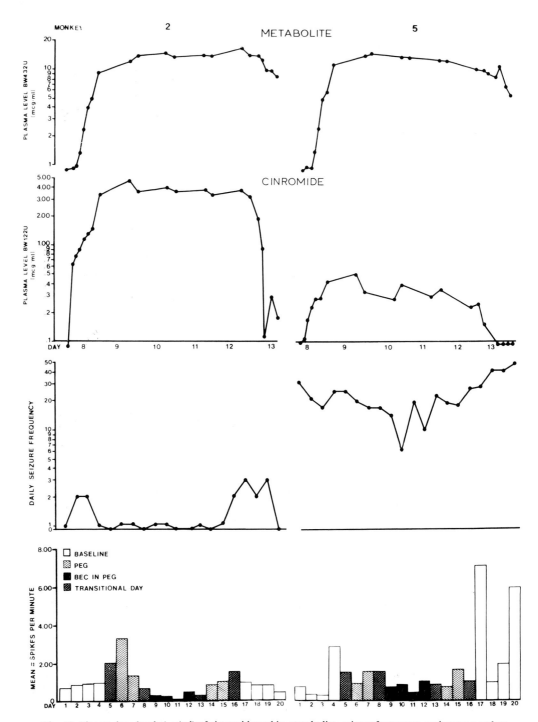

Fig. 10. Plasma drug levels (μg/ml) of cinromide and its metabolite, seizure frequency, and mean number of EEG inter-ictal spikes per minute for monkeys 2 (left) and 5 (right). Plasma levels span days 8–13 only. Drug administration by constant rate intravenous infusion in 60% PEG 400. (Adapted from Lockard et al. 1979b.)

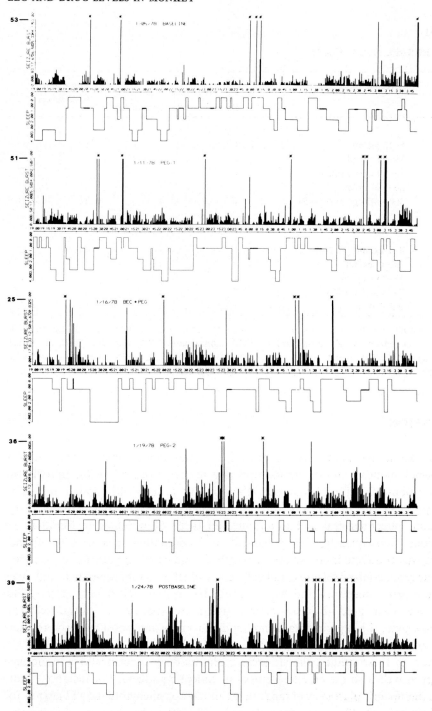

Fig. 11. EEG bursts (spikes) and seizures at night: illustrative (1 monkey) of the bursts' culmination in clinical seizures (small circles above) and their density during cinromide (BEC) or solvent alone (PEG) as compared to baselines. Sleep stages (0–4) shown below each record; REM = thickened horizontal line. Drug administration by constant rate intravenous infusion in 60% PEG 400.

TABLE II

DRUG THERAPEUTIC EFFECTS

Drug	Effective range	Seizures		Inter-ictal EEG spikes
		Partial	Generalized	
Standard				
PHT	5–12 μg/ml	↓	↓	↓
PB	13–40 μg/ml	↓	↓	↓
PRM	15–50 μg/ml (mPB)	↓	↓	↓
ESM	50–100 μg/ml	↑	↑	?
DZP	300–500 ng/ml (nDZP)	↓	↓	↓
Newer				
ABT	–	↑	↑	–
CBZ	4–8 μg/ml	↓	↓	?
CZP	30–60 ng/ml	↓	↓	↓
VPA	50–150 μg/ml	↓	↓	↓
BEC	7–14 μg/ml (BC)	?	↓	?
PGB	0.5–3.0 μg/ml	↓	↓	?

PHT, phenytoin; PB, phenobarbital; PRM, primidone; ESM, ethosuximide; DZP, diazepam; ABT, albutoin (3–11 mg/kg); CBZ, carbamazepine; CZP, clonazepam; VPA, valproate; BEC, cinromide; PGB, progabide; mPB, metabolic phenobarbital; nDZP, nordiazepam; BC, major metabolite of cinromide; –, no data; ?, ambiguous data; ↑, increase; ↓, decrease.

DISCUSSION

In the last decade a number of quantitative studies on anticonvulsants in monkey have been conducted in our laboratories (see review, Lockard 1980). Initially the clinically non-efficacious hydantoin albutoin was tested, with similar results in monkey. Then the model was further validated by testing the classical drugs phenytoin, phenobarbital and primidone, all three of which were found to be efficacious. Subsequently, the assessment of 2 compounds pertinent to absence seizures was conducted: ethosuximide which, as indicated in patients, exacerbates secondarily generalized seizures, and valproate, which was subsequently found by us to have a broad spectrum and be non-reversible in pharmacological effects. The model was next used to test newer drugs more specific to partial seizures: carbamazepine, the experimental compound cinromide and, most recently, the new GABA-mimetic drug, progabide (Lloyd et al. 1979).

In most of these studies, the efficacious plasma drug concentrations in monkey overlapped well with the effective ranges in epileptic patients. For instance (Table II), the therapeutic plasma level range in the model for phenytoin is 5–12 μg/ml, for phenobarbital, 20–40 μg/ml, for valproate, 50–150 μg/ml and for clonazepam, 30–60 ng/ml. The optimal range for carbamazepine, 4–10 μg/ml, has not been tested chronically at the higher levels because of the drug's insolubility and short half-life in monkey. The effective range for cinromide in rhesus is best indicated by its major active metabolite (Table II, BC), which is 7–14 μg/ml. These plasma level ranges decreased the frequency of EEG inter-ictal spikes and usually the number of both partial and secondarily generalized clinical seizures.

The success that we have had in utilizing the EEG as an indicant of the effectiveness of treatment in our monkey model is largely attributable to several factors: (a) the specificity of our epileptic category, namely, focal motor and secondarily generalized tonic-clonic seizures; (b) the well controlled environmental conditions under which the EEG data are gathered; (c) the strict criteria that are used to select both the EEG pages to be scored and the particular paroxysms to be counted; (d) the requirement of multiple EEG records per animal; (e) the use of each animal as its own control; (f) the control of other relevant variables such as plasma drug levels and emotional and alertness states of the animals; and, most importantly, (g) the expenditure of effort and time of well trained personnel on manual counting of individual EEG inter-ictal spikes in long-duration records (e.g., from at least 1 h per week per animal to all-night samples every 3 weeks per animal).

Since the EEG has been used primarily as a diagnostic tool in epileptic patients (e.g. Gibbs and Gibbs 1967; Klass 1970; Gastaut and Broughton 1972), its potential as a sensitive predictor of efficacy of treatment has not been explored adequately. The lack of covariation found between EEG data and seizure frequency in some patients may be a function largely of (a) the limitations in controlling the clinical setting and (b) not selecting the most appropriate patients, e.g., only those with partial seizure epilepsy (Klass 1975). The cost of serial EEGs on the same patient and the effort and time that would be expended by medical personnel to count individual EEG spikes may not seem to warrant this type of study. However, if collation of the EEG data could be automated in the future, as recent computer technology indicates (e.g., Gotman et al. 1979) and the findings of short-term samples were indicative of long-term treatment efficacy, then the cost effectiveness of such research might well be demonstrated.

The general procedure in conducting clinical studies to test the quantitative value of EEG spike data would be to standardize the conditions under which clinically prescribed EEG recording was conducted and to extend the duration of the records from their usual 30–40 min clinic sample to 1–2 h. Then, with good patient selection and strict data criteria, the EEG records would be scored by manual counts of inter-ictal spikes now (under "blind" conditions), and by computer detection and collation at a later time when the technology has been perfected. Subsequently, spike frequency could be correlated with the number of clinical seizures of the same patients over a 3–6 month period. Moreover, for an epileptic patient being seen in the clinic to initiate medication or for a drug regimen change, the first dose of the drug could be given by slow intravenous administration at the time of EEG recording so that plasma drug concentrations could be compared with the pharmacological effects (if any) on the frequency of EEG inter-ictal spikes. From these data, predictions as to the long-term efficacy of the new drug regimen could be made and follow-up studies conducted — in terms of seizure frequency (as ascertained from patient calendars), periodic EEG and plasma drug level samples and the physician's and patient's judgement as to the success of the treatment. This information could then serve to test the predictive validity of the initial EEG spike and plasma concentration data.

In this research process, a good strategy would be to first validate the EEG paradigm for a classical anticonvulsant such as phenytoin, and in partial seizure patients only, and then to use these data as a comparison standard for other antiepileptic drugs and for patients with different seizure types. It could well be that such an investment in EEG quantification may eventually turn out to be as fruitful clinically as it has been in our monkey model.

REFERENCES

Ajmone Marsan, C. and Ralston, B.L. The Epileptic Seizure: its Functional Morphology and Diagnostic Significance. Thomas, Springfield, Ill., 1957.

Brodie, B.B. and Reid, W.D. Is man a unique animal in response to drugs? Amer. J. Pharm., 1969, 140: 21–27.

Browne, T.R. Clonazepam. A review of a new anticonvulsant drug. Arch. Neurol. (Chic.), 1976, 33: 326–332.

Buchthal, F., Svensmark, O. and Simonsen, H. Relation of EEG and seizures to phenobarbital in serum. Arch. Neurol. (Chic.), 1968, 19: 567–572.

Gastaut, H. and Broughton, R. Epileptic Seizures. Clinical and Electrographic Features, Diagnosis and Treatment. Thomas, Springfield,, Ill., 1972.

Gibbs, F.A. and Gibbs, E.L. Atlas of Electroencephalography, Vol. 2: Epilepsy, 2nd Ed. Addison-Wesley, Reading, Mass., 1952.

Gibbs, F.A. and Gibbs, E.L. Medical Electroencephalography. Addison-Wesley, Reading, Mass., 1967.

Gotman, J., Ives, J. and Gloor, P. Automatic recognition of interictal epileptic activity in prolonged EEG recordings. Electroenceph. clin. Neurophysiol., 1979, 46: 510–520.

Klass, D.W. Value of the EEG to the clinician. Neurol. Neurocir. Psiquiat., 1970, 11: 197–201.

Klass, D.W. Electroencephalographic manifestations of complex partial seizures. In: J.K. Penry and D.D. Daly (Eds.), Advances in Neurology. Raven Press, New York, 1975: 133–140.

Kopeloff, L.M., Barrera, S.E. and Kopeloff, N. Recurrent convulsive seizures in animals produced by immunologic and chemical means. Amer. J. Psychiat., 1942, 98: 881–902.

Lloyd, K.G., Worms, P., Depoortere, H. and Bartholini, G. Pharmacological profile of SL 76002, a new GABA-mimetic drug. In: P. Krosgaar-Larsen, J. Scheel-Kruger and H. Kofod (Eds.), Alfred Benson Symposium 12 GABA-Neurotransmitters Pharmacochemical, Biochemical and Pharmacological Aspects. Munksgaard, Copenhagen, 1979: 308–325.

Lockard, J.S. A primate model of clinical epilepsy: Mechanisms of action through quantification of therapeutic effects. In: J.S. Lockard and A.A. Ward, Jr. (Eds.), Epilepsy: A Window to Brain Mechanisms. Raven Press, New York, 1980: 11–49.

Lockard, J.S., Uhlir, V., DuCharme, L.L., Farquhar, J.A. and Huntsman, B.J. Efficacy of standard anticonvulsants in monkey model with spontaneous motor seizures. Epilepsia, 1975, 16: 301–317.

Lockard, J.S., Levy, R.H., Congdon, W.C., DuCharme, L.L. and Patel, I.H. Efficacy testing of valproic acid compared to ethosuximide in monkey model: II. Seizure, EEG, and diurnal variations. Epilepsia, 1977, 18: 205–224.

Lockard, J.S., Levy, R.H., Congdon, W.C., DuCharme, L.L. and Salonen, L.D. Clonazepam in focal-motor monkey model: Efficacy, tolerance, toxicity, withdrawal and management. Epilepsia, 1979a, 20: 683–695.

Lockard, J.S., Levy, R.H., DuCharme, L.L. and Congdon, W.C. Experimental anticonvulsant cinromide in monkey model: Preliminary efficacy. Epilepsia, 1979b, 20: 339–350.

Lockard, J.S., Congdon, W.C., DuCharme, L.L. and Finch, C.A. Slow-speed EEC for chronic monitoring of clinical seizures in monkey model. Epilepsia, 1980, 21: 325–334.

Ojemann, G.A. Basic mechanisms implicated in surgical treatments of epilepsy. In: J.S. Lockard and A.A. Ward (Eds.), Epilepsy: A Window to Brain Mechanisms. Raven Press, New York, 1980: 261–277.

Wilkus, R.J. and Dodrill, C.B. Neuropsychological correlates of the elctroencephalogram in epileptics: Topographic distribution and average rate of epileptiform activity. Epilepsia, 1976, 17: 89–100.

Wilkus, R.J., Dodrill, C.B. and Troupin, A.S. Carbamazepine and the electroencephalogram of epileptics: A double blind study in comparison to phenytoin. Epilepsia, 1978, 19: 283–291.

Kyoto Symposia (EEG Suppl. No. 36)
Editors: P.A. Buser, W.A. Cobb and T. Okuma
© 1982, Elsevier Biomedical Press, Amsterdam

The Use of the Inter-Ictal EEG in the Study of Antiepileptic Drugs

C.D. BINNIE

Instituut voor Epilepsiebestrijding, Meer en Bosch, Achterweg 5, 2103 SW Heemstede (The Netherlands)

One of the greatest fascinations, and difficulties, of studying epilepsy, is the intermittent nature of its clinical expression. This creates difficulties for assessing drug treatment, both in the individual patient and during formal trials. The ultimate criterion of antiepileptic drug (AED) action in man is the suppression of seizures, but reliably to estimate attack frequency with a given treatment may take months. The need to measure antiepileptic effect at a point in time has therefore led many workers to study the actions of drugs on spontaneous inter-ictal epileptiform EEG events. This practice involves two assumptions: first, that a strong correlation exists, at least within patients, between seizure incidence and amount of inter-ictal epileptiform EEG activity, and secondly that the method selected for sampling the random EEG events is itself statistically reliable.

SEIZURE INCIDENCE AND INTER-ICTAL EEG DISCHARGES

In the case of absence seizures, whether classical or atypical, accompanied by generalized spike-wave activity, the first assumption is readily justified. Video monitoring of behaviour during long-term telemetric EEG registrations and continuous assessment of cognitive function by performance tests indicate that in such patients the discharges are usually accompanied by behavioural or cognitive changes and may thus virtually be equated with the seizures themselves (Binnie 1980). There appears to be much less evidence available concerning the correlation between other seizure types and inter-ictal discharges.

Table I is based on 3 years' routine referrals in which the referring physician

TABLE I

CHANGES IN AMOUNT OF EPILEPTIFORM ACTIVITY IN ROUTINE EEGs AFTER CHANGES IN SEIZURE INCIDENCE

Change in epileptiform activity	Reported change in seizure frequency	
	Increase	Decrease
Increase	75	84
No change	441	507
Decrease	40	97

specifically mentioned a change of seizure frequency since the preceding EEG. There is evidently only a very weak association between the reported alteration in seizure incidence and the change, if any, in the frequency of inter-ictal discharges.

Table II summarizes the results in a more formal study of 11 patients with therapy resistant epilepsy, investigated for 3–6 months during adjustment of medication, which was accompanied by changes in, and eventual reduction of, seizure incidence. Twice weekly EEGs were recorded during a simple task intended, so far as possible, to standardize the state of awareness, and during 15 min at rest with eyes closed. All patients had focal or multifocal discharges, all but 3 had partial seizures and the diagnosis was either partial or secondary generalized epilepsy. The patients were readily divided into 2 groups: in 6 there was a strong correlation between the amount of inter-ictal epileptiform EEG activity and seizure incidence, whether measured over a period of 48 h or 7 days symmetrically surrounding the EEG. In 5 patients, however, there was no such correlation or even a trend which might be expected to reach significance with a larger number of observations. There were no clinical features which distinguished the one group from the other. Obviously, if it is necessary to carry out a 3–6 months' study to determine whether or not a correlation exists in a particular individual, these EEG measures are of little practical use in such patients for clinical or research purposes.

SPONTANEOUS EPILEPTIFORM ACTIVITY AND AED LEVELS

This last study, and indeed any similar investigation, inevitably confounds the

TABLE II

RELATIONSHIP OF EPILEPTIFORM ACTIVITY IN TWICE WEEKLY EEGs TO SEIZURE INCIDENCE

	Sex	Age	Diagnosis	Observation (weeks)	Seizure type	Correlation of epileptiform activity with		Recording condition
						Seizures/week	Seizures/48 h	
JF	F	41	2° gen	29	PC	+ +	+ +	R > S > O
DN	F	48	2° gen	16	PC	+ +	+ +	O ≫ R = S
RF	F	58	2° gen	15	Ak.TC	+	−	O = R = S
JL	F	26	Pa	28	PE/C TC	+ +	−	S
SG	M	18	2° gen	15	Ab TC	+	+ +	R = O = S
AR	M	26	2° gen	15	TC PC	+	+	R > O
ML	M	32	2° gen	17	TC	−	−	−
HK	F	50	2° gen	16	PC	−	−	−
RD	M	21	2° gen	18	TC PC	−	−	−
MP	F	24	Pa	25	PE TC	−	−	−
VB	F	52	2° gen	28	PC TC	−	−	−

+, $P < 0.05$; + +, $P < 0.01$.
Recording condition for which correlation existed: R, rest; O, eyes open; S, eyes shut.

problem of the correlation between inter-ictal discharges and seizures with that of sampling the randomly fluctuating EEG phenomena.

Extended telemetric EEG monitoring studies highlight the problem of the fluctuations in amount of epileptiform activity from minute to minute, from hour to hour, and from day to day. The sleep-waking cycle and the effects of the different stages of sleep on epileptiform activity impose a certain consistency on the circadian rhythm but when allowance is made for these factors, there rarely remains any evidence of a consistent pattern, for instance during the hours of waking. One possibility to be considered is that this inconsistency is secondary to variations in antiepileptic drug (AED) levels.

Fig. 1 illustrates 3 typical but markedly differing 24 h profiles of serum carbamazepine concentration which we have observed with administration of this drug in 3 equal divided doses, both with and without comedication (Meijer et al. 1981). Why such variations should occur is uncertain but what is perhaps more surprising is that, even in a given individual and under carefully controlled conditions, the profiles are very inconsistent. Out of 25 patients whom we have studied for 48 consecutive hours 9 showed different patterns on the first and second days. Sodium valproate shows a similar variability, particularly when administered in enteric-coated form, as does valproic acid.

In the course of some hundreds of prolonged telemetric recordings we have obtained just 10 which met the following rather stringent criteria for a test/re-test stability study: EEG and hourly blood AED levels were monitored for 2 consecutive 24 h periods; medication was not altered; mean AED levels differed by less than

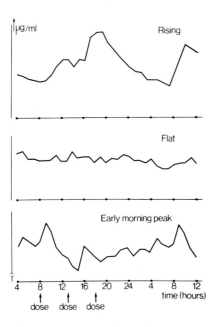

Fig. 1. Three types of 24 h carbamazepine profiles with 3 equal daily doses. Pharmacokinetic considerations predict the upper curve, rising over the day and falling at night.

TABLE III

TEST/RE-TEST STABILITY OF 24 h PRODUCTION OF EPILEPTIFORM ACTIVITY

Patient	Type of epilepsy	Epileptiform activity	Difference in amount of epileptiform activity (%)*
1	2° gen	3/s S-W	38
2	1° gen	3/s S-W	100
3	1° gen	3/s S-W	16
			100
4	2° gen	Irreg S-W	30
5	2° gen	Irreg S-W	10
6	Pa	Multifocal spikes	64
7	Pa	Temporal spikes	32
8	Pa	Temporal spikes	25
9	Pa (C.T.)	Frontal spikes	38
10	Pa	Hippocampal spikes	3
		(depth recording)	14

* $\dfrac{\text{Difference day I, day II}}{\text{day I + day II}} \times 100.$

10% and showed similar 24 h profiles; diet and activity regime were standardized; epileptiform EEG discharges were present and readily quantifiable; not less than a third of the epileptiform activity occurred during waking. The results shown in Table III indicate a highly variable degree of test/re-test stability. The inconsistencies in 24 h incidence of epileptiform activity are thus often considerable, and occur even when variations in AED levels are excluded.

On a shorter time scale too, an hour to hour correlation between epileptiform discharges and levels of chronically administered AEDs does not appear to have been established. The sleep-waking cycle imposes a periodicity on both the EEG discharges, which often increase in sleep, and on the blood levels of drugs with short half-lives, which fall at night. The correlation is nevertheless spurious, and if the time or form of administration of the drug is changed without alteration of the total dose so as to maintain a high level at night, the amount of epileptiform activity is unaffected.

EEG recording of a more or less routine nature and some tens of minutes duration forms a part of most AED trials and changes in the amount of epileptiform activity seen are sometimes interpreted as reflecting the efficacy or otherwise of the drug. Some such studies have indeed produced meaningful results. Wilkus and Green (1974), for instance, found a significant difference in waking spike counts between phenytoin and sulthiame therapy and a negative association with changes in serum phenytoin levels. Negative or inconsistent results are more usual, however. The lack of correlation between inter-ictal spike counts and seizure incidence during carbamazepine therapy is well known (Cereghino et al. 1974; Rodin and Rennick 1974; Wilkus et al. 1976) and must lead to caution in the interpretation of inter-ictal EEGs in the trial of any new drug. Paradoxically, an increase in discharges during

AED reduction in patients who are seizure free is predictive, not of relapse but of sustained remission (Overweg et al. 1981).

In the light of long-term telemetric studies it is perhaps worth considering what is the probable reliability of an estimate of discharge rate based on a short routine EEG.

In 23 patients undergoing long-term monitoring we estimated the amount of epileptiform activity per hour of 16 h of waking, divided into periods of 60 min. Fig. 2 indicates the probability of such an estimate lying between one half of and twice the mean discharge rate over the entire 16 h period. Predictably, the probability of the estimate falling within these very broad limits rises as the overall production of epileptiform activity increases. Nevertheless it is clear that in the majority of these patients a reliable estimate of the overall discharge rate was not likely to be obtained even by a sample of 60 min, which is considerably more than the running time of a typical clinical EEG in most countries. Even when the incidence of inter-ictal discharges is stationary (which is often not the case) their occurrence usually shows a Poisson distribution (Nagelkerke et al. 1982). In interpreting apparent changes in the EEG one may therefore take account of the fact that the variance of a Poisson distribution is equal to the mean. This implies, for instance, that if a control EEG contained 9 discharges within a standard recording period, to claim at a 5% level of confidence an improvement with therapy, the treatment EEG would need to contain less than 4 discharges within the same period.

It should not be supposed that the measurement of spontaneous inter-ictal EEG discharges is useless for assessment of antiepileptic drugs but rather that the limitations of the method must be recognized. Several groups of authors have clearly

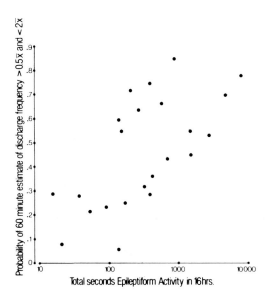

Fig. 2. Probability that production of epileptiform activity in 60 min EEG lies between half and twice the mean hourly rate over the waking day.

shown reduction of generalized spike-wave activity in long-term recordings during administration of drugs effective in absence seizures (Penry et al. 1971; Villarreal et al. 1978; Rowan et al. 1979). It should, however, be noted specifically that the phenomenon studied was generalized spike-wave activity which may be virtually equated with the seizures themselves, that the problems of EEG sampling were in part overcome by protracted telemetric or cassette recording and of course that the drugs used in absence seizures are generally very effective, commonly producing a reduction in seizure incidence and of epileptiform activity of between 90 and 100%. The test/re-test stability, even of 24 h counts, of spike-wave activity may be considerably less than seems to be generally supposed (Milligan and Richens 1982). Few pharmacological studies of focal discharges using long-term monitoring have been reported but Kellaway et al. (1978) found complete suppression of focal spikes in 6/11 patients who became seizure free on phenobarbital.

The above does not call in question the utility of pharmacological monitoring as an aid to adjusting medication. In an evaluation study of 64 consecutive investigations of this type the results led to therapeutic action in 69% with objective benefit to the patient in 35% (Aarts et al. 1982).

ACUTE STUDIES OF AED ACTIONS ON EPILEPTIFORM DISCHARGES

For the assessment of new antiepileptic drugs or studying certain pharmacokinetic aspects of established agents, acute single dose investigations using relatively stable EEG phenomena have considerable advantages.

Photosensitivity as evidenced by a classical generalized photoconvulsive response is exhibited by some 5% of persons with epilepsy. The response is obtainable over a range of flash rates, the upper and lower limits of which are fairly stable. These limits or their difference, the photosensitivity range (Jeavons and Harding 1975), provide an index for studying AEDs. Fig. 3 shows the effect of the acute oral administration of sodium valproate 900 mg: photosensitivity was demonstrated at hourly intervals during control days preceding and following administration of the drug but was abolished some 3 h after attainment of peak plasma valproate concentration. This delayed response is typically shown by valproate (Binnie et al. 1980; Milligan and Richens 1981) and also apparently by depamide and may continue for considerably longer than the half-life of the drug (Harding et al. 1978), whereas the effects of diazepam, clonazepam and progabide closely follow the plasma concentrations. The slow, prolonged action of sodium valproate despite its rapid absorption and short half-life is in accordance with the general clinical experience of this drug.

In the course of our pharmacological studies we have carried out hourly estimations of photosensitivity during 46 control days on basal medication in 26 patients. We found 2 subjects who exhibited a marked reduction in photosensitivity during the afternoon. This pattern was consistent and was demonstrated twice in one subject and 3 times in the other. A third patient showed a temporary loss of

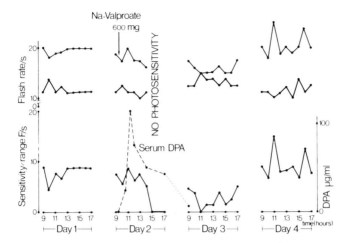

Fig. 3. Effect of single dose of sodium valproate on photosensitivity. A single oral dose of sodium valproate 600 mg given at 10.00 a.m. on the second day of the experiment produced a peak blood level within 1 h. Suppression of photosensitivity appeared only 3–4 h later but persisted throughout the following day.

photosensitivity during the morning of 1 out of 3 days studied. The remaining 23 patients were consistently photosensitive throughout. Photosensitivity thus appears to be a more stable phenomenon than spontaneous epileptiform activity. The range of AEDs with acute effects on the photosensitivity model has not yet been determined and is currently being investigated. In view of the suggestion of Myslobodsky et al. (1980) that such changes in photosensitivity range are a non-specific effect due to drowsiness it should, however, be added that we find that sodium quinalbarbitone in a dosage of 3 mg/kg does not abolish photosensitivity unless the patient is actually asleep during testing (Yamamoto et al. 1971). Caution in interpreting reduction of photosensitivity by markedly sedative drugs is nevertheless advisable (Milligan and Richens 1981).

An alternative model for acute studies of antiepileptic drugs is hyperventilation-induced spike-wave activity. The effects for instance of intravenous benzodiazepines are generally so marked as to be obvious but to study small doses or less effective agents one may need to use quantitative measures such as the latency of onset of the discharges or the total production of epileptiform activity during a standardized period of hyperventilation. Standardization of the procedure is difficult and requires at the least measurement of end-tidal pCO_2. Repeated performance of hyperventilation is considerably more demanding for the patient than photic stimulation and this model may therefore be a less convenient research tool.

Finally, and perhaps in apparent contradiction of my earlier remarks concerning spontaneous epileptiform activity, in patients in whom the discharges are extremely frequent or continuous (essentially electrical status epilepticus) intravenous administration of antiepileptic drugs may produce readily recognizable effects. Even here caution is necessary in interpreting the results. Epileptiform activity of all kinds is markedly influenced by the state of awareness and if one employs this technique under single blind conditions with a preliminary injection of saline, one of the most remarkable findings is the substantial reduction in epileptiform activity often produced by the control injection; in one study it averaged 40%.

I have confined my remarks to the effects of AEDs on epileptiform EEG phenomena because showing that a possible antiepileptic agent suppresses spikes appears to have direct face validity but it is worth while also considering the possibility of studying effects on background activity, employing techniques such as those developed so successfully for use with psychotropic agents by Fink, Itil and their colleagues and described by previous speakers. AEDs produce marked changes in the power spectrum, but how far these are specific to an antiepileptic effect remains to be seen.

In conclusion, I can only concur with the opinion expressed by most of the speakers in this symposium: the EEG appears likely to have a useful role to play in studies of antiepileptic drugs but we are still at the stage of discovering, perhaps rather belatedly, the problems, rather than exploiting the possibilities.

ACKNOWLEDGEMENT

The above includes previously unpublished results from studies carried out in collaboration with L. Bossie, C.E. Darby, D. Fung, J.W.A. Meijer and J. Overweg.

REFERENCES

Aarts, J.H.P., Binnie, C.D., Van Bentum-de Boer, P.T.E., Van de Geest, P.J.M., Kamp, A., Lopes da Silva, F.H., Meijer, J.W.A., Meinardi, H. and Van Wieringen, A. The value of telemetric EEG-monitoring in epilepsy. In: T.A. Betts, R.J. Hoeppener and V. Petersen (Eds.). Brit. J. clin. Pract. (Symp. Suppl.), 1982, 18: 5–9.

Binnie, C.D. Detection of transitory cognitive impairment during epileptiform EEG discharges: problems in clinical practice. In: B.M. Kulig, H. Meinardi and G. Stores (Eds.), Epilepsy and Behaviour '79. Swets and Zeitlinger, Lisse, 1980: 91–97.

Binnie, C.D., de Korte, R.A., Meijer, R.W.A., Rowan, A.J. and Warfield, C. Acute effects of sodium valproate on the photoconvulsive response in man. J. roy. Soc. Med., 1980, 30: 103–113.

Cereghino, J.J., Brock, J., van Meter, J., Penry, J.K., Smith, L. and White, B. Carbamazepine for epilepsy. A controlled prospective evaluation. Neurology (Minneap.), 1974, 24: 401–410.

Harding, G.F.A., Herrick, C.E. and Jeavons, P.M. A controlled study of the effect of sodium valproate on photosensitive epilepsy and its prognosis. Epilepsia, 1978, 19: 555–565.

Jeavons, P. and Harding, G.F.A. Photosensitive Epilepsy. A Review of Literature and a Study of 460 Patients. William Heineman Brooks, London, 1975.

Kellaway, P., Frost, J.D. and Hrachovy, R.A. Relationship between clinical state, ictal and interictal EEG discharges and serum drug levels: phenobarbital. Ann. Neurol., 1978, 4: 197.

Meijer, J.W.A., Aarts, J.H.P., de Beer-Pawlikowski, N.K.B., Binnie, C.D., van der Geest, P.W.M., Overweg, J., Van Parys, J.A.P. and Vermey, D. Circadian changes in serum-carbamazepine levels. In: Proc. Epilepsy International Congress, Kyoto, 1981: 97–98.

Milligan, N. and Richens, A. Ambulatory monitoring of the EEG in the assessment of antiepileptic drugs. In: F.D. Stott, E.G. Raftery, D.L. Clement and S.L. Wright (Eds.), Proceedings of 4th International Symposium on Ambulatory Monitoring, Gent, 1981. Academic Press, London, 1982: in press.

Milligan, N. and Richens, A. Methods of assessment of antiepileptic drugs. Brit. J. clin. Pharmacol., 1981, 11: 443–456.

Myslobodsky, M.S., Mintz, M. and Douglas, R. Electroencephalographic and behavioural effects of sodium valproate in patients with photosensitive epilepsy. A single dose trial. J. Neurol., 1980, 224: 111–127.

Nagelkerke, N., Binnie, C.D. and Overweg, J. The statistical properties of the occurrence of paroxysmal spike wave discharges. In: T.A. Betts, R.J. Hoeppener and V. Petersen (Eds.). Brit. J. clin. Pract. (Symp. Suppl.), 1982, 18: 75–77.

Overweg, J., Rowan, A.J., Binnie, C.D., Nagelkerke, N.J.D. and Oosting, J. Prediction of seizure recurrence after withdrawal of antiepileptic drugs. In: M. Dam, L. Gram and J.K. Penry (Eds.), Advances in Epileptology: XIIth Epilepsy International Symposium. Raven Press, New York, 1981: 503–508.

Penry, J.K., Porter, R.J. and Dreifuss, F.E. Quantification of paroxysmal abnormal discharges in the EEGs of patients with absence (petit-mal) seizures for the evaluation of antiepileptic drugs. Epilepsia, 1971, 12: 278–279.

Rodin, E., Rim, C. and Rennick, P. The effects of carbamazepine on patients with psychomotor epilepsy: Results of a double-blind study. Epilepsia, 1974, 15: 547–561.

Rowan, A.J., Meijer, J.W.A., Binnie, C.D., de Beer-Pawlikowski, N.K.B., Gutter, T., Goedhart, D., van der Geest, P. and Meinardi, H. Sodium valproate and sodium valproate-ethosuximide combination therapy: intensive monitoring studies. In: S.I. Johannessen, P. Morselli, C.E. Pippinger, A. Richens, D. Schmidt and H. Meinardi (Eds.), Antiepileptic Drug Therapy: Advances in Drug Monitoring. Raven Press, New York, 1979: 161–168.

Villarreal, H.J., Wilder, B.J., Willmore, L.J. et al. Effects of valproic acid on spike and wave discharges in patients with absence seizures. Neurology (Minneap.), 1978, 28: 886–891.

Wilkus, R.J. and Green, J.R. Electroencephalographic evaluation of the antiepileptic agent suthiame. Epilepsia, 1974, 15: 13–25.

Wilkus, R.J., Dodrill, C.B. and Troupin, A.S. Carbamazepine and the electroencephalogram epileptics: a double-blind study in comparison phenytoin. Epilepsia, 1976, 19: 283–291.

Yamamoto, J., Furaya, E., Wakamatsu, H. and Hishikawa, Y. Modification of photosensitivity in epileptics during sleep. Electroenceph. clin. Neurophysiol., 1971, 31: 509–513.

9. Effects of Psychotropic Drugs on EEG

Kyoto Symposia (EEG Suppl. No. 36)
Editors: P.A. Buser, W.A. Cobb and T. Okuma
© 1982, Elsevier Biomedical Press, Amsterdam

515

Workshop I. Psychotropic Drugs and EEG

Introductory Remarks of the Chairman

TERUO OKUMA *(Sendai, Japan)*

In recent years many of the patients who are examined in clinical EEG laboratories are under various kinds of drug medication, particularly psychotropic drugs such as benzodiazepines. Since the psychotropic drugs exert considerable influence on the human EEG, it is necessary for the clinical electroencephalographer to have enough knowledge of these effects for correct EEG interpretation.

It is well known that some psychotropic drugs induce slowing of the background activity, and others induce fast activity. Furthermore, provocation of epileptic seizure discharges or activation of pre-existing seizure discharges have been observed under the administration of some antipsychotic drugs. These facts may suggest the importance of EEG at the time of psychopharmacological treatment in clinical practice.

Another major subject in this field is the application of EEG to research in basic and clinical psychopharmacology. Recording of the EEG in experimental animals gives indispensable information on the mechanism of action of psychotropic drugs. The patterns of change in the human EEG induced by psychotropic drugs have been used for their classification. It has also been suggested that the vulnerability of the EEG of patients to psychotropic drugs seems to be related to the degree of clinical improvement in some cases. The study of the differences in sensitivity or tolerance to psychotropic drugs among individual patients, or between psychotics and normal subjects, will give us clues for the elucidation of the psychophysiological mechanisms of psychotic disorders.

With regard to developments in methodology, recent advances in computer technology have made it possible to use many sophisticated techniques such as averaging of evoked potentials and computer spectral analysis of EEG, but there are still many problems to be solved in this field.

In today's workshop we are going to discuss not only computerized quantitative analysis of pharmaco-EEG, but also more common problems such as basic neuropharmacology, paroxysmal activity in the EEG and cerebral evoked potentials, which many of the participants in this Congress may be dealing with every day. I am also expecting to be able to draw a general picture of this field of research which will contribute to the development of studies in the future.

Kyoto Symposia (EEG Suppl. No. 36)
Editors: P.A. Buser, W.A. Cobb and T. Okuma
© 1982, Elsevier Biomedical Press, Amsterdam

516

Computerized EEG in Schizophrenia and Pharmacopsychiatry

P. ETEVENON, B. PIDOUX[1], P. PERON-MAGNAN[2], P. RIOUX[3], G. VERDEAUX[1] and P. DENIKER[2]

Laboratoire d'Electroencéphalographie Quantitative, [1]Service d'Exploration Fonctionnelle du Système Nerveux, [2]S.H.U. de Santé Mentale et de Thérapeutique, Centre Hospitalier Sainte-Anne, 1, rue Cabanis, 75674 Paris Cedex 14, and [3]U194, INSERM, CHU Pitié-Salpêtrière, 93 Bd de l'Hôpital, 75013 Paris (France)

Since 1963, when Goldstein et al. discovered by quantitative EEG the hypovariability of EEG records of schizophrenic patients, 30 articles have been published confirming mainly this first result. The steady state kind of hypovariability of the time course of EEG records of chronic schizophrenic patients has been confirmed by many different laboratories (Fink et al. 1966; Marjerrisson et al. 1968; Lifshitz and Gradijan 1972, 1974; Etevenon et al. 1973, 1981; Itil 1977) which have observed this hyperstability.

Other specific features of EEG records have been described for the productive paranoid type of schizophrenic patients (Goldstein et al. 1963, 1965; Fink et al. 1966; Marjerrisson et al. 1966; Itil et al. 1972; Lifshitz and Gradijan 1972, 1974; Itil 1977; Etevenon et al. 1979b, 1981). After EEG analysis, these records present low voltage and desynchronized tracings with increased fast frequencies. In a recent publication (Etevenon et al. 1981), we described the specific features of EEGs of "paranoid type" as characterized by smaller total mean amplitude and mean frequency with higher spectral intensities for the mean amplitudes of low and high frequency rhythms. Also, specific features of the EEG of "residual type" schizophrenic patients (including deficitary hebephrenic patients, chronic undifferentiated and schizophrenia simplex) have been recently described (Etevenon et al. 1981) as presenting higher total mean amplitude and mean frequency together with a highly stable and intense alpha rhythm.

The hypovariability of EEGs of schizophrenic patients was generally expressed by low values of the coefficients of variation of the total mean amplitude as well as the specific features of quantified EEGs of the two main subtypes of schizophrenic patients. Amplitude EEG changes have also been reported (Etevenon et al. 1973, 1976, 1979b; Etevenon 1975; Flor-Henry 1976; d'Elia et al. 1977; Flor-Henry and Koles 1980). Mainly, the left/right occipital ratio was higher than 1.5 for EEGs of schizophrenic patients, around unity for control groups of normal human volunteers (d'Elia et al. 1977; Etevenon et al. 1979b), and lower than 0.5 for EEGs of depressed patients (Flor-Henry 1976; Flor-Henry and Koles 1980). Such

---

Address for reprints: P. Etevenon, INSERM, 2 rue d'Alésia, F-75014 Paris, France.

differences were not observed when dealing with relative amplitude values (or percent-time indexes) instead of absolute amplitude values (expressed in microvolts) (Pidoux et al. 1978; Kemali et al. 1980; Vacca et al. 1980).

Multivariate statistical analysis has been applied to EEGs quantified by spectral analysis followed by data reduction and parametrization. Either classification techniques (cluster analysis), discriminant analysis or factorial or constellation analysis, has been able to separate homogeneous EEG populations, especially subgroups of EEGs of schizophrenic patients (Fink et al. 1966; Etevenon et al. 1979a, b) separated from control groups and other EEG groups of psychotic patients.

Finally, the reactivity of schizophrenic patients to neuroleptic treatments (Itil et al. 1972; Etevenon et al. 1980) has been very well studied by different teams. We have also found (Etevenon et al. 1980) that therapy resistant patients present few but evident changes following intensive high dose haloperidol treatment.

PATIENTS AND CONTROL SUBJECTS

The criteria of Feighner et al. (1972) have been applied to our hospitalized patients for selecting them as schizophrenics. Complementary criteria have also been used, based on the DSM-3 manual, for differentiating 3 subgroups: "residual" type (R), characterized by presenting blunted or inappropriate affects, loosening of association, withdrawal and anergia, without delusions or hallucinations; "paranoid" type (P) characterized by minor residual features, prior paranoid episodes, persecution or grandiose delusions, hallucinations; and "other" type (O) characterized by mixed symptoms between R and P types or by other DSM-3 classifications of schizophrenia, apart from residual or paranoid types.

Exclusion criteria were defined by age limits: chronic illness longer than 6 months, onset of illness prior to the age of 40 (Feighner et al. 1972), actual age lower than 45. Patients should not have received ECT or insulin therapy for a period of 1 year preceding the EEG recording. They were withdrawn from any psychotropic medication at least 1 week before the EEG, except for chloral hydrate which was accepted at bed time as an hypnotic substitute. Of 36 schizophrenic patients, 7 required continuous mild neuroleptic treatment (2 from R, 4 from P and 1 from O type) without which their clinical condition would have aggravated. We included these patients in our study but later compared individually the patients in each group, one with another, in order to assess possible effects of such treatment. Mean age of the group was 27.3 years against 33.2 for the control group. Forty-two subjects, normal volunteers, were recorded as a control group after a session of habituation. Ten women were included in the control group, only 2 in the group of schizophrenic patients.

Following cluster analysis of quantified records of the control group two clusters were distinguished, characterized by: a high alpha amplitude type (HA) defined by $(41 \pm 11 \ \mu V)$ of total mean RMS amplitude, with $(75 \pm 10)\%$ of alpha rhythm over

P4-O2; a low alpha amplitude type (LA), defined by (19 ± 4 μV) of total mean RMS amplitude, with (53 ± 13)% of alpha rhythm over P4-O2 (% relative value measured for 100% power spectrum area computed from 1.3 to 28.2 Hz).

Table I represents the number of patients and subjects in each subgroup together with mean ages and coefficients of variation (CV) between ages.

TABLE I

	Schizophrenic patients (N = 36)			Control group (N = 42)	
	R type (n = 14 (1 F))	O type (n = 15 (1 F))	P type (n = 7)	HA type (n = 26 (7 F))	LA type (n = 16 (3 F))
Age years	28.3	25.8	28.4	32.5	33.8
CV (%)	31.2	17.8	16.1	24.4	27.0

PROTOCOL AND METHODS

Each schizophrenic patient or normal subject from the control group was recorded for 5 min, eyes closed, sitting and relaxed in a free vigilance situation. On the polygraph, a time constant of 0.3 sec was used with no filters.

The method of statistical spectral analysis developed in Paris has been previously described (Etevenon et al. 1976, 1979a, b, 1981; Etevenon 1979). Four EEG channels were recorded simultaneously: C4-P4, P4-O2, C3-P3, P3-O1. After real time A/D conversion at 200 Hz, with a frequency resolution of 0.5 Hz, on a Fourier analyser microprogrammable computer (hp 5451B), statistical spectral analysis was applied, providing repeated power spectra (for n = 120 times 2.56 sec successive epochs) and averaged power spectra. Data reduction was followed by computations of mean frequency according to the centroid formula (Lehmann and Koukkou 1980), mean amplitude in absolute and relative % values, together with their coefficients of variation (CV), for the total raw EEG and for delta (0.8–3.5 Hz), theta (3.9–7.0 Hz), alpha (7.4–13 Hz), beta1 (13.4–35 Hz) and beta2 (35.4–48.4 Hz) frequency bands. Non-parametric tests were applied to the spectral parameters for group comparisons.

Statistical multivariate analysis was made off-line on a PDP-10 from the data base of spectral parameters computed for each subject and patient. Principal component analysis was followed by cluster analysis using an arborescent hierarchical classification based on a locally adaptive clustering algorithm. Furthermore, a step by step quadratic discriminant analysis was applied to 84 or fewer spectral parameters, providing an automatic discrimination between subgroups with computed sensitivity and predictive values.

RESULTS

EEGs from the paranoid P type subgroup of patients were found to be different from the 2 other subgroups R and O. The mean RMS amplitude P4-O2 for the P subgroups was smaller than in the R, O (Table II) and HA subgroups and closer to the LA subgroup. This difference was accompanied by an increase in theta percentage for the P subgroup compared to R and O subgroups of patients (Table III).

Frequency changes have also been observed between the P subgroup and R and O subgroups (Table IV) as well as between HA and LA subgroups (Fig. 1). The total mean frequency was lower in the P subgroup compared to R and O.

When individual alpha centroid mean frequencies were plotted for the 2 subgroups of the control group, the dispersion around the mean for each EEG channel was bigger for the large amplitude HA subgroup, and smaller for the small

TABLE II

MEAN AMPLITUDE ALPHA CHANGES (μV) BETWEEN SCHIZOPHRENIC GROUPS

EEG channel	Residual type	Others	Paranoid type
C4-P4	16.0	14.5	11.7
P4-O2	22.7*	21.9*	14.1*
C3-P3	16.0	13.4	12.3
P3-O1	24.8	21.4	15.0

Mann-Whitney test: *$P \leqslant 0.05$.

TABLE III

AVERAGED THETA (PERCENTAGE) CHANGES BETWEEN SCHIZOPHRENIC GROUPS

EEG channel	Residual type	Others	Paranoid type
C4-P4	8.1*	10.2*	13.9*
P4-O2	7.6	7.3*	11.7*
C3-P3	8.6*	10.5*	14.4*
P3-O1	7.1	7.5*	12.5*

Mann-Whitney test: *$P \leqslant 0.05$.

TABLE IV

MEAN FREQUENCY CHANGES BETWEEN SCHIZOPHRENIC GROUPS (f_t Hz, raw EEG)

EEG channel	Residual type	Others	Paranoid type
C4-P4	10.8*	10.7*	9.3*
P4-O2	10.4	10.8*	9.2*
C3-P3	10.6	10.9*	9.1*
P3-O1	10.5*	10.9*	9.4*

Mann-Whitney test: *$P \leqslant 0.05$.

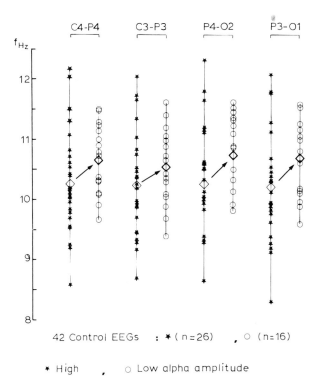

Fig. 1. Distributions of individual alpha frequencies (means indicated by diamonds).

amplitude LA subgroup. However, LA means were higher than HA means and this was statistically significant by Mann-Whitney non-parametric tests at the level of confidence of $P \leqslant 0.05$ (Fig. 1: arrows between diamond-shaped means).

Moreover, the alpha mean frequencies for the 3 subgroups R, O and P of the schizophrenic population were within the limits of the corresponding mean values of LA and HA subgroups of the control population.

Similarly, when the mean power spectra, expressed in absolute power values (μW/Hz) and then in decibels, were averaged between subjects, for each subgroup and each EEG channel, the corresponding power spectra for R, O and P subgroups of patients were within the limits of the power spectra of LA and HA subgroups of the control population.

Finally, we have applied quadratic discrimination analysis to the 5 subgroups (P, R, O and LA, HA), based on 20 mean frequencies (4 EEG channels and delta, theta, alpha, beta1 and beta2 frequency bands), and 24 mean RMS amplitude values (four EEG channels multiplied by 5 frequency bands plus raw EEG signal), for each quantified EEG (Table I). A unique combination of 10 parameters was sufficient to classify properly all the 5 groups with 99% correct recognition.

DISCUSSION

Among the 7 neuroleptic treated patients, 4 belonged to the P group, 2 were in the R group and 1 in O. The orally administered neuroleptic treatments were: 10 mg average daily dose of haloperidol (4 patients), pimozide 12 mg (1 patient), pipothiazine 10 mg (1 patient). One other patient received one injection i.m. of 50 mg of droperidol the day before the EEG recording. These treated patients presented individual EEG power spectra which were not different from the non-treated patients' spectra within the same subgroup.

After spectral analysis, the EEGs of paranoid patients presented a lowered total frequency (Table IV), as part of their specific EEG profiles. Amphetamine, acting as a psycho-stimulant in normals, produces a frequency shift towards low frequencies (Itil 1977; Kubicki et al. 1979), often with an increase of fast activities. This amphetamine profile may be considered as analogous to the power spectra obtained for the group of paranoid schizophrenics. Compared with the paranoid patients, the residual deficitary patients present a completely different EEG profile, with a highly stable alpha peak.

Besides classical EEG and computerized EEG followed by statistics, further research should be done by other means, including multicentric and multidisciplinary studies. Weinberger et al. (1981) has recently reported enlarged cerebral ventricles in chronic schizophrenic therapy resistant patients. Buchsbaum in Bethesda, NIMH, is comparing schizophrenic patients and controls by using EEG mapping and visual evoked potential mapping compared with images obtained by emission tomography, CT scans and local cerebral circulation maps. These sophisticated techniques will open new vistas for the understanding of neuropathological processes and psychotropic effects in schizophrenia.

SUMMARY

Since 1963 when Goldstein et al. discovered by quantitative EEG the hypovariability of EEG records of schizophrenic patients, 30 articles have been published confirming mainly this first result. In 36 schizophrenics and 42 normal volunteers (N group) we have recorded 5 min of EEG free of artifacts, under eyes closed conditions, from 4 derivations: C4-P4, P4-O2, C3-P3, P3-O1. After real time A/D conversion at 200 Hz on a Fourier analyser (hp 5451B), statistical spectral analysis was applied, providing repeated power spectra (for n = 120 times 2.56 sec successive epochs) and averaged power spectra. Data reduction was followed by computations of mean frequency, mean amplitude in absolute and relative % values, together with their coefficients of variation (CV), for the total EEG and delta, theta, alpha and beta frequency bands. The schizophrenic patients were separated in 3 subgroups: paranoid type (P, n = 7), residual type (R, n = 14) and "others" (O, n = 15), according to Feighner's and DSM-3 criteria.

Multivariate cluster analysis revealed 2 subgroups in the normal EEG sample: a high alpha cluster (HA, n = 26) and a low alpha (LA, n = 16) cluster, each of them being considered as homogeneous populations of quantified EEGs. Multivariate quadratic discriminant analysis confirmed the hypovariability of tracings of schizophrenics, especially for the left centro-parietal C3-P3 amplitude. Tracings of the P type presented lower alpha amplitude and mean frequency together with higher theta percentage when compared to R and O groups.

In terms of amplitudes in microvolts, averaged amplitude spectra within groups were well specified. The 3 groups R, P and O of EEGs of schizophrenics, presented spectral amplitude values between the upper limits of HA spectra and lower limits of LA spectra of normal EEGs. The amplitude spectra of R and O groups were closer to HA spectra, whereas the amplitude spectra of P group were closer to LA spectra.

Quadratic discrimination analysis between the 5 groups (P, R, O and LA, HA), based on 20 mean frequencies and 24 mean amplitudes for each quantified EEG, revealed that a unique combination of 10 parameters was sufficient to classify properly all the 5 groups with 99% of good recognition. Alpha amplitude from P3-O1 was smaller in LA (14 μV) and P (15 μV) groups when compared to HA (34 μV) and R and O groups (21 μV). This was the same for RMS amplitudes.

ACKNOWLEDGEMENTS

We wish to thank Mr. Letel for the EEG recordings and Miss S. Guillou for statistical and graphical work.

This research was supported by a French INSERM P.R.C. Grant No. 120012 "Santé mentale et cerveau" and A.T.P. INSERM Grant No. 73-79-105.

REFERENCES

d'Elia, G., Jacobsson, L., von Knorring, L., Matisson, B., Mjörndal, T., Oreland, I., Perris, C. and Rapp, W. Changes in psychopathology in relation to EEG variables and visual averaged evoked responses (V.AER) in schizophrenic patients treated with penfluridol or thiothixene. Acta psychiat. scand., 1977, 55: 309–318.

Etevenon, P. CEAN parameters in neuropsychopharmacology. In: G. Dolce and H. Künkel (Eds.), CEAN Computerized EEG Analysis. Fisher Verlag, Stuttgart, 1975: 236–250.

Etevenon, P. Etat actuel et perspectives de l'électroencéphalographie quantitative en pharmacopsychiatrie. In: P. Pichot and T. Kobayashi (Eds.), Coopération Franco-Japonaise, Colloque Psychopharmacologie. INSERM, Paris, 1979: 225–246.

Etevenon, P., Peron-Magnan, P., Rioux, P. and Littre, M.F. EEG statistical spectral analysis of schizophrenic patients. Electroenceph. clin. Neurophysiol., 1973, 34: 700.

Etevenon, P., Pidoux, B., Peron-Magnan, P., Rioux, P., Verdeaux, G., Boissier, J.R. and Deniker, P. Electroencephalography statistical spectral analysis and new trends of quantitative electroencephalography. In: P. Deniker, C. Radouco-Thomas and A. Villeneuve (Eds.), Psychopharmacology, Proc. Xth Congress C.I.N.P., 1976: 111–120.

Etevenon, P., Pidoux, B. and Rioux, P. Strategy of statistical spectral analysis in drug studies. A methodological synopsis. In: B. Saletu (Ed.), Neuropsychopharmacology. Pergamon Press, Oxford, 1979a: 383–391.

Etevenon, P., Pidoux, B., Rioux, P., Peron-Magnan, P., Verdeaux, G. and Deniker, P. Intra- and interhemispheric EEG differences quantified by spectral analysis. Acta psychiat. scand., 1979b, 60: 57–68.

Etevenon, P., Pidoux, B., Cottereau, M.J., Peron-Magnan, P., Zarifian, E., Verdeaux, G. and Deniker, P. Quantitative EEG analysis of high-dosage haloperidol effects in therapy-resistant schizophrenic patients. Adv. biol. Psychiat., 1980, 4: 175–187.

Etevenon, P., Peron-Magnan, P., Rioux, P., Pidoux, B., Bisserbe, J.C., Verdeaux, G. and Deniker, P. Schizophrenia assessed by computerized EEG. Adv. biol. Psychiat., 1981, 6: 29–34.

Feighner, J.P., Robins, E., Guze, S.B., Woodruff, R.A., Winokur, G. and Munoz, R. Diagnostic criteria for use in psychiatric research. Arch. gen. Psychiat., 1972, 26: 57–63.

Fink, M., Itil, T.M. and Clyde, D. The classification of psychoses by quantitative EEG measures. In: J. Wortis (Ed.), Recent Advances in Biological Psychiatry, Vol. 8. Plenum Press, New York, 1966: 305–312.

Flor-Henry, P. Lateralized temporal-limbic dysfunction and psychopathology. Ann. N.Y. Acad. Sci., 1976, 280: 777–795.

Flor-Henry, P. and Koles, Z.J. EEG studies in depression, mania and normals: Evidence for partial shifts of laterality in the affective psychoses. Adv. biol. Psychiat., 1980, 4: 21–43.

Goldstein, L., Murphree, H.B., Sugerman, A.A., Pfeiffer, C.C. and Jenny, E.H. Quantitative electroencephalographic analysis of naturally occurring (schizophrenic) and drug-induced psychotic states in human males. Clin. Pharmacol. Ther., 1963, 4: 10–21.

Goldstein, L., Sugerman, A.A., Stolberg, J., Murphree, H.B. and Pfeiffer, C.C. Electro-cerebral activity in schizophrenics and non-psychotic subjects, quantitative EEG amplitude analysis. Electroenceph. clin. Neurophysiol., 1965, 19: 350–361.

Itil, T.M. Qualitative and quantitative EEG findings in schizophrenia. Schizophr. Bull., 1977, 3: 61–78.

Itil, T.M., Saletu, B. and Davis, S. EEG findings in chronic schizophrenics based on digital computer period analysis and analog power spectra. Biol. Psychiat., 1972, 5: 1–13.

Kemali, D., Vacca, L., Nolfe, G., Iorio, G. and De Carlo, R. Hemispheric EEG quantitative asymmetries in schizophrenics and depressed patients. Adv. biol. Psychiat., 1980, 4: 14–20.

Kubicki, St., Herrmann, W.M., Fichte, K. and Freund, G. Reflections on the topics: EEG frequency bands and regulation of vigilance. Pharmakopsychiatrie, 1979, 12: 237–245.

Lehmann, D. and Koukkou, M. Classes of spontaneous, private experiences and ongoing human EEG activities. In: G. Pfurtscheller et al. (Eds.), Rhythmic EEG Activities and Cortical Functioning. Elsevier/North-Holland Biomedical Press, Amsterdam, 1980: 289–297.

Lifshitz, K. and Gradijan, J. Relationships between measures of the coefficient of variation of the mean absolute EEG voltage and spectral intensities in schizophrenic and control subjects. Biol. Psychiat., 1972, 5: 149–163.

Lifshitz, K. and Gradijan, J. Spectral evaluation of the electroencephalogram: Power and variability in chronic schizophrenics and control subjects. Psychophysiology, 1974, 11: 479–490.

Marjerrisson, G., Krause, A.E. and Keogh, R.P. Variability of the EEG in schizophrenia. Quantitative analysis with a modulus voltage integrator. Electroenceph. clin. Neurophysiol., 1968, 24: 35–41.

Pidoux, B., Peron-Magnan, P., Verdeaux, G. et Deniker, P. L'activité alpha dans un groupe de schizophrènes: analyse spectrale et comparaison avec un groupe témoin. Rev. E.E.G. Neurophysiol., 1978, 8: 283–293.

Vacca, L., Kemali, D., Marciano, F., Celani, T. and Pierro, C. Quantitative EEG analysis in schizophrenics and depressed patients. Adv. biol. Psychiat., 1980, 4: 111–118.

Weinberger, D.R. and Wyatt, R.J. Computer tomography (CT) findings in schizophrenia: clinical and biological implications. In: C. Perris, G. Struwe and B. Jansson (Eds.), Biological Psychiatry, 1981. Elsevier/North-Holland Biomedical Press, Amsterdam, 1981: 255–258.

Kyoto Symposia (EEG Suppl. No. 36)
Editors: P.A. Buser, W.A. Cobb and T. Okuma
© 1982, Elsevier Biomedical Press, Amsterdam

524

Computerized EEG Study on Drug-Induced Extrapyramidalism in Schizophrenic Patients

MASAMI SAITO, SHIGETOMO KITA, YOJI KAGONO, NOBUYUKI SUITSU and YOSHIHARU HONDA

Department of Neuropsychiatry, Kansai Medical University, Fumizono-cho 1, Moriguchi, Osaka 570 (Japan)

Drug-induced extrapyramidalism, such as parkinsonism, akathisia and acute dystonic reactions, is the most frequent and unpleasant side effect of major neuroleptic medication in the clinical treatment of schizophrenic patients (Toru 1981). There seems to be a close connection between the antipsychotic and the extrapyramidal actions of the major neuroleptic compounds. At present, however, this connection is believed to be less essential than was formerly considered, but to be hardly dissoluble in practice. Eventually psychiatrists have no choice but to prescribe an antiparkinsonian agent for the urgent relief of induced extrapyramidal disorders (Mizuno 1981).

Though there is not yet any decisive evidence substantiating the empirical inference that the combined use of an antiparkinsonian agent can reduce the antipsychotic effect of a neuroleptic drug, it appears to be better not to misuse antiparkinsonian agents in treatment with neuroleptic drugs for several reasons. One of them is the possible attenuation of antipsychotic action of the neuroleptic drug and another is the possible provocation of adverse reactions to the antiparkinsonian medication. Focussing on these two points, the authors have studied the therapeutic significance of induced extrapyramidalism in schizophrenic patients and the psychotropic property of antiparkinsonian agent in normal volunteers, exclusively from the computerized EEG (CEEG) point of view.

MATERIALS AND METHODS

Since there were these two different purposes in the present study the authors conducted two different series of EEG trials; schizophrenic patient trials and normal volunteer trials. For the patient trial, we selected 22 fresh patients aged 19–46 years with typical schizophrenia, of whom 8 were male and 14 were female; 17 were subdiagnosed as productive paranoid type and 5 as deficitary hebephrenic type. All the patients were treated solely with haloperidol for at least 4 weeks. The initial dose was 2.25 mg daily for the first week; for the following weeks it was left to the

---

Address for reprints and correspondence: Masami Saito, 1-7-8 Mukoyama, Takarazuka, Hyogo 665, Japan.

doctor's decision. EEG follow-up studies were done in parallel with clinical evaluations using an expanded version of Brief Psychiatric Rating Scale (EBPRS), regularly before and at the end of every week during the treatment.

For the second purpose, 5 independent single-dose oral administration trials were conducted, using a total of 30 healthy male volunteers, aged 21–26 years (mean 23.4 years), in a single blind design for 5 antiparkinsonian agents; trihexyphenidyl-HCl 2 mg, biperiden-HCl 1 mg, mazaticol-HCl 4 mg, L-DOPA 100 mg and amantadine-HCl 100 mg. Each drug trial was done using 6 volunteers according to a planned schedule for pharmaco-EEG study.

In an additional study with 6 further volunteers, aged 20 years, who received two different doses of haloperidol in two different courses, 6 received 0.75 mg haloperidol, whereas in the second course with the same subjects, only 5 of them received 2.25 mg haloperidol.

A 10 min resting EEG was recorded from the frontal, temporal, central and occipital regions with reference electrodes on the ears. In the volunteer study, for the purpose of eliminating the "first" effects of EEG recording, all the subjects had an "adaptation" recording 1 hour before the drug administration. The 4 right hemisphere to left ear leads were recorded on casette magnetic tape (SONY FRC-1402N) and were analysed off-line, using computerized (SORD M200 MARK II and III) period analysis programs. This method determined the percentage of time spent in 10 frequency bands of the primary wave (zero-crossings) and 8 bands of the first derivative measurements, the average frequency and frequency deviation for the primary wave and the first derivative, as well as integrated amplitude and amplitude variability. A total minimum of twenty 10 sec artifact-free EEGs were analysed in each evaluation, of which 24 measurements were used to compare all the time sample EEGs with the baseline EEG and to calculate t values from the differences between them.

Power spectral density analysis was also applied to illustrate the changes in the frequency domain before and after the appearance of extrapyramidalism during haloperidol medication, as well as before and after its disappearance following a biperiden-HCl injection.

RESULTS OF PATIENT STUDY

Haloperidol produced 3 different types of EEG change in the 3 h after the first single oral dose (0.75 mg): an increase of alpha activity, a decrease of it and almost no change. The first type appeared to correspond with the therapy responsive patient group, and the second and third types with the therapy resistant group, as already reported elsewhere (Saito 1979b; Kita 1980).

Twenty-two patients were divided into 5 groups based on the lag time from the beginning of haloperidol treatment to the onset of extrapyramidalism. Five patients presented extrapyramidal disorders as early as within 1 week. Fig. 1 shows the t profiles of group 1, consisting of these 5 patients. The original CEEG profile

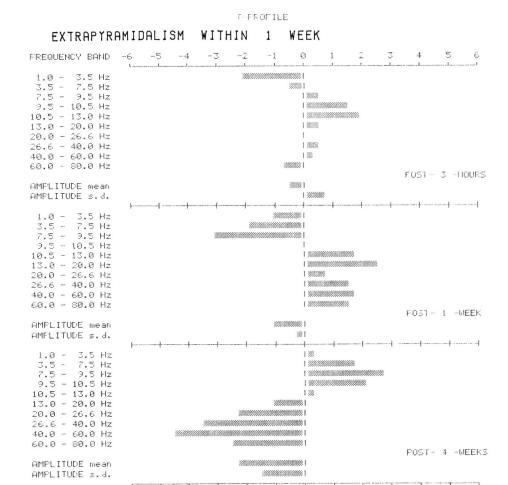

Fig. 1. *t* profiles of schizophrenic patients of group 1 (N = 5). The patients presented extrapyramidalism in the 1st week of haloperidol treatment. Upper: 3 h post- versus pre-treatment record. Middle: 1 week post- versus pre-treatment record. Lower: 4 weeks post- versus pre-treatment record. Abscissa: CEEG measurements, 10 primary wave measurements and 2 amplitude measurements. Ordinate: *t* value, zero means no change, a positive value (rightward) signifies an increase, and a negative value (leftward) signifies a decrease.

consisted of 24 measurements in terms of *t* value, as in Fig. 8, but in order to simplify the figure in the present paper the other *t* profiles show only 12 *t* values: 10 of primary wave frequency and 2 of amplitude measurements. The 3 h post-treatment profile showed a significant decrease of delta waves and a marked increase of alpha activity. The post-1 week profile indicated a marked decrease of activity slower than 9.5 c/sec and a marked increase of activity faster than 10.5 c/sec. The post-4 weeks profile showed a marked increase of 3.5–10.5 c/sec activity associated with a significant decrease of beta activity. The 5 patients (100%) in this group were markedly and quickly improved by the haloperidol treatment.

Group 2 consisted of 4 patients who developed extrapyramidalism in the 2nd week of treatment. There was a significant increase of 7.5–10.5 c/sec alpha activity and a significant decrease of fast activity above 13 c/sec in the post-3 h profile. The post-1 week profile indicated only an increase of alpha waves and an increase of 20–26.6 c/sec activity, but the post-4 weeks profile presented again a significant increase of alpha activity and a significant increase of fast activity above 20 c/sec. Of the 4 patients, 3 showed marked improvement of schizophrenic symptoms.

Fig. 2 shows *t* profiles of group 3, consisting of 6 patients who presented extrapyramidal disorders in the 3rd week. Only 2 (33.3%) of the 6 patients were clinically improved. The post-3 h profile presented a marked decrease of 7.5–9.5 c/sec and a slight increase of 20–26.6 c/sec activity. The post-1 week profile

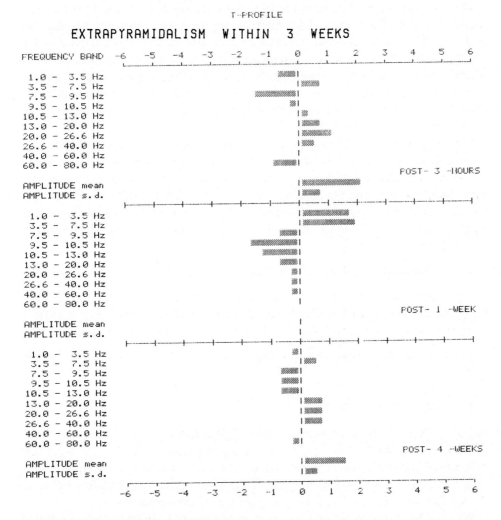

Fig. 2. *t* profiles of schizophrenic patients of group 3 (N = 6). These patients presented extrapyramidalism in the 3rd week.

indicated a marked increase of slower activity and a marked decrease of higher alpha activity. In the post-4 weeks there is very little decrease of alpha activity and increase of fast activity.

In t profiles of group 4, consisting of 2 patients who presented signs of extrapyramidalism in the 4th week the post-3 h profile indicated a significant increase of delta activity and a decrease of alpha, particularly fast alpha activity. In the post-1 week profile there was a significant decrease of alpha activity and a significant increase of fast activity, while in the post-4 weeks profile there was only a decrease of faster alpha activity. These 2 patients showed almost no improvement of clinical features.

There were 7 patients who did not present any sign of extrapyramidalism throughout the 4 week treatment with haloperidol, irrespective of the given dosage (9–40 mg/day). These 7 patients are included in group 5, of which t profiles are shown in Fig. 3. There was neither increase nor decrease in the post-3 h and the post-1 week profiles, but slight increases of delta and of slow alpha activity and a significant decrease of fast activity were seen in the post-4 weeks profile. Of the 7 patients, only 2 (28.6%) showed an increase of alpha activity and a clinical improvement. The 5 patients who were not clinically improved presented such small changes in the EEG during haloperidol treatment that they were considered to be non-responders to haloperidol.

With regard to the 15 patients who presented extrapyramidalism during the treatment period, the t values of 10 primary wave frequency measurements in the post-3 h individual profiles were used to compute Pearson product-moment correlation matrices, and the measurements were correlated with the individual lag times to the onset of induced extrapyramidalism. Based on these matrices, regressive coefficients were calculated by means of multiple regression analysis. The following expression was obtained.

$$Y = -0.4484X_4 - 0.4583X_5 + 2.2454 \tag{1}$$

Y, lag time or latency of the extrapyramidalism (week); X_4, t value for 9.5–10.5 Hz band; X_5, t value for 10.5–13 Hz band. Multiple correlation coefficient: 0.9857.

When post-1 week t values were used, the regressive expression was as follows:

$$Y = -0.1553X_4 - 0.5434X_5 + 1.3712 \tag{2}$$

or

$$Y = -0.6913X_5 + 1.4815 \tag{3}$$

and multiple correlation coefficients were 0.9984 (Eq. 2) and 0.9908 (Eq. 3). Since there were 5 patients who presented extrapyramidalism in the 1st week of haloperidol treatment, the accuracy of Eqs. 2 and 3 is the natural thing to be expected. It is interesting that there was a significant negative correlation between the lag time and the t value of particular frequency measurements.

We have attempted to see what kinds of change would be induced in the patient's EEG when an acute extrapyramidalism appeared during haloperidol treatment and

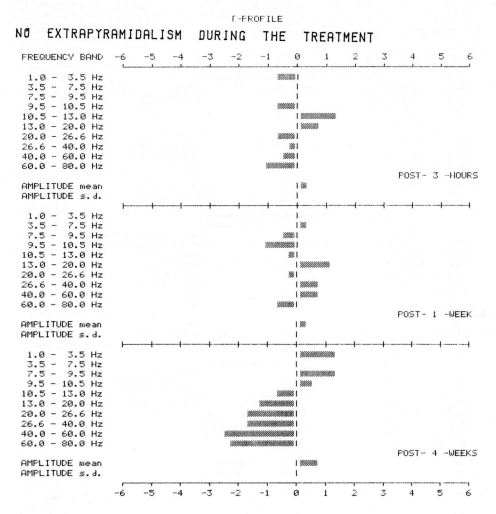

Fig. 3. *t* profiles of schizophrenic patients of group 5 (N = 7). The patients did not show any extrapyramidal disorder throughout the treatment period.

when it disappeared after the intramuscular injection of biperiden-HCl. Fig. 4 shows *t* profiles of 2 schizophrenic patients; the upper profile shows the CEEG changes before and after the appearance of extrapyramidalism, the middle one shows the changes before the appearance of extrapyramidalism and after its disappearance following biperiden-HCl injection, and the lower illustrates the change before and after disappearance of extrapyramidalism. The appearance of extrapyramidalism induced a significant decrease of delta activity and a significant increase of slow alpha activity and of fast activity. It must be noted that there was a significant increase of amplitude in spite of such an increase of fast activity. As shown in the middle profile, the disappearance of the extrapyramidalism induced a significant decrease of activity slower than 7.5 c/sec and significant increases of 7.5–10.5 c/sec alpha activity and of fast activity higher than 13 c/sec. The biperiden-HCl injection,

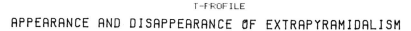

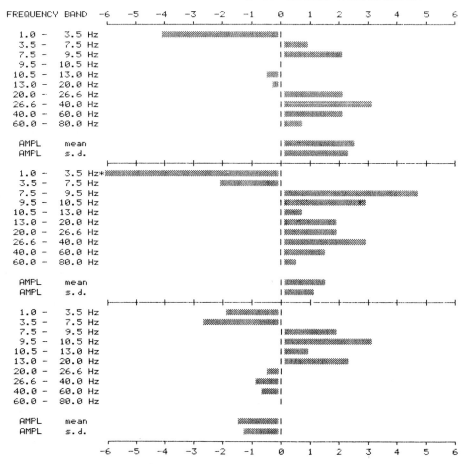

Fig. 4. *t* profiles of schizophrenic patients with acute extrapyramidalism induced by haloperidol (N = 2). Upper: pre-biperiden versus pre-extrapyramidalism. Middle: post-biperiden versus pre-extrapyramidalism. Lower: post- versus pre-biperiden.

which made the extrapyramidal disorders disappear, induced eventually a significant decrease of slow activity, significant increases of alpha activity and of intermediate fast activity, and a marked decrease of amplitude.

The EEG power spectra under 3 different conditions in 1 of the 2 patients who presented acute extrapyramidalism clearly showed that the drug-induced extrapyramidalism was accompanied by a marked increase of alpha activity at around 11 c/sec and that the biperiden-HCl injection induced a more marked increase of alpha activity as well as of slow and fast activities. The partial disagreement of the results can be attributed to the differences between the technical and theoretical bases of the two analysing methods.

Haloperidol induces a marked increase of alpha activity, associated with a marked

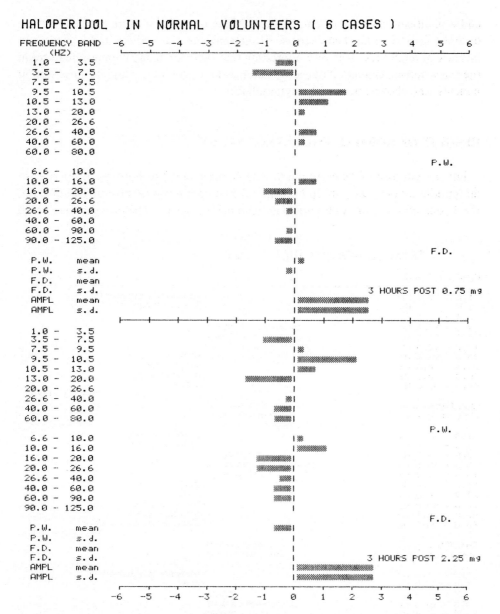

Fig. 5. CEEG profiles of haloperidol 0.75 mg and 2.25 mg in normal subjects. Upper: 3 h post- versus pre-drug record (0.75 mg, N = 6). Lower: 3 h post- versus pre-drug record (2.25 mg, N = 5). Abscissa: 24 CEEG measurements, 10 primary wave and 8 first derivative frequency measurements, their means and standard deviations, and 2 amplitude measurements. Ordinate: t values.

increase of amplitude, in normal volunteers. Fig. 5 shows the results of an additional study on haloperidol (0.75 mg and 2.25 mg single doses), using 6 normal subjects. To make these 2 profiles, all the 24 t values were used as usual. 0.75 mg of haloperidol induced a decrease of theta activity, a marked increase of alpha activity and a significant increase of amplitude. 2.25 mg produced a more marked increase of alpha activity, a marked decrease of intermediate fast activity and a significant increase of amplitude. It is very interesting that there are many common features in the characteristic changes induced by haloperidol in volunteers and in those seen in patients who showed acute extrapyramidalism.

RESULTS OF NORMAL VOLUNTEER STUDY

For the purpose of determining CEEG changes and psychotropic properties of antiparkinsonian agents, group t profiles of 5 compounds were carefully studied. Of the 5 compounds, 3 are well known anticholinergic agents. The dosages were based

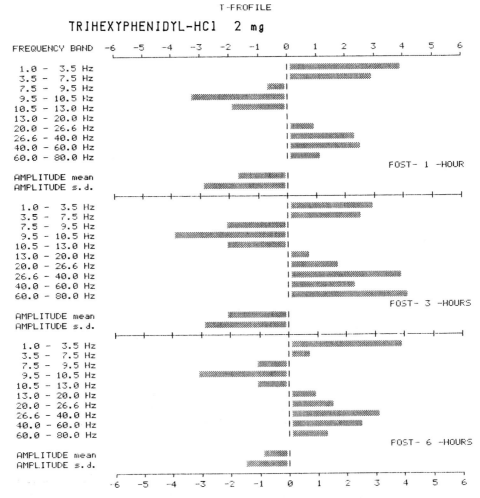

Fig. 6. CEEG profiles of trihexyphenidyl-HCl 2 mg (N = 6). Upper: 1 h post-drug versus pre-drug record. Middle: 3 h post-drug versus pre-drug record. Lower: 6 h post-drug versus pre-drug record. Abscissa: CEEG measurements, 10 primary wave (zero-crossing) and 2 amplitude measurements. Ordinate: t value.

on the ordinary therapeutic doses of each compound.

Trihexyphenidyl-HCl 2 mg produced a significant decrease of alpha activity at 9.5–13 c/sec, significant increases of slow activity and of fast activity, and a marked decrease of the integrated amplitude, accompanied by a decrease of the amplitude variability in the 1 h post-drug record. These changes were seen commonly in the 3 h and 6 h post-drug records, peaking in the 3 h post-drug one, as shown in Fig. 6.

Biperiden-HCl 1 mg induced a marked decrease of alpha activity and a significant increase of delta activity in the 1 h post-drug record, a marked increase of fast activity in addition in the 3 h post-drug record, but a marked decrease of activity slower than 10.5 c/sec and a marked increase of activity faster than 20 c/sec in the 6 h post-drug record. There were no marked changes in amplitude measurements.

Fig. 7 shows the drastic changes in the EEG induced by mazaticol-HCl 4 mg; a significant decrease of fast alpha activity and a significant increase of fast activity in

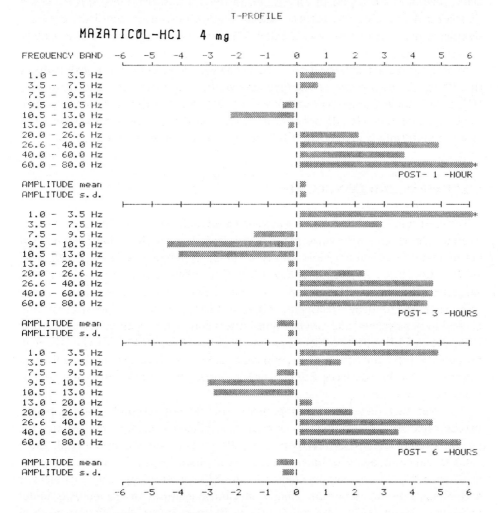

Fig. 7. CEEG profiles of mazaticol-HCl 4 mg (N = 6).

the 1 h post-drug record, and a significant decrease of alpha activity and significant increases of slow as well as of fast activity in both the 3 h and 6 h post-drug records. A slight decrease of amplitude was seen at 3 h and 6 h but did not reach the significant level.

L-DOPA (100 mg) induced a significant increase of delta waves, a marked decrease of alpha activity, a significant increase of fast activity and an increase of amplitude in the 1 h post-drug record. In the 3 h post-drug record, there were a significant increase of slow waves, a marked decrease of alpha activity, a marked increase of fast activity and an increase of amplitude. In the 6 h post-drug record a marked decrease of theta and alpha activities, a significant increase of fast activity and a slight increase of amplitude were seen.

Amantadine-HCl 100 mg produced an entirely different change in the EEG from those described above. In the 1 h post-drug record there were a marked decrease of delta waves and a decrease of amplitude. In the 3 h post-drug record there was a significant decrease of fast activity, and in the 6 h post-drug record there were a significant decrease of slow waves below 7.5 c/sec and an increase of fast activity above 20 c/sec.

According to Itil's classification of EEG changes induced by psychotropic drugs (Itil 1974), CEEG profiles of trihexyphenidyl-HCl, biperiden-HCl and mazaticol-HCl are of anticholinergic type and those of L-DOPA are of thymoleptic type, while those of amantadine-HCl do not conform to any particular type because it does not produce uniformly characteristic EEG changes, as the other compounds do.

DISCUSSION AND CONCLUSION

The predictability of the clinical outcome based on EEG changes induced by drug treatment in patients with schizophrenia and depressive psychosis has been pointed out by many investigators (Goldstein et al. 1963; Etevenon et al. 1973, 1980; Aoki 1977; Saito 1979a, b, 1981a; Tsuda 1979; Kita 1980). Particularly, Kita (1980) suggested the close relationships between EEG responsiveness and clinical responsiveness to drug treatment, between extrapyramidal responsiveness and clinical responsiveness, and EEG responsiveness and extrapyramidal responsiveness in his detailed EEG study on schizophrenic patients. Tsuda (1979) revealed the high probability in the prediction of the clinical outcome of depressive patient solely on the basis of the 3 h post-drug EEG changes produced by the first single oral dose of antidepressant drug.

It is true that there are a few patients who do not respond to some potent psychotropic drug, either clinically or electroencephalographically, and also that the patient's responsiveness or reactivity is not always constant (Goldstein et al. 1963; Lifshitz and Gradijan 1974; Etevenon et al. 1980; Saito 1981a). However, it appears most probable that a massive change in the EEG induced by drug treatment is accompanied by an important change in clinical features in the patients under treatment. Tsuda (1979) and Saito (1979a, b) stressed the elasticity of cerebral functioning as an important factor in determination of the patient's responsiveness. In the present study, the patients who produced an EEG change similar to that of normal volunteers presented early onset of extrapyramidalism and rapid improvement of clinical features. A late onset of extrapyramidalism seemed to correspond with an EEG change in the opposite direction and also with resistance to therapy.

Two out of 7 patients, who did not show any sign of extrapyramidalism during the treatment period, presented clinical improvement; therefore, it suggests that the extrapyramidal insensitivity does not correspond with the clinical resistance.

The appearance of extrapyramidalism was associated with an expected increase of fast activity but it was also associated with increases of alpha activity and of amplitude, which had not been expected. If the most characteristic EEG change induced by haloperidol is an increase of alpha activity, this increase accompanied by the appearance of extrapyramidalism has to be interpreted that the intrinsic action of haloperidol was released or facilitated by a certain change due to the functional blockade of postsynaptic receptors in the strio-nigral dopaminergic pathway in the brain. Furthermore, the disappearance of an extrapyramidal disorder was accompanied by an increase of alpha activity and a decrease of amplitude. The former can be regarded as an influence of haloperidol and the latter as that of biperiden-HCl. It is interesting that an increase of alpha activity was induced in spite of the acute application of an anticholinergic agent, which would produce a marked decrease of alpha activity, as shown in the present study.

Three anticholinergic agents (trihexyphenidyl-HCl, biperiden-HCl and mazaticol-HCl) and L-DOPA produced apparently similar CEEG profiles as far as frequency is concerned. The only but important difference is the change of amplitude, decreased or unchanged for the anticholinergic agents and increased for L-DOPA. Amitriptyline is a well known potent anticholinergic and thymoleptic agent which induces a decrease of alpha activity and increases of slow and fast activity and of amplitude (Fink 1969; Itil 1974; Tsuda 1979; Saito 1981a, b). Moskovitz et al. (1978) drew attention to the psychoactive property of L-DOPA. It is quite probable that L-DOPA has a mild but certain thymoleptic effect in patients with depression.

The EEG changes induced by anticholinergic agents suggest the potent psychotropic effects of the antiparkinsonian medication (Porteous and Ross 1956; Nakamura and Shimazono 1964). In our experience, some antiparkinsonian agents at higher doses produce important psychic changes such as illusions, hallucinations, delusional ideas, clouding and altered consciousness and so forth, in normal persons. They appear to correspond with the acute delirious state which is provoked by tricyclic antidepressant drugs on some occasions. Thus, the EEG changes of anticholinergic type are likely to be interpreted as representing a psychotropic property to derange consciousness or have a psychedelic action (Porteous and Ross 1956; Bolin 1960; Nakamura and Shimazono 1964; Fink 1969; Itil 1974; Saito 1981a, b). This may cause some confusion with the psychodysleptic properties of hallucinogenic agents such as ditran and LSD25. We should like to stress that anticholinergic actions do not immediately correspond to psychodysleptic actions but do produce different effects between normal and psychotic subjects.

As Tsuda (1979) pointed out, tricyclic antidepressants induce a different type of EEG change in depressive patients from those of thymoleptic type in normal volunteers. Anticholinergic agents seem to produce a different type of EEG change in patients with extrapyramidal disorders from that in normal subjects; accordingly a different type of psychotropic effect. Therefore, even in the case of psychotic patients, the application of antiparkinsonian medication, particularly with anticholinergic agents, should be conducted with prudence. It is needless to say that an abuse of the antiparkinsonian agents must be avoided.

SUMMARY

A CEEG study was conducted on 22 fresh schizophrenic patients under haloperidol treatment and the relationship between extrapyramidal and EEG responsiveness was investigated.

Another CEEG study was also conducted using normal volunteers to determine the psychotropic properties of 5 antiparkinsonian agents; trihexyphenidyl-HCl, biperiden-HCl, mazaticol-HCl, L-DOPA and amantadine-HCl. The first 4 compounds produced a decrease of alpha activity and an increase of slow and fast activities but amantadine did not induce any particular type of EEG change. Based on the changes of amplitude 3 anticholinergic agents were allocated to the anticholinergic type and L-DOPA to the thymoleptic type, according to Itil's classification (Itil 1974).

The appearance of extrapyramidalism and its influence on the EEG were discussed and the possibility of its therapeutic effect was suggested with regard to the haloperidol action. The lag time from the beginning of the haloperidol treatment to the onset of extrapyramidal disorders appeared to correlate closely with the t value indicating a change in the higher alpha frequency band in the 3 h post-drug EEG.

It must be noted that the acute application of an anticholinergic agent produced an almost opposite type of EEG change in a case of haloperidol-induced extrapyramidalism compared with the EEG change seen in normal subjects. Finally, it was suggested that potent antiparkinsonian agents may present psychedelic effects in subjects without extrapyramidal disorders and the application of anticholinergic agents should be conducted with prudence.

REFERENCES

Aoki, T. EEG changes in the course of perphenazine treatment of schizophrenia. (In Japanese.) J. Kansai med. Univ., 1977, 29: 235–261.
Bolin, R.R. Psychiatric manifestations of Artane toxicity. J. nerv. ment. Dis., 1960, 131: 256–259.
Etevenon, P., Peron-Magnan, P., Rioux, P. and Littre, M.F. EEG statistical spectral analysis of schizophrenic patients. Electroenceph. clin. Neurophysiol., 1973, 34: 700.

Etevenon, P., Pidoux, B., Cottereau, M.J., Peron-Magnan, P., Zarifian, E., Verdeaux, G. and Deniker, P. Quantitative EEG analysis of high-dosage haloperidol effects in therapy-resistant schizophrenic patients. Adv. Biol. Psychiat., 1980, 4: 175–187.

Fink, M. EEG and human psychopharmacology. Ann. Rev. Pharmacol., 1969, 9: 241–258.

Goldstein, L., Murphree, H.B., Sugerman, A.A., Pfeiffer, C.C. and Jenny, E.H. Quantitative electroencephalographic analysis of naturally occurring (schizophrenic) and drug-induced psychotic states in human males. Clin. Pharmacol. Ther., 1963, 4: 10–21.

Itil, T.M. Quantitative pharmaco-electroencephalography. In: T.M. Itil (Ed.), Psychotropic Drugs and the Human EEG: Mod. Prob. Pharmacopsychiat., Vol. 8. Karger, Basel, 1974: 43–75.

Itil, T.M. Qualitative and quantitative EEG findings in schizophrenia. Schizophr. Bull., 1977, 3: 61–78.

Kita, S. An electroencephalographic study on the treatment of schizophrenia with haloperidol. (In Japanese.) J. Kansai med. Univ., 1980, 32: 384–432.

Lifshitz, K. and Gradijan, J. Spectral evaluation of the electroencephalogram: Power and variability in chronic schizophrenics and control subjects. Psychophysiology, 1974, 11: 479–490.

Mizuno, Y. Drug treatment of extrapyramidal diseases. (In Japanese.) Jap. J. Neuropsychopharmacol. (Shinkei-seishin-yakuri), 1981, 3: 707–716.

Moskovitz, C., Moses, H. and Klowans, H.L. Levodopa induced psychosis: a kindling phenomenon. Amer. J. Psychiat., 1978, 135: 669–675.

Nakamura, T. and Shimazono, Y. On the therapeutic effects of biperiden-HCl (Akineton) and its action to normal subjects. (In Japanese.) J. Psychiat. (Seishin-igaku), 1964, 6: 213–221.

Porteous, H.B. and Ross, D.N. Mental symptoms in parkinsonism following benzhexol hydrochloride therapy. Brit. med. J., 1956, 21: 138–140.

Saito, M. Drug-induced EEG changes studied on two-dimensional rectangular coordinates using principal component analysis. Pharmacopsychiatry, 1979a, 12: 59–68.

Saito, M. CEEG study on patients under the psychiatric drug treatment: The correlation between EEG alteration and clinical evolution. In: Obbiols, Ballus and Gonzales Monclus (Eds.), Biological Psychiatry Today. Elsevier/North-Holland, Amsterdam, 1979b: 1306–1311.

Saito, M. Psychotropic drugs and EEG. (In Japanese.) J. Neuropsychopharmacol. (Shinkei-seishin-yakuri), 1981a, 3: 323–348.

Saito, M. EEG changes induced by psychotropic drugs: Their contributions in clinical psychiatry. (In Japanese.) J. Psychiat. (Seishin-igaku), 1981b, 23: 538–549.

Toru, M. Extrapyramidal side effects of antipsychotic drugs. (In Japanese.) J. Neuropsychopharmacol. (Shinkei-seishin-yakuri), 1981, 3: 717–725.

Tsuda, T. An electroencephalographic study on the drug treatment of endogenous depression. (In Japanese.) J. Kansai med. Univ., 1979, 31: 548–578.

Kyoto Symposia (EEG Suppl. No. 36)
Editors: P.A. Buser, W.A. Cobb and T. Okuma
© 1982, Elsevier Biomedical Press, Amsterdam

538

Psychotropic Drugs and Evoked Potentials*

CHARLES SHAGASS, JOHN J. STRAUMANIS and RICHARD A. ROEMER

Temple University Medical Center and Eastern Pennsylvania Psychiatric Institute, Philadelphia, Pa. (U.S.A.)

We have studied the effects of psychotropic drugs on evoked potentials (EPs) in conjunction with our EP investigations of psychiatric patients. The ultimate aim of the drug studies is to obtain information that may help to elucidate CNS mechanisms related to their psychiatric therapeutic actions. More immediately, the drug data are important for the interpretation of EP differences between clinical groups; knowledge of the EP changes produced by psychotropic drugs should help us to determine the extent to which variations in drug history may be responsible for EP differences.

Although psychotropic drug effects have been studied since the EP recording method became generally available, the literature concerning changes produced by the major psychiatric drugs in treated patients is relatively sparse and incomplete (see Shagass and Straumanis 1978, for a recent review). Most of the studies have dealt with EPs in one sensory modality and records have usually been made from few electrode locations, often only one. The drug studies reported here utilized a comprehensive EP recording procedure (Shagass et al. 1977), developed to deal with similar limitations in EP investigations of psychiatric patients. This procedure employs 4 kinds of stimuli in 3 sensory modalities, and provides EPs from 15 locations. We shall present here data bearing on the effects of antipsychotic and antidepressant drugs and lithium carbonate; comparative findings for a group of hospitalized patients retested after receiving no drug treatment will also be reported.

In assessing the relationship between EP changes and clinical therapeutic effects of a drug, a critical question is whether or not the drug shifts previously abnormal EP characteristics toward normal. To help answer this question, we shall present results to illustrate the kinds of EP deviation from normal that we have found in psychiatric patients ordinarily treated with a particular class of drugs. By relating drug effects to pre-treatment deviations from normal, it may be possible to assess the relevance of the EP changes to the clinical effects of the drugs. It may be noted that clinically relevant EP effects should be distinguished from those secondary to drug-induced alterations of alertness and also from non-specific "tissue" effects, apparently unrelated to the drug's actions on either symptoms or consciousness (Shagass 1972).

---

*Research supported (in part) by U.S.P.H.S. Grant MH12507.

For reprint requests: Charles Shagass, M.D., Eastern Pennsylvania Psychiatric Institute, Henry Avenue and Abbottsford Road, Philadelphia, Pa. 19129, U.S.A.

METHODS

Recording procedure

Details of the EP recording procedure have been described (Shagass et al. 1977). Electrode locations are shown in the head diagram of Fig. 1; 6 leads are non-standard — F3X, F4X, C3X, C4X are 2 cm posterior and 1 cm lateral to the F3, F4, C3 and C4 locations in the 10-20 system, and O3 and O4, respectively, are midway between T5 and O1 and T6 and O2. All are referred to linked ears. Stimuli are: electrical pulses (1 msec duration; 10 mA above sensory threshold) applied over left and right median nerves at the wrist to elicit somatosensory EPs (SEPs); a brief flash of a checkerboard pattern on the television (TV) monitor for visual EPs (VEPs); binaural auditory clicks, 50 dB above a steady 75 dB white noise level applied through earphones, to evoke auditory EPs (AEPs). The seated subject is instructed to fixate a spot in the center of the TV screen. The order of stimuli and interstimulus intervals are pseudorandomized. Two recording montages each contain 7 scalp leads and a lead (E) to monitor the electro-oculogram (EOG). Each average EP (512 data points, sampled at 1 msec intervals) contains 192 sweeps. Fig. 1 shows group mean SEPs, AEPs, and VEPs for 16 normal subjects.

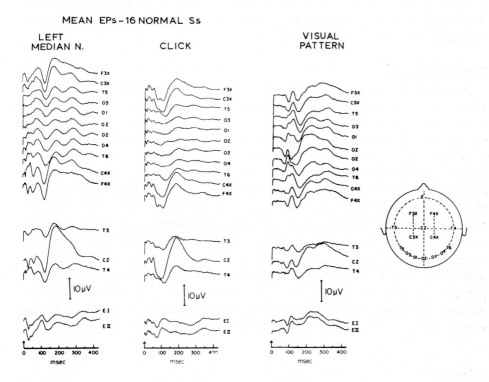

Fig. 1. Grand mean EPs of 16 normal subjects evoked by left median nerve, binaural click and visual checkerboard flash stimuli. Scalp lead referred to linked ears; in this and subsequent figures, scalp positivity gives upward deflection. EI and EII are E lead (EOG) records for first and second montage.

Subjects

Clinical considerations made it necessary to conduct these studies in a "naturalistic" manner. We attempted to test the patients initially after at least 7 days freedom from medication; we succeeded for about 90% of the patients, who were drug free for a median interval of 10 days, but the remainder had had drugs from 4 to 6 days before testing. After testing, the patient entered treatment and was solicited to undertake a second EP test when there was significant clinical change, or when discharge from hospital was imminent. The interval between first and second tests varied considerably, ranging from 18 to 300 days (median, 39) for antipsychotic drugs, 22 to 60 days (median, 39) for antidepressants, 23 to 56 days (median, 28) for lithium, and 13 to 110 days (median, 30) for the no drug group. Drug dosage also varied; antipsychotics, 50–3000 mg daily chlorpromazine equivalent (median, 805 mg); tricyclics, 100–300 mg daily amitriptyline equivalent (median, 175 mg); serum lithium levels ranged from 0.51 to 1.88 mg/l (median, 0.92). Most of the 28 patients receiving antipsychotic drugs were diagnosed as schizophrenic, most of the 10 receiving tricyclic antidepressants were diagnosed as suffering from major depressive disorder, and the 12 patient lithium group was also composed of depressive patients (Straumanis et al. 1981). The 15 patients in the no medication group included 6 schizophrenics, 4 personality disorders, 2 drug psychoses, 2 brain syndromes, and 1 neurosis. Although it can be stated that the average patient was clinically improved upon retest, the detailed data relating EP changes to degree of clinical improvement will not be presented here.

Treatment of data

To demonstrate gross differences between grand mean EPs of groups, we have computed *t* tests for significance of mean differences between consecutive data points; the computer program plots a line of *t* test values in which only those that achieve the 0.05 level of significance (2-tailed) rise above baseline (Fig. 2). To demonstrate drug effects we used matched pair *t* tests. The *t* test results should be regarded as primarily descriptive, since differences in both amplitude and latency could lead to significant *t* tests and the overall level of significance is uncertain with multiple *t* tests. However, we have analysed the data in other ways to verify findings; these include visual detection of peaks by means of a cursor program to obtain specific amplitude and latency measures (Shagass et al. 1979), and automatic computation of an amplitude measure that reflects the area under the curve for selected portions of the EP (Shagass 1972). Although the data presented here will be primarily the group mean EPs, the conclusions have been verified by the other methods. The illustrations presented here are derived from key leads, selected to be representative of the main findings yielded by the 4 sets of 14 scalp records.

RESULTS

Antipsychotic drugs

Fig. 2 shows the group mean EPs (6 selected leads) of 32 schizophrenic patients

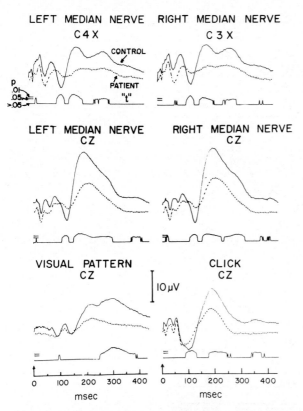

LEFT MEDIAN NERVE   RIGHT MEDIAN NERVE
C 4 X   C 3 X

CONTROL
PATIENT
"t"

p
.01
.05
>.05

LEFT MEDIAN NERVE   RIGHT MEDIAN NERVE
CZ   CZ

VISUAL PATTERN   CLICK
CZ   CZ

10 µV

0   100 200 300 400   0   100 200 300 400
msec   msec

Fig. 2. Grand mean EPs from selected leads for 32 schizophrenic patients and 16 controls of same age and sex, *t* tests between means of corresponding data points displayed below EPs; *t* line deflects from baseline only when *t* gives *P* of 0.05 or less (2-tailed).

and of 16 non-patient controls matched with them for age and sex (Shagass et al. 1977). Several zones of major difference between the 2 groups are evident. SEPs to both left and right median nerve stimulation were of smaller amplitude in the schizophrenics at time points corresponding to peaks N130, P185, and P290. The main VEP difference was contributed by a smaller amplitude P300 wave in the schizophrenics. The AEP means differed at N100 (smaller amplitude and earlier peak in schizophrenics), P180 (smaller amplitude in schizophrenics), and P360 (also smaller in patients). Although not obvious in Fig. 2, generally reduced SEP activity after 100 msec in schizophrenics was accompanied by little difference in the amplitude of earlier activity, and even a tendency for greater amplitude, particularly of peak N60 (Shagass et al. 1978a, 1979).

Fig. 3 shows the selected lead group means for 28 patients before and during treatment with antipsychotic drugs (mainly phenothiazines, 16 cases, and thioxanthenes, 8 cases). For SEPs, particularly with left median nerve stimulation, the largest changes consisted of a reduction of amplitude in the zone of P30 and greater negativity, i.e., increased amplitude, at N130. With right median nerve stimuli, there was also an increase of P90 amplitude at the Cz lead. In VEPs, P300

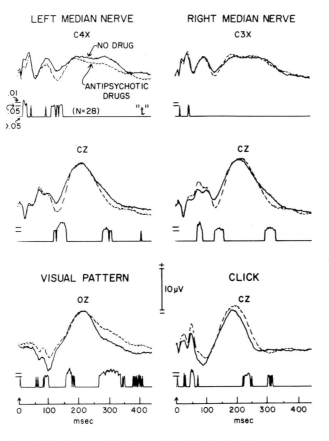

Fig. 3. Grand mean EPs from selected leads for 28 patients tested pre-drug and while receiving antipsychotic medication; *t* line based on test for paired observations.

amplitude tended to be increased with drugs, whereas earlier peaks showed amplitude decrease. AEP peaks P30 and P50 were increased in amplitude with the drugs, and there was a tendency for both N100 and P180 to be shifted backward in time.

Comparing the group mean EPs of normals in Fig. 2 with those of drug-treated patients in Fig. 3, it will be evident that the EPs of the treated patients were still markedly deviant from normal. However, most of the changes associated with antipsychotic drugs in Fig. 3, such as augmentation of SEP N130, were in the direction of more normal group mean EPs. Thus, while the EPs of patients treated with antipsychotic drugs did not differ greatly from those recorded before treatment, the changes that did occur were in the direction of normality.

Tricyclic antidepressants

Fig. 4 shows group sum EPs of 27 patients with major depressions (psychotic depression; manic-depressive, depressed) and 27 non-patient controls matched for age and sex (Shagass et al. 1980). It will be seen that the main zones of significant

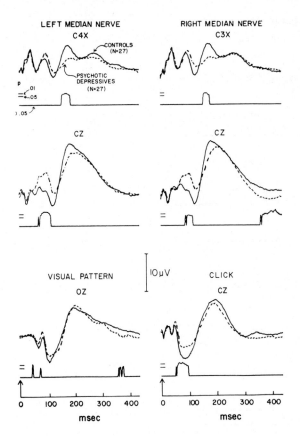

Fig. 4. Grand mean EPs from selected leads for 27 psychotic depressives and 27 controls of same age and sex.

differences in SEPs were the larger amplitude P90 (Cz leads) and smaller amplitude P185 (C4X, C3X leads) in the depressives. The VEP differences were minimal, while N100 amplitude was considerably lower in the depressives' than in the controls' AEPs.

Fig. 5 displays group mean EPs before and during treatment with tricyclic antidepressant drugs (amitriptyline in 9 cases) for a group of 10 patients. The t tests suggest relatively few statistically significant effects, but both kinds of SEP did show reduced amplitude in peak P30 and increased amplitude (greater negativity) for peak N130. The mean VEP tended to be of smaller amplitude from 150 to 200 msec and after 300 msec during drug treatment. In the mean AEP, peak N100 was increased in amplitude. The tendencies for reduced amplitude of SEP peak P30 and increased amplitude of SEP peak N130 suggest that the tricyclics produced SEP effects similar to those observed with antipsychotic drugs. Although relatively minor in magnitude, these changes, together with the tendency for the AEP N100 to increase, were in the direction of greater normality.

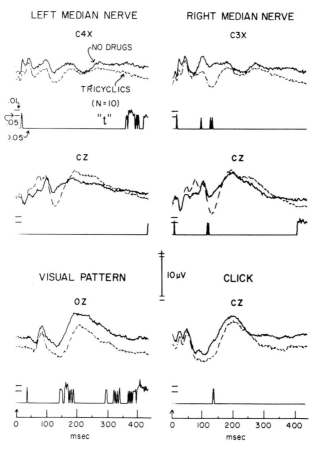

Fig. 5. Grand mean EPs from selected leads for 10 patients tested pre-drug and while receiving tricyclic antidepressant medication.

Lithium carbonate

Although lithium (Li) is customarily used to treat mania, it also has antidepressant properties, and the data reported here were obtained from a group of depressive patients who volunteered for a placebo-controlled study of the antidepressant effects of lithium. However, EPs of manic patients tend to resemble those of depressives in a number of respects (Shagass et al. 1978a), and the EP effects of Li are similar in both kinds of patient. Until recently, it appeared that the sole EP effect of lithium consisted of augmentation of SEP P30 amplitude (Shagass and Straumanis 1978). Subsequent observations indicated that Li produced additional changes, both in SEPs and AEPs, so that the notion of a specific CNS effect of Li on the "primary" somatosensory cortex required modification.

Fig. 6 illustrates, in EPs from selected leads, the main changes that we found with Li (Straumanis et al. 1981). Both kinds of SEP show greatly augmented amplitude of peak P30. SEP peaks P90 and P185 also tended to increase in amplitude; in contrast, N60 and N130 amplitudes tended to be reduced (less negativity). VEP

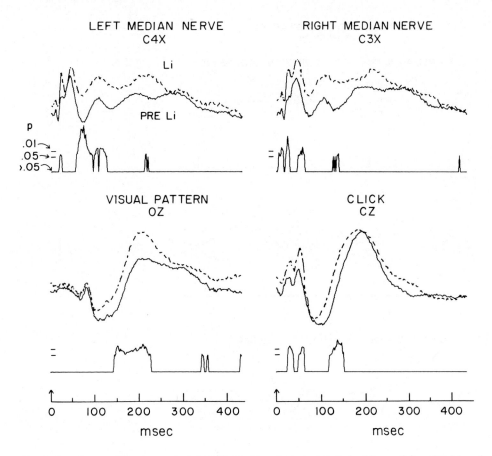

Fig. 6. Grand mean EPs from selected leads for 12 patients tested first while receiving placebo and subsequently during lithium carbonate therapy.

amplitude was increased in the zone of P200. In AEPs, Li therapy was associated with increased amplitudes of P30 and P50, while P180 appeared to occur earlier. The overall data indicated that Li increased the amplitudes of positive EP peaks and decreased those of negative peaks. We also found that the magnitudes of these EP changes were poorly correlated with clinical change in depressive symptoms, as reflected in the Hamilton Depression Scale. However, the EP changes were significantly related to serum Li levels; the greater the EP changes, the higher the serum Li level.

Comparing Figs. 3, 5 and 6, it will be seen that Li produced greater alterations in EP characteristics than the antipsychotic and tricyclic antidepressant drugs, and that the nature of the changes was different. Whereas the relatively small effects of the antipsychotics and tricyclics could be interpreted as normalization, some of the more striking Li effects, e.g., the higher SEP P30 and lower N130 amplitudes, cannot be so interpreted, as greater P30 and lower N130 have been associated with psychopathology.

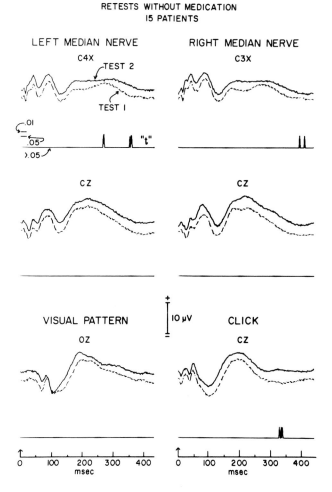

Fig. 7. Grand mean EPs from selected leads for 15 patients retested after receiving no psychotropic drugs.

Retests without medication

Fig. 7 shows the group mean EPs for the 15 patients whose second test was performed after a period of hospitalization without pharmacotherapy. It will be seen that the 2 sets of mean EPs were very similar to one another, and that significant *t* tests were virtually absent. The lack of consistent changes in repeat EPs when no medication was administered suggests that the changes found with drugs can probably be attributed to the pharmacotherapy.

DISCUSSION

There is now much evidence that EP characteristics of patients with schizophrenic and affective psychoses differ from normal (Figs. 2, 4; Shagass et al. 1978a, b, 1979,

1980). However, the possibility that the EP differences in patients could result from previous or current intake of psychotropic drugs has clouded the interpretation of these findings. Although our own data came from patients who had not received drugs for an average of 10 days, and although other workers have found no relation between EP measurements and drug dosage in patients tested while receiving drugs (e.g., Roth et al. 1981), the possibility that the EP findings represent a pharmacological artifact remained. Our patients could still be manifesting effects of drugs known to be long acting, or be in a state of drug rebound, and EP changes need not necessarily be dose related. Consequently, the present findings, showing that both antipsychotic and antidepressant drugs produce relatively small changes in EPs (Figs. 3, 5), and that those changes that they do elicit are in the direction of normalization, are very reassuring. If previous drugs were responsible for EP deviations from normal, then administration of drugs should make EPs more, not less, deviant. The drug effect results strongly imply that the EP deviations found in the psychoses are not secondary to antipsychotic or antidepressant drugs. Furthermore, the fact that the drugs produce only modest shifts toward normal EP patterns suggests that EP recording from patients receiving these drugs will provide results that are not too different from those that might be obtained in the drug-free state. Also, errors will be conservative, in the sense that the EPs will be less abnormal than they might be without drugs.

The relatively minor EP changes with antipsychotics and antidepressants cannot be attributed to the reduced alertness that may accompany these agents, as they were opposite in direction to those seen with drowsiness (Shagass 1972).

The reassurance about contamination of EP findings that present data provide for antipsychotic and antidepressant drugs does not extend to lithium, which clearly produces major changes in EP characteristics in directions away from normal (Fig. 6). However, it seems reasonably certain that Li is entirely excreted in 14 days (Baer 1973), so that EPs recorded after this time should be unaffected by previous Li therapy.

The fact that Li augments SEP P30 amplitude while both antipsychotics and antidepressants reduce it suggests that the CNS effects of Li are rather different from those of the other drugs. The only agent known to us that augments SEP P30 like Li is triiodothyronine (Straumanis and Shagass 1976), a hormone with behavioural effects unlike those of Li. The observation that the magnitude of EP changes with Li is correlated with the serum level of the ion suggests that the EP alteration could be a "tissue" effect, with no direct relationship to the effect of Li on mood or consciousness.

Although we hope ultimately to relate the findings concerning effects of psychotropic drugs on EPs to concepts of CNS mechanisms underlying the therapeutic actions of these drugs, a serious attempt to do so is probably premature and beyond the scope of this paper.

SUMMARY

Effects of antipsychotic and antidepressant drugs and lithium carbonate (Li) on somatosensory, visual and auditory EPs were studied in psychiatric patients under treatment with those agents. A comparison group of patients treated without medication was also examined. The no medication group showed fewer EP changes on retest than the drug-treated groups. The effects of Li were greater than, and differed from, those of antipsychotics and antidepressants. EP changes with antipsychotics and antidepressants were relatively small and in the direction of normalization; these findings indicate that the pre-treatment EP differences from normal found in psychotic patients are probably not secondary to previous treatment with these drugs.

ACKNOWLEDGEMENTS

We thank the following for assistance: I. Chung Hung, J. Kline, M. Kormanik, A. McGrath, W. Nixon and S. Slepner.

REFERENCES

Baer, L. Pharmacology — lithium absorption, distribution, renal handling, and effect on body electrolytes. In: S. Gershon and B. Shopsin (Eds.), Lithium: its Role in Psychiatric Research and Treatment. Plenum Press, New York, 1973: 33–50.

Roth, W.T., Pfefferbaum, A., Kelly, A.F., Berger, P.A. and Kopell, B.S. Auditory event-related potentials in schizophrenia and depression. Psychiat. Res., 1981, 4: 199.

Shagass, C. Evoked Brain Potentials in Psychiatry. Plenum Press, New York, 1972.

Shagass, C. and Straumanis, J.J. Drugs and human sensory evoked potentials. In: M.A. Lipton, A. DiMascio and K.F. Killam (Eds.), Psychopharmacology: a Generation of Progress. Raven Press, New York, 1978: 699–709.

Shagass, C., Straumanis, J.J., Roemer, R.A. and Amadeo, M. Evoked potentials of schizophrenics in several sensory modalities. Biol. Psychiat., 1977, 12: 221–235.

Shagass, C., Roemer, R.A., Straumanis, J.J. and Amadeo, M. Evoked potential correlates of psychosis. Biol. Psychiat., 1978a, 13: 163–184.

Shagass, C., Ornitz, E.M., Sutton, S. and Tueting, P. Event related potentials and psychopathology. In: E. Callaway, P. Tueting, S. Sutton and S. Koslow (Eds.), Event-Related Brain Potentials in Man. Academic Press, New York, 1978b: 443–496.

Shagass, C., Roemer, R.A., Straumanis, J.J. and Amadeo, M. Spatial distribution of sensory evoked potentials in psychiatric disorders. In: E. Callaway and D. Lehmann (Eds.), Human Evoked Potentials: Applications and Problems. Plenum Press, New York, 1979: 347–362.

Shagass, C., Roemer, R.A., Straumanis, J.J. and Amadeo, M. Topography of sensory evoked potentials in depressive disorders. Biol. Psychiat., 1980, 15: 183–207.

Straumanis, J.J. and Shagass, C. Electrophysiological effects of triiodothyronine and propranolol. Psychopharmacologia (Berl.), 1976, 46: 283–288.

Straumanis, J.J., Shagass, C., Roemer, R.A., Ramsey, T.A. and Mendels, J. Cerebral evoked potential changes produced by treatment with lithium carbonate. Biol. Psychiat., 1981, 16: 113–129.

Kyoto Symposia (EEG Suppl. No. 36)
Editors: P.A. Buser, W.A. Cobb and T. Okuma
© 1982, Elsevier Biomedical Press, Amsterdam

Abnormal EEG Activities Induced by Psychotropic Drugs

R. SPATZ and J. KUGLER

Psychiatrische Klinik der Universität München, Nussbaumstrasse 7, D 8000 Munich 2 (F.R.G.)

PROBLEM

The EEG during the course of psychopharmacological treatment varies largely according to the effects of many factors and depends upon the age of the patient, the type of his illness, his individual constitution, the kind of application (i.v., i.m., orally) and the dosage of the drug (Bente 1963; Fink 1964; Itil 1974; Longo 1975; Verdaux and Nery-Filho 1977; Kugler et al. 1979). Generally speaking, one can distinguish 4 main types of reaction in the EEG, commonly associated with different groups of psychoactive drugs: (1) fast activity (anxiolytics, tranquilizers); (2) slow activity (neuroleptics, hypnotics); (3) changes in alpha activity (psychostimulants, psychoenergizers, nootropics); (4) paroxysmal activity (antidepressants, lithium salts).

By visual inspection of EEG records these changes, when only slight changes of background activity, are often difficult to discern, but they can be detected better at relatively early stages by quantitative electronic analysis (Bente and Pfeiffer 1964; Künkel and Westphal 1970; Matejcek and Schenk 1975; Saletu 1976; Hermann et al. 1981). In the more advanced stages the drug-induced abnormalities may appear with paroxysmal EEG activity and combined with slow and fast EEG activity. Paroxysmal activity consists of groups of two or more waves or complexes, which can be distinguished clearly from the background by their form, amplitude and sudden appearance.

Paroxysmal EEG activity of this type is a manifestation of abnormally synchronous neuronal discharge, which may also, but not necessarily, occur in epilepsy; nor is every paroxysmal EEG activity epileptic. Convulsants (metrazol, picrotoxin, bicuculline) by intravenous injection very often induce paroxysmal EEG activity. It is also seen relatively frequently following parenteral and prolonged oral treatment with antidepressant drugs (Table I).

To the drugs which elicited paroxysmal EEG activities in our therapeutic trials belong reserpine, cycloserine, promaxine (Protactyl), promethazine (Atosil), amitriptyline (Laroxyl, Sarotan, Tryptizol), maprotiline (Ludiomil), bemigride, clozapine (Leponex), perazine (Taxilan), laevomepromazine (Neurocil) and lithium salts (Fink 1964; Spatz et al. 1978; Kugler et al. 1979).

In animal experiments, when rats were given 30–50 mg/kg imipramine (Tofranil) i.v., it was possible to elicit recruited EEG wave patterns which were accompanied by an increase in spike discharges in the amygdala and hippocampus (Van Meter et al. 1959). An increase in irritability in the amygdaloid nucleus has also been

TABLE I

PAROXYSMAL EEG ACTIVITIES AND PSYCHOACTIVE DRUG TREATMENT

Author	Year	Drug	Dose (mg)	EEG
Delay	1952	Imipramine	75 i.v.	S-W complexes
Van Meter et al.	1959	Imipramine	30–50 mg/kg i.v.	Recruited spikes
Fink	1959	Imipramine	40–150 i.v.	Slow sharp waves
Zappoli	1959	Imipramine	300–400 orally	Spikes, S-W, 25%
Kiloh et al.	1961	Imipramine	75 i.v.	Sharp waves
Bente and Pfeiffer	1964	Amitriptyline	150–300 orally	Spikes, S-W, 28%
Mayfield and Brown	1966	Lithium salts	0.76 mval/l	Delta groups
Helmchen and Kanowski	1971	Lithium salts	536–1608 orally	S-W complexes
Isermann and Haupt	1976	Clozapine	200–300 orally	S-W complexes 20%
Kugler et al.	1979	Clozapine	200–250 orally	S-W complexes 13%

TABLE II

CEREBRAL SEIZURES BY TREATMENT WITH PSYCHOACTIVE DRUGS

Author	Year	Drug	Dose (mg)	
Davison	1965	Amitriptyline	1000–1500	orally
Helmchen and Kanowski	1971	Lithium salts	536–1608	orally
Schulze	1972	Dibenzepine	240	orally
Mueller and Heipertz	1977	Clozapine	400	orally
Porter and Jick	1977	Chlorpromazine	125	orally
		Perazine	40	orally
Kugler et al.	1979	Maprotiline	150	orally
		Clozapine	200–400	orally
		Amitriptyline	150	orally

produced by the use of MAO inhibitors (Gloor 1960). Other authors only observed a decrease in amplitude and an increase in slow wave activity (anticholinergic reaction type, according to Itil 1974), following the intravenous administration of 40–150 mg imipramine (Fink 1959).

The extent of paroxysmal EEG activity with orally administered psychoactive agents is influenced by the duration of administration, the dose, the bioavailability of the drug and by the individual metabolic reactions, which not only occur in the neurones. The reports in the literature show, moreover, generalized tonic-clonic seizures with varying incidence during treatment with the whole range of psychoactive drugs (Table II).

On the other hand, there are observations on amitriptyline poisoning without seizures (Davis and Allaye 1963).

In the light of our current knowledge the 4 following questions may be raised. (1) Is there a relation between paroxysmal EEG activity produced by drugs and the occurrence of seizures? (2) Are systematic EEG examinations of patients receiving psychoactive drugs useful? (3) Is there a relation between the activation of EEG changes and the psychological signs and symptoms of the patient? (4) Can any conclusions be drawn as to the pharmacodynamic efficiency of the substances in question? To answer these questions we have reviewed our EEG findings and, in doing so, selected records which showed paroxysmal activity.

OBSERVATIONS

In recent years we have observed abnormal EEG activities in a large number of

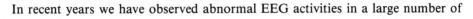

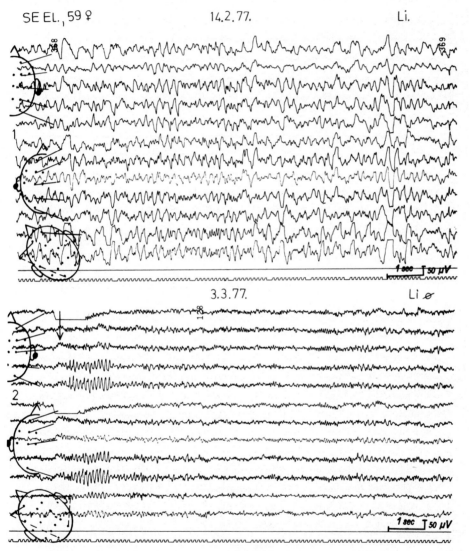

Fig. 1. Woman, 59 years, affective psychosis (depression) on 14-2-77 after 40 weeks on 3 × 536 lithium acetate daily (Quilonum). Abnormal background activity, generalized 4–6 c/sec waves. Severe ataxic signs. Lithium treatment interrupted next day. On 3-3-77 normalized EEG background activity; transient drowsiness. Ataxic signs had disappeared 10 days earlier.

patients whose psychoses were treated with different psychoactive drugs. However, the proportions of records showing abnormal EEG activity varied between the treated groups. In one of our studies involving 680 investigations of 593 inpatients abnormal background activities were seen more frequently in the EEGs of patients treated with a combination of several psychoactive drugs (Table III, Figs. 1 and 2).

The proportions of abnormal EEG activities (Figs. 1 and 2) in the various groups

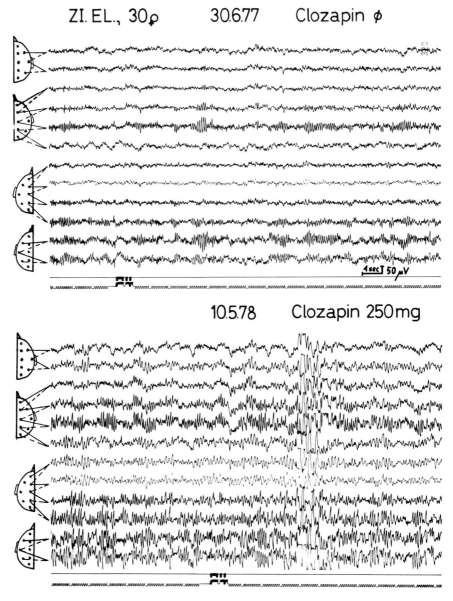

Fig. 2. Woman, 30 years, paranoid psychosis on 30-6-77, before clozapine treatment. Normal 11–12 c/sec alpha activity. On 10-5-78 after 27 days of treatment with 50–250 mg clozapine daily. Irregular background activity, paroxysmal groups of 3–5 c/sec waves.

TABLE III

PSYCHOACTIVE DRUG TREATMENT (1973–1974) AND EEG RECORDS

N = 608.

Drug	Mean dosage (mg/day)	EEG records	Abnormal EEG (%)	Generalized transient disturbances	
				Paroxysmal	Non-paroxysmal
Clozapine	250	181	59	17	51
Lithium salts	1000	92	50	4	30
Laevomepromazine	500	88	31	1	18
Diazepam	30	85	4	–	2
Amitriptyline	150	57	31	1	3
Butyrophenone	12	54	44	4	13
Imipramine	300	51	9	–	2
		608	32.5	27	119

were, in descending order: clozapine 59%, lithium salts 50%, butyrophenone 44%, maprotiline 37%, dibenzepine 32%, laevomepromazine 31%, amitriptyline 31%, imipramine 9% and diazepam 4%. The proportions of paroxysmal EEG activities (13%) and generalized transient disturbances with groups of slow waves (30.5%) were also greatest in the clozapine group. However, paroxysmal EEG activity was also seen in patients undergoing treatment with other drugs such as butyrophenones, laevomepromazine and imipramine.

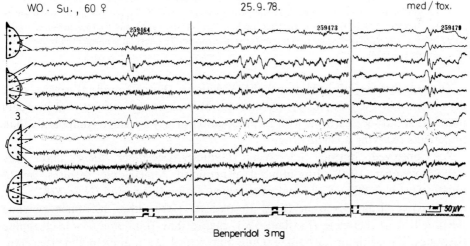

Fig. 3. Woman, 60 years, affective psychosis (chronic paranoid schizophrenia). After 17 days of treatment with 3 mg benperidol daily appearance of bilateral irregular groups of slow waves, partly paroxysmal. The EEG before treatment on September 8 and 15, 1978, showed regular background activity without transient disturbances. Also later records without benperidol showed normal EEG background activity.

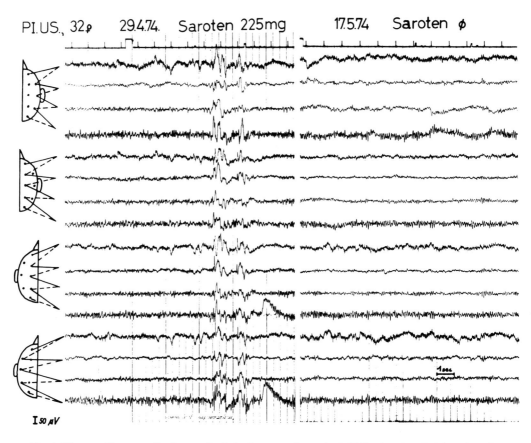

Fig. 4. Woman, 32 years, affective psychosis (endogenous depression). Following the administration of 225 mg daily of amitriptyline for 1 week bilateral paroxysmal groups of 3–4 c/sec waves with sharp waves and S-W complexes (29-4-74). Two weeks later, on May 7, 1974, the patient suffered a generalized tonic-clonic seizure after sleep deprivation. Treatment was interrupted. Ten days later normalized background EEG activity (17-5-74).

The appearance of paroxysmal EEG activity (Figs. 3 and 4) seems dose dependent, like the non-paroxysmal changes of background activity, and it occurs more often during treatment with a combination of psychoactive compounds than in patients receiving a single drug.

We observed during 3.5 years (January–December 1974 and May 1979–November 1980) drug-induced generalized tonic-clonic seizures in 16 inpatients, i.e. 0.28% of all inpatients treated during this period (N = 5785). The psychoactive drugs given in these 16 patients were either laevomepromazine (Neurocil, 4×), perazine (Taxilan, 3×), maprotiline (Ludiomil, 3×), clozapine (Leponex, 2×), lithium carbonate (Quilonum retard, 2×), amitriptyline (Saroten, 2×) alone, or, in 8 cases, in combination with butyrophenone (3×), fluphenacine (2×) or biperiden (3×). We observed no seizures in patients treated with lithium salts at therapeutic levels; this complication occurred in 2 patients with intoxication.

On the basis of these observations it is impossible to decide with certainty whether clozapine and lithium salts activate paroxysmal EEG activity to a greater extent than other substances. The small number of patients observed during treatment with other medications prevents conclusions being made with regard to differences in pharmacodynamic effects. However, it is apparent that in those groups with sufficient numbers of observed patients they occurred more frequently during treatment with clozapine than during treatment with lithium salts.

DISCUSSION

We now try to answer the 4 questions which we posed in the initial section.

(1) There is no reliable relationship between the paroxysmal EEG activity induced by a given psychoactive drug and the appearance of generalized tonic-clonic seizures. So the appearance of a paroxysmal EEG activity in a patient whose EEG was previously normal is not necessarily a reason for breaking off drug treatment. However, the patients whose EEG records showed paroxysmal activity had certain noticeable characteristics. Some of them exhibited an unusual degree of autonomic lability and of personality change with unusual behaviour. The activation of paroxysmal EEG activities seems to be associated with instability of central regulation of the autonomic nervous system and can probably be mediated via the medial thalamic nucleus and systems of neurones in the lower brain stem and in the limbic structures. It would be reasonable and prudent to assess the common risks ensuing from activation of paroxysmal EEG activities in the same manner as other risk factors in internal medicine are assessed: the presence of a single risk factor cannot on its own be a sufficient reason for interrupting a treatment. On the other hand, if several risk factors are simultaneously present in a given patient, the occurrence of paroxysmal EEG activity may be interpreted as a warning sign to which one should react by reducing the dosage of the drug (with careful measurement of the serum concentration) or by changing to another drug. Paroxysmal EEG activity does not usually appear unless the patient has been taking the drug for several days or weeks. The unusually early occurrence of paroxysmal EEG activity in isolated cases can be regarded as an expression of individual hypersensitivity, or of an epileptic predisposition, and caution should be exercised during the subsequent treatment of these patients.

Moreover, in earlier investigations we were able to show that the occurrence of paroxysmal EEG activities and of generalized non-paroxysmal EEG activities are dose dependent (Spatz et al. 1978). Thus high serum concentrations of lithium salts, which were well within the therapeutic range, were accompanied twice as frequently by EEG changes as low serum concentrations.

(2) The results of the foregoing observations suggest that systematic pharmacotherapy of hospitalized patients may usefully be monitored by regular EEG examinations at intervals of approximately 7 days. If several risk factors are operative in the same patient, examinations at more frequent intervals may be necessary.

(3) Analysis of the relationships between the frequency of activation of paroxysmal EEG activities and the subjective symptoms of the patients reveals that the proportions of patients who experience subjective relief of their depression or schizophrenia are not only dependent on the absence or presence of paroxysmal EEG activity. Our experience has shown that the clinical state of patients with paroxysmal EEG activity improves just as often as that of patients without such activity. However, our impression was that EEG records with stable, relatively unchanged alpha activity following several weeks of treatment with neuroleptics were as a whole less often associated with clinical improvement than EEG records with transient irregularities or transient abnormal synchronization during the first few weeks of treatment. Generalized or focal paroxysmal theta or delta bursts are regarded by some authors as a sign of successful antipsychotic treatment (Helmchen and Kanowski 1971).

(4) For the time being, conclusions regarding the pharmacodynamic effects of psychoactive drugs can only be drawn by analogy with animal experiments and by observation of side effects in humans. Neuroleptics elicit a marked reduction in the activity of the ascending reticular activating system and inhibit motor action. The irritability of the neostriatum and the median thalamic nucleus are increased. The metabolism of serotonergic, adrenergic and dopaminergic systems are influenced. In addition, the effects of various psychoactive drugs on ion exchange through the membranes of neurones and glial cells may be of importance. Changes of this kind can promote the appearance of paroxysmal EEG activity. However, if the neocortical brain function is sufficiently intact and the vigilance of the subject not reduced, paroxysmal EEG activities are not necessarily followed by manifestations of motor disinhibition leading to myoclonus or tonic or clonic seizures.

SUMMARY

In a retrospective study involving 680 EEG investigations in 593 patients the effects of various psychopharmaceutical agents were examined by visual interpretation of the EEG. The drugs were given singly in the majority of cases and were combined in others, and special attention was paid to the occurrence of paroxysmal EEG activity. The proportions of abnormal EEGs in the various groups were (in descending order): clozapine 59%, lithium salts 50%, butyrophenone 44%, maprotiline 37%, dibenzepine 32%, laevomepromazine and amitriptyline 31%, imipramine 9% and diazepam 4%. The proportions of paroxysmal discharges (13%) and generalized transient disturbances with groups of slow waves (16%) were also greatest in the clozapine group.

During 3.5 years (1973–1974, May 1979–November 1980) we observed drug-induced generalized seizures in 16 inpatients = 0.28% of all inpatients (N = 5785) in that time. The psychotropic drugs given to these patients were either laevomepromazine (Neurocil 4×), perazine (Taxilan 3×), maprotiline (Ludiomil 3×), clozapine (Leponex 2×), lithium carbonate (Quilonum retard 2×) and amitriptyline (Saroten 2×) alone or partly in combination with butyrophenone (3×), fluphenazine (2×) and biperiden (3×).

The appearance of paroxysmal EEG activity seems dose dependent and occurs more often during treatment with a combination of psychoactive compounds, than in patients receiving a single drug.

REFERENCES

Bente, D. EEG changes after acute and chronic application of psychotropic drugs. Electroenceph. clin. Neurophysiol., 1963, 15: 133–137.

Bente, D. und Pfeiffer, W.M. Verlaufsdynamische Besonderheiten der Amitriptylin-Medikation unter besonderer Berücksichtigung elektroenzephalographischer Befunde. Arzneimittel-Forsch., 1964, 14: 523–527.

Davis, D.M. and Allaye, R. Amitriptyline poisoning. Lancet, 1963, ii: 543, 643.

Davison, K. EEG activation after intravenous amitriptyline. Electroenceph. clin. Neurophysiol., 1965, 19: 298–300.

Delay, J.T. 38 cas de psychoses traités par la cure prolongée et continue de 4568 R.T. Ann. Méd. Psychol., 1952, 110: 364.

Fink, M. Electroencephalographic and behavioural effects of Tofranil. Canad. psychiat. Ass. J., 1959, Suppl. 4: 166–171.

Fink, M. A selected biography of electroencephalography in human psychopharmacology 1951–1962. Electroenceph. clin. Neurophysiol., 1964, Suppl. 23.

Gloor, P. Amygdala. In: J. Field, H.W. Magoun and V.E. Hall (Eds.), Handbook of Physiology, Section I: Neurophysiology, Vol. II. American Physiological Society, Washington, D.C., 1960.

Helmchen, H. und Kanowski, S. EEG-Veränderungen unter Lithium-Therapie. Nervenarzt, 1971, 42: 144–148.

Herrmann, W.M., Fichte, K. und Kubicki, St. Beispiele für die Projektion von Substanzwirkungen typischer Psychopharmaka auf eine elektrophysiologische Messebene. Z. EEG-EMG, 1981, 12: 21–32.

Isermann, H. und Haupt, R. Auffällige EEG-Veränderungen unter Clozapin-Behandlung bei paranoid-halluzinatorischen Psychosen. Nervenarzt, 1976, 47: 268.

Itil, T.M. Quantitative pharmaco-electroencephalography. In: T.M. Itil (Ed.), Psychotropic Drugs and the Human EEG, Mod. Probl. Pharmacopsychiat., Vol. 8. Karger, Basel, 1974: 43–75.

Kiloh, L.G., Davison, K. and Osselton, J.W. An electroencephalographic study of the analeptic effects of imipramine. Electroenceph. clin. Neurophysiol., 1961, 13: 216–223.

Kugler, J., Lorenzi, E., Spatz, R. and Zimmermann, H. Drug-induced paroxysmal EEG-activities. Pharmakopsychiatrie, 1979, 12: 165–172.

Künkel, H. and Westphal, M. Quantitative EEG analysis and pyrithioxine action. Pharmakopsychiatrie, 1970, 3: 41–49.

Longo, V.G. Effect of drugs on the EEG. In: A. Rémond (Ed.), Handbook of Electroencephalography and Clinical Neurophysiology, Vol. 7, Part C. 1975: 1–132.

Matejcek, M. and Schenk, G.K. Quantitative analysis of the EEG methods and applications. In: Proc. 2nd Symposium of the Study Group for EEG-Methodology. AEG-Telefunken, Konstanz, 1975: 119–395.

Mayfield, D. and Brown, R.G. The clinical laboratory and electroencephalographic effects of lithium. J. psychiat. Res., 1966, 4: 207–219.

Mueller, P. und Heipertz, R. Zur Behandlung manischer Psychosen mit Clozapin. Fortschr. Neurol. Psychiat., 1977, 45: 420–424.

Porter, J. and Jick, H. Drug induced anaphylaxis, convulsions, deafness, and extrapyramidal symptoms. Lancet, 1977, i: 587–588.

Saletu, B. Psychopharmaka, Gehirntätigkeit und Schlaf. Neurophysiologische Aspekte der Psychopharmakologie und Pharmakopsychiatrie. Karger, Basel, 1976.

Schulze, B. Zur Frage medikamentös induzierter zerebraler Reaktionen: Ein Fall von myoklonischem Status unter Behandlung mit trizyklischen Antidepressiva. Nervenarzt, 1972, 43: 332–336.

Spatz, R., Kugler, J., Greil, W. und Lorenzi, E. Das Elektroencephalogramm bei der Lithium-Intoxikation. Nervenarzt, 1978, 49: 539–542.

Spatz, R., Lorenzi, E., Kugler, J. und Ruether, E. Häufigkeit und Form von EEG-Anomalien bei Clozapin-Therapie. Arzneimittel-Forsch., 1978, 28: 1499–1500.

Van Meter, W.G., Owens, H.F. and Himwich, H.E. Effects of tofranil, an antidepressant drug, on electrical potentials of rat brain. Canad. psychiat. Ass. J., 1959, 4: 113–119.

Verdeaux, J. et Nery-Filho, A. Images électroencéphalographiques au cours des traitements par les drogues psychotropes et en particulier neuroleptiques. J. EEG Technol., 1977, 3: 302–312.

Zappoli, R. Electroencephalographic study of patients affected by depressive state treated with imipramine hydrochloride. Electroenceph. clin. Neurophysiol., 1959, 11: 849.

Kyoto Symposia (EEG Suppl. No. 36)
Editors: P.A. Buser, W.A. Cobb and T. Okuma
© 1982, Elsevier Biomedical Press, Amsterdam

Psychoactive Drugs, Animal ECoG and Behaviour*

A. ROUGEUL**

Laboratoire de Neurophysiologie Comparée, Université Pierre et Marie Curie, 9, Quai Saint Bernard, 75005 Paris (France)

In this workshop, the effects of psychoactive drugs were discussed, using several distinct features of the CNS activity, human EEG alpha rhythm, evoked potentials and paroxysmal phenomena, as well as animal hippocampal theta rhythm, arousal reaction, recruiting and augmenting responses. Our own contribution was also based on animal data, but our interest was centered on a rather different set of activities, namely synchronized cortical rhythms with restricted spatial extent that can be characterized within the sensorimotor and anterior parietal cortex during immobility in cat and monkey. They are homologous to human mu and beta rhythms, as often described since Jasper and Penfield (1949) and Gastaut et al. (1957).

These rhythms are of particular interest since (1) they consist in several subsets with distinct frequencies and precise localizations over the fronto-parietal cortex; (2) the development of each subset of rhythms is correlated with a specific level of vigilance; (3) each of these subsets is under the control of a specific monoaminergic system (Bouyer et al. 1979); (4) these activities are very sensitive to the action of various psychoactive drugs that simultaneously alter the animal's behaviour. In this way the correlation between ECoG and behaviour remains unchanged under the effect of these substances.

We shall here take a few examples to illustrate how these ECoG studies, in correlation with observations of the animal's behaviour, can contribute to our knowledge of the mode of action of psychoactive drugs. Our records were taken from animals left free in a recording space; a large number of electrodes were implanted above the sensorimotor and parietal cortex. The recorded ECoG activities were inspected visually (especially in order to identify sleep and drowsiness) and, at least in part of these studies, computer processed, using the fast Fourier transform algorithm, and then displayed as "evolutive" power spectra.

(1) BETA RHYTHMS IN CAT, A DOPAMINE CONTROLLED SYSTEM

Let us first consider the case with the fastest set of rhythms (beta band). These develop for instance when the cat is in a phase of exploration of a new environment,

---

* This study was supported by DRET (Contract No. 79/352), CNRS (ERA 411) and INSERM (ATP 80.79.112).

** With collaboration of J.J. Bouyer and M.F. Montaron.

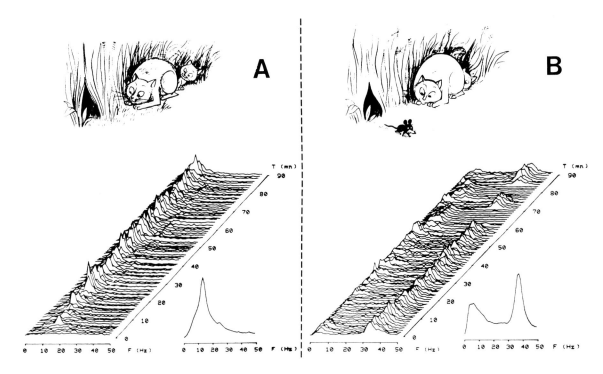

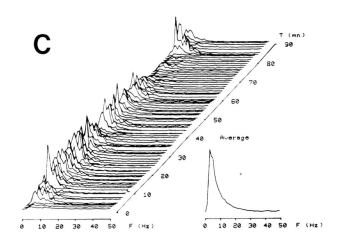

Fig. 1. Evolutive spectra, minute after minute, of the ECoG recorded from the cat anterior cortex during 90 min. A: during expectancy, note quasi-permanent peak around 14 c/sec (mu rhythms). B: in a situation of attention focussed on a mouse. The peak now developed around 40 c/sec (beta rhythms) during about 60 min. C: after a VMT lesion, there were no more beta rhythms. The cat developed restless behaviour, as indicated by movement artifacts in the low frequency band. Added to each set of evolutive spectra is the average spectrum computed over 90 min recording time.

with periods of immobility, or when it is motionless watching a prey. In our experiments, the prey was a mouse in a perspex box: the cat could see it, but could not catch it. The corresponding evolutive spectra displayed, minute after minute, a peak around 40 c/sec for about 1 h (Fig. 1B), during which the animal gazed at the mouse. We could establish that the beta rhythms are favoured by a certain number of drugs known to increase cerebral dopaminergic activity. This is the case with DOPA (dihydroxyphenylalanine), a precursor of dopamine: in Fig. 2N it can be noticed that the 40 c/sec rhythms this time persist uninterruptedly for 90 min, during which time the animal remains completely immobile, displaying visual exploration (even in the absence of a visual target). After apomorphine (8 mg/kg), a substance directly acting on dopaminergic receptors, beta rhythms and immobile phases also occurred, interrupted by well known stereotyped movements (producing low frequency artifacts in the spectrum). Conversely, with drugs like neuroleptics

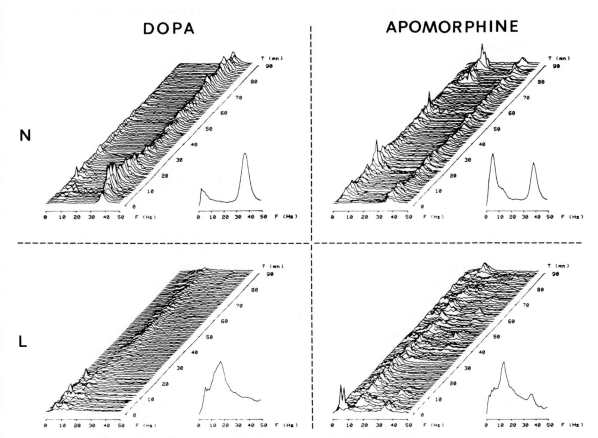

Fig. 2. Evolutive spectra from the cat anterior cortex after administration of DOPA (left spectra) and of apomorphine (right spectra). N: in the normal animal, DOPA induced an uninterrupted peak around 40 c/sec; under apomorphine notice coexistence of the 40 c/sec peak and of low frequency peaks due to the stereotyped movements alternating with periods of immobility with beta rhythms. L: in the same animal after a VMT lesion, DOPA no longer induced beta rhythms. After administration of apomorphine some beta rhythms reappeared although not as abundantly as in the normal subject.

(haloperidol, chlorpromazine) which are known to decrease cerebral dopamine activity, beta rhythms were reduced or even suppressed. Chlorpromazine induced a quasi-permanent state of sleep with spindles and slow waves, interrupted by short phases of wakefulness, but no beta rhythm could ever be observed.

A step further was made when we could show that after an electrolytic lesion of the ventral mesencephalic tegmentum (VMT), which contains perikarya of the meso-cortico-limbic dopaminergic system, beta rhythms were suppressed and the animal became at the same time restless when it was placed in a situation inducing a high level of arousal, for instance in the presence of the mouse (Fig. 1C). Correspondingly, focussed attention and immobility completely disappeared from the behavioural repertoire of the subject (Bouyer et al. 1980). Moreover, in these animals with lesions, DOPA was no longer effective to restore normal ECoG and behaviour (Fig. 2L). On the other hand, apomorphine was still active, even at doses lower than in controls (4 mg/kg); this finding supports the hypothesis that dopamine receptors were not destroyed by VMT lesions, but instead displayed denervation sensitization.

(2) MU AND DROWSINESS RHYTHMS IN CATS

Contrasting with the beta rhythms, activities at lower frequencies developed in distinct behavioural conditions.

One set of rhythms are the 14 c/sec mu rhythms (see also Roth et al. 1967); these appear while the cat is in a position of "expectancy" (e.g. waiting for an absent mouse to get out of its hole (Fig. 1A). These 14 c/sec mu rhythms, and the associated expectancy behaviour, seem to be under the control of a noradrenergic system: both are favoured by dihydroxyphenylserine (DOPS), a substance known to produce directly noradrenaline without dopamine as an intermediary step. After DOPS administration (30 mg/kg i.p.), the animal remains lying quietly in a sphinx position during the 90 min recording. During all this time, the evolutive spectra only display the 14 c/sec rhythm.

Conversely, diethyldithiocarbamate (DDC), which blocks the synthesis of noradrenaline from dopamine, as well as neuroleptics known to block the noradrenergic receptors, suppressed the mu rhythms and induced a behaviour of visual exploration.

Finally, the third, 8 c/sec rhythmic system was shown to develop during states of drowsiness. Indications were obtained that this third subset is modified by drugs affecting the serotoninergic system. 5-HTP administered in small doses thus enhanced these rhythms while at the same time inducing a state of prolonged drowsiness.

(3) RHYTHMS IN MONKEY: EFFECTS OF BENZODIAZEPINES

Other data were obtained on the monkey (Bouyer et al. 1978). For these studies, we used a different method for EEG data compression. Instead of the evolutive spectra as above, we computed the time occupied during each minute by each type of rhythm (Fig. 3). In this representation the oblique axis is time (90 min); each calibration vector corresponds to 10 sec of a given type of central rhythm: the horizontal ($-x$) vector to the left for the beta rhythm (18 c/sec in this species), the

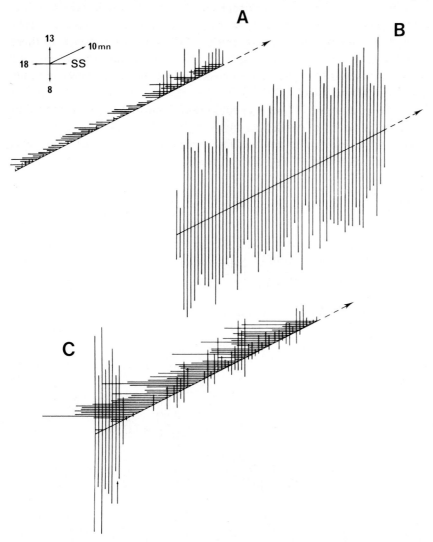

Fig. 3. Distribution of rolandic rhythms in a baboon during 1 h recording. Calibrations: oblique vector: 10 min recording time. $-x$, $+y$, $-y$ vectors: 10 sec duration of 18 c/sec (beta), 13 c/sec (mu) and 8 c/sec (slow) rhythms respectively; $+x$ (SS) vector: 10 sec duration of sleep spindles. A: normal baboon free to move in a large cage. B: same subject kept in restraining chair with hands fastened. C: same animal, still restrained in a chair, after administration of diazepam (vertical arrow indicates time of injection).

vertical vector up ($+y$) for mu rhythm (13 c/sec) and the vertical vector down ($-y$) for the slow rhythms (8 c/sec).

When the animal could move in a large cage it developed intense motor activity like climbing, drinking, looking at different items, etc. ... and the only visible immobility rhythms were those of the beta range (18 c/sec) (Fig. 3A).

On the other hand, when the monkey was placed in a primate chair, with its hands fastened or with its head maintained in painless fixation in a stereotaxic apparatus, it became almost immediately unreactive, closed its eyes and developed a state of "withdrawal of attention" from its environment; it looked as if it were sleeping. However, the ECoG *never* displayed sleep activities but instead, slow 8 c/sec and mu (13 c/sec) rhythms over the rolandic cortex (Fig. 3B). These activities were those characteristic of drowsiness; however, they occupied almost the whole recording time (90 min), which never happened in normal conditions, in which drowsiness only represents a short-lasting stage.

Administration of diazepam (2 mg/kg) could restore normal attentive behaviour and, simultaneously, an ECoG with beta rhythms (Fig. 3C), similar to those which develop during active life in a large cage. Other benzodiazepines, like nitrazepam (Fig. 4A) and lorazepam (Fig. 4B) displayed the same effect during the first 20 min

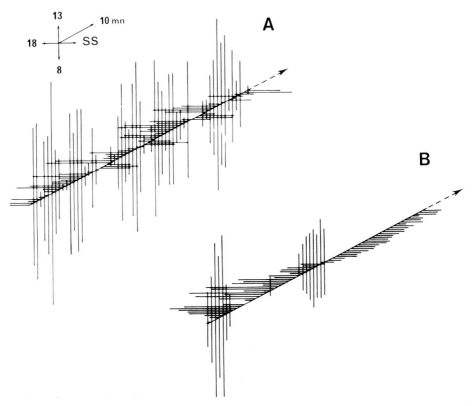

Fig. 4. Distribution of rolandic rhythms in a baboon kept in restraining chair with hands bound for 1 h of recording after administration, at time 0, of nitrazepam (A) or lorazepam (B) (see Fig. 3 for further explanation).

(Bouyer and Rougeul 1980). Afterwards these two drugs induced signs of sleep (see horizontal +x lines in the figure, corresponding to sleep spindles), which seemed rather specific of each substance. This record of fronto-parietal rhythms in the monkey in a chair represents an interesting model to study anxiolytic drugs, together with their secondary hypnogenic effects.

Finally, these examples illustrate how a study of focal cortical rhythms in the animal can bring up information to understand some mechanisms of action of psychotropic drugs in man.

REFERENCES

Bouyer, J.J. and Rougeul, A. Comparative anxiolytic and hypnotic effects of 3 benzodiazepines on baboons. Electroenceph. clin. Neurophysiol., 1980, 49: 401–405.

Bouyer, J.J., Dedet, L., Debray, O. and Rougeul, A. Restraint in primate chair may cause unusual behaviour in baboons; electrographic correlates and corrective effects of diazepam. Electroenceph. clin. Neurophysiol., 1978, 44: 562–567.

Bouyer, J.J., Dedet, L., Joseph, J.P. and Rougeul, A. Modification of spontaneous ECoG and behavior in cat by monoamine precursors. Psychopharmacology, 1979, 65: 49–54.

Bouyer, J.J., Montaron, M.F., Rougeul-Buser, A. and Buser, P. A thalamocortical rhythmic system accompanying high vigilance levels in the cat. In: Pfurtscheller et al. (Eds.), Rhythmic EEG Activities and Cortical Functioning. Elsevier/North-Holland, Amsterdam, 1980: 63–77.

Gastaut, H., Jus, A., Jus, C., Morrell, F., Storm van Leeuwen, W., Dongier, S., Naquet, R., Regis, H., Roger, A., Bekkering, D., Kamp, A. et Werre, J. Etude topographique des réactions électroencéphalographiques conditionnées chez l'homme. Electroenceph. clin. Neurophysiol., 1957, 9: 1–34.

Jasper, H.H. and Penfield, W. Electrocorticograms in man: effect of voluntary movement upon the electrical activity of the precentral gyrus. Arch. Psychiat. Z. Neurol., 1949, 183: 163–174.

Roth, S.R., Sterman, M.B. and Clemente, C.D. Comparison of EEG correlates of reinforcement, internal inhibition and sleep. Electroenceph. clin. Neurophysiol., 1967, 23: 509–520.

Kyoto Symposia (EEG Suppl. No. 36)
Editors: P.A. Buser, W.A. Cobb and T. Okuma
© 1982, Elsevier Biomedical Press, Amsterdam

The Influence of Psychotropic Drugs on the Animal EEG: Electrophysiological Analysis of the Effects of Psychotropic Drugs

NARIYOSHI YAMAGUCHI[1], HIROAKI YOSHIMOTO[1], MIKIO KUBOTA[1], TATSUHIKO ITO[1] and KEISUKE NAKAMURA[2]

[1]*Department of Neuropsychiatry, Kanazawa University School of Medicine, Kanazawa 920, and* [2]*Department of Psychology, Fukui University Faculty of Education, Fukui 910 (Japan)*

For a physiological interpretation of the clinical effects of psychotropic drugs, we have investigated the influence of such drugs on the functional systems in the central nervous system. As shown in Fig. 1, there are many of these systems, such as the ascending reticular activating system, the diffuse thalamo-cortical projection system, the specific thalamo-cortical projection system, the limbic system, the nigro-striatal system and so on.

The above functional systems have individual electrophysiological features. For example, as shown in Table I, the ascending reticular activating system induces the EEG arousal reaction (Moruzzi and Magoun 1949). The diffuse thalamo-cortical projection system produces the recruiting response (Morison and Dempsey 1942). The specific thalamo-cortical projection system induces the augmenting response (Dempsey and Morison 1943). The limbic system, especially the hippocampus, exhibits the hippocampal rhythmic slow activity (RSA) (Green and Arduini 1954). And, the nigro-striatal system, especially caudatum, produces the caudate spindle (Buchwald et al. 1961).

We have investigated the influences of psychotropic drugs on the above-mentioned electrophysiological characteristics of each functional system in the central nervous system by using unanaesthetised, unrestrained cats with electrodes chronically implanted in the brains.

METHODS

Adult cats were used in this study. As the surgical procedures of implantation of electrodes were previously described (Yamaguchi et al. 1964), the particulars are omitted here.

Stainless steel screws were placed bilaterally on the cranial dura mater for recording electrical activities from the anterior (motor area) and posterior sigmoid gyri (somatosensory area). Concentric electrodes were implanted into the head of caudatum, the thalamus, the dorsal hippocampus and the mesencephalic reticular formation. The nucleus centralis lateralis (CL) of the thalamus was chosen for

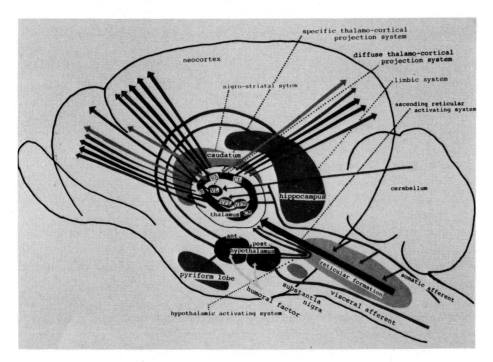

Fig. 1. Various functional systems in the central nervous system.

TABLE I

FUNCTIONAL SYSTEMS IN THE CENTRAL NERVOUS SYSTEM AND THEIR
ELECTROPHYSIOLOGICAL CHARACTERISTICS

Functional systems in the central nervous system	Electrophysiological characteristics
Ascending reticular activating system	EEG arousal reaction
Diffuse thalamo-cortical projection system	Recruiting response
Specific thalamo-cortical projection system	Augmenting response
Limbic system (hippocampus)	Hippocampal rhythmical slow activity
Nigro-striatal system (caudatum)	Caudate spindle

producing recruiting responses and the nucleus ventralis lateralis (VL) was used for augmenting responses.

Chronic experiments usually started not earlier than 2 weeks after the surgery. A cat was placed in a sound-reducing viewing box. Continuous polygraphic recording of the EEG, ECG, EMG, EOG and respiration curve, observation of the animal's behaviour and electrical stimulation of the caudatum, the thalamus and the mesencephalic reticular formation were carried out during various stages of wakefulness and sleep. We analysed the recruiting response, the augmenting response and the caudate spindle by means of a medical data processing computer and analysed the dorsal hippocampal activity by using an automatic frequency analyser. Psychotropic drugs were administered intravenously.

RESULTS

(1) Influence of psychotropic drugs on the EEG arousal reaction induced by electrical stimulation of the ascending reticular activating system

Fig. 2 shows the EEG arousal reaction induced by high frequency stimulation of the ascending reticular activating system during slow wave sleep before the application of haloperidol, one of the butyrophenone derivatives. As demonstrated in Fig. 3, after the application of haloperidol, the EEG arousal reaction was prolonged as compared with control.

After the application of imipramine, one of the tricyclic antidepressants, the EEG arousal reaction was reduced in contrast with the control, and sometimes disappeared.

After the intravenous injection of chlorpromazine, one of the phenothiazine derivatives, the EEG arousal reaction was sometimes reduced in its duration. The effect of diazepam, one of the benzodiazepine derivatives, on the EEG arousal reaction was not definite.

(2) Influence of psychotropic drugs on the recruiting response induced by electrical stimulation of the diffuse thalamo-cortical projection system

Fig. 4 shows the recruiting responses induced by low frequency stimulation of the

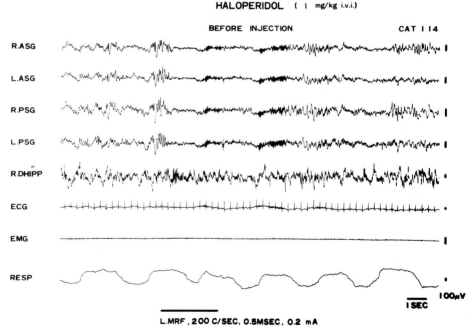

Fig. 2. EEG arousal reaction induced by high frequency electrical stimulation of the ascending reticular activating system during slow wave sleep before the application of haloperidol. R, right; L, left; ASG, anterior sigmoid gyrus; PSG, posterior sigmoid gyrus; DHIPP, dorsal hippocampus; ECG, electrocardiogram; EMG, electromyogram of neck muscle; RESP, respiration curve.

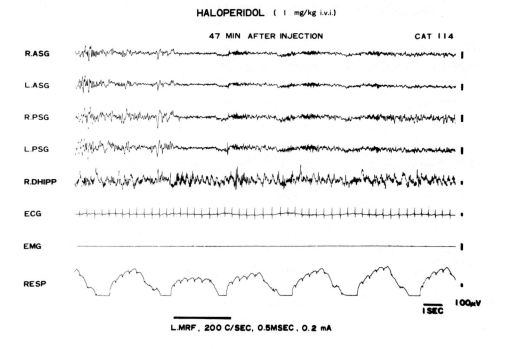

Fig. 3. After the intravenous application of haloperidol of 1 mg/kg, the EEG arousal reaction prolonged as compared with Fig. 2.

n. centralis lateralis (CL) belonging to the diffuse thalamo-cortical projection system, before and after the application of imipramine. Imipramine resulted in a decrease in amplitude of the long latency, negative wave of the recruiting response. It was also decreased in amplitude by intravenous injection of diazepam.

Fig. 5 shows the recruiting responses before and after the application of oxypertine, which causes a depletion of norepinephrine in the presynaptic vesicles. After oxypertine, the long latency, negative wave of the recruiting response increased in amplitude.

(3) Influence of psychotropic drugs on the augmenting response induced by electrical stimulation of the specific thalamo-cortical projection system

Fig. 6 shows the augmenting responses induced by low frequency stimulation of the n. ventralis lateralis (VL) belonging to the specific thalamo-cortical projection system, before and after the application of diazepam. The short latency, biphasic positive-negative wave of the augmenting response increased in amplitude, but its long latency, negative phase disappeared for a long while after the injection of diazepam.

On the contrary, both amitriptyline and imipramine resulted in an increase in amplitude of the long latency, negative wave of the augmenting response.

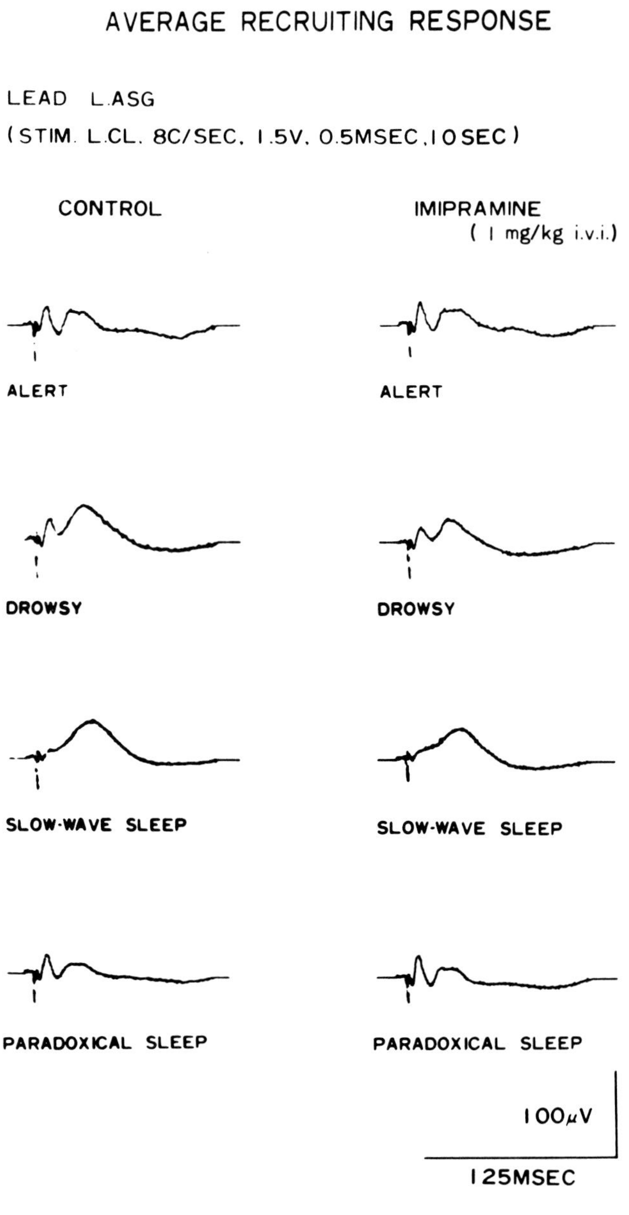

AVERAGE RECRUITING RESPONSE

LEAD L.ASG

(STIM. L.CL. 8C/SEC. 1.5V, 0.5MSEC,10SEC)

CONTROL   IMIPRAMINE
                                       (1 mg/kg i.v.i.)

ALERT   ALERT

DROWSY   DROWSY

SLOW-WAVE SLEEP   SLOW-WAVE SLEEP

PARADOXICAL SLEEP   PARADOXICAL SLEEP

100μV

125MSEC

Fig. 4. Computed average of 80 recruiting responses elicited from the left anterior sigmoid gyrus by low frequency electrical stimulation of the left CL before and after the intravenous administration of imipramine (1 mg/kg).

(4) Influence of psychotropic drugs on the hippocampal rhythmic slow activity (RSA)

In 1954, Green and Arduini reported that the hippocampal electrical activity of rabbits showed rhythmic slow waves (RSA) during wakefulness. Afterwards, Jouvet et al. (1959) observed the hippocampal RSA during the paradoxical sleep in cats.

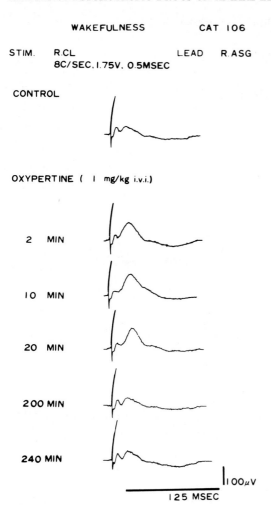

WAKEFULNESS   CAT 106

STIM.   R.CL   LEAD   R.ASG
            8C/SEC. 1.75V. 0.5MSEC

CONTROL

OXYPERTINE (1 mg/kg i.v.i.)

2 MIN

10 MIN

20 MIN

200 MIN

240 MIN

100μV

125 MSEC

Fig. 5. Computed average of 80 recruiting responses elicited from the right anterior sigmoid gyrus by electrical stimulation of the right CL before and after the intravenous administration of oxypertine (1 mg/kg).

The automatic frequency analysis of hippocampal RSA was carried out continuously for 24–48 h following the intravenous injection of the benzodiazepine derivatives. As shown in Fig. 7, the frequency of hippocampal RSA in paradoxical sleep diminished from 5 c/sec to about 3 c/sec after the application of diazepam. The slowing of the hippocampal RSA induced by the application of the benzodiazepine derivatives returned gradually to the original frequency during a period of 24 or 48 h. On the other hand, there were no changes in the frequency of hippocampal RSA in the paradoxical sleep after the application of imipramine, chlorpromazine and haloperidol.

Contrariwise, as shown in Fig. 8, after the application of methamphetamine the frequency of hippocampal rhythmic slow activity during wakefulness and also during paradoxical sleep slightly increased.

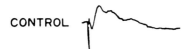

DIAZEPAM (0.5 mg/kg i.v.i.)

STAGE   WAKEFULNESS
LEAD   L.ASG
STIM.   8C/SEC. 0.5MSEC
    L.VL. 6.5 V

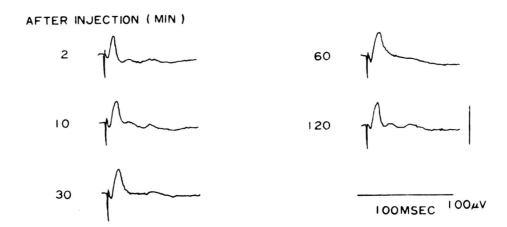

Fig. 6. Computed average of 80 augmenting responses elicited from the left anterior sigmoid gyrus by low frequency electrical stimulation of the left VL before and after the intravenous administration of diazepam (0.5 mg/kg).

(5) Influence of psychotropic drugs on the caudate spindle initiated by single shock stimulation of the caudate nucleus

The effect of psychotropic drugs on the caudate spindle initiated by single shock stimulation of the caudate nucleus was compared with the effect on the thalamic spindle elicited by single shock stimulation of the non-specific thalamic nuclei.

Fig. 9 shows the caudate spindle and thalamic spindle which were initiated by single shock stimulation of the caudate and of the non-specific thalamic nuclei delivered at 3 sec intervals before and after the application of chlorpromazine. After the application of chlorpromazine, both the caudate spindle and thalamic spindle increased their amplitudes. After the injection of imipramine, both spindles decreased in amplitude. Haloperidol increased the caudate spindle, but the thalamic spindle did not definitely change. Diazepam also increased the caudate spindle, but decreased the thalamic spindle.

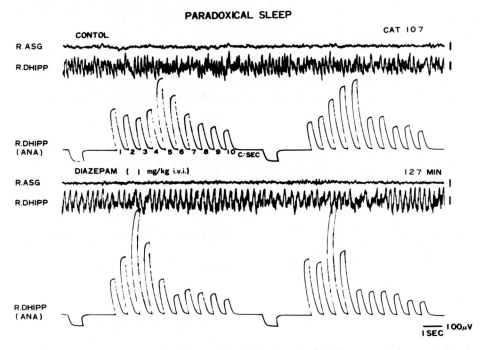

Fig. 7. The hippocampal rhythmical slow activity during paradoxical sleep stage before and after the intravenous application of diazepam of 1 mg/kg. R. ASG, right anterior sigmoid gyrus; R. DHIPP, right dorsal hippocampus; ANA, frequency analysis by an automatic frequency analyzer.

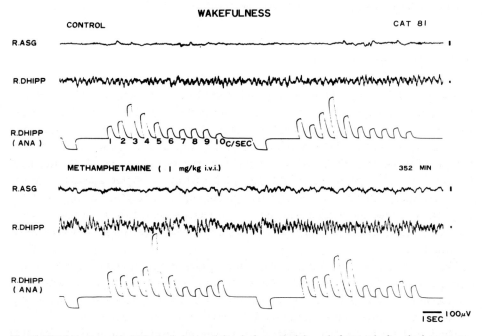

Fig. 8. The hippocampal rhythmical slow activity during wakefulness before and after the intravenous application of methamphetamine (1 mg/kg).

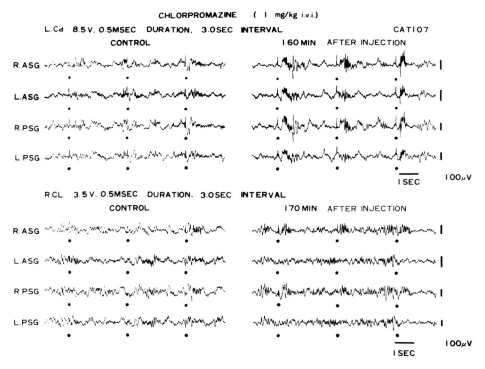

Fig. 9. Caudate spindle and thalamic spindle which were initiated by single shock stimulation of the head of caudate nucleus and of the non-specific thalamic nucleus (CL) delivered at 3 sec interval before and after the intravenous application of chlorpromazine (1 mg/kg).

DISCUSSION AND CONCLUSION

It is generally known that the psychotropic drugs have various effects on the human and animal EEGs. Based on the visual evaluation of human EEG records, Itil (1961) first classified the clinically useful phenothiazines into 4 groups and in his later classification (Itil 1968), psychotropic drugs were placed in 6 groups according to their EEG patterns. Fink (1978) classified the psychotropic drugs into 4 categories by EEG criteria. In recent years, Itil (1974) has carried out systematic quantitative, pharmacoencephalographic studies with digital computer analysis; he believes that it may be possible to predict the clinical effectiveness of new drugs if their computerized EEG (CEEG) profiles are compared with those of drugs with known clinical effects.

The above results of our animal experiments are summarized as follows.

After haloperidol, the EEG arousal reaction induced by electrical stimulation of the ascending reticular activating system is prolonged as compared with control. On the other hand, after imipramine, the EEG arousal reaction is reduced.

The long latency, negative phase of the recruiting response induced by electrical stimulation of the diffuse thalamo-cortical projection system is decreased in amplitude by intravenous diazepam. On the contrary, after oxypertine, it is increased in amplitude.

The short latency, biphasic positive-negative waves of the augmenting response induced by electrical stimulation of the specific thalamo-cortical projection system increased in amplitude, but its long latency, negative phase disappeared for a long while after the injection of diazepam. Both amitriptyline and imipramine resulted in an increase in amplitude of the long latency, negative phase of the augmenting response.

The frequency of hippocampal rhythmic slow activity (RSA) in wakefulness and in paradoxical sleep diminished from 5 c/sec to 3 c/sec after the application of benzodiazepine derivatives. We think that the stronger the slowing effect of benzodiazepine derivatives on the hippocampal RSA, the longer and deeper will be the clinical hypnotic effect of the same drugs (Yamaguchi 1981). On the other hand, there was no change in frequency of hippocampal RSA in paradoxical sleep after imipramine, chlorpromazine and haloperidol. Contrariwise, the frequency of the hippocampal RSA during wakefulness and during paradoxical sleep increased slightly after methamphetamine.

After chlorpromazine, haloperidol and diazepam, the caudate spindle initiated by single shock stimulation of the caudate nucleus increased in amplitude. On the contrary, after the injection of imipramine, the caudate spindle decreased in amplitude.

Haloperidol and chlorpromazine are believed to block dopamine receptors, imipramine and amitriptyline inhibit cellular re-uptake of norepinephrine and serotonin, and benzodiazepine derivatives have an affinity for GABAnergic receptors. Therefore, on the basis of our results, it is assumed that the dopaminergic receptor may be involved mainly in the nigro-striatal system, noradrenergic and serotonergic receptors in the non-specific and specific thalamo-cortical projection systems, dopaminergic, noradrenergic and serotonergic receptors in the ascending reticular activating system and the GABAnergic receptor in the limbic system.

REFERENCES

Buchwald, N.A., Wyers, E.J., Okuma, T. and Heuser, G. The "caudate-spindle". I. Electrophysiological properties. Electroenceph. clin. Neurophysiol., 1961, 13: 509–518.

Dempsey, E.W. and Morison, R.S. The electrical activity of a thalamocortical relay system. Amer. J. Physiol., 1943, 138: 283–296.

Fink, M. EEG and psychopharmacology. In: W.A. Cobb and H. van Duijn (Eds.), Contemporary Clinical Neurophysiology, EEG Suppl. No. 34. Elsevier, Amsterdam, 1978: 41–56.

Green, J.D. and Arduini, A.A. Hippocampal electrical activity in arousal. J. Neurophysiol., 1954, 17: 533–557.

Itil, T.M. Elektroencephalographische Befunde zur Klassifikation neuro- und thymoleptischer Medikamente. Med. Exp., 1961, 5: 347–363.

Itil, T.M. Electroencephalography and pharmacopsychiatry. In: F.A. Freyhan, N. Petrilowitch and P. Pichot (Eds.), Modern Problems of Pharmacopsychiatry, Vol. 1. Karger, Basel, 1968: 163–194.

Itil, T.M. Quantitative pharmaco-electroencephalography. In: T.M. Itil (Ed.), Modern Problems of Pharmacopsychiatry, Vol. 8. Karger, Basel, 1974: 43–75.

Jouvet, M., Michel, F. et Courjon, J. Sur un stade d'activité électrique cérébrale rapide au cours du sommeil physiologique. C.R. Soc. Biol. (Paris), 1959, 153: 1024–1028.

Morison, R.S. and Dempsey, E.W. A study of thalamo-cortical relations. Amer. J. Physiol., 1942, 135: 281–292.

Moruzzi, G. and Magoun, H.W. Brain stem reticular formation and activation of the EEG. Electroenceph. clin. Neurophysiol., 1949, 1: 455–473.

Yamaguchi, N. Psychotropic drugs and the animal EEG. In: N. Yamaguchi and K. Fujisawa (Eds.), Recent Advances in EEG and EMG Data Processing. Elsevier/North-Holland Biomedical Press, Amsterdam, 1981: 237–246.

Yamaguchi, N., Ling, G.M. and Marczynski, T.J. Recruiting responses observed during wakefulness and sleep in unanesthetized chronic cats. Electroenceph. clin. Neurophysiol., 1964, 17: 246–254.

10. Data Reduction in Intensive Care and Long-term Surveillance of Patients

Kyoto Symposia (EEG Suppl. No. 36)
Editors: P.A. Buser, W.A. Cobb and T. Okuma
© 1982, Elsevier Biomedical Press, Amsterdam

Long Term Monitoring of the EEG: the Challenge of the Future

P. GLOOR

Montreal Neurological Institute and Department of Neurology and Neurosurgery, McGill University, Montreal, Que. H3A 2B4 (Canada)

At the outset of this review of data reduction in long term monitoring of the EEG it is useful to consider some general principles underlying the present state of the art and to try to define the premises on which future development should be based. This introduction will not deal, except briefly in the form of some illustrative examples, with specific applications and modalities of long term EEG monitoring and data reduction. It will instead emphasize why these methods represent one of the most important challenges for the future of the art and science of clinical electroencephalography.

Among clinical laboratory procedures in neurology, electroencephalography holds the unique distinction of being the only method capable of monitoring uninterruptedly over long periods of time the physiological state of the brain and its alterations by pathological processes. There is no other laboratory method that offers this opportunity. There are certainly other ways of getting information on brain function and its derangements, as opposed to obtaining information on brain structure and its alteration by pathological processes. There is first the clinical examination, then biochemical measurements on cerebrospinal fluid and even the cerebral angiogram or the CT scan can give functional in addition to anatomical information. There is radio-isotope scanning and most recently positron emission tomography which for the first time will give us the opportunity of obtaining a pictorial representation of the topographical profile of cerebral metabolism and blood flow on the surface as well as in the depth of the brain. None of these methods, however, can be used continuously over a long period of time, and even their frequent repetition is impossible, mostly because of inherent risks, not the least that of exposing the patient to unacceptable doses of radiation. In any case with these methods one obtains only momentary "snap-shots" of the brain's functional state, often at purely random points in time, and one cannot follow a process that evolves over many hours or days. These limitations do not exist for electroencephalography which is non-invasie, riskless, painless and can be used in continuity virtually for as long as one wishes. Long term monitoring of cerebral function by means of the EEG appears therefore to be the ideal clinical application of this type of laboratory investigation. The question arises of why only now, more than 50 years after the discovery of the EEG, the great potential of using it in this manner is slowly beginning to be realized.

There are a number of reasons for this, principally two: (i) firstly, until the advent of the CT scan, when all neuroradiological procedures, except for the plain skull X-ray, carried distinct risks, the EEG was a very easy, convenient and often quite effective way of providing localizing information on pathological lesions of the brain. The EEG was and still is being used in a way as a substitute for neuroradiology, i.e. as an anatomical, rather than a physiological diagnostic tool. There is really nothing wrong with this; in fact for localizing an epileptogenic focus, the EEG still beats the CT scan hands down. However, this fixation on anatomical localization rather than on disordered physiology exploits only some of the opportunities offered by electro-encephalography and wastes its main potential, namely that of providing functional in addition to anatomical information.

(ii) The second reason is a more practical one: it is obviously possible to record the EEG for many hours or even days, but the paper which accumulates if such recording is done in the traditional manner by making a continuous record on paper is enormous. If it takes about as long to read the paper record as to record it, nothing is being gained for the sheer abundance of data defies effective analysis by the unaided human reader. Obviously the continuous flow of this overabundance of information, which contains enormous redundancy, has to be handled in some intelligent way by using data reduction methods that do not bring us back to the level of the other methods of investigating brain function, namely the more or less random collection of "snap-shots."

Let us now consider what at the present time can be achieved and what are the requirements for making full use of the EEG as a long term monitoring device. When considering the application of long term monitoring to a given problem it is important to devise intelligently conceived data reduction methods that can effectively deal with the question asked in an accurate and reliable fashion. One should, however, always be mindful of the late Grey Walter's prophetic adage, that "data reduction is data destruction," in other words there is always a price to pay with every method of data reduction. If one cones in on a certain set of data, let us say, e.g., one follows by spectral analysis the shifts in the frequency content of the EEG over time, one will inevitably, by doing so, miss random, non-stationary events. This may be quite acceptable as long as one is not interested in detecting them.

Now let us look at some of the questions that can be asked. One may, for instance, be interested in studying changes in brain function which occur slowly over relatively long periods of time. For instance, one may want to follow the normal (or abnormal) sleep cycle, or one may want to monitor cerebral function and its changes during the evolution of a metabolic disorder or during a certain form of treatment. Obviously hours or even days of recording are needed and the data must be compressed in some form. One can, for instance, use power spectrum analysis and compress the data by stacking successive spectra encompassing successive EEG epochs on top of each other as Bickford et al. (1972) have done with their compressed spectral arrays. Another interesting and imaginative application of data reduction in long term monitoring is a recent study by Friedman and Jones (1981) on the normal sleep cycle of cats and its derangement by brain stem lesions. By combining data from surface EEG, EMG and PGO spikes in cats and using trivariate cluster analysis a graphic display of a 24 h sleep-wakefulness cycle can be produced and displayed on a TV monitor screen. The sequential changes in sleep stages can be played back on the video screen in accelerated motion. This allows one to detect not only the dynamics of change and the sequential patterns in the shifts from one sleep stage to another, but also how such patterns are disrupted and, for instance, become truly chaotic when a lesion is placed in a specific part of the reticular formation. The aim in this first group of applications is thus to monitor brain activity continuously over many hours and to compress the data, telescoping time without losing essential information, and to obtain an easily readable picture of the changes of brain function over time which, as the need may be, can be correlated with some time-dependent biological variable such as a circadian rhythm, or with some evolving structural, functional or biochemical pathology.

The second type of application aims at detecting randomly occurring events, such as inter-ictal epileptiform discharges, whenever they occur over a prolonged time span, to count them, classify them if necessary, for instance with regard to their localization, and to produce at the end of the period of analysis a quantitative picture of how many events have occurred over a given period of time, in what region of the brain and in what kind of temporal order. Thus, one may ask questions of localization, consistency of localization and whether seemingly random events were indeed random, or in fact occurred in cycles and, if so, what were the physiological or pathological correlates of periods of high versus low incidence of such cyclic events. The effects of therapy on the occurrence and temporal pattern of such events can also be studied, using such methods. What one asks the monitoring system and the computer to do in this kind of application is to monitor brain activity continuously, but to pick out only those sporadically occurring events, for instance epileptic spikes, that one is interested in, record the time of their occurrence, their localization and their relation to the sleep cycle, therapy, etc., and to disregard the rest of the EEG information. One may say that this is also tantamount to taking just "snap-shots," a defect discussed above that limits the usefulness of all methods other than the EEG of obtaining functional information on the brain. One must concede that this type of data reduction indeed produces only "snap-shots," but "snap-shots" of a very special kind. They are not random or occasional "snap-shots;" they represent a carefully collected inventory of *all* the sporadic events that have occurred over a long period of time during which the EEG has been *continuously* monitored and scrutinized for their occurrence. Such a method of detecting epileptiform discharges in the EEG developed by Gotman and Gloor (1976) is in fact in use in our clinical laboratory and has proved very useful: instead of having to sift through a big pile of paper and arrive at best only at an impressionistic and certainly non-quantitative assessment of inter-ictal epileptiform activity occurring over a given time span, it now becomes possible to glance at a few pages of paper and derive quantitative information from it in less than a minute or two. There is a catch to this, however: computer analysis is still not fool-proof in the sense that it is not yet able always to distinguish between a true epileptic sharp wave or spike and an artefact, although it can recognize a wide range of the latter. The only way to circumvent this problem effectively at present is to use very strict and limiting criteria of spike recognition, e.g., the requirement of conforming to a template. Such a method will pick up only those spikes that conform to the chosen template. This method can be made virtually artefact-free, but is clinically not very useful, because it will reject all of the genuine epileptic discharges that do not conform to the template. With our system, by writing out on paper each event that the computer has recognized as a spike, it is possible to obtain a very compressed traditional looking EEG. If it is full of artefacts one cannot, of course, trust the quantitative computer generated display and must discard it; if there are only a few, it is easy to remove them from the data analysis by human intervention through interaction with the computer, and produce a reliable display of quantitative information.

The third application is the search for the unique unpredictable, salient clinical event that may occur at any time of the day or night without forewarning. The best known application is the detection and full recording from its very start of a patient's habitual clinical epileptic seizure (Ives et al. 1976). Ives covers this subject in some detail in the last paper of this Symposium, to which the reader is referred. These then are some examples of the applications of data reduction methods in long term monitoring of the EEG, methods which we can already apply and which show the promise of this approach. However, to advance further we need to come to grips with some technological and fundamental scientific problems.

On the technological front, besides devising new and even more sophisticated computational methods of data analysis, we need a more concerted effort in confronting the problem of artefacts. No surface EEG is ever free of either unwanted biological signals such as EMG, eye movements, etc. or of extraneous artefacts of some kind, although the latter are more easily preventable. The tremendous variability of these unwanted signals and the overlap of their spectral or other quantifiable properties with those of true cerebral potentials have so far prevented anyone from developing a data reduction system of the EEG that is fully automatic in the sense that it can deal successfully, in an open-ended clinical situation, with EEG records under all circumstances met in clinical practice, in such a way that the raw EEG data can be completely ignored. No specific suggestions will be offered here as to how this difficult problem of artefacts ought to be tackled and solved, but unless it is solved there will be serious obstacles to the ready application of data reduction in the kind of realistic clinical settings where EEG monitoring is most often needed.

There is one final point worth making: it is important to realize that if we want to obtain meaningful information about the pathophysiological significance of changes in brain function as reflected in alterations of the EEG, we must know what the underlying neurophysiological, neuropathological and biochemical correlates of abnormal EEG patterns are. For epileptic discharges we are no longer ignorant of many of these correlates, particularly those within the realm of electrophysiology at the unitary and synaptic level. The fundamental mechanisms involved in the non-epileptic pathology of the EEG, however, which express themselves mostly by slow waves, remain largely unexplored territory. We know that some relationship exists between EEG frequency and cerebral blood flow (Ingvar et al. 1965), but in pathological states when autoregulation of cerebral blood flow breaks down, this relationship no longer holds (Ingvar 1967). We know something about the nature and the distribution of structural pathology responsible for polymorphic delta activity. It has been shown, for instance, that white matter lesions, brain stem lesions, but not purely cortical lesions or vasogenic oedema, produce polymorphic delta activity (Gloor et al. 1977). We know that the generators of delta waves are pyramidal cortical neurones (Ball et al. 1977). Thus, the generators of this kind of slow wave activity seem to be the same as those generating the normal EEG. But by virtue of what derangement do pyramidal neurones of the cortex produce the very slow potential oscillations that underly delta waves when the brain is subjected to either a structural or biochemical insult? Which transmitters or neuromodulators are involved or missing? What about the slow wave activity seen, for instance in renal failure, hepatic encephalopathy, electrolyte imbalances, diffuse encephalopathies like CNS lupus, etc.? What is the basic pathophysiology of slow wave production in these conditions? Do some of the abnormal metabolites switch off or activate some neuromodulator system, or do they themselves act as false neurotransmitters or false neuromodulators? There is a whole world here waiting to be explored, a field that has remained fallow for the whole 50 years of the history of electroencephalography and it is high time that we start tilling it. Until we do know more about these mechanisms, monitoring changes of the EEG over time in conditions of deranged brain function caused by structural damage or by biochemical changes will have only limited clinical value. Electroencephalography will only fully live up to its potential if we devote time and effort to clarifying the basic mechanisms of the pathological EEG at the single cell, synaptic and biochemical levels. We must know how pathological changes in brain structure and brain biochemistry can alter the EEG at the basic neurophysiological level. It is the necessary prerequisite for future progress.

REFERENCES

Ball, G.J., Gloor, P. and Schaul, N. The cortical electromicrophysiology of pathological delta waves in the electroencephalogram of cats. Electroenceph. clin. Neurophysiol., 1977, 4: 346–361.

Bickford, R.G., Billinger, T.W., Flemming, N.I. and Stewart, L. The compressed spectral array (CSA). A pictorial EEG. Proc. San Diego biomed. Symp., 1972: 365–370.

Friedman, L. and Jones, B.E. Computerized classification by cluster analysis of sleep-waking states in the cat. Sleep Res., 1981, 10: 275.

Gloor, P., Ball, G. and Schaul, N. Brain lesions that produce delta waves in the EEG. Neurology (Minneap.), 1977, 27: 326–333.

Gotman, J. and Gloor, P. Automatic recognition and quantification of interictal epileptiform activity in the human scalp EEG. Electroenceph. clin. Neurophysiol., 1976, 41: 513–529.

Ingvar, D.H. The pathophysiology of the stroke related to findings in EEG and to measurements of regional cerebral blood flow. In: Thule International Symposia. Nordiska Bokhandels Förlag, Stockholm, 1967: 105–122.

Ingvar, D.H., Baldy-Moulimier, M., Sulg, I. and Hörman, S. Regional cerebral blood flow related to EEG. Acta neurol. scand., 1965, Suppl. 14: 179–182.

Ives, J.R., Thompson, C.J. and Gloor, P. Seizure monitoring: a new tool in electroencephalography. Electroenceph. clin. Neurophysiol., 1976, 41: 422–427.

Kyoto Symposia (EEG Suppl. No. 36)
Editors: P.A. Buser, W.A. Cobb and T. Okuma
© 1982, Elsevier Biomedical Press, Amsterdam

584

Technical Aspects of Long-Term Monitoring

MASAO SAITO

*Institute of Medical Electronics, Faculty of Medicine, University of Tokyo, Bunkyo-ku, Tokyo 113
(Japan)*

With the recent development of electronic technology, automatic processing of EEGs has been an object of study for more than 30 years. There have already been published many excellent review articles, such as those by Kellaway, Rémond and others (Wakabayashi and Fujimori 1957; Suhara et al. 1971; Kellaway and Petersen 1973; Rémond 1977; Barlow 1979; Gevins 1980), on the state of the art in EEG data processing.

With the emerging need for long-term monitoring of EEGs, a change seems to be occurring in the technology, since most data processing in the past was directed toward short-term processes, such as quantitative representation of information or detection of particular wave forms.

Processing of long-term EEG data should of course be considered according to particular requirements from the medical aspect but, generally speaking, it should be considered as follows: (i) data acquisition; (ii) pre-processing; (iii) transmission; (iv) processing; (v) storage and retrieval; (vi) representation.

In the discussion of these aspects from the technical point of view, 2 time scales should be differentiated. In other words, long-term monitoring of several hours is quite different from that of several days or weeks, in terms of stabilization of electrodes, number of data, etc. This point must be kept in mind in the discussion of technologies.

Recent advances in engineering, such as those in electronics, materials and information processing, will have significant effects on the utilization of technologies in EEG data processing. Some of the technologies that will be combined with EEG processing technology are microprocessors, new materials for electrodes, implant electronics, data transmission technologies, memory devices and display terminals. The choice of methodology from the medical point of view is of course the essential factor in determining the design of the system, but the available hardware is also a decisive factor in actual realization of the system.

DATA ACQUISITION

It should be noted that even if the interest is in EEG data processing, a satisfactory result cannot be arrived at without paying attention to the peripheral technologies such as electrodes and display. In data acquisition, major factors for the success of the system are convenient devices and stable electrodes.

Development of low-noise, low-powered electronics is now making it possible to realize tiny data acquisition devices that can be attached to the subject or implanted, with batteries and telemetering functions. A goal in this direction may be an implanted transmitter or a helmet with electronics to acquire multichannel EEG data, which can be sent to a near-by relay-station by a wireless channel. Several examples have been published.

It is well known that it is very important to use an appropriate electrode for EEG data acquisition. Depending on the choice of the metal and the electrolyte, a noise greater than the amplitude of the EEG may easily be produced, making the observations meaningless. The efforts made in the past to design electrodes for long-term observation of a patient have mostly been on the realization of a stable mechanical contact and a stable electrode characteristic. It is often observed, however, in the long-term use of electrodes, that gradual changes in its characteristics, movement artefacts and inflammation of the skin are apt to occur.

Some new ideas have been published to improve these properties, such as spray electrodes, organic conductive compounds and dry insulated semi-conductor electrodes. Some organic materials seem to be effective to prevent inflammation of the skin, and recently developed silicon-nitride electrodes with built-in input circuitry may prove to be useful in reducing the artefacts.

Implant electronics is also a recently developed notion. Technologies for implant materials and electronics will progress very rapidly in the near future. The final problem will be the power supply. Because of the inability to design a device of appropriate size, implants will only be used for a certain period for animal experiments, where they will undoubtedly become a very powerful tool.

PRE-PROCESSING

The general tendency in medical data processing is to execute data reduction in as early a stage as possible, since redundant data will burden every stage of data handling, such as transmission, storage, retrieval and display. In the case of the EEG, data reduction is required at every stage of data processing. The need for data reduction is obvious if one considers the information quantity contained in observed EEG wave forms compared to the amount of information actually needed in medical decision-making.

For the modest assumption of a 20 Hz bandwidth and signal-to-noise ratio of 30 dB, 1 h of EEG wave forms contains 720 k bits of information, which is too much for transmission and storage. Using a low-speed, 300 band channel, it will take 40 min to transmit that amount of information. One may use analogue transmission and compress the time scale, based on the difference of bandwidth, but it is still practically uneconomical to transmit all the data. In addition, the possible presence of artefacts will complicate the problem, since a larger dynamic ratio is required if whole data are to be transmitted and the artefacts are to be rejected at a later stage of processing.

The advent of microprocessors and other related electronic devices is making pre-processing possible, which is more sophisticated than it has been. Immediate requirements are rejection of artefacts and reduction of data, but the requirement from the medical point of view must be specified at this point.

One might argue that by fabricating dedicated devices by large-scale integration techniques, a handy data acquisition and pre-processing terminal could be produced with abundant processing functions. But the size of the expected market for such technology is too small to permit custom-designed electronics, and the general purpose devices must be used, at least for some period.

In order to check and remove, if necessary, the artefacts due to movement of the subject or incomplete contact of electrodes, the recently developed notion of a self-checking mechanism should be used. Some indications of artefacts outside the range of EEG signals, such as high-frequency impedance or unusual change in the statistical property of the observed wave forms, may be used to detect the artefact.

The scheme for pre-processing and data reduction should depend on the particular medical requirements, but typical examples are extraction of statistical parameters such as the spectrum, detection of particular wave forms and of non-stationarity. Since complete processing of EEG data cannot be expected from simple processing functions, typical raw data of wave forms should also be sent for final processing. The detection of wave forms is a difficult task for a machine at the present stage; even a clearly specified wave form such as a spike cannot be detected with 100% accuracy. From this point of view, it is advisable to send intermediate or analog data as the result of wave form detection, so that the degree of certainty can be used in later stages of processing.

The essential notion of data reduction in long-term monitoring is that it is not necessary to send statistical parameters so long as the phenomenon is stationary. Only in the case of a change in statistical properties should new data be added. From this point of view, the testing of stationarity is a very important item in long-term data reduction. Extracted parameters or sample wave forms should be recorded at regular intervals or when any non-stationarity is indicated.

There are various ways to test the stationarity. A kind of test of the hypothesis may be used in which, for example, an analysis method for a stationary process is applied (Blackman and Tukey 1958), and fluctuation of the result is observed. If the fluctuation fits with the theory for stationary processes, the phenomenon is regarded as stationary as far as the tested parameters are concerned. A typical example is seen in the estimation of the power spectrum and correlation functions.

TRANSMISSION

There can be various schemes for data transmission and processing. The data may be pre-processed by the terminal device and then transmitted through a normal transmission channel, such as that using telephone lines.

Although the notions of a computer network, centralized processing etc. are becoming quite usual, and the shortage of EEG specialists to make clinical reports may seem to necessitate such a scheme of data transmission, the actual situation will not justify this. The situation may vary in different countries, but the cost of using a large-scale computer and the cost of data transmission will often be prohibitive. For example, in Japan, the use of a telephone line for a distance of some 200 km for 20 min will cost approximately 10 dollars, which is comparable with the fee for EEG examination.

From such a point of view, pre-processing before transmission is mandatory, and the central processor should refine the result of pre-processing or supplement the data for representation.

Although it may seem primitive, transportation of the storage media such as magnetic tape can be effected by car or mail to transmit the raw data to the central station. This will sometimes be very practical.

PROCESSING, STORAGE AND RETRIEVAL

The data processing in the centralized facility may have several goals: (i) refinement of the result of pre-processing; (ii) aiding medical decision-making; and (iii) editing of received data and retrieved data for representation.

Because of the physical limitations of the terminal devices, a complete processing executed at the terminal cannot be expected, but refinements should be made in the centralized large-scale system after transmission. The sample wave forms transmitted will be used at this stage to check and refine the results. Refinement of the pre-processed result may be done following the same items, but various tests for the accuracy and testing of hypotheses may be added, or methods of analysis which have not been applied at the pre-processing stage can be applied.

Taking the example of power spectra, in addition to the classical Fourier analysis, various methods to enhance the apparent resolution of visual observations have been published. Examples are parallel representation of short-term data or extraction of fine structure by the maximum entropy method, etc. It should be kept in mind that the result of such analysis strongly depends on the model assumed before analysis. If the assumed model does not apply to the actual situation, the result is not appropriate, even if it may seem so. Non-stationarity, linearity and presence of remarkable frequency components are examples which one must carefully consider before determining the method of analysis.

Although there has been a considerable development in automatic analysis of the EEG (Japan EEG Soc. and Japan Soc. MEBE 1964), its function has not reached the point to replace human intuition. In some cases such as wave form detection, it is still advisable to represent the data in analogue format, leaving the final decision to the doctor.

The major storage medium for EEG at this stage of technology is the magnetic tape. Reduction of data before storage is again an absolute requirement. Otherwise, a whole reel of magnetic tape may be used up for 1 or 2 patients. Suitable labelling is needed to store the incoming data which are not necessarily arranged in the order of patient number or date.

Since the requirements for presentation of data may be different for different users, a flexible structure for the data retrieval and representation will be required. The notion here is close to that of a data base, in which a unified set of data is edited at each representation to fit the need of each user.

Aids to medical decision making can be made in various ways. Presentation of data to fit the human intuition is the first thing. Even though the amount of information contained in the display is the same, the display can be improved by, for example, interpolating or extrapolating the data, or by indicating a particular portion by a mark, etc. The performance of human judgement is not governed only by the amount of information, but is closely related to the characteristics of human recognition, for which plenty of data can be furnished from psychology.

A technique to combine the numerical analysis with litteral data or representation will be important, although not very difficult. A conversational mode to take what the doctor has felt into the system to improve the method of analysis or modify the logical way of processing will be a new problem in medical decision making.

CONCLUSION

In conclusion, I would like to emphasize the following points.

(i) Various methods of analysis are available, but their performance depends entirely on their appropriateness, viewed from the actual situation. In this regard, it is important that the medical point of view should strongly affect the determination of the actual system of analysis.

(ii) One should always be aware of the development of technologies in the near future. If one develops a system based on present technical knowledge, the system when realized will already be obsolete.

(iii) Not only the methodology of analysis, but also peripheral techniques such as electrodes are important in the actual system.

(iv) One should not ignore the economical aspects of the system. Even though it is true that by standardization the cost of the system becomes lower, it will be meaningless if one discusses a system which will be 1 or 2 orders of magnitude more expensive than the economical limit.

(v) The final result of analysis should be fully acceptable to the doctor. On each side, man and machine, there are limitations as well as prospects. For example, a method of analysing a non-linear system that takes too much time compared with the degree of non-stationarity, has its own limitation on the machine side. Or, furnishing too much information to the doctor and expecting him to select the correct information would also be a nuisance.

The technique of long-term monitoring has just started at this stage. There can be various degrees of performance in the actual requirement. One should not aim only at a very high performance sophisticated system, but rather look for the applications of various kinds of system, from relatively low to high performance.

REFERENCES

Barlow, J. Computerized clinical electroencephalography in perspective. IEEE Trans. biomed. Engng, 1979, BME 26: 377–391.

Blackman, R.B. and Tukey, J.W. The Measurement of Power Spectra from the Point of View of Communication Engineering. Dover, New York, 1958.

Gevins, A.S. Pattern recognition of human brain electric potentials. IEEE Trans., 1980, PAMI 2: 383–404.

Japan EEG Soc. and Japan Soc. MEBE. Standards for Clinical Standard EEG Frequency Analyzers, 1964.

Kellaway, P. and Petersen, I. Automation of Clinical Electroencephalography. Raven Press, New York, 1973.

Rémond, A. EEG Informatics, a Didactic Review of Methods and Applications of EEG Data Processing. Elsevier, Amsterdam, 1977.

Suhara, K. et al. A review of the progress and present situation of study of EEG analysis in Japan, presented at the 9th ICMBE, Melbourne, 1971.

Wakabayashi, T. and Fujimori, B. Analysis of EEG and its Application (in Japanese). Igaku-shoin, Tokyo, 1957.

Kyoto Symposia (EEG Suppl. No. 36)
Editors: P.A. Buser, W.A. Cobb and T. Okuma
© 1982, Elsevier Biomedical Press, Amsterdam

Automatic Recognition of Abnormal EEG Activity during Open Heart and Carotid Surgery

R.A.F. PRONK* and A.J.R. SIMONS**

*Institute of Medical Physics TNO, Utrecht, and **Department of Clinical Neurophysiology, St. Antonius Hospital, Utrecht (The Netherlands)*

The main objective of continuous monitoring of brain function during open heart and carotid surgery is to check whether the metabolism of the brain is influenced adversely by these operations. This can be done by monitoring the electrical activity of the brain, i.e., by recording the EEG. It is assumed that EEG monitoring during these operations should provide the necessary information to the surgical team for rapid intervention should a dangerous situation for brain function tend to develop. Thus it may be possible to limit irreversible brain damage which could result in postoperative neurological and psychopathological complications.

Brain damage may be caused by hypoxia or inadequate perfusion of the brain, e.g. owing to low blood pressure, when a heart-lung machine is applied for artificial blood oxygenation and circulation or when a carotid artery is clamped.

If hypoxia occurs or cerebral perfusion is insufficient, the EEG activity will change in such a way that initially low frequency (slow waves) and, thereafter, small amplitude activity will appear. These changes in EEG activity must be distinguished from other EEG changes which may take place during the usual evolution of the anaesthetic procedure and which are caused by general anaesthesia, drugs, cooling or rewarming. Therefore, the EEG has to be monitored simultaneously with blood pressure and temperature and in relation to information regarding anaesthetic procedures.

The aim of the study described here was to develop an *automatic procedure* for detecting patterns of abnormal EEG activity which may occur during open heart or carotid surgery. The key problem is the selection of the most relevant EEG features. In the present investigation, we computed EEG features using different methods of analysis (spectral, period-amplitude, autoregressive filtering computed by way of a Kalman filter, Hjorth's descriptors). The capacity of these features to classify in a reliable way the EEG patterns which were judged normal or abnormal by several EEGers was determined by using linear discriminant analysis.

The performance of different sets of features is discussed, keeping in view the application of the automatic recognition procedure in the operating room.

In this article, we shall first give an account of different approaches to EEG monitoring during open heart surgery; secondly we shall give a description of our automated EEG monitoring system and some aspects of its evaluation in clinical practice; thirdly we shall describe an investigation concerning the automatic recognition of abnormal EEG activity.

BRAIN DAMAGE DURING CARDIO-PULMONARY BYPASS

In the past years, several authors (Björk and Hultquist 1960; Brierly 1967; Arfel et al. 1968; Aguilar et al. 1971; Stockard et al. 1973; Skagseth et al. 1974; Åberg and Kihlgren 1977; Kinichi et al. 1978; Kolkka and Hilberman 1980) have written about brain damage in patients who underwent cardio-pulmonary bypass (CPB). Most authors reported that the brain damage was mainly caused by factors such as microembolism, a low perfusion pressure or a largely reduced blood flow through the brain. Other factors which enhanced the probability of brain damage were length of perfusion time, age of the patient, cerebrovascular disease and previous neurological damage.

Brain damage resulted postoperatively in neurological dysfunction, motor defects (e.g. hemiplegia), psychiatric abnormalities, impairment in intellectual functions or subclinical neurological complications. The study of Kolkka and Hilberman (1980) indicated that monitoring of blood pressure during CPB is not a reliable method to predict the postoperative neurological outcome.

Because of the existence of many influencing factors, e.g. microembolism, hypoxia, hypotension, patient's age, etc., a more precise method of evaluating brain function and thus predicting neurological complications is direct monitoring of electrical brain activity.

In the last decades, several reports on EEG monitoring during open heart surgery have appeared (Arfel et al. 1961; Storm van Leeuwen et al. 1961; Fischer-Williams and Cooper 1964; Prior et al. 1971; Wright et al. 1972; Branthwaite 1973; Simons 1973; Stockard et al. 1973; Witoszka et al. 1973; Weiss et al. 1975; Kinichi et al. 1978; Salerno et al. 1978; Prior 1979). Nearly all these reports are concerned with the factors which cause abnormal EEG activity.

A clinical evaluation of EEG monitoring during open heart surgery in our clinic (Dijkstra 1979) was carried out on a group of 1000 patients who were operated from November 1978 to November 1979. In 77 patients, messages about the occurrence of abnormal EEG activity during cardio-pulmonary bypass were given to the anaesthetist. In 33 of the 77 patients, the EEG was still abnormal at the end of the operation. In those cases, postoperative EEG recording was indicated.

EEG monitoring during anaesthesia requires rapid interpretation of EEG strip chart records. The need to make this interpretation more reliable has led several investigators to the development of computer-assisted methods. The main characteristic of these methods is to reduce the EEG data to a small number of features which permit rapid detection of abnormalities and trends in the EEG. Bickford et al. (1971) developed a spectral analysis system which transforms the ongoing EEG into a series of autospectra, called a "compressed spectral array" (CSA). This method was adapted by Fleming and Smith (1974) to produce so-called "density spectral arrays" (DSA) and was built into a microprocessor system. Uhl et al. (1977) also used Bickford's method for the development of a system for EEG monitoring during anaesthesia. The Berg Fourier analyser (Bricolo et al. 1978) was one of the first commercially available EEG spectral analysis systems to be used for monitoring purposes.

Computerized EEG monitoring using period-amplitude analysis was employed by Tönnies (1969), Klein (1976), Klein and Davis (1981), Pronk et al. (1975), Cohen (1976) and Demetrescu (1975).

Other techniques used for this purpose are that of Hjorth (1970) who introduced the normalized slope descriptors: activity, mobility and complexity, and that of Prior et al. (1971) who developed an EEG monitoring device, the cerebral function monitor (CFM). This device was made commercially, making possible its use in a number of hospitals. Several reports on the use of the CFM during open heart surgery were published (Branthwaite 1973; Kinichi et al. 1978; Maynard 1979; Prior 1979). Recently, Levy et al. (1980) compared several EEG monitoring methods (spectral analysis (CSA and DSA), cerebral function monitor, period-amplitude analysis) and found that spectral analysis with DSA presentation was the most useful for monitoring during anaesthesia.

A COMPUTER-ASSISTED EEG WARNING SYSTEM

All the monitoring methods mentioned above consist in transforming the EEG record into a set of numbers by means of which the representation of the EEG in a synoptical way can be achieved. However, the interpretation of the data presented, e.g. spectra, has to be done visually by the user. This has meant an important obstacle to routine use of EEG monitoring in the operating room because the anaesthetist is in general not trained to interpret the presented data.

Therefore, in our computer-assisted EEG monitoring system we included automatically generated warning or alarm signals if abnormal EEG activity was detected. In this way, the anaesthetist can be alerted that the patient's EEG activity has gone below accepted limits. In such a situation, corrective measures can be taken immediately. Our system has been implemented for routine use at the St. Antonius Hospital in Utrecht.

Based on preliminary experience with a first system for EEG monitoring (Pronk et al. 1975), we developed a small, stand-alone, computer-based EEG monitoring system which should fulfil the following requirements: (1) artefact-free recording of the EEG of both hemispheres; (2) recording of patient data, such as blood pressure, temperature and anaesthetic information; (3) EEG data reduction and extraction of clinically relevant features; (4) automatic warning or alarming at the occurrence of abnormal EEG activity; (5) synoptic presentation of long-term patient data; (6) numerical display of short-term patient data; (7) interactive use by the anaesthetist; (8) documentation of patient and anaesthetic data.

The system was provided with a new type of electrically isolated EEG preamplifier/filter designed to amplify and low-pass filter the EEG signals and in particular to suppress electrocautery interference (Van der Weide and Pronk 1979).

Two symmetrical bipolar EEG derivations were used (F4-O2 and F3-O1). In our system, the durations of zero-crossing intervals (full wave length) are converted to frequency; wave length data measured during periods of 1 min are displayed above

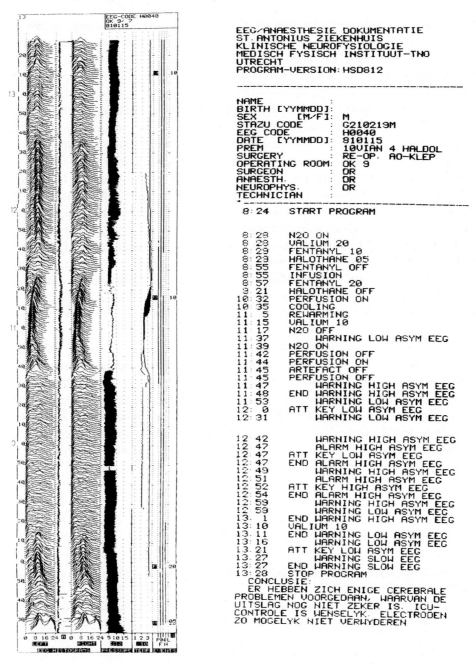

Fig. 1. Patient data during an open heart operation. At far left real time is indicated from 8.24 to 13.28 h. In the 3 left columns the zero crossing histograms and mean EEG amplitude (middle) of 2 symmetrical derivations are given. The histograms were computed every minute; the 3 columns to the right of the histograms indicate arterial blood pressure, temperature values and anaesthetic data respectively (P is a symbol for Perfusion on, F for Fentanyl, N for Nitrous oxide/oxygen, H for Halothane, L for Lidocaine). At the right side, next to the graphical display, the text of the operation protocol is presented. Notice in the text that at 11:47 h a warning was given about an asymmetry in the EEG which occurred a few minutes after stopping the artificial perfusion and persisted till the end of the operation.

each other on a video monitor as a series of histograms (Fig. 1). Values of blood pressure and temperature are also digitized and displayed. A keyboard with special function keys is used for input of anaesthetic data. To signal fast changes instantaneous values of all parameters are displayed every 15 sec on the video monitor.

A warning and alarm program was developed to assist the user in interpreting distinct EEG abnormalities. The warning program uses data on EEG wave length and amplitude in combination with blood pressure, temperature and anaesthetic values. Based on empirical experience about the relations between EEG and these variables, a number of criteria were programmed for detecting low frequency (SLOW EEG), low frequency + low voltage (LOW EEG) and asymmetry (ASYM EEG). The warning program has a logical decision tree structure. It checks the EEG data against data of blood pressure, temperature and type and dosage of drugs every 15 sec. Warning and alarm messages are given in the following order of priority: SLOW EEG, LOW EEG, ASYM EEG. Unilateral low frequency EEG activity may be detected as constant slight asymmetry or as severe asymmetry. At the end of an operation, the patient data are read from mass storage (floppy disk) and written in graphical and alpha-numerical form on a hard copy device. Fig. 1 shows a typical video display.

An evaluation of our monitoring system was carried out on a group of 145 heart patients who were operated on from May to October 1981. Table I presents how many warnings and alarms were generated by the occurrence of abnormal EEG activity in different situations during open heart surgery. Although alarms were given in 49 cases, in only 6 patients was the EEG still abnormal at the end of the operation. In 35 cases, there were no warnings or alarms. In 23 patients, false warnings or alarms were generated by signal artefacts and missing anaesthetic data. In only 1 patient, abnormal EEG activity (asymmetry) was not detected.

TABLE I

EVALUATION OF EEG MONITORING DURING OPEN HEART SURGERY IN A GROUP OF 145 PATIENTS OPERATED IN 1981

The vertical columns indicate how many warnings and alarms at the occurrence of abnormal EEG activity before, during and after cardio-pulmonary bypass (CPB) were generated.

Operation period	Warnings (no. of patients)	Alarms (no. of patients)
Preperfusion	3	4
After starting CPB	14	11
During rewarming	28	43
After stopping CPB	7	13
Postperfusion	4	6
Total number of patients	38	49

AUTOMATIC RECOGNITION OF ABNORMAL EEG ACTIVITY

Several research studies have been carried out to assess the possibility of automatic interpretation by means of pattern recognition and trend analysis techniques. For determining the depth of anaesthesia, McEwen (1975) performed an EEG feature extraction and classification study. Spectral analysis and period-amplitude features were used to classify EEG patterns which were recorded during different levels of anaesthesia. Barlow and Dubinsky (1976) evaluated some methods for the detection of suddenly occurring low frequency activity or sharp waves in the EEG during carotid surgery. Jansen (1979) used a clustering procedure for the classification of 1.28 sec EEG epochs, which were characterized by a set of 5 autoregressive coefficients computed by a Kalman filtering technique.

In the study described here, we compared the performance of several methods currently available using the same patient population. The aim of this study was to increase our empirical knowledge of the recognition of abnormal EEG patterns by means of statistical classification methods in order to improve the automatic classification procedure of our EEG monitoring system.

MATERIAL

EEG, blood pressure and temperature data of 30 patients recorded for several hours (3–5) during open heart surgery with artificial perfusion were stored on magnetic tape. There were 8 female and 22 male patients varying in age from 30 to 75 years. The EEG was recorded from the right (F4-O2) and the left hemispheres (F3-O1). Blood pressure was measured by means of a catheter placed in the left radial artery. The nasopharyngeal temperature and the temperature of the perfusion blood of the heart-lung machine were also continuously measured.

The patient data used in this study were recorded under as far as possible a standardized anaesthetic technique. Premedication, usually thalamonal, was administered 1–1.5 h before surgery. Induction of anaesthesia was carried out most commonly with 20 mg diazepam and 5 ml fentanyl and, after tracheal intubation, continued with a gas mixture of nitrous oxide/oxygen (40% N_2O, 60% O_2). In a number of patients, halothane was administered to suppress a blood pressure increase due to intubation. Fentanyl (10–20 ml) was given to cause analgesia; higher dosages of fentanyl (> 20 ml) were used to maintain a stable blood pressure. For regulating cardiac rhythm of a number of patients, lidocaine was administered. A written record was kept of the type and dosage of anaesthetics and other drugs.

The patient data base consisted of 10 records containing EEG patterns which were interpreted as *normal* under the given circumstances and 20 records in which the EEG presented moderately or severely *abnormal* activity during surgery. To classify the EEGs into normal and abnormal epochs, reliable a priori labelling was required; the judgement of a panel of 3 electroencephalographers with experience in EEG monitoring during open heart surgery was used. Visual interpretation was done by each of the 3 EEGers separately by reading the records written with a paper speed of 1.5 or 0.6 cm/sec. On the strip chart additional information had been written by an EEG technician concerning anaesthesia, blood pressure, starting and stopping of the cardio-pulmonary bypass (CPB) and temperature values during cooling and rewarming.

It is known that in EEG interpretation a large interrater variability is usually encountered. However, in this study the EEGers showed a good measure of agreement concerning the type of abnormal EEG activity, probably because they had acquired clinical experience of EEG monitoring in the same hospital. Besides, EEGs recorded during anaesthesia present more common features than routine EEGs recorded in the waking state. EEG pattern changes directly related to anaesthetic drugs and hypothermia were interpreted as normal changes. The occurrence of low frequency/low voltage activity owing to low blood pressure, air embolism or unknown cause was interpreted as abnormal EEGs activity. The interpretation of the EEG epochs was made according to the type and to the degree of abnormality. Criteria for the detection of severely low frequency and low voltage were mean values of respectively 2 c/sec and 15 μV.

The following types of abnormal EEG activity were distinguished by the panel: (1) low frequency (or slow EEG); (2) low frequency EEG occurring with low voltage; (3) unilateral low frequency or low voltage EEG (asymmetry).

The visual inspection of the EEGs of the group of 30 patients (see Table II) revealed that critical situations with respect to brain function occurred in relation to starting CPB (13 patients), to rewarming to normothermia (19 patients) and to stopping the perfusion (17 patients). At the end of the operation slow waves were present in the EEGs of 13 patients and too low voltages in one EEG. In 3 patients, the occurrence of slow waves appeared to be related to a low blood pressure, i.e., less than 7 kP$_a$ (50 mm Hg). In 4 patients, an EEG asymmetry was signalled, being caused by unilateral air embolism.

TABLE II

NUMBER OF PATIENTS WITH ABNORMAL EEG ACTIVITY

20 EEG records of a group of 30 patients were interpreted by 3 EEGers as abnormal in different situations during open heart surgery. At the end of the operation (usually 1 or 2 h after stopping of CPB), the EEG was still abnormal in 14 patients.

Probable cause	Preperfusion period	Cardio-pulmonary bypass			End of operation
		Starting	During	Stopping	
Low blood pressure	4	7	7	5	3
Air embolism	–	1	4	4	4
Unknown	1	5	8	8	7
Total number of patients	5	13	19	17	14

ANALYSIS METHODS

EEGs and blood pressure signals were read from magnetic tape and were fed into a computer after sampling at 102.4 Hz. The digitized EEGs were divided into 10 sec epochs. After visual inspection, the digitized signals were labelled with an artefact code whenever artefacts occurred within a 10 sec epoch. The EEG epochs were analysed by 4 methods.

(1) Period-amplitude analysis. Zero crossings of the EEG signal and of its first derivative were detected and used for measuring the following features: wave durations and mean, variance and peak-to-peak values of the waves, as described previously (Pronk et al. 1978). An approximation of the first derivative was computed by bandpass filtering of the EEG signal.

(2) Spectral analysis. A Fast Fourier Transform algorithm was used to estimate autospectra. The spectra were smoothed by filtering with a $\cos^2$ filter, resulting in a frequency resolution of 1 Hz; the 95% confidence interval in the estimated power values was ± 3 dB.

(3) Autoregressive filtering by means of Kalman filtering. The Kalman filtering technique of Jansen (1979) was used for estimating the filter coefficients of a 5th order autoregressive model; the coefficients were averaged over epochs of 10 sec.

(4) Computation of normalized slope descriptors. The normalized slope descriptors activity, mobility and complexity, introduced by Hjorth (1970), were determined in the time domain over 10 sec epochs of the EEG signal and its first and second derivatives.

The features extracted by period and spectral analysis were computed within frequency bands (0.5–4, 4–8, 8–12, 12–24 Hz) and for the total frequency band (0.5–24 Hz). Based on previously obtained results (Pronk et al. 1980), the following period-amplitude features were selected: the number of zero crossings in the EEG and in the first derivative, the sum of the peak-to-peak amplitudes of the waves and a quotient of zero crossing rates in the alpha + beta band and delta + theta band. The selected spectral features were the mean frequency, the total power computed from the autospectrum, the relative delta power, and a quotient of alpha + beta power and delta + theta power. In Fig. 2, an example is given representing the evolution of a few features at starting and stopping the artificial perfusion.

Feature evaluation and classification were carried out for the periods after rewarming and stopping CPB. The EEG epochs of this period were chosen in order to evaluate the influence of the last phase of CPB and of stopping CPB on the electrical activity. The total set of EEG epochs of 30 patients was split into a learning set (LI) containing the data from 15 even-numbered patients and a test set (TI) containing those from 15 odd-numbered patients. The classification of the EEG epochs was done by means of a statistical pattern recognition program ISPAHAN developed by Gelsema (1980).

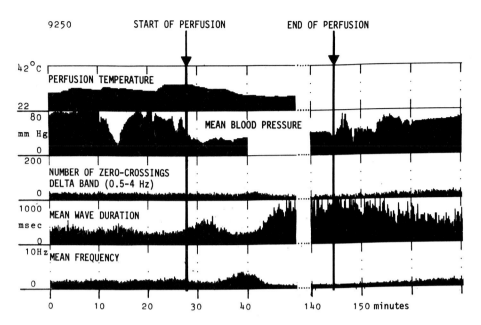

Fig. 2. Feature values for perfusion temperature, mean (arterial) blood pressure and 3 EEG parameters of consecutive 10 sec intervals during the start and end of artificial perfusion. Notice the abnormal evolution of EEG activity at the end of perfusion as indicated by high values of the mean wave duration and low values of the mean frequency.

RESULTS

The EEG features of the learning set were ranked as a function of their discriminatory power for the classification of the EEG epochs into normal and abnormal EEGs, using a stepwise linear discriminant method. In the ranking procedure, the most relevant feature is first determined, then the feature with the highest amount of uncorrelated discriminatory power is added, and so on. At first, feature ranking was done separately for each analysis method. Later ranking of all features was performed. Fisher's linear discriminant method was applied for the classification of the EEG epochs (Duda and Hart 1973). An index of merit was calculated in order to present the classification result; it consists of the total percentage of correctly classified EEG epochs.

Classification results of the EEG epochs recorded after rewarming and stopping cardio-pulmonary bypass are presented in Fig. 3. The learning set LI consisted of 306 normal and 432 abnormal EEG epochs. The test set TI consisted of 434 normal and 384 abnormal epochs. The feature ranking results obtained when using separate EEG analysis methods show that mean frequency, total number of zero crossings, mobility and the 4th Kalman filter coefficient came in the first place. The indices of merit for the learning set were comparable when using spectral features, period-amplitude features or Hjorth parameters, and were slightly worse using Kalman filter coefficients. The test set results using Hjorth parameters were better than the

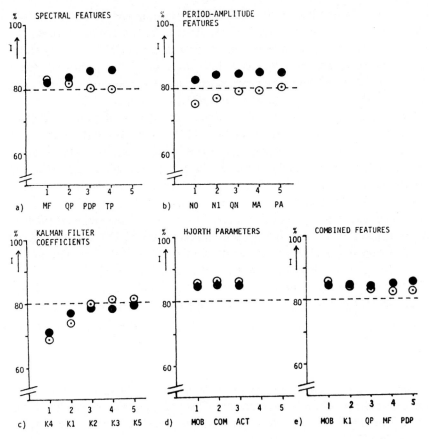

Fig. 3. Results of classification for learning set LI (●) and test set TI (○) of 10 sec EEG epochs recorded in 30 patients after rewarming to normothermia and after stopping cardio-pulmonary bypass by using EEG features as a function of their discriminatory power. The index of merit I is the total percentage of correctly classified epochs into normal and moderately or severely slow EEG epochs. The learning set consists of 306 normal and 432 abnormal epochs, the test set of 434 normal and 384 abnormal epochs. The feature ranking results are: *spectral features:* (1) mean frequency (MF); (2) quotient of powers (alpha + beta) (delta + theta) (QP); (3) relative delta power (PDP); (4) total power (TP). *Period-amplitude features:* (1) number of zero crossings (N0); (2) number of zero crossings in first derivative (N1); (3) quotient of number of zero crossings (alpha + beta) (delta + theta) (QN); (4) mean rectified amplitude (MA); (5) mean peak-to-peak amplitude (PA). *Kalman filter coefficients:* (1) 4th filter coefficient (K4); (2) 1st filter coefficient (K1); (3) 2nd filter coefficient (K2); (4) 3rd filter coefficient (K3); (5) 5th filter coefficient (K5). *Hjorth parameters:* (1) mobility (MOB); (2) complexity (COM); (3) activity (ACT). *Combination of features:* (1) mobility (MOB); (2) 1st Kalman filter coefficient (K1); (3) quotient of powers (QP); (4) mean frequency (MF); (5) relative delta power (PDP).

results obtained with other features. After feature ranking of all measured EEG features, mobility came in first place.

The indices of merit for the learning set LI and test set TI were respectively 85% and 86% when using only mobility and 90% and 82% when using 17 EEG features. A combination of 5 features (Fig. 3e) yielded learning and test set results which were comparable to results obtained using separate EEG analysis methods.

Important aspects in interpreting the classification results are the percentages of false negative and false positive classifications. In our EEG warning method, the aim is to get a low percentage of missed warnings for abnormal EEG activity (false negatives) and an acceptable percentage of false warnings (false positives). After testing with set TI, these percentages were respectively 10% and 20% using Hjorth parameters, and 7% and 30% using all measured EEG features.

It should be noted that the variance of the indices of merit is unknown as long as the results of new test sets are not available. Although a new test set was not available, we used set TI as a learning set and set LI as a test set. After feature ranking of all EEG features mobility came again in the first place. The indices of merit of learning set TI and test set LI were respectively 85% and 84% when using only mobility and 89% and 83% when using 17 EEG features.

It may be concluded that the test set results using Hjorth parameters were the best results (index of merit: 85%) and that the test set results using EEG features derived from the other analysis methods were nearly similar (80–83%). Combination of features of different methods did not improve the classification results.

This finding indicates that even a simple method such as period-amplitude analysis gives satisfactory results for EEG monitoring in the operating room.

SUMMARY

During open heart and carotid surgery, brain function may be disturbed owing to inadequate cerebral perfusion or oxygenation. This may result in irreversible brain damage and, subsequently, in postoperative neurological or psycho-pathological dysfunction. Therefore, it is useful to monitor brain function by means of continuous recording of the EEG. For reliable interpretation it is essential to monitor the EEG in relation to other patient data (blood pressure, temperature, anaesthesia).

Based on period-amplitude features and neurophysiological criteria we developed a computer-assisted EEG monitoring system. Part of the system is an EEG warning program which assists the anaesthetist in detecting abnormal EEG activity during open heart and carotid surgery.

In a study concerning the applicability of several EEG quantification techniques for monitoring during open heart surgery, 4 methods were compared: spectral analysis, period-amplitude analysis, autoregressive filtering, and Hjorth's analysis based on time domain descriptors. EEGs recorded from 30 heart patients were analysed by these methods. The results were used for EEG feature extraction and classification by way of linear discriminant functions. This study revealed that the recognition of abnormal EEG activity may be obtained in approximately the same way by using features computed according to different methods. Thus even such a simple method as period-amplitude analysis gives satisfactory results as an EEG data reduction method for the purpose of long-term monitoring.

REFERENCES

Åberg, T. and Kihlgren, M. Cerebral protection during open heart surgery. Thorax, 1977, 32: 525–533.

Aguilar, M.J., Gerbode, F. and Hill, J.D. Neuropathologic complications of cardiac surgery. J. thorac. cardiovasc. Surg., 1971, 61: 676–685.

Arfel, G., Weiss, J. and DuBouchet, N. EEG findings during open heart surgery with extra-corporeal circulation. In: J.S. Meyer and H. Gastaut (Eds.), Cerebral Anoxia and the Electroencephalogram. Thomas, Springfield, Ill., 1961: 231–249.

Arfel, G., Passelecq, J., Casanova, C. et Dubost, Ch. L'embolie gazeuse en chirurgie cardiaque (étude électro-encéphalographique de 8 observations). Anesth. Analg. Réanim., 1968, 25: 175–202.

Barlow, J.S. and Dubinsky, J. Some computer approaches to continuous automatic clinical EEG monitoring. In: P. Kellaway and I. Petersen (Eds.), Quantitative Analytic Studies in Epilepsy. Raven Press, New York, 1976: 319–327.

Bickford, R.G., Fleming, N. and Billinger, Th. Compression of EEG data. In: S.A. Trufant (Ed.), Transaction of the American Neurological Association, Vol. 96. Springer, New York, 1971: 118–122.

Björk, V.O. and Hultquist, G. Brain damage in children after deep hypothermia for open heart surgery. Thorax, 1960, 15: 284–291.

Branthwaite, M.A. Factors affecting cerebral activity during open heart surgery. Anaesthesia, 1973, 28: 619–625.

Bricolo, A., Turazzi, S., Faccioli, F., Odorizzi, F., Sciarretta, G. and Erculiani, P. Clinical application of compressed spectral array in long-term EEG monitoring of comatose patients. Electroenceph. clin. Neurophysiol., 1978, 45: 211–225.

Brierly, J.B. Brain damage complicating open heart surgery: a neuropathological study of 46 patients. Proc. roy. Soc. Med., 1967, 60: 858–859.

Cohen, B.A. Period analysis of the electroencephalogram. Comput. Progr. Biomed., 1976, 6: 269–276.

Demetrescu, M. The aperiodic character of the electroencephalogram (EEG): a new approach to data analysis and condensation. Physiologist, 1975, 18: 189.

Duda, R.O. and Hart, P.E. Pattern Classification and Scene Analysis. John Wiley, New York, 1973: 114–118.

Dijkstra, Y. Evaluation of EEG monitoring. In: Automated EEG/Anesthesia Monitoring and Documentation during Open Heart and Carotid Surgery (in Dutch). Symposium Report, Utrecht, 1979: 22–26.

Fischer-Williams, M. and Cooper, R.A. Some aspects of electroencephalographic changes during open heart surgery. Neurology (Minneap.), 1964, 14: 472–482.

Fleming, R.A. and Smith, N.Ty. An inexpensive EEG processor for operating room and intensive care use. In: Proc. San Diego Biomed. Symp., 1974: 13.

Hjorth, B. EEG analysis based on time domain properties. Electroenceph. clin. Neurophysiol., 1970, 29: 306–310.

Gelsema, E.S. Ispahan; an interactive system for pattern analysis: structure and capabilities. In: E.S. Gelsema and L.N. Kanal (Eds.), Pattern Recognition in Practice. North-Holland Publ., Amsterdam, 1980: 481–491.

Jansen, B.H. EEG Segmentation and Classification: an Explorative Study. Ph.D. Thesis, Amsterdam, 1979.

Kinichi, S., Vijaya, K., Keshav, K., Vajubhai, S. and Vibhavary, S. Detection of neurological abnormalities during open heart surgery. In: Anesth. Congress, San Francisco, Calif., 1978.

Klein, F.F. A waveform analyzer applied to the human EEG. IEEE Trans. biomed. Engng, 1976, BME-23: 246–252.

Klein, F.F. and Davis, D.A. A further statement on automated EEG processing for intraoperative monitoring. Anesthesiology, 1981, 54: 433–434.

Kolkka, R. and Hilberman, M. Neurological dysfunctions following cardiac surgery with low flow, low pressure cardiopulmonary bypass. J. thorac. cardiovasc. Surg., 1980, 79: 432–437.

Levy, W.J., Shapiro, H.M., Maruchak, G. and Meathe, E. Automated EEG processing for intraoperative monitoring. Anesthesiology, 1980, 58: 223–236.

Maynard, D.E. Development of the CFM: the cerebral function analysing monitor (CFAM). Ann. anesth. franç., 1979, 3: 253–255.

McEwen, J.A. Estimation of the Level of Anesthesia during Surgery by Automatic Pattern Recognition. Ph.D. Thesis, Vancouver, 1975.

Prior, P.F. Monitoring Cerebral Function. Elsevier/North-Holland Biomedical Press, Amsterdam, 1979.

Prior, P.F., Maynard, D.E., Sheaff, P.C., Simpson, B.R., Strunin, L., Weaver, E.J.M. and Scott, D.F. Monitoring cerebral function: clinical experience with new device for continuous recording of electrical activity of the brain. Brit. med. J., 1971, 2: 736–738.

Pronk, R.A.F., Simons, A.J.R. and de Boer, S.J. The use of the EEG for patient monitoring during open heart surgery. In: IEEE Proc. Computers in Cardiology, Rotterdam, 1975: 77–82.

Pronk, R.A.F., de Boer, S.J., Cornelissen, R.E.M., Doornbos, P., Lasance, H.A.J., Simons, A.J.R. and Van der Weide, H. Computer-assisted patient monitoring during open heart surgery with the aid of the EEG. In: B. van Eijnsbergen, and F.H. Lopes da Silva (Eds.), Progress Report, No. PR6, Institute of Medical Physics TNO/Utrecht, 1978: 85–91.

Pronk, R.A.F., Doornbos, P., Hengeveld, S.J., Cornelissen, R.C.M., Ackerstaff, R.G.A., Simons, A.J.R. and Lopes da Silva, F.H. Automatic recognition of abnormal EEG patterns during open heart surgery. In: B. van Eijnsbergen and F.H. Lopes da Silva (Eds.), Progress Report, No. PR7, Institute of Medical Physics TNO/Utrecht, 1980, 61–66.

Salerno, T.A., Lince, D.P., White, D.N., Beverly, L.R. and Charette, E.J.P. Monitoring of electroencephalogram during open heart surgery. A prospective analysis of 118 cases. J. thorac. cardiovasc. Surg., 1978, 76: 97–100.

Simons, A.J.R. Aspects of EEG control during open heart surgery. Electroenceph. clin. Neurophysiol., 1973, 35: 105–106.

Skagseth, E., Froysaker, T. and Refsum, S.B. Disposable filter for microembolism in cardiopulmonary bypass. J. cardiovasc. Surg., 1974, 15: 318–322.

Stockard, J.J., Bickford, R.G. and Schauble, J.F. Pressure-dependent cerebral ischemia during cardiopulmonary bypass. Neurology (Minneap.), 1973, 23: 521–529.

Storm van Leeuwen, W., Mechelse, K., Kok, L. and Zierfuss, E. EEG during heart operations with artificial circulation. In: J.S. Meyer and H. Gastaut (Eds.), Cerebral Anoxia and the Electroencephalogram. Thomas, Springfield, Ill., 1961: 268–278.

Tönnies, J.F. Automatische EEG-Intervall-Spektrumanalyse (EISA) zur Langzeitdarstellung der Schlafperiodik und Narkose. Arch. Psychiat. Nervenkr., 1969, 212: 423–445.

Uhl, R.R., Meathe, E.A., Maruschak, G.F., Saidman, L.J. and Ozaki, G.T. Correlative monitoring of brain activity and perfusion during anesthesia. In: Proc. San Diego Biomed. Symp., 1977: 425–428.

Van der Weide, H. and Pronk, R.A.F. Interference suppression for EEG recording during open heart surgery. Electroenceph. clin. Neurophysiol., 1979, 46: 609–612.

Weiss, M., Weiss, J., Cotton, J., Nicolas, F. and Binet, J.P. A study of the electroencephalogram during surgery with deep hypothermia and circulation arrest in infants. J. thorac. cardiovasc. Surg., 1975, 70: 316–329.

Witoszka, M.M., Tamura, H., Indeglia, R., Hopkins, R.W. and Simeone, F.A. Electroencephalographic changes and cerebral complications in open heart surgery. J. thorac. cardiovasc. Surg., 1973, 66: 855–864.

Wright, J.S., Lethlean, A.K., Hicks, R.G., Torda, T.A. and Stacey, R. Electroencephalographic studies during open heart surgery. J. thorac. cardiovasc. Surg., 1972, 63: 631–638.

Kyoto Symposia (EEG Suppl. No. 36)
Editors: P.A. Buser, W.A. Cobb and T. Okuma
© 1982, Elsevier Biomedical Press, Amsterdam

Long-Term Monitoring during Sleep – a High-Speed Automatic Processing System for Human All-Night Sleep Scoring and Statistical Data Analysis

HATAO HIRAGA[1], SADAO ICHIJO[2] and TERUO OKUMA[3]

[1]*EEG and Computer Section, Central Clinical Laboratories, Tohoku University School of Medicine, Sendai;* [2]*Neuropsychiatric Clinic, Sendai Hospital of Japanese National Railways, Sendai; and* [3]*Department of Neuropsychiatry, Tohoku University School of Medicine, Sendai (Japan)*

Continuous monitoring of the state of consciousness or sleep provides us with varied valuable information on cases of organic brain diseases and sleep disorders. Sleep is one of the most important subjects in the field of long-term surveillance, and data reduction by means of computer analysis is of the upmost importance in this field of research.

Since the early works of Itil (1969), Smith and Karacan (1971), Martin et al. (1972) and others (Itil et al. 1969; Gaillard et al. 1972), many researchers have reported on computer analysis of sleep polygrams, and several kinds of system are already in the stage of clinical application (Naitoh 1981). With regard to the use of computers, however, some differences are seen among these systems. For example, comparing on-line systems with off-line systems, on-line systems are good for monitoring continuously changing data and for handling them, but the computer is occupied by one study only. On the other hand, off-line systems cannot be used for simultaneous monitoring, but by using high-speed processing many data for many patients can be handled.

We are of the opinion that the characteristics of a system which is intended for clinical use should be as follows: (1) data collection is best done by using telemetry, which keeps subjects unhindered and safe; (2) easy handling is necessary and is best realized with a one push-button automatic system; (3) compatibility between machine scoring and human scoring of sleep stages is needed; (4) in addition to scoring, the system should be able to count and print out sleep parameters in statistical figures; (5) it should allow for overall high speed processing; (6) it should have a high resistance to artifacts; (7) the system should be characterized by a good balance between general performance and low running cost.

We have done research into setting up our off-line system (Matsuo et al. 1977; Okuma et al. 1977; Nonaka et al. 1978; Hiraga et al. 1980, 1981) which is mainly designed for the purpose of analysing all-night sleep polygrams in clinical work and experimental sleep studies. We would like to present an outline of our system and show cases of clinical application.

METHOD

The system includes a 4-channel telemeter (Saneisokki), an analog data recorder (Sony), a hybrid pre-processor (designed by Tohoku University School of Technology, and made by Oki Electric Co.) and a multiprogramming minicomputer system (OKITAC-4300; cpu 24 kilowords, disc 2.5 megawords, Oki Electric Co.). It has 4 main characteristics. The first is obtainability of sleep stage scoring as well as analysed parameters for statistics. The second characteristic, high speed data processing, was achieved by using a hybrid pre-processor and a multiprogramming minicomputer system. The third characteristic, the scoring of sleep stages, is according to the manual edited by Rechtschaffen and Kales (1968). And the fourth characteristic, measurement of EEG activity, is based on a method of EEG analysis reported by Fujimori et al. (1958) which is often used in Japan.

The first and second channels of the 4-channel telemeter are for the left and right EOGs; there is also one channel for EMG and another for EEG. These are according to Rechtschaffen and Kales (1968) and the EEG is recorded from the central region with the contralateral ear lobe as reference. For the detection of rapid eye movement (REM), 2 channels are used so that phase reversals can be detected. For the scoring of stage 2, only spindle components are counted.

Fig. 1 shows a diagram of our system. Recorded tape is reproduced at 10 times the speed of real time, and for data suppression we use a pre-processor. This includes hybrid microprocessors. Peaks of EEG wave forms are detected by the pre-processor, and detected values are sent to the computer for recognition of frequency and amplitude of the EEG. REMs are detected by using parameters of amplitude, differentiated values, phase reversal and synchronization (the threshold of REM

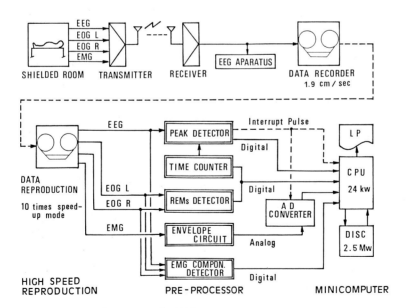

Fig. 1. Diagram of the system (in 1980).

detection can be changed by adjustments on the front panel of the apparatus). Tonic EMGs are smoothed to an envelope curve for measuring the tonic EMG level. Transient EMG artifacts on the EEG and EOG channels are also detected by the pre-processor, and are excluded from EEG measurement. Noisy EMG data on the EOG channels are also omitted from REM detection. This information about EMG artifacts is used for the determination of the critical points of stage shifts.

When we use Fujimori's method each wave is represented by a triangular form. The duration of a wave is measured as the interval between adjacent bottom peaks. The amplitude is measured vertically from the upper peak to the base of the triangle. The threshold for measurement depends on the frequency categories of the wave. Superimposed waves and the basal wave are measured in a similar manner (Fig. 2).

In our system the procedure of scoring of sleep stages involves 3 decision steps. The first is independent or static scoring of each 20 sec epoch. We call it "preliminary scoring." In the second step the preliminary scores are revised so as to correlate with the scores of neighbouring epochs. We call it "revision scoring." These 2 steps are according to the scoring rules described by Rechtschaffen and Kales (1968). In the third step of our system, the "final scoring" for minute-by-minute epochs is made from the scores of 3 sub-epochs of 20 sec, according to the rules of decision by majority. These procedures were reported on at the Third International Congress of Sleep Research held in Tokyo in 1979 (Hiraga et al. 1981). Recently, however, we have slightly modified the criteria for discrimination between stage W and stage 1 to improve the scoring in the cases with poor alpha activity. Fig. 3 shows our new flow chart used for preliminary scoring. This modification has proven to be successful (Hiraga et al. 1980).

RESULTS

Results of the automatic scoring and statistics of sleep parameters are printed by the line printer in two routine output modes. In the first, sequential output format, data for 1 min epochs are written in a line and include the following: time; an analog display of tonic EMG levels and percent-time of beta, alpha, theta and delta activity of EEG; a digital display of percent-time of EEGs; the percent-time of delta waves (0.5–2 Hz, higher than 75 μV); number and average frequency of spindles; number of REMs; and percent-time of transient increase of EMG appearing on the EEG and EOG channels. On the right side the results of stage scoring are shown graphically by numbers or letters indicating their stage names (e.g. 4, 3, 2, 1, R, W and MT). The second output format is a statistical one. The routine output items are divided into 2 categories which are sleep stages and sleep parameters. The items printed out for sleep stages are the distribution of stages in total record time (TRT), in total sleep time (TST) and in thirds of the night; the value of sleep latency; the number of stage shifts; and the number of nocturnal awakings. The following statistics of sleep parameters are printed out: the percent-time of delta waves; the integrated value of delta and beta activities; various parameters of spindles, REMs and EMGs.

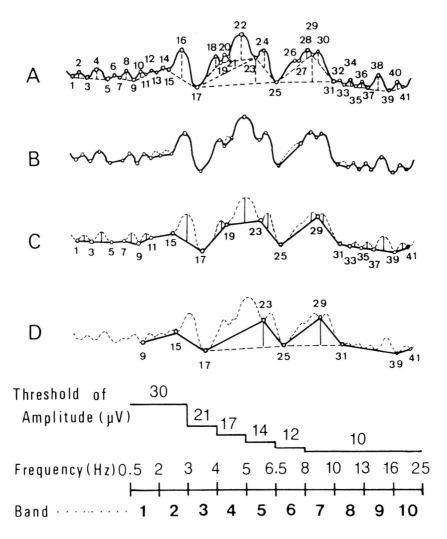

Fig. 2. Procedure for measurement of EEG activity based on Fujimori's method. (A) Original EEG consists of superimposed waves and basal waves. Small dots (circles) on the waves indicate the peak points detected by the pre-processor. The broken lines show triangular formation for measurement of the amplitude and duration (frequency) of waves. (B) Omitted waves (Nos. 12, 14 etc.) are indicated by the broken lines, because they have an amplitude below threshold. (C) Broken lines indicate measured superimposed waves and solid lines indicate remaining basal waves. (D) The basal waves having points Nos. 23 and 29 are measured, but the wave having point No. 15 is not computed, because its amplitude is below threshold. At the bottom of the diagram, the thresholds of amplitude for each frequency band are indicated.

As to the operation, this system is very easy to handle. After preparation of calibration, the procedure is begun by pushing one button, and the input procedure automatically ends when the recorded tape data are finished. Printouts are started automatically, immediately after the end of the recorded tape. For an 8 h sleep

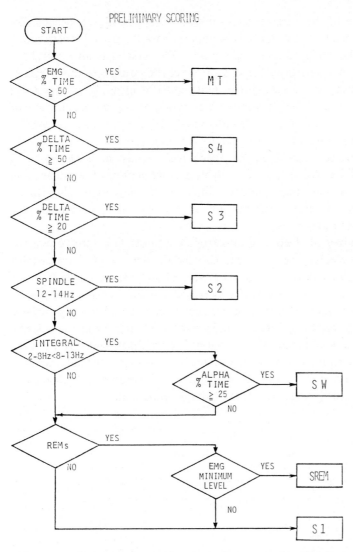

Fig. 3. A new flow chart of our system for preliminary scoring, slightly modified to improve scoring in cases with poor alpha activity (in 1980).

polygram, total run time of our system is about 70 min; 50 min are for reproduction of tape and analysis, and 20 min are taken for a delayed printout.

Results of the automatic analysis were tested in 7 healthy young adults, including 2 cases with poor alpha activity and 3 cases with 50 Hz artifacts or much EMG activity. Overall performance for stage scoring was 84.0% for the final score.

CLINICAL APPLICATION

Although our system is not designed for on-line analysis, it can be used for the continuous observation of the state of sleep for several days or nights, because the total run-time of the system for the analysis of data for each 8 h period is very short, and we can observe the analysed data successively. This system is also useful for longitudinal observation of nocturnal sleep, as in the case of studies of the effects of hypnotic drugs. We investigated an experimental model of insomnia (Okuma and Honda 1978; Okuma et al. 1980; Okuma 1981) produced by administration of central stimulant drugs such as methylphenidate and caffeine, and the recovery in such cases of model insomnia after hypnotic drug medication.

The experimental protocol covered 12 nights with 7 day intervals. After 2 adaptation nights and 1 baseline (placebo) night, a combination of stimulant and hypnotic drugs was given to normal volunteer subjects in random order. These drugs were methylphenidate (10 mg), caffeine (150 mg) and a new benzodiazepine hypnotic, temazepam (15 and 30 mg).

Fig. 4 shows 3 examples of sleep diagrams from 1 subject. The upper one is the baseline record. Three sleep cycles are seen. The middle diagram shows a caffeine night; the sleep latency and slow wave sleep latency, S3 and S4, are longer than the baseline. The number of sleep stage shifts increased remarkably and splitting of stage REM is seen. The diagram at the bottom shows the sleep when both caffeine and temazepam were given. Sleep latency became shorter than that of the caffeine night and the sleep as a whole recovered to that of the baseline night. Over 8 h the administration of caffeine increased the percentage of stage W remarkably, without significant change of stage $3+4$ and stage REM. Administration of temazepam restored almost all the sleep stages to those of the baseline night.

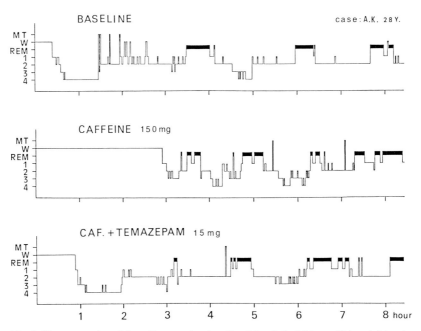

Fig. 4. Three examples of sleep diagrams in a baseline (placebo) night, a caffeine night and a caffeine plus temazepam night, from one model insomnia subject.

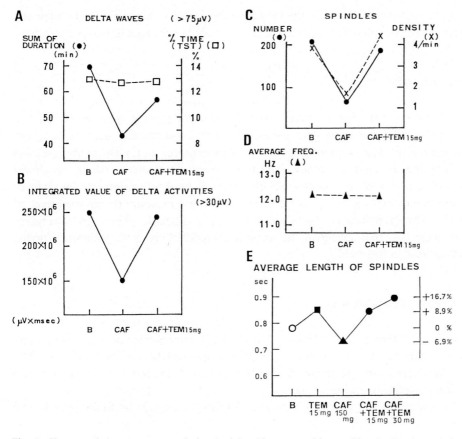

Fig. 5. Changes of sleep parameters during 3 nights (the same subject as Fig. 4). Graph symbols are defined near the vertical scales.

Besides the automatic determination of sleep stages, the automatic analysis of various sleep parameters can give us much information on the quality of sleep. For example, we think that the amount of delta activity will be useful as an indicator of quantity and quality of sleep in a night. In Fig. 5A, the solid circles show the sum of the durations of delta waves of 0.5–2 c/sec and larger than 75 μV in amplitude, during baseline, caffeine and caffeine + temazepam nights. The value in the caffeine night decreased from that of the baseline night, but in the caffeine and temazepam night the value recovered to that of the baseline night. On the other hand, the percent-time of the delta waves in total sleep time did not change. In the lower graph (Fig. 5B), integrated values of delta activities of 0.5–2 c/sec and of more than 30 μV are shown by solid circles in μV × msec. These changes are seen in the same way as the sum of the durations of delta waves.

Fig. 5C shows the number and average density of spindles in total sleep time. By giving caffeine the total number and average density per minute of spindles are both decreased but, as shown in Fig. 5D, no changes in the mean frequency of individual waves in spindles are observed.

Fig. 5E shows the change in the length of the spindles. After giving the hypnotic the length of the spindles becomes longer. This change is probably dose dependent.

CONCLUSION

As reported in the present paper, by using this computer system we can analyse sleep polygrams and determine the sleep stages automatically with an accuracy comparable to that of manual analysis. Furthermore, computer analysis makes possible the analysis of many important sleep parameters, which is almost impossible with manual analysis. Sleep is one of the most important functions of human beings and the study of sleep will contribute not only to the treatment of patients with sleep disorders but also to the benefit of healthy people. In this regard, it is expected that progress in computer technology will promote further development in this field.

ACKNOWLEDGEMENTS

We wish to thank Prof. Matsuo (Tohoku University School of Technology) and many collaborators: Mr. Shimizu (Tohoku University School of Medicine), Mr. Nonaka (NHK), Mr. Teshigawara and Mr. Nagai (Oki Electric Co.), who helped and supported this study.

This study was supported by a grant from the government of Japan in 1974 and 1975.

REFERENCES

Fujimori, B., Yokota, T., Ishibashi, Y. and Takei, T. Analysis of the electroencephalogram of children by histogram method. Electroenceph. clin. Neurophysiol., 1958, 10: 241–252.

Gaillard, J.M., Krassoievitch, M. et Tissot, R. Analyse automatique du sommeil par un système hybride: nouveaux résultats. Electroenceph. clin. Neurophysiol., 1972, 33: 403–410.

Hiraga, H., Okuma, T., Ichijo, S. and Teshigawara, T. High speed automatic analyzing system for all-night sleep polygram: for improvement of performance and statistical procedure. In: The 10th Japanese Congress of EEG and EMG, Nagoya, 1980 (Japanese abstr.). Jap. J. EEG EMG, 1981, 9: 25.

Hiraga, H., Ichijo, S. and Okuma, T. High-speed automatic sleep stage scoring and data analysis. In: I. Karacan (Ed.), Psychophysiological Aspects of Sleep: Proceedings of the Third International Congress of Sleep Research. Noyes Medical Publications, Park Ridge, 1981: 176–182.

Itil, T.M. Effects of psychotropic drugs on computer "sleep prints" in man. In: A. Cerletti and F.J. Bové (Eds.), The Present Status of Psychotropic Drugs: Proceedings of the Sixth International Congress of the CINP, Tarragona, 1968. Excerpta Medica, Amsterdam, 1969: 211–227.

Itil, T.M., Shapiro, D.M., Fink, M. and Kassebaum, B.A. Digital computer classifications of EEG sleep stages. Electroenceph. clin. Neurophysiol., 1969, 27: 76–83.

Martin, W.B., Johnson, L.C., Viglione, S.S., Naitoh, P., Joseph, R.D. and Moses, J.D. Pattern recognition of EEG-EOG as a technique for all-night sleep stage scoring. Electroenceph. clin. Neurophysiol., 1972, 32: 417–427.

Matsuo, M., Nonaka, S., Shimizu, Y., Okuma, T., Hiraga, H. and Ichijo, S. High-speed processing system of all-night sleep polygram. Jap. J. MEBE, 1977, 15: 214–215 (abstr., in Japanese).

Naitoh, P. Wated: a Cookbook (Chairman's Review). In: I. Karacan (Ed.), Psychophysiological Aspects of Sleep: Proceedings of the Third International Congress of Sleep Research. Noyes Medical Publications, Park Ridge, 1981: 196–202.

Nonaka, S., Shimizu, Y., Matsuo, M., Okuma, T., Hiraga, H. and Ichigo, S. High-speed processing system of all night sleep EEG. Bull. appl. Inform. Study, 1978, 4: 1–11 (in Japanese).

Okuma, T. Model insomnia – for testing hypnotic medication. In: I. Karacan (Ed.), Psychophysiological Aspects of Sleep: Proceedings of the Third International Congress of Sleep Research, Noyes Medical Publications, Park Ridge, 1981: 133–138.

Okuma, T. and Honda, H. Model insomnia, noise and methylphenidate, used for the evaluation of hypnotic drugs. Psychopharmacology, 1978, 57: 127–132.

Okuma, T., Hiraga, H., Ichijo, S., Matsuo, M., Shimizu, Y. and Nonaka, S. High-speed automatic system for analyzing all-night sleep polygram, by using a minicomputer. Jap. J. EEG EMG, 1977, 5: 58 (abstr., in Japanese).

Okuma, T., Matsue, T., Wagatsuma, S., Matsuoka, H. and Toyomura, K. Comparison of sleep disturbance induced by methylphenidate and caffeine – for an improvement of "model insomnia technique." Ann. Rep. Pharmacopsychiat. Res. Found., 1980, 12: 160–167.

Rechtschaffen, A. and Kales, A. (Eds.) A Manual of Standardized Terminology, Techniques and Scoring System for Sleep Stages of Human Subjects. Public Health Service, U.S. Government Printing Office, Washington, D.C., 1968.

Smith, J.R. and Karacan, I. EEG sleep stage scoring by an automatic hybrid system. Electroenceph. clin. Neurophysiol., 1971, 31: 231–237.

Kyoto Symposia (EEG Suppl. No. 36)
Editors: P.A. Buser, W.A. Cobb and T. Okuma
© 1982, Elsevier Biomedical Press, Amsterdam

Long-Term Monitoring in Epileptic Patients

J.R. IVES

Montreal Neurological Hospital and Institute, 3801 University Street, Montreal, Que. H3A 2B4 (Canada)

Until recently the long-term monitoring of epileptic patients was not a widespread routine EEG service. Long-term monitoring was, and still is in some instances, an expensive, time-consuming, labour intensive, technically difficult and usually logistically frustrating special procedure.

For a specific group of epileptic patients with intractable focal epilepsy who were being investigated for the surgical removal of their epileptic focus, the interictal epileptic activity has generally played the major EEG role in determining whether surgery was possible and to what extent and at which location the removal should be made (Gloor 1975; Rasmussen 1980). Compared to the ictal activity, the interictal activity has always been relatively easy to obtain without artefacts in routine EEGs. The epileptic interictal spike and sharp wave have been well documented and extensively studied since the discovery of the human EEG itself. However, the ictal activity has not been studied to any comparable extent.

There has always been one basic reason for pursuing the documentation in the EEG of the patient's spontaneous clinical seizure: the major complaint or symptom that brings an epileptic patient to seek medical attention is his seizure. Based on this, it seemed that documentation of the seizure would provide information that was relevant to the diagnosis and treatment of the epileptic patient and, in particular, to the intractable patient considered for surgical intervention.

With the development of special electrodes, telemetry, computer, video and miniature cassette systems over the past 10 years and their application to a large series of epileptic patients on a routine basis where the main purpose was to document their spontaneous seizures, a preliminary insight into the pertinent diagnostic value and possible importance of the ictus during the EEG has been obtained.

RECENT RELEVANT TECHNICAL DEVELOPMENTS

(A) Cassette

The 4-channel 24 h cassette recorder, when adapted to record EEGs via neck-mounted amplifiers (Ives and Woods 1975, 1980b; Ives 1976) has permitted ambulatory EEG recording to take place for many days on outpatients. It has either proved useful or demonstrated possible applications in dealing with some of the following situations: (1) evaluating the effectiveness of treatment of patients with

3/sec spike and wave-type attacks; (2) diagnosis of patients with questionable seizure activity (Ives et al. 1981); (3) lateralizing temporal lobe seizures (Ives and Woods 1980a); (4) studying the time relationships of epileptic spikes, electrographic and clinical seizures recorded from surface, sphenoidal and depth electrodes.

(B) Chronic sphenoidal electrode

The development of this very useful electrode has permitted its extensive routine application to all patients now investigated for possible focal epilepsy (Ives and Gloor 1977a, 1978a). Table I illustrates its impact in the EEG department at the M.N.I.

TABLE I

USE OF CHRONIC SPHENOIDAL ELECTRODES

	Total* EEGs	With sphenoidals	With pharyngeals
Before (1972) Chronic sph.	2851	83 (3%)	22 (0.8%)
After (1976) Chronic sph.	3086	281 (9%)	22 (0.7%)
After (1980) Chronic sph.	3089	501 (16%)	3 (0.1%)

*Equivalent 9 month periods (September–May).

(C) Cable-telemetry

The development of the 16-channel cable-telemetry EEG monitoring system (Ives et al. 1974, 1976) and the parallel introduction of the chronic stereotaxic depth electrode investigation of bitemporal epileptic patients at the M.N.I. in the early 1970s greatly complemented one another (Olivier et al. 1980). The depth electrode protocol called for the repeated and consistent documentation of the spontaneous clinical seizures. The cable telemetry unit, when coupled to a digital computer, efficiently met this requirement.

The computer generated a 2 min delay of the EEG and thus the system could automatically monitor for clinical seizures over periods lasting days or weeks with minimal human intervention or supervision. The average recording time for a patient with depth electrodes was 3 weeks (range: 1–5 weeks).

On-going development, particularly in the implementation of a larger, dedicated mini computer (PDP-11/60), a second patient monitoring option and advanced software has greatly expanded the seizure monitoring capability.

Table II outlines in point form some of its present features.

PRELIMINARY FINDINGS AND COMMENTS OF SEIZURE MONITORING

(A) The intact recording in the EEG of a spontaneous clinical seizure is usually the most significant factor contributing to the diagnosis and treatment of an epileptic patient. In the hierarchy of diagnostic information the "trump card" is the

TABLE II

SEIZURE MONITORING SYSTEM

1.	(a) Two patients, each wearing a 16-channel cable-telemetry unit or (b) 1 patient (with stereotaxic depth electrodes) wearing a 32-channel cable-telemetry unit (Ives et al. 1981).
2.	Patients can be monitored from any of 35 hospital locations.
3.	Time-lapsed audio/video tape recording which is time-locked to the EEG* (Ives and Gloor 1978b).
4.	Clinical seizures fully recorded (2 min pre and 2 min post) by using a 2 min delay of the EEG which is activated by the patient or nursing staff pushing a button.
5.	Random sampling of the background EEG, e.g., a 20 sec sample every 10 min (Ives and Gloor 1977b).
6.	Automatic detection of epileptic spikes and sharp waves** (Gotman et al. 1979).
7.	Automatic detection of electrographic seizures** (Gotman et al. 1982).
8.	Digital filtering of seizure onsets contaminated with muscle artefact (Gotman et al. 1982).
9.	Monitoring operates automatically for more than 24 h before requiring intervention.
10.	Fast computer relay ($2\times$) of any stored or processed EEG.

*Limited to 1 patient since only 1 unit is available.
**Computer software and hardware limitations permit monitoring of only 1 patient.

recording of a clear focal seizure onset. This information will either overrule other contradictory localizing information or mean that more extensive studies with implanted depth electrodes are required to resolve the conflict.

(B) Several seizures recorded from the same patient with the same montage demonstrate very similar patterns in terms of location, amplitude, frequency and time course.

This "seizure signature" is illustrated in Fig. 1A and B and could also be used in the automatic detection of seizures.

(C) The onset EEG frequency of the seizure is probably related to: (i) the type of seizure and its localization, e.g., focal or generalized; (ii) underlying cortical or subcortical pathology, e.g. tumour or non-tumour.

This distinct rhythmical epileptic discharge which is well organized must contain more information than just that of localization. In an attempt to extract more relevant relationships from the seizures themselves, the seizure onset frequency was analysed, in patients suspected of having temporal lobe epilepsy, with surface and sphenoidal electrodes and recorded either on the 16-channel cable-telemetry system or the 4-channel, 24 h cassette recorder (Ives and Woods 1980a).

Fig. 2A illustrates the initial analysis, using the 4-channel cassette, of 24 highly selected temporal lobe epileptic patients who demonstrated clear unilateral seizures from either the left or right temporal lobe. The lower frequency distribution of the 5 patients with tumours was an interesting and provocative finding.

Fig. 2B illustrates a more extensive study of all temporal lobe patients (47) who had a seizure recorded on the cassette while Fig. 2C was obtained from a group of epileptic patients suspected of having temporal lobe seizures (48) who were recorded on the 16-channel cable-telemetry system. In the distinct bimodal distribution shown

TELEMETRY RECORDINGS OF SPONTANEOUS SEIZURES RECORDED FROM DEPTH ELECTRODES

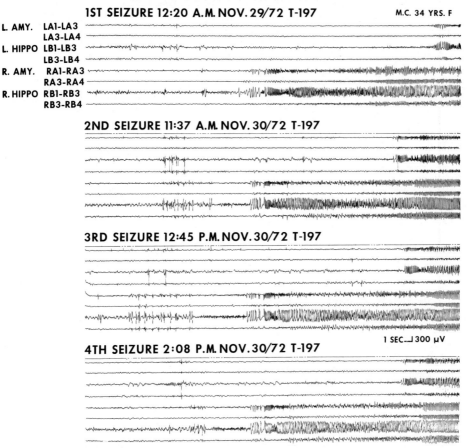

1ST SEIZURE 12:20 A.M. NOV. 29/72 T-197   M.C. 34 YRS. F

L. AMY.   LA1-LA3
          LA3-LA4
L. HIPPO LB1-LB3
          LB3-LB4
R. AMY.   RA1-RA3
          RA3-RA4
R. HIPPO RB1-RB3
          RB3-RB4

2ND SEIZURE 11:37 A.M. NOV. 30/72 T-197

3RD SEIZURE 12:45 P.M. NOV. 30/72 T-197

1 SEC 300 µV

4TH SEIZURE 2:08 P.M. NOV. 30/72 T-197

Fig. 1A. Illustration of 4 seizures recorded from the same patient with depth electrodes demonstrating the repetitive pattern of the onset and the development of this patient's "seizure signature". This shows that the amplitude/time relationship is very similar.

in Fig. 2C, in particular, the higher frequency group was caused by a subgroup of patients whose seizures were generalized at onset.

In Fig. 2D a more extensive study of a group of 34 patients with temporal lobe epilepsy due to confirmed tumours was investigated. A summary of the above findings is shown in Table III.

(D) Patients who are considered to have bitemporal involvement on the basis of interictal findings usually have exclusively or predominantly unilateral discharges if the ictal activity is evaluated.

During our investigation, using chronic stereotaxic depth electrodes (Olivier et al. 1980; Gloor et al. 1980), of patients who were initially diagnosed as bitemporal, and thus not surgical candidates, on the basis of traditional surface and sphenoidal studies, it was found that the ictal records from the depth electrodes were

Instantaneous EEG Frequency VS Seizure Length

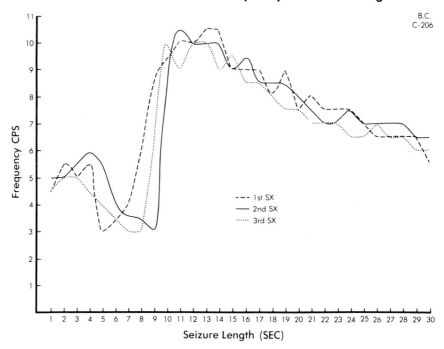

Fig. 1B. Illustration of 3 seizures recorded from the same patient with surface and sphenoidal electrodes (not the same patient as Fig. 1A) using the 4-channel cassette recorder. This demonstrates that the instantaneous frequency for 1 sec epochs vs. the seizure length is also very similar.

predominantly or exclusively unilateral, as shown in Table IV.

Subsequent surgery of the offending temporal lobe, based solely on the localization of seizure onset, and a >2 year follow-up revealed very favourable results (Olivier et al. 1980), similar to those obtained with the larger M.N.I. temporal lobectomy series (Rasmussen 1980). These results are shown in Table V.

(E) The lateralization of the ictal onset does not always correlate with the predominance of the bitemporal interictal activity.

In this same group of 18 "bitemporal" epileptic patients studied with implanted

TABLE III

COMPARISON OF THE SEIZURE ONSET FREQUENCY OF TEMPORAL LOBE EPILEPTIC PATIENTS WITH AND WITHOUT TUMOURS

	Onset frequency (c/sec) of seizure discharge		
	0–2	2–3	>3
Number of patients with a tumour	21	8	5
Likelihood that the TLE is due to a tumour	100%	38%	6%
Number of patients with non-tumoural lesions	0	13	82
Likelihood that the TLE is due to a non-tumoural lesion	0%	62%	94%

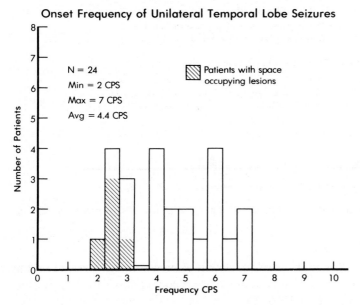

Fig. 2A. In a series of 24 patients with temporal lobe epilepsy who had unilateral seizures, the onset EEG frequency of the seizure was determined.

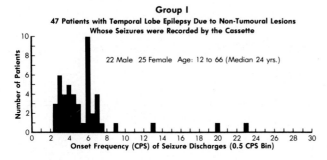

Fig. 2B. In a larger series of 47 temporal lobe patients recorded with the cassette, the onset frequency of the seizure was analysed.

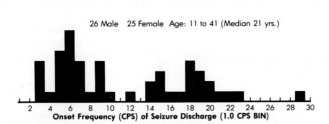

Fig. 2C. Documents of a similar group from an independent study of the seizure onset frequency of patients with temporal lobe epilepsy recorded on the 16-channel cable telemetry system.

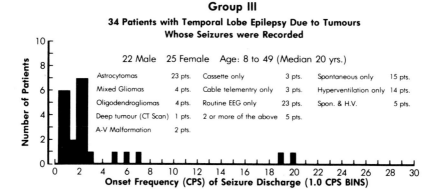

Fig. 2D. Illustrates the seizure onset frequency of a third group of patients with temporal lobe epilepsy due to a tumour.

depth electrodes, it was found that the correlation of predominant interictal spiking with the side of clinical seizure onset was not 100% (Gloor et al. 1980). The statistics of this finding are presented in Table VI.

(F) The prognostic value of the preoperative ictal finding is probably more significant than the interictal finding.

TABLE IV

BILATERAL INTERICTAL VS. UNILATERAL ICTAL

Number of patients demonstrating bitemporal interictal activity with surface/sphenoidal recording	18
Number of clinical and electrographic seizures recorded with depth electrodes	(clin 555, 1122; elect 567; range 4–115, avg. 30.8/pt)
100% of the ictal events unilateral	7
>90% of the ictal events unilateral	6 } 89%
>80% of the ictal events unilateral	3
>60% of the ictal events unilateral	1
50/50	1

TABLE V

FOLLOW-UP RESULTS OF 'BITEMPORAL' EPILEPTIC PATIENTS STUDIED WITH STEREOTAXIC DEPTH ELECTRODES

Total number of patients investigated	18	
Number of patients operated for removal of temporal lobe	15	
Number of patients with > 2 year follow-up	13	
Results		
Group A seizure free or 1–3 minor attacks/year	6	(46%)
Group B > 50% reduction	7	(54%)
Group C no change	0	

TABLE VI

BITEMPORAL INTERICTAL PREDOMINANCE VS. ICTAL LATERALIZATION

Number of patients with bitemporal interictal activity	18
Number of patients with no interictal predominance	2
Number of patients with definite interictal predominance	16
Number of patients where the ictal localization did not correlate with the predominant interictal activity	3 (19% of 16)

In a group of 57 patients who were operated on for the removal of their epileptic temporal lobe between 1975 and 1977 (inclusive) and who also had a spontaneous clinical seizure documented prior to surgery, a study was made concerning ictal and interictal localization vs. >2 year follow-up.

Table VII demonstrates the follow-up results in relationship to the preoperative interictal findings of surface and sphenoidal records. Table VIII demonstrates the follow-up results in relationship to the preoperative ictal findings of surface and sphenoidal records. Table IX was obtained by combining both ictal and interictal preoperative results and comparing these with the follow-up results.

Although these data are preliminary and cover only small patient subgroups, it appears that patients demonstrating a focal seizure onset with no contralateral spread have a strong possibility of being completely seizure free after removal of the offending temporal lobe. This cannot be said of unilateral interictal activity.

(G) The general pattern of a localized temporal lobe seizure recorded by surface and sphenoidal electrodes consists of an organized rhythmic epileptic discharge which may or may not be preceded by a focal or generalized flattening. In most

TABLE VII

INTERICTAL EPILEPTIC ACTIVITY VS. THE RESULTS OF A > 2 YEAR FOLLOW-UP OF 57 TEMPORAL LOBE EPILEPTIC PATIENTS WHO HAD A SPONTANEOUS CLINICAL SEIZURE DOCUMENTED PRIOR TO THE SURGICAL REMOVAL OF THE TEMPORAL LOBE

The "unilateral only" refers to the preoperative EEGs which never revealed any independent contralateral epileptic activity or any generalized epileptic activity.

	Unsatisfactory result	Good result			Ratio good/ unsatisfactory
	Moderate or less reduction >1–2%	Marked reduction <1–2%	Became + remained SX free	SX free	33:24
Unilateral only (39%)	5	5	1	11	17:5
Unilateral + independent (35%)	10	7	1	2	10:10
Unilateral + independent + generalized (26%)	9	1	0	5	6:9

TABLE VIII

ICTAL EPILEPTIC ACTIVITY VS. THE RESULTS OF A > 2 YEAR FOLLOW-UP OF 57
TEMPORAL LOBE EPILEPTIC PATIENTS WHO HAD A SPONTANEOUS CLINICAL SEIZURE
DOCUMENTED PRIOR TO THE SURGICAL REMOVAL OF THE TEMPORAL LOBE

The "focal no spread" refers to patients whose seizures did not spread to or involve the contralateral
temporal lobe. The "focal with spread" refers to patients whose seizures were focal at onset but spread
to the contralateral temporal lobe.

	Unsatisfactory result	Good result			Ratio good/ unsatisfactory
	Moderate or less reduction $> 1-2\%$	Marked reduction $< 1-2\%$	Became + remained SX free	SX free	33:24
Focal no spread (25%)	0	1	0	13	14:0
Focal with spread (35%)	10	4	1	5	10:10
Generalized or bi-lateral (25%)	7	7	0	0	7:7
Unreadable (15%)	7	1	1	0	2:7

cases, the EEG frequency at the onset may range from 2 to 8 c/sec.

This frequency distribution is shown in Fig. 2B and C and corresponds to other
investigations (Gotman et al. 1981).

(H) A distinct rhythmic epileptic discharge is not always present during a clinical
event when the surface and sphenoidal electrodes are used.

In a study of 100 patients (Ives et al. 1980a) with temporal lobe epilepsy, using the
4-channel 24 h cassette, summarized in Table X, the results indicated that 94% of
the auras and 20% of the clinical seizures showed no epileptic activity in the EEG
during the reported or witnessed clinical event.

(I) Electrographic seizures occur frequently in a significant number of temporal
lobe epileptic patients.

Also, from Table X, it can be seen that of the 273 epileptic EEG events recorded,
41% of them were electrographic.

From a separate study of the 18 depth electrode cases outlined in Table IV, of the
1122 epileptic discharges recorded, 51% were electrographic.

CONCLUSION

The preceding has taken you from an idea that recording the spontaneous clinical
seizures of epileptic patients might be beneficial, through the development and
implementation of specialized techniques to realize the goal of routinely,
consistently and "easily" documenting this most elusive event. It has not only

TABLE IX

A COMBINATION OF ICTAL AND INTERICTAL VS. THE RESULTS OF A < 2 YEAR FOLLOW-UP OF 57 TEMPORAL LOBE EPILEPTIC PATIENTS WHO HAD A SPONTANEOUS CLINICAL SEIZURE DOCUMENTED PRIOR TO THE SURGICAL REMOVAL OF THE TEMPORAL LOBE

	Unilateral + independent + generalized	Unilateral + independent	Unilateral only
Focal no spread	0 0 0 0	0 0	0 0 0 0
		3	0 0 0
	0		0 0 0 0
Focal with spread		1	
		3 3 3	
		4 4 4	3
	4	4 4 4	4 4
Generalized or bilateral	3		
	4 4 4 4	3 3	3 3 3 3
	4 4 4		
			1
Unreadable		3	
	4	4 4 4	4 4 4

0, SX free; 1, became SX free; 3, marked reduction (< 1–2%); 4, moderate or less reduction (> 1–2%).

TABLE X

CLINICAL/EEG RESULTS FROM 100 PATIENTS WITH TEMPORAL LOBE EPILEPSY

EEG events	Clinical events			
	Auras	Clinical seizures	Electro-graphic	Total
Lost or unreadable	0	19	unknown	19
No epileptic activity	48 (94% of 51)	31 (20% of 157)	N.A.	79
Definite epileptic activity	3	157	113 (41% of 273)	273
Total	51	207	113	371

demonstrated that the results are of an immediate benefit to the diagnosis and treatment of epileptic patients but also reveals preliminary results indicating that the seizure itself contains significant basic information that warrants further, more detailed investigations.

REFERENCES

Gloor, P. Contribution of electroencephalography and electrocorticography to the neurosurgical treatment of the epilepsies. In: D.P. Purpura, J.K. Penry and P.D. Walter (Eds.), Advances in Neurology. Raven Press, New York, 1975: 59–105.

Gloor, P., Olivier, A. and Ives, J.R. Prolonged seizure monitoring with stereotaxically implanted depth electrodes in patients with bilateral interictal temporal lobe epileptic foci: how bilateral is bitemporal epilepsy? In: J. Wada and J.K. Penry (Eds.), Advances in Epileptology: The Xth Epilepsy International Symposium. Raven Press, New York, 1980: 83–88.

Gotman, J., Ives, J.R. and Gloor, P. Automatic recognition of interictal epileptic activity in prolonged EEG recordings. Electroenceph. clin. Neurophysiol., 1979, 46: 510–520.

Gotman, J., Ives, J.R. and Gloor, P. Frequency content of EEG and EMG at seizure onset: possibility of removal of EMG artefact by digital filtering. Electroenceph. clin. Neurophysiol., 1981, 52: 626–639.

Ives, J.R. EEG monitoring of ambulatory epileptic patients. Postgrad. med. J., 1976, 52 (Suppl. 7): 86–91.

Ives, J.R. and Gloor, P. New sphenoidal electrode assembly to permit long-term monitoring of the patient's ictal or interictal EEG. Electroenceph. clin. Neurophysiol., 1977a, 42: 575–580.

Ives, J.R. and Gloor, P. Automatic nocturnal sleep sampling: a useful method in clinical electroencephalography. Electroenceph. clin. Neurophysiol., 1977b, 43: 880–884.

Ives, J.R. and Gloor, P. Update: chronic sphenoidal electrodes. Electroenceph. clin. Neurophysiol., 1978a, 44: 789–790.

Ives, J.R. and Gloor, P. A long-term time-lapse video system to document the patient's spontaneous clinical seizure synchronized with the EEG. Electroenceph. clin. Neurophysiol., 1978b, 45: 412–416.

Ives, J.R. and Woods, J.F. 4-Channel 24-hour cassette recorder for long-term EEG monitoring of ambulatory patients. Electroenceph. clin. Neurophysiol., 1975, 39: 88–92.

Ives, J.R. and Woods, J.F. A study of 100 patients with focal epilepsy using a 4-channel ambulatory cassette recorder. In: F.D. Stott, E.B. Raftery and L. Goulding (Eds.), ISAM 1979: Proceedings of the Third International Symposium on Ambulatory Monitoring. Academic Press, London, 1980a: 383–392.

Ives, J.R. and Woods, J.F. The contribution of ambulatory EEG to the management of epileptic patients. In: W.A. Littler (Ed.), Clinical Ambulatory Monitoring. Chapman and Hall, London, 1980b: 122–147.

Ives, J.R., Thompson, C.J., Gloor, P., Olivier, A. and Woods, J.F. Multichannel EEG telemetry-computer monitoring of epileptic patients. In: P.A. Neukomn (Ed.), Biotelemetry II (2nd International Symposium on Biotelemetry, Davos, 1974). Karger, Basel, 1974: 216–218.

Ives, J.R., Thompson, C.J. and Gloor, P. Seizure monitoring: a new tool in electroencephalography. Electroenceph. clin. Neurophysiol., 1976, 41: 422–427.

Ives, J.R., Hausser, C., Woods, J.F. and Andermann, F. Contribution of 4-channel cassette EEG monitoring to differential diagnosis of paroxysmal attacks. In: M. Dam, L. Gram and J.K. Penry (Eds.), Advances in Epileptology, XIIth Epilepsy International Symposium. Raven Press, New York, 1981: 329–336.

Olivier, A., Gloor, P. et Ives, J.R. Investigation et traitement chirurgical de l'épilepsie bitemporale. Union méd., 1980, 109: 1–4.

Rasmussen, T.H. Surgical aspects of temporal lobe epilepsy: results and problems. Acta neurochir. (Wien), 1980, Suppl. 30: 13–24.

11. EEG Polygraphy in Respiratory Disorders and other Risk Conditions in Infancy

Kyoto Symposia (EEG Suppl. No. 36)
Editors: P.A. Buser, W.A. Cobb and T. Okuma
© 1982, Elsevier Biomedical Press, Amsterdam

Mechanisms of Respiratory Control during Sleep and Wakefulness: Implications in Newborn Sleep Apnoea

ANDRÉ HUGELIN

Laboratoire de Physiologie, CHU Saint-Antoine, 27, rue Chaligny, 75571 Paris Cedex 12 (France)

Pulmonary ventilation is the only vegetative function entirely controlled by striated muscles. Alternate contraction of inspiratory and expiratory thoracic and abdominal muscles is responsible for motion of the air column, while laryngeal and pharyngeal muscles coordinate the traffic of air and alimentary bolus at the upper airway level. However, in addition to the ventilatory function, the respiratory muscles are also engaged in a variety of motor behaviours either involving air motion, such as breath holding or deep breathing, phonation, coughing, sniffing and laughing, or which do not necessitate air motion, such as posture, locomotion, ballistic movements, deglutition or defaecation. This dual function — metabolic and behavioural — explains the organization of respiratory motoneurone command.

ANATOMICAL AND PHYSIOLOGICAL ORGANIZATION OF CENTRAL CONTROL OF RESPIRATION

The final common path to muscles is driven by separate inspiratory and expiratory pathways located in the spinal cord at the most ventral part of the lateral funiculus. In addition, motoneurones receive direct inputs from the pyramidal and extrapyramidal systems and from segmentary reflex afferents (Fig. 1).

Localization (Fig. 1) of the cell bodies of neurones giving rise to bulbo-spinal respiratory axons can only be accomplished by using electrophysiological methods; stimulation of descending inspiratory and expiratory pathways in the spinal cord triggers antidromic invasion of units firing spontaneously in phase with inspiration or expiration. These antidromically invaded respiratory neurones lie in two separate regions of the medulla, dorsally in the infrasolitarius nucleus and ventrally in the ambiguus and retro-ambigualis nuclei. In 95% of cases, the axons decussate below the obex; this explains the erroneous localization of the respiratory centre close to the midline reported by earlier authors who used lesions and stimulation methods.

The somata of bulbo-spinal neurones are surrounded by units phase-related to respiration which are not invaded antidromically; this leads to the conclusion that they represent respiratory interneurones. Other respiratory interneurones are widespread in the reticular formation where their density is lower than that of bulbo-spinal neurones and varies markedly according to the anaesthetic level. In the chronic or semichronic preparation, inspiratory and expiratory interneurones

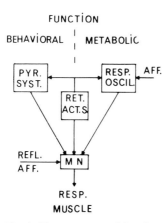

Fig. 1. Diagram summarizing the various inputs to motoneurones (MN) supplying respiratory muscle. PYR. SYST., pyramidal system; REFL. AFF., reflex afferents; RESP. OSCIL., respiratory oscillator(s); RET. ACT. S., reticular activating system.

constitute two separate uninterrupted columns of cells extending among non-respiratory units in the reticular formation from the caudal part of the bulb to the ponto-mesencephalic junction. The respiratory columns there reach the region of the pneumotaxic centre.

The pneumotaxic centre is located in the latero-dorsal tegmentum in the parabrachialis medialis and Kölliker-Fuse nuclei. At this level, the respiratory unit density increases markedly. Electrophysiological and anatomical studies using anterograde and retrograde transport of tracers have demonstrated direct connections between pneumotaxic and dorsal and ventral bulbar respiratory nuclei.

Although there is as yet no direct demonstration of the mechanism generating respiratory oscillation, indirect arguments strongly suggest that the origin of respiratory rhythm results from interaction of at least 4 subsystems of interneurones: (1) a trigger mechanism which switches on inspiration; (2) a ramp generator responsible for the increment of inspiratory discharge; (3) a cut off system which switches off inspiration and starts expiration; (4) one or several expiratory systems activating expiratory discharge and simultaneously keeping silent inspiratory neurones. Respiratory oscillation depends upon the segmental activation of these systems by operational oscillators.

The work of any neural oscillator critically depends on 2 components: a tonic input and a non-linear system which introduces periodicity. As a matter of fact, there is evidence for the existence of at least 3 non-linear systems responsible for respiratory oscillation. They are interrelated but have different characteristics. The first system is made up of the bulbo-spinal respiratory neurones and the Hering-Breuer reflex loop; it stops after opening of the reflex circuit or when the amplitude of respiratory movements is low. The second comprises the bulbo-spinal neurones and the pneumotaxic system; it can be eliminated by pontine lesions. The third system is made up of bulbo-spinal neurones and reticular interneurones; it is excluded by light anaesthesia and probably during slow wave sleep (SWS). These 3 oscillators normally work simultaneously, the observed respiratory frequency

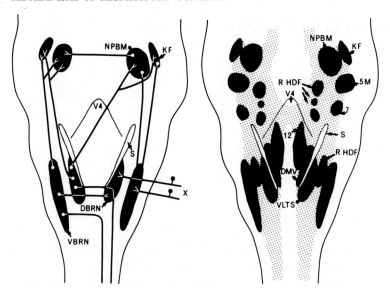

Fig. 2. Schematic representation of respiratory neurone (firing with a respiratory rhythm) topography as it appears from studies in deeply anaesthetized animals (left) and without anaesthesia (right). Neurones projecting onto spinal motoneurones and interconnections between the main respiratory nuclei are represented in the left diagram. Black areas: high density regions; dotted area: region of moderate density corresponding to the reticular core. In unanaesthetized preparations, high density regions are found widespread in the reticular formation and in the cranial nuclei having a respiratory function. DBRN, dorsal bulbar respiratory nucleus (n. infrasolitarius); DMV, dorsal motor nucleus of the vagus; KF, Kölliker-Fuse nucleus; NPBM, nucleus parabrachialis medialis; R HDF, reticular high density foci; S, tractus solitarius; VBRN, ventral bulbar respiratory nucleus (ambiguus); V4, fourth ventricle; 5M, motor trigeminal nucleus; 7, facial nucleus; 12, hypoglossal nucleus.

resulting from their coupling. However, in experimental or pathological conditions, each of them may oscillate alone.

Respiratory rhythmicity critically depends on tonic input influences which converge on the bulbar neurones and drive oscillation (Fig. 2). (1) The peripheral chemoreceptors located in the carotid and aortic bodies are sensitive to changes in blood CO_2 and O_2 content and pH level. (2) The central chemoreceptors located close to the ventral surface of the medulla are excited by H^+ ion concentration in the cerebrospinal fluid. (3) The reticular activating system activity depends upon the general level of excitation in both exteroceptive and interoceptive fields. (4) In addition, it has been shown recently that the pneumotaxic system itself possesses an intrinsic tonic activity contributing to the respiratory drive. The main characteristic of the tonic drive that came to light recently is that the various driving influences must summate to produce oscillation. For instance, decrease in reticular activity produced by very light pentobarbital anaesthesia leads to apnoea when associated with either decrease in central chemoreceptor drive due to metabolic alkalosis, or suppression of pneumotaxic drive by a lesion.

RESPIRATION DURING WAKEFULNESS AND SLEEP

The most convenient experimental situations for physiologists studying respiration consist in working with the awake human subject in a quiet stable environment, or with animals either deeply anaesthetized or decerebrate. Results of studies carried out in these oversimplified conditions brought a considerable body of knowledge in the past. However, it has recently become evident that respiration is markedly different in sleep and wakefulness and that the neural control of sleep states is a crucial determinant of respiratory activity. Several factors must be considered: (1) ventilation variations; (2) changes in respiratory reflexes according to the sleep-wakefulness state; (3) intensity of respiratory facilitation and (4) changes in respiratory reflexes resulting from arousal induced by asphyxia.

Ventilation changes and resulting variations in blood gas composition are currently observed during sleep. In SWS, breathing deepens and decreases in frequency. The rise in $PaCO_2$ observed simultaneously indicates that respiratory chemostat sensitivity decreases. When the animal shifts from SWS to rapid eye movement sleep (REMS), profound respiratory changes are observed. Erratic rapid shallow breathing replaces the regular large amplitude low frequency rhythm, leading to hyperventilation. The appearance of the REM respiratory rhythm is associated with the phasic motor outbursts characteristic of REMS.

At the same time, the respiratory system responds poorly to inhalation of CO_2 and to hypoxic stimuli. These observations raise the question of whether the respiratory pattern generator prevailing during the waking state and SWS is replaced or driven by the still unknown brain stem structure responsible for phasic movements during REMS.

An arousal reaction due to reticular activating system excitation produces a typical respiratory response. It consists of decreased expiratory duration with

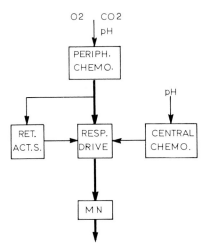

Fig. 3. Origin of the respiratory drive to motoneurones (oscillatory loop not represented). The respiratory centre itself is supposed to be inherently tonically excited.

inhibition of expiratory discharge, resulting in acceleration of respiratory rate, increased instantaneous air flow during inspiration due to increased recruitment of inspiratory neurones and a variable effect on inspiration amplitude according to its initial value. The inspiratory facilitatory response to arousal is characteristically different from the respiratory response to hypercapnia or asphyxia, which always associates facilitation of inspiration and expiration.

The threshold and intensity of respiratory, as well as other somatic and vegetative, components of arousal vary markedly with the sleep state. Arousal is easily induced during drowsiness and – to a lesser extent – during SWS. In contrast, during REMS, the threshold of arousal is increased several-fold. It is noteworthy that arousal is produced by changes in external environment and *milieu intérieur* composition as well. Thus a rise in $PaCO_2$, hypoxia, lowering of blood pH and asphyxia all induce a general arousal reaction with resultant respiratory arousal. Consequently, apnoea, which always results in transient asphyxia, ends when asphyxic arousal occurs.

Respiratory reflexes normally coordinate mutually exclusive acts such as breathing and swallowing. The most important reflexes are triggered by irritant receptors located in the nose, larynx, pharynx and trachea. Irritant receptor stimulation in the larynx typically produces an apnoeic response with closure of the glottis and bradycardia, reminiscent of the diving reflex. The sleep-wakefulness state profoundly influences these reflexes. The apnoeic reflex to laryngeal stimulation does not occur in the waking state: in the awake subject weak stimulation of irritant receptors induced by water or instillation of certain chemicals in the larynx, triggers an expiratory reflex followed by coughing. Similarly, during SWS, weak stimulation produces an expiration reflex, whereas strong stimulation produces arousal followed by coughing. In contrast, strong stimuli occurring during REMS do not induce an expiration reflex, arousal and coughing but apnoea associated with bradycardia. In the case of very strong stimulation apnoea persists, sometimes until death, unless the arousal reaction and coughing occur.

IMPLICATIONS IN NEWBORN SLEEP APNOEA

Through active research carried out during recent years, the mechanisms of sleep apnoea are now well documented. Schematically there exist two main causes of apnoea during sleep. When the respiratory rhythm generator stops, cessation of breathing is referred to as "central respiratory apnoea." Alternatively, in "upper airway obstructive apnoea," the air traffic is interrupted, while activity of the respiratory rhythm generator is on-going.

Central respiratory apnoea generally occurs during SWS, when the reticular respiratory drive decreases. It may be terminated by a shift from SWS to either arousal or REMS. As stated above, several driving influences summate to set in action the respiratory rhythm generator. Oscillation stops when several (at least two) driving influences are withdrawn. This occurs typically in Ondine's curse: in the case of chronic alteration of chemoreceptor sensitivity to carbon dioxide and pH, the additional decrease in reticular driving influence during SWS induces hypo-ventilation and apnoea. In the newborn, chronic hypoxaemia – due, for instance, to narrow airways – produces lesions of the lateral upper pons in the region where the pneumotaxic system is located. A deficit in the tonic drive exerted normally by the pneumotaxic system, associated firstly with a decrease in the driving influence of the reticular formation during SWS and secondly with a lower responsiveness of the reticular formation to hypoxic stimuli may explain the occurrence of central sleep apnoea in neonates.

Obstruction of the pharynx by the tongue due to the drastic decrease in muscle tone during REMS, explains apnoea in adults sleeping in the supine position. In newborns, obstructive sleep apnoea is most frequently produced by the apnoeic reflex originating in the upper airway. An interesting point is that the apnoeic reflex is particularly pronounced in newborn animals and is still stronger in preterm subjects. After birth its magnitude diminishes with age. These facts may suggest the decline of a normal reflex appropriate to an intrauterine liquid environment. In newborn lambs, in which reflex asphyxial death is readily observed, it occurs always during REMS, when the threshold to arousal markedly increases. Death occurs when asphyxia fails to produce arousal and coughing.

Kyoto Symposia (EEG Suppl. No. 36)
Editors: P.A. Buser, W.A. Cobb and T. Okuma
© 1982, Elsevier Biomedical Press, Amsterdam

Respiratory Pauses in Normal Infants and in Siblings of Victims of the Sudden Infant Death Syndrome

R. FLORES-GUEVARA[1], L. CURZI-DASCALOVA[2], M.F. RADVANYI[2],
P. PLOUIN[3], B. STERNBERG[4], R. PERAITA[5], S. GUIDASCI[6] and
N. MONOD[7]

Centre de Recherches de Biologie du Développement Foetal et Néonatal, INSERM U 29, Hôpital Port-Royal, 123, boulevard de Port-Royal, 75014 Paris (France)

In recent years interest in polygraphic studies of apnoea in normal infants has been growing (Parmelee et al. 1972; Monod et al. 1976; Gould et al. 1977; Hoppenbrouwers et al. 1977; Stein et al. 1979; Ellingson et al. 1982), partly as a result of the hypothesis that sleep apnoea plays a role in the sudden infant death syndrome (SIDS) (Steinschneider 1972). Siblings of infants who have been victims of the sudden infant death syndrome are at a 4–5 times increased risk of SIDS (Froggatt et al. 1970).

Hoppenbrouwers et al. (1976) reported that at 3 months of age a group of siblings exhibited a decreased total incidence of central apnoea during night-time recording. Conversely Nogues and Samson-Dollfus (1979) and Guilhaume et al. (1981) have found a higher incidence of central apnoea in siblings than in controls during half-night or all-night studies. The present study focussed on a comparison between respiratory pauses in control babies and SIDS siblings during daytime polygraph recording sessions, and an attempt was made to assess the risk of severe apnoeic episodes or death in the group of siblings.

MATERIAL AND METHODS

Daytime polygraphic records were made from 57 normal infants and from 100 siblings of victims of SIDS, studied at different ages: during the first 5 weeks of life, 6th–9th, 10th–13th, and 14th–17th weeks. Most infants were subjected to only one recording. The total number of records was 68 for controls and 130 for siblings.

This work was supported by Grants C.L. 77.5.034-4 from INSERM and CRL CNAMTS, 1980.

[1]Maternité de Port-Royal.
[2]Chargé de Recherche INSERM.
[3]Hôpital St. Vincent-de-Paul.
[4]Hôpital International de la Cité Universitaire.
[5]Boursière du Gouvernement Français.
[6]Technicienne INSERM.
[7]Maître de Recherche INSERM.

Daytime records from 69 SIDS siblings were compared to all-night records (20.00–08.00) from 51 other SIDS siblings.

All infants were full-term: 38–42 weeks gestational age (GA). GAs were determined precisely according to criteria described in a previous paper (Flores-Guevara et al. 1982).

Polygraphic records were made with babies dressed normally and in their cribs at room temperature of 25–26°C. Records were made either in the morning or around noon between 2 feeds with the babies sleeping in the supine or prone position. The polygraphic recording technique has already been described by Flores-Guevara et al. (1982). All records included at least one full sleep cycle with periods of active sleep (AS) and quiet sleept (QS) of more than 10 min duration. Most included 2 or more sleep cycles.

Interpretation of the records focussed on analysis of the sleep states and quantification of respiratory apnoeas. Sleep was scored every 20 sec and differentiated according to the method already described (Monod et al. 1976; Flores-Guevara et al. 1982).

Sleep analysis

Percentage of total sleep time (TST) with respect to total recording time (TRT) and percentages of AS, QS and transitional or indeterminate sleep (IS) with respect to TST were studied.

Apnoea analysis

Central respiratory apnoea (simultaneous interruption of the signals in all respiratory channels) was measured in seconds from the end of expiration until the signal resumed (Fig. 1). We considered apnoeas of 2 sec and longer duration. Measurements of obstructive apnoea were based on the common arrest of the nasal, oral and laryngeal flow signals, while thoracic and abdominal respiration signals persisted. The measurement of mixed apnoea included the length of the central apnoea and that of the obstructive part of the non-breathing episode. The numbers and the durations of the apnoeas were counted by 20 sec epochs.

Three different measurements were obtained on central apnoea in AS, QS, IS and in TST: (1) apnoea index (AI) represents the percentage of non-breathing time and is calculated by dividing the total minutes of central apnoea (≥ 2 sec) during a sleep stage by the total minutes of the sleep stage and multiplying the result by 100; (2) number of apnoeas (NA) per 100 min of the sleep stage was determined for apnoeas of 2–4.9 sec, ≥ 5 sec, ≥ 6 sec, and ≥ 10 sec duration; (3) the percentage time spent in periodic breathing (PB) (defined as 2 apnoeas of 3 sec or more per 20 sec of recording during one continuous minute) was also determined for each stage of sleep.

Statistical studies

The non-parametric Mann-Whitney test was used to compare control babies and SIDS siblings at various ages. Comparisons were also made on the basis of GA

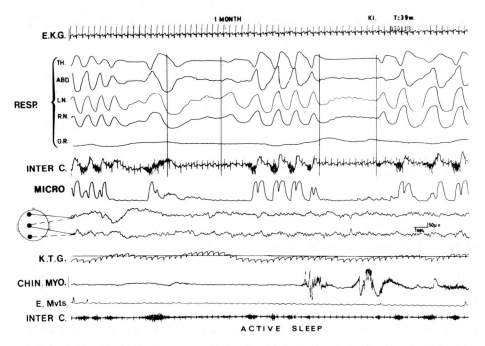

Fig. 1. Two central respiratory pauses in active sleep (AS) seen in all respiratory channels. RESP., respiration; TH., thoracic movements; ABD., abdominal movements; L.N., left nasal flow; R.N., right nasal flow; O.R., oral flow; INTER C., intercostal electromyogram; MICRO, microphone; K.T.G., instantaneous heart rate; Chin MYO., chin electromyogram; E. Mvts, rapid eye movements; INTER C. (lower channel), filtered intercostal electromyogram activity.

during the first 5 weeks. In each age group only one record per infant was considered.

RESULTS

(1) Normative studies

Preparatory to studying pathological children normative data are essential. A study of the first 52 control infants has been published elsewhere (Flores-Guevara et al. 1982).

The AI and the numbers of apnoeas of < 5 sec were higher in AS than in QS during the period studied. A decrease of AI and NA occurred before the end of the 2nd month both in AS and QS. During the first 5 weeks of life the AI, the NA, and the per cent time of PB were higher in infants born at 38–39 weeks GA than in infants born at 40–42 weeks.

Apnoeas ≥ 10 sec were infrequent, and were an exception beyond the first month. No apnoea longer than 14 sec was observed. A positive correlation between short apnoeas (< 5 sec) and apnoeas ≥ 5 sec was found in AS and in TST. Obstructive and mixed apnoeas were very infrequent. There was great interindividual variability of NA, particularly during the 1st month of life.

Our present results, including 57 infants, confirm the previous study. In addition, the present study has yielded normative data for the 4th month of life (see below).

(2) Comparative study of siblings of victims of SIDS

The results obtained in control babies are compared to those of SIDS siblings born at the same GAs.

Sleep analysis

TST of control babies and SIDS siblings is not different except for infants born at ⩾ 40 weeks of GA during the first week of life when siblings sleep less than control infants. There is no significant difference in percentages of AS and of QS between the 2 groups of infants at any age.

Apnoea analysis

(1) Apnoea index. In AS during the first 5 weeks the mean AIs in controls and SIDS siblings are nearly identical (Table I). If GA is taken into consideration siblings born at 38–39 weeks have significantly lower AIs than control subjects, and those born at 40 weeks and over have significantly higher AIs than control babies (Fig. 2). Moreover, in contrast with control infants there is no significant AI difference between SIDS siblings born at < 40 weeks and those born at ⩾ 40 weeks.

As shown in Table I, siblings have 4 times higher AIs than do control infants between the 6th and 9th weeks. The AI remains slightly higher in siblings at 10–13 weeks but this difference disappears in the group at 14–17 weeks.

In QS, AI is not significantly different in controls vs. siblings except for the group at 6–9 weeks ($P < 0.004$) with higher AIs in siblings.

(2) Number of apnoeas. In AS there is no significant difference in NA (all

TABLE I

APNOEA INDEX IN ACTIVE SLEEP IN CONTROLS AND SIBLINGS

For all tables: n, number of subjects; x̄, mean; S.E.M., standard error of the mean; *P,* degree of significance.

Infants	1st − 5th week				6th − 9th week				10th − 13th week				14th − 17th week			
	n	x̄	S.E.M.	*P*	n	x̄	S.E.M.	*P*	n	x̄	S.E.M.	*P*	n	x̄	S.E.M.	*P*
Controls	35	5.7	± 1		15	0.9	± 0.2		11	1.6	± 1		7	4.5	± 2	
				NS				0.0001				0.04				NS
Siblings	70	5.4	± 0.5		37	4.1	± 0.8		14	2.7	± 0.7		9	3	± 0.9	

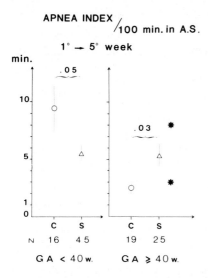

Fig. 2. Apnoea index (mean and standard error of the mean) in active sleep (AS) during the first 5 weeks of life. Difference according to gestational age. Controls (C) born at 38–39 weeks GA have a higher apnoea index than siblings (S) of the same GA. On the contrary controls born at or after 40 weeks GA have a lower apnoea index than siblings of the same GA. N, number of infants recorded in each group. Stars indicate the apnoea index of 2 siblings who subsequently had severe apnoeic episodes.

TABLE II

NUMBER OF APNOEAS OF DIFFERENT DURATIONS IN ACTIVE SLEEP IN CONTROLS AND SIBLINGS

Age	Infants	n	< 5 sec			≥ 5 sec			≥ 10 sec		
			$\bar{x}$	S.E.M.	P	$\bar{x}$	S.E.M.	P	$\bar{x}$	S.E.M.	P
1st − 5th week	Controls	35	63	± 8		27	± 7		0.7	± 0.3	
					NS			NS			NS
	Siblings	70	70	± 6		21	± 3		0.6	± 0.2	
6th − 9th week	Controls	15	13	± 3		1.6	± 1		0	0	
					0.0002			0.001			−
	Siblings	37	60	± 8		13.8	± 2		0	0	
10th − 13th week	Controls	11	26	± 10		4.2	± 4		0.3	± 0.3	
					0.03			NS			NS
	Siblings	14	51	± 11		5.6	± 2		0	0	
14th − 17th week	Controls	7	58	± 20		11	± 5		0	0	
					NS			NS			−
	Siblings	9	50	± 12		13	± 7		0	0	

TABLE III

NUMBER OF < 5 SEC AND ⩾ 5 SEC APNOEAS IN ACTIVE SLEEP ACCORDING TO GESTATIONAL AGE (GA) DURING THE FIRST 5 WEEKS OF LIFE IN CONTROLS AND SIBLINGS

GA	Infants	n	< 5 sec apnoea			⩾ 5 sec apnoea		
			$\bar{x}$	S.E.M.	P	$\bar{x}$	S.E.M.	P
< 40 weeks	Controls	16	94	± 12	NS	51	± 13	0.05
	Siblings	45	75	± 7		21	± 3	
⩾ 40 weeks	Controls	19	38	± 6	0.03	8	± 3	0.02
	Siblings	25	63	± 9		22	± 5	

categories considered) during the first 5 weeks (Table II). But if GA and duration of apnoea are taken into consideration: (1) siblings born at < 40 weeks have significantly lower scores for NAs of ⩾ 5 sec than do controls; (2) siblings born at ⩾ 40 weeks GA have significantly much higher NAs of all durations, < 5 sec and ⩾ 5 sec (Table III).

As shown in Table II, between the 6th and 9th weeks a highly significant difference is found for respiratory pauses of any category under 10 sec duration between controls and siblings, the higher incidence being for siblings. At 10–13 weeks a significant difference persists only for pauses < 5 sec, but not at 14–17 weeks.

In QS there is no significant difference in NA at any age except for the 6–9 week group. At this age respiratory pauses are significantly more frequent in siblings than

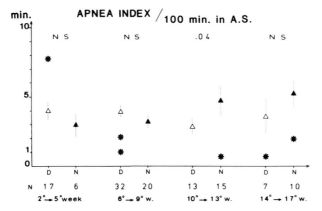

Fig. 3. Comparison between apnoea index (mean and standard error of the mean) of day time (white triangle, D) and night time recording (black triangle, N) in siblings. Stars represent the apnoea index of 5 children recorded between 2 and 17 weeks who subsequently had severe apnoeic episodes. The 2 stars at the right part of the figure belong to the same child recorded in a morning nap and the following night; a severe apnoeic episode occurred 1 month later.

in control babies for < 5 sec apnoeas ($P < 0.004$) and for $\geqslant 5$ sec apnoeas ($P < 0.01$).

(3) *Periodic breathing and obstructive apnoea.* The 2 groups of infants show no significant differences in the mean incidence of periodic breathing (less than 3% TST) nor in obstructive apnoea (less than 2 per 100 min of AS) at any age and at any state of sleep.

Day/night recording comparison in SIDS siblings (Fig. 3)

During the first 2 months, AI and NA are not significantly higher during the daytime than during night time recording. On the contrary, during the 3rd month AI is significantly higher in overnight recording ($P < 0.04$). All categories of pauses are more frequent in night records than in day records at this age. Particularly, pauses $\geqslant 6$ sec are significantly more frequent ($P < 0.01$) in night records (7.03 ± 10) than in day records (1.95 ± 2.5). During the 4th month a significant difference is not found. As shown in Fig. 3, daytime or night time AIs of 5 siblings that subsequently had severe apnoeic episodes were not very different from AIs of the other siblings or from AIs of control babies in daytime records (see Table I).

DISCUSSION

Our results show that between the 6th and 13th weeks of life respiratory pauses are significantly more frequent during morning naps in SIDS siblings than in control subjects. This difference seems to disappear after the 13th week, but these results must be confirmed as our last age group (14–17 weeks) was small, because infants at this age do not sleep sufficiently long in the morning.

It is interesting to note that in control babies AI shows an evolution with a fall between 1–5 weeks and 6–9 weeks, and a progressive increase beyond the last age. On the contrary, there is a remarkable stability of AI in siblings during all the periods studied (Table I). NA also evolves differently in the 2 groups of infants.

It is known that polygraphic recording involves an increase in peripheral afferent stimulation. Does such stimulation decrease, at a certain level of maturation, the number of respiratory pauses by triggering a central respiratory mechanism? Are SIDS siblings less sensitive to such stimulation than control infants during the 2nd and 3rd months of life? These hypotheses could explain the significant differences in AI and NA between control babies and siblings at 6–13 weeks.

On the other hand, why does the number of respiratory pauses increase in control babies after this age? Is the depth or shallowness of AS modified at this age? This could be tested by determining whether the number of micro-awakenings and crying episodes during sleep are different before and after 13 weeks. Such a study has not been done. Another possible explanation is that an inhibitory mechanism effecting respiratory pauses appears between 6 and 13 weeks and then becomes less effective after 13 weeks. In a recent study Haddad et al. (1981) compared control infants and aborted crib death infants. They showed that maximum differences in tidal volume and in other ventilatory variables are seen at 2 months and disappear by 3 months. This would support the last hypothesis.

Whatever the explanation, it is notable that this difference between the 2 groups of infants occurs at the same age at which sleep spindles appear. We have also seen previously that other parameters of sleep change at this age, for example the distribution of spontaneous skin galvanic responses in sleep (Curzi-Dascalova and Dreyfus-Brisac 1976).

In another regard, Fig. 2 shows that control infants born at < 40 weeks GA, recorded between their 1st and 5th weeks of life, have significantly higher AI than SIDS siblings. Infants born at ⩾ 40 weeks GA show the opposite result.

Some maturational change in respiratory mechanisms may occur during the 2 last weeks of gestation in controls which does not occur in SIDS siblings. We have no hypothesis as to why SIDS siblings at 38–39 weeks GA show fewer pauses than controls of the same GA.

Our results, as far as NA are concerned, are in contradiction to those of Hoppenbrouwers et al. (1976, 1980), who found no difference between overnight records of control babies and SIDS siblings of the same ages, or even fewer apnoeas in siblings than in controls. It must be noted that there were differences in the recording techniques and the methods of analysis between the Hoppenbrouwers et al. study and ours. Could circadian organization of sleep respiratory pauses be responsible for this contradiction? As noted in Fig. 3, during the first 2 months AIs in siblings are not significantly higher during the daytime than during overnight records. After the 2nd month, on the contrary, AIs are higher during night records than during day records. Thus, circadian organization of sleep respiratory pauses is not responsible for these conflicting results. However, the distribution of respiratory pauses during the nycthemer in control infants is not known. On the contrary, our results are consistent with those of Nogues and Samson-Dollfus (1979), who also found more respiratory pauses in siblings than in controls during the first third of the night between 2 and 12 months of age. Perhaps this difference could diminish during the rest of the night or even become inverted. Thus, this could be in accordance with Hoppenbrouwers' results. However, Guilhaume et al. (1981) also found more apnoeas in siblings than in controls during overnight recording, between 1 and 5 months of age.

Concerning PB, we have found no difference between controls and SIDS siblings at any age. This is different from the results of Kelly et al. (1980). They found more PB in SIDS siblings than in controls. It must be pointed out that they recorded overnight cardiorespirograms at home, which involves less afferent stimulation than does polygraphy.

Six babies had, after their records, more or less severe apnoeic episodes, but only 2 required resuscitation manoeuvres. The nature of the events in the others was not clearly specified. No baby in this study died from SIDS.

Our conclusions from these preliminary results are that:

1. Between the 6th and 13th weeks of life respiratory pauses are significantly more frequent in sudden infant death syndrome siblings than in control subjects. This

difference seems to disappear after the 13th week but further studies of infants after this age are needed.

2. No difference was found between SIDS siblings who subsequently presented with an apnoeic episode and SIDS siblings who did not. To date, it appears that polygraphic records do not yield information which permits accurate estimation of the risks of future apnoeic episodes, regardless of whether day or night records are considered.

SUMMARY

Sleep polygraphic recording was carried out on 57 normal infants and on 100 SIDS siblings during morning naps between birth and the 4th month of life. Total sleep time and duration of sleep stages were determined.

Central apnoeas of 2 sec and longer duration were analysed in AS, QS and IS.

Apnoea index and number of apnoeas per 100 min of sleep stage were determined. Obstructive and mixed apnoeas were tabulated separately. Percentage of periodic breathing was also determined.

Control babies and SIDS siblings were compared on these parameters, using the Mann-Whitney test.

Between the 6th and 13th weeks of life respiratory pauses were significantly more frequent in SIDS siblings than in control subjects. The difference disappeared after the 13th week.

The roles that peripheral afferents and the circadian organization of respiratory pauses play in determining the results are discussed.

This technique does not appear to permit estimation of the risk of subsequent apnoeic episodes.

REFERENCES

Curzi-Dascalova, L. and Dreyfus-Brisac, C. Distribution of skin potential response according to states of sleep during the first months of life in human babies. Electroenceph. clin. Neurophysiol., 1976, 41: 399–407.

Ellingson, R.J., Peters, J.F. and Nelson, B. Respiratory pauses and apnea during daytime sleep in normal infants during the first year of life: longitudinal observations. Electroenceph. clin. Neurophysiol., 1982, 53: 48–59.

Flores-Guevara, R., Plouin, P., Curzi-Dascalova, L., Radvanyi, M.F., Guidasci, S., Pajot, N. and Monod, N. Sleep apnea in normal neonates and infants during the first 3 months of life. Neuropediatrics, 1982, 13 (Suppl.): 21–28.

Froggatt, P. The contribution of epidemiology to the study of the sudden infant death syndrome. In: A.B. Bergman et al. (Eds.), Sudden Infant Death Syndrome. Univ. of Washington Press, Seattle, Wash., 1970: 25–31.

Gould, J.B., Lee, A.F.S., James, O., Sander, L., Teager, H. and Fineberg, N. The sleep state characteristics of apnea during infancy. Pediatrics, 1977, 59: 182–194.

Guilhaume, A., Navelet, Y. et Benoit, O. Les pauses respiratoires dans le sommeil nocturne du nourrisson. Arch. franç. Pédiat., 1981, 38: 673–677.

Haddad, G.G., Leistner, H.L., Lai, T.L. and Mellins, R.B. Ventilation and ventilatory pattern during sleep in aborted sudden infant death syndrome. Pediat. Res., 1981, 15: 879–883.

Hoppenbrouwers, T., Hodgman, J.E., Harper, R.M., McGinty, D.J. and Sterman, M.B. Incidence of apnea in infants at high and low risk for sudden infant death syndrome (S.I.D.S.). Pediat. Res., 1976, 10: 425

Hoppenbrouwers, T., Hodgman, J.E., Harper, R.M., Hofman, E., Sterman, M.B. and McGinty, D.J. Polygraphic studies of normal infants during the first six months of life. III. Incidence of apnea and periodic breathing. Pediatrics, 1977, 60: 418–425.

Hoppenbrouwers, T., Hodgman, J.E., McGinty, D., Harper, R.M. and Sterman, M.B. Sudden infant death syndrome sleep apnea and respiration in subsequent siblings. Pediatrics, 1980, 66: 205–214.

Kelly, D.H., Walker, A.M., Cahen, L. and Shannon, D.C. Periodic breathing in siblings of sudden infant death syndrome victims. Pediatrics, 1980, 66: 515–520.

Monod, N., Curzi-Dascalova, L., Guidasci, S. et Valenzuela, S. Pauses respiratoires et sommeil chez le nouveau-né et le nourrisson. Rev. E.E.G. Neurophysiol., 1976, 6: 105–110.

Nogues, B. et Samson-Dollfus, D. Etude comparative de la respiration pendant le sommeil chez des bébés témoins et des bébés à risque de mort subite (enfants de 2 mois à 1 an). Waking Sleeping, 1979, 3: 263–271.

Parmelee, A.H., Stern, E. and Harris, M.A. Maturation of respiration in prematures and young infants. Neuropädiatrie, 1972, 3: 294–304.

Stein, I.M., White, A., Kennedy, Jr., J.L., Merisalo, R.L., Chernoff, H. and Gould, J.B. Apnea recordings of healthy infants at 40, 44 and 52 weeks postconception. Pediatrics, 1979, 63: 724–730.

Steinschneider, A. Prolonged apnea and the sudden infant death syndrome: Clinical and laboratory observations. Pediatrics, 1972, 50: 646–654.

Kyoto Symposia (EEG Suppl. No. 36)
Editors: P.A. Buser, W.A. Cobb and T. Okuma
© 1982, Elsevier Biomedical Press, Amsterdam

Near Miss Sudden Infant Death Infants: a Summary of Findings (1972–1981)

CHRISTIAN GUILLEMINAULT and SUSAN COONS

Stanford Sleep Disorders Center, Stanford University School of Medicine, Stanford, Calif. (U.S.A.)

During the past 10 years, great attention has been given to infants who present breathing problems of unexplained origin during sleep. These infants have been called "near miss for sudden infant death syndrome" or "NMSIDS" infants. This label is based not only on objective criteria, but also on the belief of an observer (usually the parent) that the infant had experienced an episode in which its death was imminent and was "nearly missed." The hypothesis that sleep apnoea may play a significant role in SIDS has been considered by several authors and has led to specific evaluations of NMSIDS infants with the hope of gaining more insight into this syndrome.

Our own group has studied NMSIDS infants since 1972. Over 200 full-term infants have been monitored polygraphically for 24 h sessions during the past 9 years. The results are presented here.

STUDY POPULATION

All NMSIDS infants were referred to the SIDS research team at the Stanford University Medical Center. We considered an infant to be NMSIDS if an event was reported by a caretaker during which the infant was apnoeic, pale or cyanotic, limp, and requiring either vigorous stimulation or cardiopulmonary resuscitation. Most infants were thought to be asleep at the time of the event. Sixty-eight percent had been given mouth-to-mouth resuscitation by a parent before reaching a hospital.

All infants were evaluated initially in an emergency room or by their family paediatrician soon after the event. They were hospitalized and had blood count, blood glucose, electrolytes, calcium and phosphate estimations, chest X-rays, electrocardiograms (ECG) and electroencephalograms (EEG). If no obvious clinical cause such as sepsis, seizure, hypoglycaemia, primary pulmonary or cardiac abnormality could be found, the babies were referred to the SIDS research team for further evaluation. We have systematically eliminated from this report infants who were premature, regardless of the age at which the "near miss" event occurred. All infants were full term and had experienced no problems before the second week of

Address correspondence to: Christian Guilleminault, M.D., Stanford Sleep Disorders Center, TD114, Stanford University Medical Center, Stanford, Calif. 94305, U.S.A.

life at the earliest. Infants presented near miss episodes between 3 weeks and 8 months of age. The mean age was 7.8 weeks, the median age was 6.2 weeks. Depending on the year in which the infant was seen by us, various research protocols were used for evaluation. Thus, data obtained from some of the infant groups have already been published.

METHODS

Recording procedures

After informed consent had been obtained from the parents and approval from the referring physician, all infants were monitored under similar conditions. Mothers slept in the recording area and were present during the monitoring to give their infant routine care. Initial monitoring lasted 24 h for 79% of the infants, between 16 and 21 for 20%, and 12 h in 1% of the cases.

Variables monitored included: EEG (C_3/A_2-C_4/A_1 of the 10-20 system); electro-oculogram (EOG); chin EMG; ECG, lead II; respiration, measured by abdominal and thoracic strain gauges (respiratory effort) and oral and nasal thermistors (airflow). Depending on the protocol used and the year in which the study was performed, the following variables were sometimes monitored: percentage expired CO_2 by means of a nasal or oral catheter (Beckman $LBCO_2$ analyser); blood oxygen saturation (Waters Instrument Co. ear oximeter or Litton Co. transcutaneous pO_2 electrode); oesophageal pH obtained with a probe placed well above the gastro-oesophageal sphincter under fluoroscopy. A 24 h "ambulatory" Holter ECG recording was used in many cases.

Behaviour was systematically coded on the record in all cases. Notations were made of jerks, twitches, eye movements, vocalizations, snores, sucking, gross body movements, etc. Artifacts were checked systematically at all times.

Neurological evaluation

At the time of the recording, a developmentally oriented neurological evaluation was performed (St. Anne Dargassies 1974). We used the neurological assessment form described by Amiel-Tison (1976) for all evaluations performed after 1976. Four physicians were involved in the neurological evaluation of the NMSIDS infant group.

CONTROL POPULATION

A control population was gathered in relation to 2 specific research protocols. The monitoring techniques used in both cases were the same as those described for the NMSIDS infants. The first control group, studied between 1974 and 1976, included 12 full-term infants. The second group, studied between 1977 and 1979, included 31 infants. The data obtained from the second group were placed on a PDP 11/34 computer and subsequently were used in several research protocols. All normal controls were full-term infants. The parents of the control infants were residents of the San Francisco Bay area and were in the lower-middle to upper-middle income bracket, coincidentally equivalent to the income range among the majority of the NMSIDS infants' parents. Criteria for controls included that the family history for hereditary diseases or SIDS siblings was negative, that the parents were in good health, that pregnancy and delivery had been normal, and that the infant's growth and development had been within normal range. These infants were followed, and in most cases underwent several (2–3) recordings. They continued to be classified as "flow risk controls" regardless of monitored findings and their health status at follow-up consultations.

RESULTS

One hundred and ninety-eight NMSIDS infants were tabulated. Nine infants, seen between 1972 and 1975, were not included in the analysis because too little information about them was available.

Number of deaths in the studied group

We are aware of 5 deaths in the NMSIDS group and none in the control group. The 5 deaths all occurred between 1972 and 1977. Since that time, not a single death has been reported. Of the 5 deaths, only one was given an extensive research evaluation just prior to death and a very thorough anatomical investigation, involving special techniques and a serial brain section, after death (Guilleminault et al. 1979a). None of the other autopsy protocols were performed at Stanford. Two infants had an anatomical examination with samples (particularly brain) sent to specialists for examination. Two infants underwent a general autopsy protocol performed by the county coroner. All infants were classified as having died from sudden infant death syndrome.

Home monitoring and death

Between 1972 and mid-1977, our infants were not systematically sent home with a monitoring system. The attitude of private paediatricians in our community toward home monitoring varied greatly during that period. Since 1977, 99% of the NMSIDS infants have been placed under home monitors. The home monitor prescribed for our population is both a cardiac and respiratory monitoring system. The criteria for use of home monitors and the protocol for follow-up of infant and family have not changed since we began using them. Three physicians only have been involved in prescribing these home monitors since 1972.

One of the 5 NMSIDS infants who subsequently died of SIDS was under a home monitor. When the monitor alarm sounded, the parents initiated cardiopulmonary resuscitation (CPR), a technique taught to all parents whose infants we placed under home monitor. The emergency paramedical team noted that the infant presented repetitive apnoea. The infant died during transport.

Home monitoring and severe, repetitive near miss events*

We have reliable data for the period of 1977 to the present only. Of 103 infants, 39% presented a repeat near miss event, noted by either parents or health-related personnel, which necessitated immediate intervention and CPR. These severe repeat near miss episodes were noted within 5 weeks of the original event in 32% of the cases; the other 7% presented their repeat event up to 3.5 months after the initial event. In all cases but one, the infants presented monitored alarms regularly between the initial near miss event and the second severe episode. However, none of these alarms had required CPR.

Polygraphic monitoring results

(1) General results

Apnoea was seen during sleep in all NMSIDS infants at the time of recording; however, when comparisons with normal control infant groups were made, there was an overlap between the results in the control group and 17% of the NMSIDS group. We have already reported that "periodic breathing" – as defined by Parmelee et al. (1972) – and central apnoea do not help in statistically differentiating control and NMSIDS infant groups (Guilleminault et al. 1979b). In some cases, very long central apnoeas were seen in several NMSIDS infants, but we emphasize that these were too few to have statistical impact on group differentiation. Mixed and obstructive apnoea did differentiate the 2 populations. This finding is still accurate at the present time; however, it is the groups and not the individuals which are differentiated.

If we consider the subsequent SIDS death group, and the severe repeat near miss group, the following results are seen.

(A) SIDS (deceased infants)

One infant had a normal polysomnogram. The other 4 were considered to be abnormal, compared to normative data. One of these 4 presented long central apnoea of up to 30 sec duration (30 sec is the limit tolerated for apnoea during polysomnographic recording before intervention is initiated). The 3 others presented a predominance of mixed and obstructive apnoeic events, none of which was longer than 15 sec.

(B) Severe repeat near miss episodes

All had abnormal polygraphic records compared to controls, but most of them

---

*We are greatly indebted to M. Owen-Boeddiker, R.N., who obtained these data.

did not present particularly long apnoeic events. Rather, they presented a greater number of events than did controls.

(2) Results of sleep analyses

In all our group comparisons, total sleep time (TST) has never shown statistical differences. However, NMSIDS infants always appeared to be behaviourally more "sleepy" than controls. Analysis of body movement time indicated that a statistically significant difference ($P < 0.01$, paired t test) existed between NMSIDS infant and control groups.

(3) Results from study of the development of the longest sleep period over age

A recent study (Coons and Guilleminault 1982) was performed in which the progressive development of wakefulness and sleep over several months in normals and NMSIDS infants was examined, using the accumulated polygraphic data. During the first 4.5 months of life there is normally a progressive coalescence of sleep, with the development of NREM sleep stages and wakefulness. The longest sleep period becomes progressively nocturnal; by 4.5 months this pattern is established clearly in normals but is still lacking in NMSIDS infants (see Fig. 1).

The results obtained from studies of body movement and circadian development of the sleep-waking pattern indicate a significant developmental difference between NMSIDS and normal control infants.

(4) Results from study of apnoea distribution during sleep

When all sleep periods over 24 h are considered, and an analysis is made of the apnoea distribution in each independent period, it appears that there is an increase in the number of apnoeas seen per sleep hour over time; i.e., the greater the amount of preceding sleep within a sleep period, the greater the number of apnoeas seen.

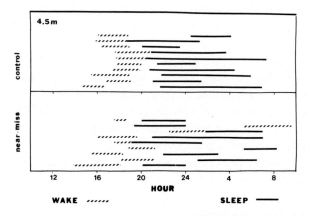

Fig. 1. Distribution of longest sleep and waking periods at 4.5 months of age in an NMSIDS group compared to a normal control group. As is clearly shown in the figure, NMSIDS infants still present a scattered distribution of their longest sleep and waking periods, as would normally be seen in younger infants. In control infants patterns have stabilized by the age of 4.5 months.

When apnoea did not appear to be distributed evenly, an analysis was performed to discover the relationship between arousal from sleep and apnoea distribution. All sleep periods were again considered, having been normalized to their terminal awakening. By definition, all infants were asleep before arousal, and the percentage of the population asleep decreases with time from awakening. The distribution of apnoeic pauses is again noted to be uneven over the sleep period, with a sharp increase just prior to awakening. If one compares the apnoeas in the last 10 min before awakening with those in the remaining TST by a matched pairs t test, a statistically significant difference ($P \leqslant 0.01$) is seen. The frequency of mixed and obstructive apnoeic events is significantly higher within the 10 min before any awakening than during the remaining sleep (Guilleminault et al. 1981).

(5) Negative results

Interestingly, polygraphic monitoring never revealed a long Q-T syndrome in any NMSIDS infant. Also, there was no frequent association between gastro-oesophageal reflux and apnoea. Of 52 cases, only one presented an association between central apnoea and reflux. Furthermore, there was no correlation between the severity or the total number of apnoeic events and gastro-oesophageal reflux (Ariagno et al. 1981).

(6) Results from the developmental neurological examinations

We have already reported (Korobkin and Guilleminault 1979) that 41 NMSIDS infants, studied under one research protocol and seen when under the age of 3 months, consistently presented abnormalities of muscle tone, particularly shoulder hypotonia. These abnormalities disappeared with maturation. Systematic developmental neurological examinations were performed at the end of the research protocol and the results confirmed the initial findings: full-term NMSIDS infants presented abnormalities in their developmental scores. These abnormalities involved hypotonia of the limbs, particularly of the shoulders.

(7) Summary

When full-term NMSIDS infants were analysed as a group, results of polygraphic recording and developmental neurological examinations were concordant. Body movement scores, development of the longest sleep period during the nocturnal period, development of NREM sleep stages, and development of muscle tone in NMSIDS infants were all inappropriate for age, independent of the age at which the near miss event occurred. The infants had scores appropriate to a younger age group. A maturational delay is noted at the time of evaluation for the near miss event.

Long term follow up of full-term NMSIDS infants

1. Rationale for research protocol

The relationship between NMSIDS infants and SIDS victims is not clear cut. At times, controversy has arisen between those who believe in the usefulness of studying NMSIDS infants as a valid model of the sudden infant death syndrome and their opponents who believe that NMSIDS infants are a poorly defined group. The latter maintain that there are no objective criteria to delineate the limits of the NMSIDS population, no objective tests available to ascertain the initial diagnosis in this group, and no obvious links between the NMSIDS and SIDS groups, only a few NMSIDS infants become SIDS victims.

We cannot answer all these objections. However, it would appear that long term, unbiased follow-up study of NMSIDS infants is absolutely mandatory in the light of the emphasis placed on these infants during the past 10 years. More information on this group is needed because of the anxiety experienced by the parents after the reported near miss event. In cases where home monitoring is prescribed, the funds used to rent the equipment and to perform adequate medical follow up during the home monitoring period are important. However, both federal and private agencies within the United States have been reluctant to fund these long term follow-up studies (we hope that other international research groups will remedy this deficiency). To our knowledge, the following results are the first of their kind to be reported, incomplete though they are.

(2) Protocol (see acknowledgements)

Our protocol was not designed as part of a definitive study, but rather was performed as a preliminary study to discover whether a significant problem existed and needed to be investigated more extensively.

We recontacted the parents of NMSIDS infants seen at Stanford by mail. Not all infants' parents were re-contacted; only those who met the following criteria were included: (a) the infant had been full-term; (b) the infant had had a complete clinical and polygraphic examination, the results of which were complete and had been entered in the chart at the time of the near miss event; (c) the infant and parents were located in the San Francisco Bay area at the time of the near miss event.

These selection criteria were based upon the following considerations: (a) we had to have a clear picture of the initial problem, and (b) should we need to see the infant again to perform an adequate study, or to speak with the parents directly, distance from Stanford would be a consideration (particularly if no funds for travel reimbursement were available).

Fifty infants who had been seen between 1977 and 1979 were selected. All letters were sent on the same day at the same post office, and included a stamped return envelope and a one page, simple questionnaire. The parents' current phone number was requested, and each positive response was followed by a telephone contact and, if the parents agreed, a visit to the clinic. However, follow-up polygraphic records were not obtained systematically.

(3) Results

Of the 50 letters mailed, 6 were returned "Addressee unknown." Twenty-four failed to elicit a response, and we have no further information on these cases. We assume that none of these 24 infants had presented sufficient problems to lead their parents to respond to the questionnaire; this at least has the advantage of avoiding the error of positive overinterpretation.

Of the 20 responses received, 10 reported normal infants and 10 reported infants with some health problems. The latter group was re-evaluated and the following problems were found.

Two children (2 and 3 years of age) had episodic loss of consciousness which had appeared after 22 months of age, with questions of seizure disorder (their EEGs were normal). One child (25 months) presented with mental retardation. One child (23 months) had language acquisition delay. One child (24 months) had a mild right-left asymmetry of muscle tone and abnormal left plantar flexor reflexes with an upgoing left toe. One child (15 months) had ataxia of the lower extremities. Three children (15, 27 and 27 months) had recurrent, unexplained cyanotic spells, particularly associated with fever in one case. One child (30 months) had a moderate obstructive sleep apnoea syndrome confirmed by polygraphic recording.

Even if we consider the ratio of abnormal to normal follow-up findings in this population to be 10/50, the fact that 20% of the children presented problems is unexpected.

COMMENTS

There is no doubt that SIDS still baffles the medical community. Several different disorders may be masked by this term. "Near miss" SIDS infants do not die at the time of the initial event, and in fact appear to be long term survivors for the most part. The question of the usefulness of studying NMSIDS infants in an attempt to understand SIDS has been raised regularly; our goal has not been to resolve this issue. Unquestionably, some NMSIDS infants subsequently die of SIDS. However, our own results indicate that although NMSIDS infants may become victims of SIDS more often than the general population, nonetheless this occurs in only 0.25–0.30% of the NMSIDS population – not an impressive number. It is also true that, during polygraphic monitoring, life-threatening cardiorespiratory events may be observed, particularly during sleep (Guilleminault and Ariagno 1978), and dramatic recurrences of these severe episodes are noted during home monitoring periods. However, in more than 50% of the NMSIDS infants studied at Stanford, no such severe episodes were documented. Some of the infants who presented life-threatening events during their initial polygraphic monitoring, occurring soon after their near miss event, never presented serious subsequent episodes under home monitoring; on the other hand, some of the infants who presented only minor abnormalities during their initial recording later experienced dramatic events while being monitored at home. It is possible to argue that "NMSIDS" may cover several different types of disorder, as does "SIDS." Apnoea is common final pathway for many disorders, particularly in infants. However, we wish to emphasize that NMSIDS events, which are frequently equated with "unexplained respiratory disorders in an infant at a time when the infant supposedly is asleep,'' and NMSIDS infants themselves, need to be investigated further. Our preliminary data seem to indicate that death per se may not be the only problem deserving consideration; neurological sequelae may be seen in NMSIDS infants. We hope that our preliminary study will encourage investigation of the long term risks to NMSIDS infants.

If we consider the polygraphic results obtained on NMSIDS infants by different research groups (Steinschneider 1972; Kelly and Shannon 1979; Hoppenbrouwers et al. 1980) the findings appear to be contradictory. Some of these contradictions may be related to patient selection procedures; very often, premature and full-term infants have been included in the same study group. This, in our view, renders understanding of the problems difficult. In addition, the duration of the polygraphic recording varies and this may be a source of error (Guilleminault et al. 1981). However, even within our own patient population, all of whom were full term and received extended monitoring, infants presented different types of apnoea, although only mixed and obstructive apnoea allowed statistically significant differentiation of the NMSIDS group from the control group.

The major findings from our studies are: (a) a delayed maturational change, noted for many variables, is found in NMSIDS infants as compared to normal controls. These maturational delays disappear progressively, as noted in follow-up consultations, after the age of 6 months (Guilleminault et al. 1979a; Korobkin and Guilleminault 1979). (b) The distribution of respiratory pauses with respect to sleep onset and arousal during sleep follow a specific pattern in NMSIDS infants. The longer the preceding sleep within a given sleep period, the greater the chance of apnoeic events and, when apnoea occurs repetitiously, the greater the chance of a resulting arousal. (c) The type of apnoea monitored may change, depending on how long after the near miss event the monitoring is performed. If a mild "runny nose" is noted at the time of the initial event, the apnoea seen at that time is more likely to be mixed and obstructive; later, more frequent central pauses may be seen (Guilleminault et al. 1975). (d) Mixed and obstructive apnoea lead to more severe oxygen desaturation and have more effect on cardiovascular variables than do central apnoeic episodes of the same duration (Guilleminault et al. 1975).

These findings need to be integrated with the results reported by Phillipson et al. (1980) in dogs, and our own studies in man (Guilleminault and Rosekind 1981) on changes in the arousal threshold in relation to sleep fragmentation and sleep deprivation. "Near miss" episodes may result from a conjunction of several factors, perhaps including an "immature" central nervous system, a slightly impaired arousal threshold, a moderate sleep disturbance with resulting mild sleep fragmentation and sleep deprivation, and perhaps the presence of a "runny nose" − all may combine to cause mixed and obstructive apnoea during sleep in NMSIDS infants. When all these factors are present − and, quite possibly, there are other factors of which we are as yet unaware − they may lead to near miss events and even to SIDS. Challenges designed to evaluate the arousal threshold, such as those proposed by Hunt et al. (1981) using specific respiratory gases, may allow better understanding of near miss SIDS events and may also shed new light on SIDS.

SUMMARY

One hundred and ninety-eight full-term infants were referred to and studied by the Stanford group for a "near miss for sudden infant death" event between 1972 and 1981. All infants received extended polygraphic monitoring soon after the time of the reported near miss event. Five infants died subsequently of SID, and 39% of infants seen after 1977 suffered a second near miss event requiring resuscitation soon after the initial referral. In addition, a preliminary long term follow-up study is reported.

Findings indicated that infants who have suffered a near miss event present with delayed maturational changes. Polygraphic monitoring showed that near miss infants present central, obstructive, or mixed apnoea; only the latter 2 types serve to differentiate the near miss group from the control group. In near miss infants, the frequency of apnoeic episodes increases with the duration of preceding sleep within a given sleep period. The role of arousal from sleep appears to be an important variable.

Fifty infants seen between 1977 and 1979 were chosen for a long term follow-up study; the parents of 20 of them were contacted successfully. Assuming that the 30 infants about whom we have no further information are healthy, 20% of the studied population still presented subsequent problems. Detailed investigation of near miss events and large scale, long term follow-up studies of infants who have suffered them are indicated.

ACKNOWLEDGEMENTS

These studies were supported in part by National Institute of Child Health and Human Development Grant No. HD 08339 from 1974 to 1979; Public Health Service Grant Nos. R-R-70 and R-R-81 from the General Clinical Research Centers Program, Division of Human Resources, from 1975 to 1981; by INSERM to C. Guilleminault. The preliminary data on long term follow up were obtained with the support of a gift from the Pacific Firefighters' Wives Association.

Many researchers were involved in the collection and analysis of the data reported. We wish to acknowledge the help of R. Ariagno, R. Baldwin, M. Owen-Boeddiker, M.J. Challamel, W. Flagg, R. Korobkin, L. Nagel, M.R. Paraita, D. Raynal, J. Skinner and M. Souquet.

REFERENCES

Amiel-Tison, C. A method for neurological evaluation within the first year of life. Curr. Probl. Pediat., 1976, 7: 1–50.

Ariagno, R.L., Guilleminault, C., Boeddiker, M. and Baldwin, R. Evaluation of gastro-esophageal reflux and apnea in near miss for SIDS infants. Clin. Res., 1981, 29: 146A (abstr.).

Coons, S. and Guilleminault, C. Maturing sleep structures in the first year: state proportion and circadian distribution. Sleep Res., 1982, in press (abstr.).

Guilleminault, C. and Ariagno, R.L. Why should we study the infant "near miss for sudden infant death"? Early hum. Develop., 1978, 2/3: 207–218.

Guilleminault, C. and Rosekind, M. The arousal threshold: sleep deprivation, sleep fragmentation, and obstructive sleep apnea syndrome. Bull. Europ. Physiopath. Resp., 1981, 17: 341–349.

Guilleminault, C., Peraita, R., Souquet, M. and Dement, W.C. Apneas during sleep in infants: possible relationship with SIDS. Science, 1975, 190: 677–679.

Guilleminault, C., Ariagno, R.L., Forno, L.S., Nagel, L., Baldwin, R. and Owen, M. Obstructive sleep apnea and near miss for SIDS: 1. Report of an infant with sudden infant death. Pediatrics, 1979a, 63: 837–843.

Guilleminault, C., Ariagno, R., Korobkin, R., Nagel, L., Baldwin, R., Coons, S. and Owen, M. Mixed and obstructive sleep apnea and near miss for sudden infant death syndrome: 2. Comparison of near miss and normal control infants by age. Pediatrics, 1979b, 64: 882–891.

Guilleminault, C., Ariagno, R., Korobkin, R., Coons, S., Owen-Boeddiker, M. and Baldwin, R. Sleep parameters and respiratory variables in "near miss" sudden infant death syndrome infants. Pediatrics, 1981, 68: 354–360.

Hoppenbrouwers, T., Hodgman, J.A., McGinty, D., Harper, R. and Sterman, M.B. Sudden infant death syndrome: sleep apnea and respiration in subsequent siblings. Pediatrics, 1980, 66: 205–214.

Hunt, C.E., McCulluch, K. and Brouillette, R.T. Diminished hypoxic ventilatory responses in near-miss sudden infant death syndrome. J. appl. Physiol., Resp. Environm. Exercise Physiol., 1981, 60: 1313–1317.

Kelly, D.H. and Shannon, D.C. Periodic breathing in infants with near miss sudden infant death syndrome. Pediatrics, 1979, 63: 355–361.

Korobkin, R. and Guilleminault, C. Neurologic abnormalities in near miss for sudden infant death syndrome infants. Pediatrics, 1979, 64: 369–374.

Parmelee, A.H., Stern, E. and Harris, M.A. Maturation of respiration in prematures and young infants. Neuropaediatrie, 1972, 3: 294–299.

Phillipson, E.A., Bowes, G., Sullivan, C.E. and Woolf, G.M. The influence of sleep fragmentation on arousal and ventilatory responses to respiratory stimuli. Sleep, 1980, 3: 281–289.

St.-Anne Dargassies, S. Le Développement Neurologique du Nouveau-né à Terme et Prématuré. Masson, Paris, 1974: 340 pp.

Steinschneider, A. Prolonged apnea and the SIDS: Clinical and laboratory observation. Pediatrics, 1972, 50: 646–652.

Kyoto Symposia (EEG Suppl. No. 36)
Editors: P.A. Buser, W.A. Cobb and T. Okuma
© 1982, Elsevier Biomedical Press, Amsterdam

652

Some Aspects of EEG Polygraphy in Newborns at Risk from Neurological Disorders

CESARE T. LOMBROSO

Seizure Unit and Division of Neurophysiology, Department of Neurology, Children's Hospital Medical Center, and Harvard Medical School, Boston, Mass. 02115 (U.S.A.)

A comprehensive review of the EEg polygraphy in newborns "at risk" neurologically is outside the scope of this symposium. Thus, only somewhat eclectic topics will be briefly presented, the aim being to outline "the state-of-the-art" rather than to cover the vast repertoire available from past and ever increasing contributions by world-wide experts. This arbitrary selection will include some information ripened by time and generally agreed upon and some not yet firmly established but offering potential directions for future clinical research.

As is known, clinical electrophysiology in this age group differs considerably from that applicable to older populations, both in techniques and in valid interpretations. To the neophyte in this complex field I suggest consulting a few basic publications (Monod et al. 1972; Parmelee 1972; Petre-Quadens 1972; Prechtl 1974; Dreyfus-Brisac and Monod 1975; Werner et al. 1977; Watanabe 1978; Ellingson 1979; Tharp 1980; Lombroso 1982a).

Historically, the modern era of EEG polygraphy in the newborn developed along two main directions: (1) the *ontogenesis* of the EEG and of the newborn behavioural "states"; and (2) studies of one of the most frequent morbid events in the biography of a neonate, namely, *seizure* phenomena.

SOME GENERALIZATIONS FROM EARLY STUDIES ON EEG ONTOGENESIS

They established that conceptional age (CA) rather than gestional age (GA) dictates maturation and that cerebral maturation proceeds along similar schedules outside the uterus; hence, a newborn of 29 weeks GA after 10/11 weeks of life will exhibit the same EEG and state organization* as a newborn born at term.

As we know now, some exceptions to these rules occur, both for normal preterms and for those "at risk" (Schulte et al. 1971; Monod et al. 1972; Theorell et al. 1974; Lombroso 1975, 1979).

Abnormalities in EEG and in behavioural "states" cover a large spectrum. We have tentatively adopted a classification based on 3 broad categories for the

---

*For definition of state see Prechtl (1974) and Lombroso (1982a).

interpretation of EEG polygraphs of the neonate: (1) abnormalities of background; (2) ictal abnormalities; and (3) abnormalities in organization of states and of EEG maturation.

Each carries a different message. At times they overlap. Nonetheless, this simple classification allows more precise identification and quantification of EEG/states deviations. It may also facilitate better semantic interchanges among investigators. I shall start with data from a group of about 300 newborns with seizures, followed prospectively for about 15 years. The following main conclusions in general confirm and extend those of previous investigators.

EEG POLYGRAPHY IN NEWBORNS WITH SEIZURES

(A) It is *not* a powerful tool for aetiological diagnosis.

Exceptions: detection of subtle, tonic, apnoeic ictal phenomena vs. non-ictal ones. A few patterns suggest diagnostic clues: interhemispheric asymmetry; positive sharp waves; delta-, theta-, alpha- and beta-like discharges.

(B) It may be a powerful tool for making long-term prognostic profiles.

Seizures in the newborn are frequent and often indicate serious assaults upon the developing brain (Monod et al. 1972; Theorell et al. 1974; Dreyfus-Brisac and Monod 1975; Dennis 1979; Tharp 1980; Lombroso 1981, 1982a, b). About one-half will die or develop serious sequelae, but the others appear to escape with no obvious deficits (Rose and Lombroso 1970; Dennis 1979; Lombroso 1981, 1982b). Over the past few years the trend has been towards a mildly improved outcome. Clinical and laboratory data during the newborn period at times fail to provide reliable long-term prognosis. EEG polygraphy in the newborn has shown statistically high "group" correlations with long-term outcomes (Monod et al. 1972; Dreyfus-Brisac and Monod 1975; Ellingson 1979; Lombroso 1982b). Utilizing the classification mentioned, we can examine briefly these correlations. First, according to *background abnormalities* (Table I); next, the correlations with the second parameter of the above classification, or *ictal abnormalities* (Table II).

Thus far, although some aspects of our classification differ from those of previous authors, the general conclusions seem to agree (Monod et al. 1972; Dreyfus-Brisac and Monod 1975; Ellingson 1979).

Next, we extended these prospective investigations to other cohorts of neonates neurologically "at risk" to determine whether the EEG classification used in convulsing babies had general validity. Involved were: hypoxic-ischaemic encephalopathies (stages 2 and 3); intracranial haemorrhages; CNS infections; inborn errors of metabolism.

Table III summarizes the patterns of background abnormalities we met in this mixed group of neonates with their correlations for long-term outcome.

From Table III it is evident that, although these populations were different, the abnormal EEG patterns and their prognostic "group" reliabilities were about identical to those observed for the convulsive newborn. The only significant

TABLE I

BACKGROUND ABNORMALITIES IN CORRELATION WITH LONG-TERM OUTCOMES

| Neonatal EEGs | Clinical outcome at 4–7 years | | | | |
Background abnormalities	Normal	Abnormal	Dead	Totals	Level of significance by chi-square test
Isoelectric	–	4	6	10	$P < 0.002$
Paroxysmal or "burst suppression"	3	23	11	37	$P < 0.002$
Low voltage throughout REM and NREM sleep	1	7	1	9	$P < 0.04$
Persistent severe dysmaturity for CA	6	12	–	19	N.S.
Rolandic positive sharp transients	2	2	2	6	N.S.
Normal EEGs	92	10	1	103	$P < 0.001$
Total	160	131	44	335	

N.S., not reaching level of significance.

TABLE II

ICTAL ABNORMALITIES IN CORRELATION WITH LONG-TERM OUTCOMES

| Neonatal EEGs | Clinical outcome at 4–7 years | | | | |
Ictal abnormalities	Normal	Abnormal	Dead	Totals	Level of significance by chi-square test
Focal discharges (spikes or sharp waves) with normal background	43	22	2	67	N.S.
Multifocal discharges with abnormal background	13	19	8	41	$P < 0.002$
Beta-, alpha-, theta-, delta-like discharges	7	13	8	25	$P < 0.005$
Repeated low frequency sharp waves usually on a low voltage background	3	8	3	14	$P < 0.05$
No recordable discharges during clinical ictus	–	2	3	5	N.S.*
Total	66	64	22	152	

N.S., not reaching level of significance.
*The test did not reach a significant level because of the small N, although none of the children are normal.

TABLE III

BACKGROUND ABNORMALITIES IN CORRELATION WITH LONG-TERM OUTCOMES IN A MIXED GROUP OF NEONATES

Neonatal EEGs	Clinical outcome at 6 years			
Background abnormalities	Normal	Abnormal	Dead	Level of significance by chi-square test
Isoelectric or profound depression	3*	19	12	$P < 0.001$
Low voltage through state III, REM, NREM	5**	17	8	$P < 0.01$
Burst suppression	5	24	6	$P < 0.001$
Transient dysmaturity	18	3	–	$P < 0.01$
Severe (> 2 weeks) persistent dysmaturity	10	17	4	$P < 0.05$
Positive sharp waves	8	4	5	N.S.
Normal EEGs	73	11	1	$P < 0.001$
Total	122	95	36	

*One baby had 3 EEGs, all with high levels of diazepam.
**One had persistent scalp oedema: his third EEG was normal.

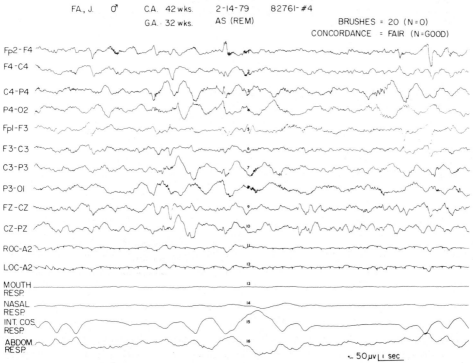

Fig. 1. For legend see next page.

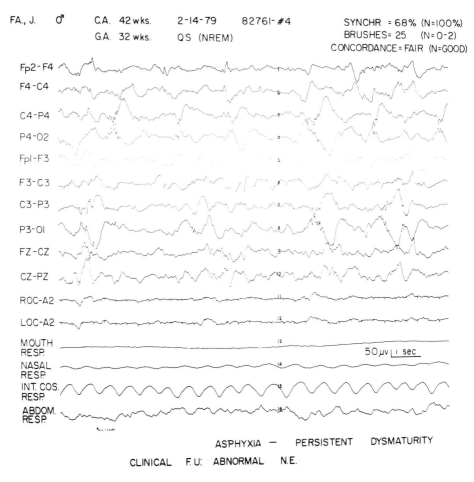

Figs. 1 and 2. FA.J. was born at 32 weeks GA and had paranatal evidence of marked asphyxia, and developed focal clonic seizures lasting a few days. CT scan revealed grade 1 intraventricular haemorrhage. He had 6 EEGs from 35 to 44 weeks CA. All showed lag in maturational indices (Lombroso 1979, 1982a). We show here only samples of EEGs obtained at 42 weeks. In the upper right corner are the indices measurable at this time vs. the norms for this CA. At 44 weeks there were still significant lags in these EEG maturational parameters. At 18 months the baby exhibited global retardation and quadriparesis.

difference here involved the pattern of *persistent severe dysmaturity* (Lombroso 1975, 1982a, b). This pattern did not reach statistical validity for prognosis in the group of convulsive newborns, but it did in those babies with other morbidities. By the term "persistent dysmaturity" is meant that gross quantifiable indices of maturation in a given EEG correspond to those found at an earlier CA. Further, that this lag persists in serial records obtained up to or past the newborn period. These quantified EEG indices in normative controls have been published (Lombroso 1975, 1982a, b). One example of this pattern is illustrated by Fa.J. who had an uneventful pregnancy but was born at 32 weeks of GA. During delivery his foetal heart monitor showed type 2 deceleration; he was severely acidotic and developed a few seizures. An EEG obtained then exhibited exaggerated *tracé discontinu* throughout waking and sleep. One done at 36 weeks CA exhibited 10 times more spindle-delta (brushes) complexes (a hallmark of dysmaturity) than expected, and complete asynchrony between hemispheres of episodic high voltage runs during *tracé alternant*. In the EEG obtained at 42 weeks CA (Fig. 1) during REM sleep the background was mildly discontinuous; there were 20 brushes during 5 min instead of none as expected at this CA. In NREM (Fig. 2), the interhemispheric synchrony during *tracé alternant* was only 68% instead of 100%; there were 25 brushes instead of two. It should be noted that otherwise there were no other EEG abnormal features and there was good organization of sleep states.

These dysmature features persisted into early infancy. At 4 years, the child was quadriparetic and had significant delay in language development. A similar positive correlation between persistent dysmaturity and poor outcome was observed in a group of neonates with intracranial haemorrhages (DaCosta and Lombroso 1980; Lombroso 1982a). A recent paper (Tharp et al. 1981) confirmed that some of these dysmature features, if persisting, are poor prognostic indices also in prematures.

Further refinement in selection and quantification of maturational parameters that will include "waking" states and correlate with behavioural indices should be more effective in anticipating less severe neurological sequelae. Pressing is the need to move from what, so far, are "group" prognostic profiles to individual ones.

The value of extending the period of EEG polygraphic recording beyond the newborn into infancy has been stressed by some investigators. Perhaps one of the best recent examples to mention in this respect are the studies by Ellingson and Peters (1981); they first established normative data for maturational schedules in both preterm and full-term normal controls followed into early infancy. They were then able to demonstrate that babies with Down's syndrome, although not exhibiting abnormalities during the neonatal epoch, showed statistically significant deviations in several EEG parameters in early infancy. Table IV lists some maturational delays in a group of neonates with trisomy-21.

We have confirmatory data, as yet unpublished, in a series of newborns with this chromosomal defect followed prospectively.

TABLE IV

EXAMPLE OF DELAYED MATURATION OF BRAIN ELECTRICAL INDICES DURING EARLY INFANCY*

	Trisomy-21 (mean age in days)	Controls (mean age in days)	Level of significance
Tracé alternant disappears	55.6	33.4	$P < 0.001$
Sleep spindles appear	62.0	43.8	$P < 0.01$
Frontal sharp waves disappear	64.6	39.1	$P < 0.001$

*Modified after Ellingson and Peters, *Electroenceph. clin. Neurophysiol.*, 1981, 51: 165.

TABLE V

ABNORMALITIES IN ORGANIZATION OF STATES AND IN EEG MATURATIONAL INDICES

Neonatal EEGs	Outcome at 4 years		
	Normal	Abnormal*	Level of significance by chi-square test
No recognizable states	1	40	$P < 0.001$
Lability of states	4	23	$P < 0.001$
Persistence of early neonatal states into infancy (1–61 weeks CA)	16	61	$P < 0.001$
Transient EEG dysmaturity indices	19	3	$P < 0.001$
Persistent EEG dysmaturity indices	9	25	$P < 0.01$

*Includes: death, neuro-sensory deficits, epilepsy, D.Q. < 80.

Coming now to the third parameter of our classification: *abnormalities in organization of states and in EEG maturational indices,* we have already discussed briefly all subgroups except that of "lability of states" (Table V).

Several investigators in the past have stressed that often babies neurologically affected cannot develop or maintain "states" (Schulte et al. 1971; Prechtl 1974; Theorell et al. 1974; Watanabe 1980). It is known also that in normal neonates there is inter-subject variability in the time spent in various waking and sleeping states. Thus such variations, unless quite marked, have not been very useful for clinical correlations.

A systematic investigation across a significant period of time on individual babies with less marked variations in their "states" has not been performed to my knowledge. We can report on a pilot study that shows potentially promising results (Lombroso and Matsumiya 1982). It involved 14 full-term newborns: 6 of these were assessed as being "at risk" neurologically, 8 were thought to be normal. We selected 5 states: awake and crying; awake and quiet; awake and drowsy; asleep in REM; asleep in NREM. EEG recording and behavioural observation were carried out for 7 consecutive hours at the same time of day at about 1 week intervals over a span of approximately 5 weeks. Each state for each baby was scored and expressed as a percentage of the total observation time. Thus, we obtained percentages for each selected state and for each subject during 4 prolonged recordings 1 week apart. It was then feasible to calculate a "*consistency profile*" for each baby. An F value was used to express the profile, which was obtained from observation × state analysis of variance. (F = mean square for observation/error term.) In this analysis, the higher the F value, the more consistent the profile. Lastly, we could correlate (using the Mann-Whitney U tests) these profiles both with the initial assessment and with the eventual clinical outcome. The latter was obtained by standard neurological and developmental measures carried out at various intervals up to ages varying from 2.2 to 3.6 years (mean 2.9). Of the 8 newborns assessed as normal, 7 showed highly consistent profiles, though these varied from baby to baby. All 8 were normal on follow-up. The one exception was a neonate who showed a very inconsistent weekly distribution in percentages of the 5 states. At 8 months he developed seizures of unknown aetiology. These were controlled, but at age 2.9 years he exhibited poor motor control and a D.Q. of 70. Conversely, of the 6 newborns considered to be "at risk," 5 had a low F value or a notable variability in percentages of states during the first 5 weeks of life. All had poor clinical outcomes on follow-up. Here, too, there was an exception: 1 newborn thought to be "at risk" because of tonic seizures in his first 2 days and a grade I intraventricular haemorrhage, exhibited a high F value; namely, a relatively stable week-to-week distribution of various state times. However, at 2.2 years he had a normal neurological examination and a D.Q. of 90. Thus, it appears that prolonged, weekly recording of a given baby's state percentages might become a useful tool for more individual prognosis, in spite of the notable inter-subject variability in times spent in the various states by normal babies. Clearly, larger populations will have to be studied to validate these initial data.*

Two of the most common problems in intensive care nurseries now are encephalopathies from hypoxic-ischaemic insults and from intracranial haemorrhages. While in the latter, "positive sharp waves" may occur as a distinctive though not pathognomonic pattern, I am not aware of any distinctive EEG pattern correlated with asphyxia. The ensuing encephalopathies vary greatly in severity. Also, though there may be a history of asphyxia, the underlying main morbid event can be a different one; for example, a haemorrhage, a congenital CNS defect or an infectious problem.

In this context, the simultaneous use of evoked potentials (DaCosta and Lombroso 1980; Lütschg et al. 1980) may add to the information obtainable by EEG polygraphy alone. I will discuss only the brain stem auditory evoked potentials (BAEP) as adjuncts for diagnostic and prognostic clues (cf. as general reference Stockard and Stockard 1981). The two examples that will be given are from a series of 10 newborns, all considered to have suffered from severe asphyxia and included in an ongoing investigation involving a large group. What distinguished these 10 babies was that they died early and, thus, careful autoptic data became available for correlations with their electrophysiological data.

Baby McL. was a male of 36 weeks GA, born by caesarian section because of transverse position and signs of foetal distress. Apgar scores were 4 and 5 at 5 min. He was acidotic with low blood pressure and required assisted ventilation. Neurologically he was hypertonic, with depressed suck and Moro reflexes. Chemistries, spinal fluid and CT scan were negative. An EEG at 5 days showed an invariant "burst suppression" pattern alternating with long periods of diffuse low voltage background. The BAEPs exhibited mild latency prolongation of wave III and complete loss of waves IV and V. At autopsy 5 days later there were mild changes in the telencephalic white matter. Serial sections of the brain stem showed: normal VIII nerves; mild neuronal loss in cochlear nuclei and superior olivary

---

*A recent paper by Thoman et al. (1981) also indicates that inconsistent state organization during the neonatal period may be predictive of later neurological dysfunction.

complexes. The inferior colliculi in the midbrain, however, were devastated, with no nerve cells left and marked gliosis.

Baby Le. was full term, born with his cord tightly wrapped around his neck. Apgars were 1 and 3, blood pH 6.7, and he had severe hypoglycaemia. Resuscitation was required after 5 min. At 12 h he developed seizures and apnoea. Neurologically he showed no suck, no doll's eye movements, no grasp reflexes. He was thought to be too ill to get a CT scan at this time. A portable EEG showed no differentiation between states and a continuous interhemispheric asymmetry with depressed voltages over the left anterior quadrant. Sharp discharges were present intermittently. The BAEP showed mild asymmetry, but all waves were present and with normal latencies. A day later the CSF showed blood, and the scan demonstrated a haemorrhage in the left frontal lobe. At autopsy a week later, a large frontal lobe clot was found. Serial brain stem sections showed no abnormalities in any of the auditory nuclei or pathways. Hence: (1) some newborns thought to have had severe asphyxia showed at autopsy other pathologies. The EEGs, while abnormal, could not offer clear diagnoses. The BAEPs showed good correlations between their abnormalities and autoptic findings in the brain stem; (2) an abnormal EEG accompanied by clear BAEP abnormalities suggests severe asphyxia and poor survival prognosis.

Even combined EEG polygraphy and evoked potentials may fail to detect significant insults in newborns. A recently developed technique, *brain electrical activity mapping,* or *BEAM,* may be useful in some of these cases (Duffy et al. 1979). This technique mainly presents in a concise manner a topographic map of the EEG spectral bands and a similar topographic display of evoked potentials, in

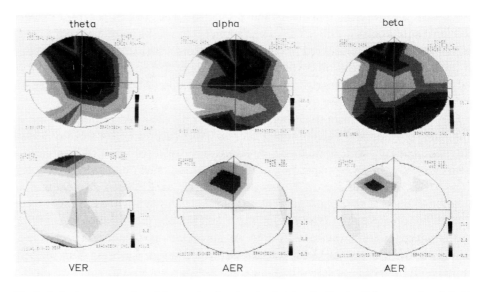

Fig. 3. In the top row are few of the spectra showing clearly lateralization in all frequency bands to the left anterior quadrant. In the lower row are just a few pictures taken between 100 and 502 msec following flashes (VER) or clicks (AER). These also show abnormal responses with left frontal lateralization.

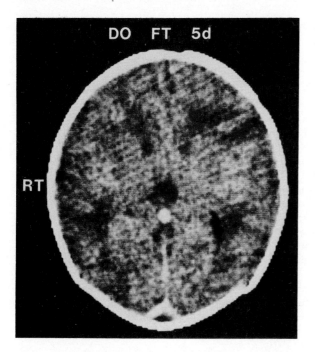

Fig. 4. Shows the CT scan obtained a few days later showing the attenuation over the left frontal lobe, due to a vascular insult, likely ante- or paranatal in origin.

continuous sequences of time, frequency and space. By the use of graded colours, polarities and power can be displayed also and, through the use of a cartoon-like technique, these maps can be displayed on a colour TV screen. For those interested in further details of this technique and its application to clinical problems, we refer to a recent publication (Lombroso and Duffy 1982).

Baby boy Dow was born at 41 weeks GA with uneventful pregnancy and delivery, but with early onset of seizures. An EEG obtained at this time showed mild asymmetry over the left anterior quadrant, which was intermittent. There were some "dysmature" features. Possibly most significant but missed at this time was the relative lack of "brushes" over the left hemisphere. Some salient illustrations of his BEAM (Fig. 3) showed a clearly abnormal spectral display, with delta, theta, as well as alpha and beta bands strikingly focal over the left frontal region, both with the eyes open and closed.

The BEAM to light flashes showed early occipital evoked components that were within normal limits. However, late VER and AER components exhibited significant asymmetry in both negative and positive activities over the left anterior quadrant, clearly abnormal and usually indicative of atrophic underlying lesions. A CT scan (Fig. 4) a few days later demonstrated an area of decreased density within the left frontal lobe, interpreted as the result of a vascular insult, probably antenatal in origin.

In conclusion, we have touched upon various neurophysiological techniques and their usefulness in the multi-faceted examination of neonates neurologically at risk.

Some can add significantly to the process of diagnosis, others seem most pertinent to delineate prognosis.

REFERENCES

DaCosta, J.C. and Lombroso, C.T. Neurophysiological correlations of neonatal intracranial haemorrhages. Electroenceph. clin. Neurophysiol., 1980, 50: 183P.

Dennis, J. The implications of neonatal seizures. In: R. Korobkin and C. Guilleminault (Eds.), Advances in Perinatal Neurology. S.P. Medical Scientific Books, Vol. 1. New York, 1979: 205–222.

Dreyfus-Brisac, C. and Monod, N. Neonatal status epilepticus. In: G. Lairy (Ed.), Handbook EEG clin. Neurophysiology, Vol. 15B. Elsevier, Amsterdam, 1972: 38–52.

Dreyfus-Brisac, C. and Monod, N. The EEG in full-term and premature infants. In: G. Lairy (Ed.), Handbook EEG clin. Neurophysiology, Vol. 6B. Elsevier, Amsterdam, 1975: 6–23.

Duffy, F.H., Burchfiel J.L. and Lombroso, C.T. Brain electrical activity mapping (BEAM): a new method for extending the clinical utility of EEG and evoked potential data. Ann. Neurol., 1979, 5: 309–321.

Ellingson, R.J. The EEGs of premature and full-term newborns. In: D.W. Klass and D.D. Daly (Eds.), Current Practice in Clinical Electroencephalography. Raven Press, New York, 1979: 149–169.

Ellingson, R.J. and Peters, J.F. Development of EEG and daytime sleep patterns in Trisomy-21 infants during the first year of life: longitudinal observations. Electroenceph. clin. Neurophysiol., 1980, 50: 457–466.

Lombroso, C.T. Neurophysiological observations in diseased newborns. Biol. Psychiat., 1975, 10: 527–558.

Lombroso, C.T. Quantified electroencephalographic scales on 10 preterm healthy newborns followed to 40–43 wk CA by serial polygraphic recordings. Electroenceph. clin. Neurophysiol., 1979, 46: 460–474.

Lombroso, C.T. Prognosis of neonatal seizures. In: V.A. Delgado-Escueta, C. Wasterlain, D.M. Treiman and R.J. Porter (Eds.), Status Epilepticus: Mechanisms of Brain Damage and Treatment. Raven Press, New York, 1982: 103–115.

Lombroso, C.T. Neonatal electroencephalography. In: E. Neidermeyer and P. Lopes de Silva (Eds.), Electroencephalography. Basic Principles, Clinical Application and Related Fields, Part III. Urban and Schwatzenburg, Baltimore, Md., 1982a: 232–259.

Lombroso, C.T. Neonatal seizures. In: T.R. Browne and R.G. Feldman (Eds.), Epilepsy: Diagnosis and Management. Little, Brown and Co., Boston, Mass., 1982b: 244–277.

Lombroso, C.T. and Duffy, F.H. Brain electrical activity mapping in the epilepsies. In: H. Akimoto, H. Kazamatsuri, M. Seino and A. Ward (Eds.), Advances in Epileptology. Raven Press, New York, 1982: 173–179.

Lombroso, C.T. and Matsumiya, J. States consistency profiles of individual newborns and outcomes. Amer. EEG Soc. Ann. Meeting Proc., Phoenix, 1982: 20–21.

Lütschg, J., Bina, M., Matsumiya, Y. and Lombroso, C.T. Brain stem auditory evoked potentials in asphyxiated and neurologically abnormal newborns. Electroenceph. clin. Neurophysiol., 1980, 49: 27P.

Monod, N., Pajot, N. and Guidasci, S. The neonatal EEG: statistical studies and prognostic value in full-term and preterm babies. Electroenceph. clin. Neurophysiol., 1972, 32: 529–544.

Parmelee, A.H. Development of states in infants. In: C.D. Clemente, D.P. Purpura and P.E. Meyer (Eds.), Sleep and the Maturing Nervous System. Academic Press, New York, 1972: 200–228.

Petre-Quadens, O. Sleep in mental retardation. In: C.D. Clemente, D.P. Purpura and P.E. Meyer (Eds.), Sleep and the Maturing Nervous System. Academic Press, New York, 1972: 383–396.

Prechtl, H.F.R. The behavioral states of the newborn (a review). Brain Res., 1974, 76: 185–212.

Rose, A.L. and Lombroso, C.T. Neonatal seizures states: A study of clinical, pathological and electroencephalographic features in 137 full term babies with long term follow-up. Pediatrics, 1970, 45: 404–425.

Schulte, F.J., Hinze, G. and Schrempf, G. Maternal toxemia, fetal malnutrition and bioelectric brain activity of the newborn. Neuropädiatrie, 1971, 2: 439–446.

Stockard, J.E. and Stockard, J.E. Brainstem auditory evoked potentials in normal and otoneurologically impaired newborns and infants. In: C.E. Henry (Ed.), Current Clinical Neurophysiology: Update on EEG and Evoked Potentials. Elsevier, Amsterdam, 1980: 421–465.

Tharp, B.P. Pediatric electroencephalography. In: M. Aminoff (Ed.), Electrodiagnosis in Clinical Neurology. Churchill-Livingston, New York, 1980: 67–117.

Theorell, K., Prechtl, H.F.R. and Vos, J.E. A polygraphic study of normal and abnormal newborn infants. Neuropädiatrie, 1974, 5: 279–317.

Thoman, E.B., Denenberg, V.H., Sievel, J. et al. State organization in neonates: Developmental inconsistency indicates risk for developmental dysfunction. Neuropediatrics, 1981, 12: 45–54.

Watanabe, K. Neurophysiological approaches to the normal and abnormal development of CNS in early life. Asian med. J., 1978, 21: 421–450.

Werner, S.S., Stockard, J.E. and Bickford, R. Atlas of Neonatal Electroencephalography. Raven Press, New York, 1977.

12. Human Factors and Hazards in Industrial Work: EEG and EMG Contributions

Kyoto Symposia (EEG Suppl. No. 36)
Editors: P.A. Buser, W.A. Cobb and T. Okuma
© 1982, Elsevier Biomedical Press, Amsterdam

Introduction: The Need for Neurophysiological Methods in Studies of Human Factors and Hazards in Industrial Work

INGEMAR PETERSÉN

Department of Clinical Neurophysiology, Sahlgrenska Hospital, S-413 45 Göteborg (Sweden)

The 6th International Congress of Electromyography, organized by IFSECN, was held in Stockholm, 1979. This congress included 2 symposia concentrated partly upon studies of environmental problems: "Muscle fatigue" and "Environmental and toxic hazards. Neurophysiological methods for early detection of neuropathies." The present, "Human factors and hazards in industrial work: EEG and EMG contributions," is, however, the federation's first real symposium of its kind.

This symposium gives reports on research done with the aid of EEG and EMG, and deals with such problems as environmental toxic hazards, muscular strain in industrial work, sleep disturbances in shift workers, biological effects of electromagnetic fields, and whole-body and local vibrations.

The time limits of such a symposium make it necessary to restrict the range of the review to studies using EEG and EMG; clinical neurophysiology represents many other methods for the study of human factors and hazards in industrial work.

A few of the areas left uncovered due to lack of time were neurophysiological studies of the significance of climatic factors in industrial work, stress in industrial work and the philosophy of limit values. This latter area includes safe limit threshold, from the point of view of clinical neurophysiology, comparisons of different effects of arduous work on men and women, studies with neurophysiological methods, and the epidemiology of neurophysiological results in studies of industrial work, transferred effects of, for instance, solvents from mother to child.

Some of the less well-known methods of interest should be mentioned here. Blomberg (1959) developed a method for the objective evaluation of glare recovery or readaption time of the eye. This method was further developed (Tengroth et al. 1976; Högman et al. 1977; Linde 1980) and proved to be a very sensitive instrument to show certain effects, for example, of welding fumes on the central nervous system. Also of interest is a recently published method for the measurement of vibration threshold (Goldberg and Lindblom 1979) and its use for screening for neurological symptoms and signs after exposure to jet fuel (Lindblom and Goldberg 1979).

The interaction of one strain with others, whether occurring sequentially or simultaneously, is another important aspect. The effects may in some cases be additive and in other cases counteracting, and the effect may be dependent on the context of the strain, or of the individual.

An additional factor of interest in neurophysiological studies of industrial environments using, for example, the EEG, is that a successive adaptation to the environment may cause a successive diminution in physiological and psychological response patterns (Frankenhaeuser et al. 1962, 1967; Monat et al. 1972).

Changes in the EEG pattern have been found to remain after predominantly mental activity (Sickel 1962; Rogge 1972), but also subsequent to predominantly physical activity (Sickel 1962). The interaction between physical and psychological strains in industrial work and the adaptation factor is of great interest when studying hazards in these environments. Within this area also lies an interest in studying the importance of individual alertness variations in industrial works by using the EEG (Petersén et al. 1981).

The study of injurious effects of an industrial environment often necessitates cooperative efforts in order to reach beyond the normal limits of expertise. Such efforts have proved to be of great value in the application of neurophysiological methodology. Clinical neurophysiologists have, in cooperation with neurologists, psychologists, orthopaedic surgeons, physicists, mathematicians and medical technologists, contributed to the knowledge and understanding of a number of problems associated with working environments, a few examples of which are given in this symposium.

Interest in normative data has increased steadily in recent years. A summary of certain such data within clinical EEG was recently published by Petersén and Selldén (1981). It is obvious that this knowledge is extremely useful as a tool in epidemiological investigations of functional disturbances in man caused by harmful factors, such as chemicals, in the working environment. These agents can be measured by determining the amounts found in the air by physical and chemical methods. A further evaluation can be made by calculating the amount of the agent found in the blood or urine, for instance, of the exposed population. With methods such as these, knowledge can be gained of the occurrence of hazardous factors in man's environment and of the subsequent presence in the body. The functional effects of strain or overloading by these agents can in many cases be studied effectively with neurophysiological methods, particularly in combination with neurological, psychological and sociological analyses.

It is evident from the symposium that recent years have seen a great interest in the possibility of using neurophysiology in the study of the learning process in industrial work. This process in itself can have medical consequences in the industrial environment. If one learns an unsuitable work technique, one may still be able to perform work of good quality, but in such a way that, over a long period, the work implies a risk for injury, for example to tendons or ligaments. The interest in this new type of research becomes broader when considering its suitability as an aid to rehabilitating individuals who have suffered injury and who will return to and be trained for their previous work or for another type of industrial work.

It is even possible that neurophysiology can be of assistance in judging the particular risk for an individual to take up a certain type of industrial work. In applying neurophysiological methods in the study of industrial work, it is not possible for the clinical neurophysiologist only to work undisturbed in his "ivory tower" on registrations and analyses. Rather, it is necessary for him to visit the industrial setting in question to discuss suitable forms for the investigation, and often also in order to ascertain which other types of investigations – neurological, cardiological and psychological, for example – might be required to set the neurophysiological results in the proper perspective of the total picture of the work studied.

Registration of electrophysiological signals such as EMG and EEG at the working site can involve significant technical difficulties in terms of different sources of disturbance, demands on telemetric registration, etc. Planning, registration and analysis all require particular technical expertise. Should the neurophysiologist be content to perform his work in isolation in his laboratory – while technicians, psychologists and others work instead at the industrial site – his contribution to the investigation will decrease in value.

Such a discussion must include more than traditional industrial work on land. Industries at sea – for instance, the oil and fishing industries – involve many factors and actions in the framework of the working environment which require analysis by neurophysiological methods.

Neurophysiological research and development within industrial work demands not only knowledgeable researchers to perform the planned studies, but also education of different types and on a variety of different levels. The education of neurophysiologists should include particular instruction to familiarize the student with certain basic features of different types of industrial work and to give certain basal ergonomic knowledge. Education is also needed so that neurophysiology will not be limited only to large industrialized nations with advanced technology so that they may use and receive the benefits of such methodology in improving their work environments. Finally, education of another type is needed in order to facilitate communication between researchers and workers; this is valuable and necessary in several of the stages of neurophysiological investigations discussed here. In order for investigations of this kind to be successfully performed, it is important that workers are given such knowledge so that they are able themselves to take responsibility for questions of priority and for directing research.

In summary, human factors and hazards in industrial work represent a challenge for clinical neurophysiology to contribute – via research, development and education – to the establishment of preventive medical measures, toward motivating the development of improved techniques in the performance of work tasks and furnishing politicians with valuable information to be used as a basis for decisions concerning actions for improved working environments.

REFERENCES

Blomberg, L.-H. A simple objective method for determination of the glare effect. Experientia (Basel), 1959, 15: 358.

Frankenhaeuser, M., Sterkey, K. and Jaerpe, G. Psychophysiological reactions in habituation to gravitational stress. Percept. Mot. Skills, 1962, 15: 63–72.

Frankenhaeuser, M., Fröberg, J., Hagdal, R., Rissler, A., Björkvall, C. and Wolff, B. Physiological, behavioral and subjective indices of habituation to psychological stress. Physiol. Behav., 1967, 2: 229–237.

Goldberg, J.M. and Lindblom, U. Standardized method of determining vibratory perception thresholds for diagnosis and screening in neurological investigation. J. Neurol. Neurosurg. Psychiat., 1979, 42: 793–803.

Högman, B., Bergman, H., Borg, S., Eriksson, T., Goldberg, L., Linde, C.-J. and Tengroth, B. Readaption time after photo stress: alcohol induced acute and postalcohol "hangover" changes in ocular readaption time. Psychopharmacology, 1977, 53: 165–167.

Lindblom, U. and Goldberg, J.M. Screening for neurological symptoms and signs after exposure to jet fuel. In: A. Persson (Ed.), Symposia – Sixth International Congress of Electromyography in Stockholm, Sweden, 1979. Department of Clinical Neurophysiology, Huddinge Hospital, Huddinge, Sweden.

Linde, C.-J. The effect of welding fumes on ocular readaption time. Scand. J. Work environm. Hlth, 1980, 6: 135–145.

Monat, A., Averill, J.R. and Lazarus, R.S. Anticipatory stress and coping reactions under various conditions of uncertainty. J. Personality soc. Psychol., 1972, 24: 237–253.

Persson, A. (Ed.) Symposia – Sixth International Congress of Electromyography, Stockholm, Sweden, 1979. Department of Clinical Neurophysiology, Huddinge Hospital, Huddinge, Sweden, 1979.

Petersén, I. and Selldén, U. On the Need to Collect EEG Data from So-Called Normal Individuals. Butterworths International Medical Reviews, Neurology I. Butterworths, London, 1981.

Petersén, I., Herberts, P., Kadefors, R., Persson, J., Ragnarsson, K. and Tengroth, B. The measurement, evaluation and importance of electromyography and electroencephalography in arduous industrial work. In: L. Levi (Ed.), Society, Stress and Disease – Working Life. University Press, Oxford, 1981; in press.

Rogge, K.-E. EEG-Veränderungen nach verzögerten akustischen Rückmeldung der Lautsprache, 3. Exp. Angew. Psychol., 1972, 19: 641–670.

Sickel, W. Über das menschliche Electroenzephalogram nach mehrstündiger psychischer Aktivität. Arch. ges. Psychol., 1962, 114: 1–54.

Tengroth, B., Högman, B., Linde, C.-J. and Bergman, H. Readaption time after photo stress: readaption as a function of oxygen concentration. Acta ophthal. (Kbh.), 1976, 54: 507–516.

Kyoto Symposia (EEG Suppl. No. 36)
Editors: P.A. Buser, W.A. Cobb and T. Okuma
© 1982, Elsevier Biomedical Press, Amsterdam

Neurophysiological Studies of *n*-Hexane Polyneuropathy in the Sandal Factory

MITSUO IIDA

Section of Neurology, First Department of Internal Medicine and Section of Electromyography, Central Laboratory of the Nagoya University Hospital, Nagoya University School of Medicine, Nagoya (Japan)

Intoxication by organic solvents of the human nervous system has been emphasized and studied in the neurological field all over the world. *n*-Hexane was long believed to be an organic solvent with extremely low toxicity, and widely used in the fields of printing, extraction of vegetable oils and cleaning processes. However, its neurotoxic property had gradually become apparent and in Japan, in 1967 and 1968, a large outbreak of polyneuropathy due to *n*-hexane intoxication occurred among manufacturers of sandals in a small district 30 km from Nagoya City (Yamamura 1969; Sobue et al. 1978). By questionnaire and medical, especially neurological, examination 93 cases of polyneuropathy were found, who had engaged in the work for more than 8 h per day with very poor ventilation conditions, in which the gas concentration of *n*-hexane in the work room ranged from 500 to 2500 ppm (5–25 times the maximal allowable concentration in Japan in those days). Recently the maximal allowable concentration of *n*-hexane in Japan has been fixed below 100 ppm and the ventilation conditions have been considerably improved, without definite nervous system complaints among the sandal workers. In order to clarify the condition of the neurological deficit in recent workers, re-screening, medical re-examination and neurophysiological studies have been performed.

MATERIAL AND METHOD

Symptoms and signs among 93 cases in 1968 found by neurological examination are summarized in Table I, showing numbness of the distal portion of the extremities in 82 cases (88.2%) as the initial symptom. Similarly, a chief finding on neurological examination was sensorimotor involvement of the extremities, symmetrically and distally with glove and stocking distribution. All cases are classified in Table II in 3 groups by mode and degree of disability: (I) sensory polyneuropathy 53 cases (57.0%); (II) sensorimotor polyneuropathy 32 cases (34.4%); (III) sensorimotor polyneuropathy with amyotrophy 8 cases (8.6%). The grade of the neurological disorder was dependent on the hygienic conditions at work, that is, the working hours and work load and the conditions of room ventilation. Among these patients 44 cases were picked out and underwent conventional electromyography and conduction velocity studies of distal peripheral

TABLE I

SYMPTOMS AND SIGNS (1968)

	Number of cases	Percentage of total, 93 cases
Cranial nerve involvement		
Anosmia	5	5.4
Blurring of vision	13	14.0
Constriction of visual field	7	7.5
Optic nerve atrophy	2	2.2
Retrobulbar neuritis	1	1.1
Numbness over the face	5	5.4
Weakness of facial muscles	2	2.2
Sensory disturbance		
Numbness	93	100.0
Dysaesthesia	21	22.6
Pain or tenderness	5	5.4
Muscle weakness	40	43.0
Muscle atrophy	8	8.6
Reflexes		
Hypoactive	36	38.7
Hyperactive	10	10.8
Pathological reflexes	0	0
Micturition disturbance	1	1.1
Skin changes		
Coldness, redness, roughness	55	59.2
Emaciation	14	15.1
Anaemia	3	3.3

TABLE II

CLASSIFICATION BASED ON THE MODE OF INVOLVEMENT AND CLINICAL COURSE OF POLYNEUROPATHY

	III	II	I	R	Missing	Death
Spring, 1968	8(8.6)	32(34.4)	53(57.0)			
Summer, 1970	0	5(5.5)	34(37.8)	51(56.7)	3	
Spring, 1972	0	0	7(7.9)	82(92.1)		1*

Group I, sensory polyneuropathy; group II, sensorimotor polyneuropathy; group III, sensorimotor polyneuropathy with amyotrophy; R, completely recovered case.

* Died of gastric cancer.

nerves; the results were previously reported in detail (Iida et al. 1969). In the present series 21 cases were picked out through the same procedure; among these there were 20 cases of sensory polyneuropathy and only one of sensorimotor polyneuropathy, as shown on Table III. These were cases with mild motor and sensory deficits, especially 5 cases in group I of sensory polyneuropathy of a plexus neuropathy or peripheral neuropathy type. This is further shown in Table IV, that is, a slight

TABLE III

CLASSIFICATION OF n-HEXANE POLYNEUROPATHY DURING RESCREENING IN SPRING, 1981

	Number of cases
Group I, sensory polyneuropathy	20* (95.2%)
Group II, sensorimotor polyneuropathy	1 (4.8%)
Group III, sensorimotor polyneuropathy with amyotrophy	0

* Including 5 cases with asymmetrical distribution.

TABLE IV

SYMPTOMS AND SIGNS (1981)

	Number of cases	Percentage of total, 21 cases
Cranial nerve involvement		
Tinnitus	1	4.8
Floating by postural change	5	23.8
Sensory disturbance		
Numbness	12	57.1
Dysaesthesia	6	28.6
Pain or tenderness	1	4.8
Muscle weakness	6	28.6
Muscle atrophy	0	0
Reflexes		
Hypoactive	10	47.6
Hyperactive	3	14.3
Pathologic	0	0
Micturition disturbance	0	0
Skin change		
Coldness, redness, roughness	4	19.0

floating sensation on postural change was detected in 23.8% of the cases, numbness of the limbs in 57.1% and dysaesthesia in 28.6%, but slight muscle weakness in 28.6% and hypoactive deep tendon reflexes in 47.6% and 14.3% having hyperreflexia. Similarly, autonomic nervous dysfunction in the distal portion of the extremity was seen only in 4 cases (19.0%), showing coldness, redness and roughness. The concentration of *n*-hexane was simultaneously measured in the small rooms during sandal manufacture and was under 50 ppm in all cases.

In the next section the results of the neurophysiological studies on *n*-hexane involvement will be reported briefly for the large outbreak in 1968 and mainly for the rescreening of the present series (1981).

For the neurophysiological studies conventional electromyography of both extremities, motor nerve conduction velocity, compound nerve conduction velocity (evoked potentials) and sensory nerve conduction velocity of the distal segment of the extremities were performed. Furthermore, a course study of those studies was done in a few cases.

RESULTS

(1) Study of 44 cases during the large outbreak in 1968

(a) Conventional electromyogram

Fourty-four cases with *n*-hexane polyneuropathy included 10 males and 34 females. Electromyography was done in 4 muscles, m. flexor pollicis brevis and m. abductor digiti quinti of the upper limb; and m. tibialis anterior and m. gastrocnemius of the lower limb; the findings are summarized in Table V. Fibrillation potentials and positive sharp waves as signs of denervation were detected in about 20% in both extremities, without a high frequency of fasciculation potentials. Large amplitude potentials and polyphasic potentials, considered to be a sign of regeneration, appeared twice as often in the upper extremity (26.1% and 55.7%) as in the lower (10.2% and 33.3%), showing a reverse relation to reduced interference pattern and low voltage potentials, suggesting different courses of regeneration in the two extremities. On the other hand, these electromyographic findings indicate a good correspondence with the severity according to the group classification.

(b) Measurement of conduction velocities

Conduction velocities of the ulnar, median, peroneal and tibial nerves in *n*-hexane polyneuropathy are plotted in Fig. 1. In each column a small bar shows the average value. The averages in each group in Table VI show good correlations with the severity of the disorders; group III with amyotrophy had the slowest velocity for each measurement, with greatest reduction in the lower extremity in each group, of

TABLE V

NUMBER OF MUSCLES WITH ABNORMAL FINDINGS IN ELECTROMYOGRAPHY (1968)

Muscles	Upper extremity, flexor poll. brev., abductor digit. V	Lower extremity, tibialis anter., gastrocnemius	Total
Number of muscles examined	88	88	176
Fibrillation potentials	18 (20.5)	9 (10.2)	27 (15.3)
Positive sharp waves	16 (18.2)	19 (21.6)	35 (19.9)
Fasciculation potentials	5 (5.7)	1 (1.1)	6 (3.4)
Reduced interference pattern	19 (21.6)	38 (43.4)	56 (31.9)
Low amplitude potentials	3 (3.4)	7 (8.0)	10 (5.7)
Large amplitude potentials	23 (26.1)	9 (10.2)	32 (18.2)
Polyphasic potentials	49 (55.7)	29 (33.0)	78 (44.3)

( ): %

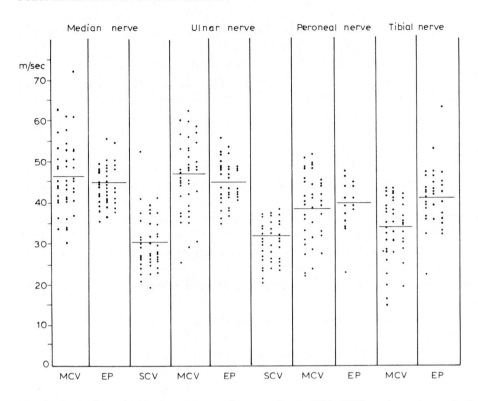

Fig. 1. Conduction velocities in *n*-hexane polyneuropathy in 1968. MCV, motor nerve conduction velocity; SCV, sensory nerve conduction velocity; EP evoked potential.

TABLE VI

AVERAGE CONDUCTION VELOCITIES IN ALL GROUPS (m/sec)

	Number of cases	MCV				EP				SCV	
		U	M	P	T	U	M	P	T	U	M
Group I	11	50.2	51.1	39.5	35.2	47.1	47.8	40.5	44.2	32.1	32.7
Group II	25	47.6	45.8	39.0	35.4	44.4	42.8	39.0	40.4	30.5	29.6
Group III	8	42.7	40.1	30.8	29.1	44.2	45.2	–	36.4	30.7	30.7

MCV, motor nerve conduction velocity; EP, evoked potentials; SCV, sensory nerve conduction velocity; U, ulnar nerve; M, median nerve; P, peroneal nerve; T, tibial nerve (1968).

which sensory nerve conduction velocity (SCV, finger to wrist) was the most remarkable. Pathological reduction of motor nerve conduction velocity (MCV) below 45 m/sec in the ulnar and median nerves (elbow to wrist) was observed in 16 cases (36.4%) and 22 cases (50.0%), respectively. Reduction below 40 m/sec of MCV in the tibial and peroneal nerves (knee to ankle) was present in 21 cases (47.7%) and 31 (70.5%), respectively, the former including 5 cases with no response, indicating an advanced pathology. Compound nerve conduction velocity and evoked potentials (EP), measured by antidromic stimulation in the same segment as the MCV, detected pathologic reduction below 40 m/sec in 7 cases (15.9%) of both ulnar and median nerves, 10 cases (22.7%) of the peroneal and 15 cases (34.1%) of the tibial. SCV of the ulnar and median nerves revealed pathological reduction below 40 m/sec in most cases.

(c) Follow-up study along clinical course

Since the large outbreak in 1968, hygienic and environmental conditions have been improved under the direction of the Health Center of K City and the clinical course of 93 cases has been followed up from spring, 1968 to spring, 1972. As shown in Table II, after 2 years there were 51 cases (56.7%) of complete recovery and after a further 2 years, 82 cases (92.1%), the remaining 7 cases (7.9%) being in group I.

In the neurophysiological follow-up study many cases of groups I and II had revealed remarkable improvement of both the conventional EMG and the conduction velocity. Even in the severe cases with amyotrophy (group III) the electromyographic findings corresponded well with the course of the clinical signs and symptoms, with disappearance of denervation activity and polyphasic potentials and appearance of interference patterns and high voltage potentials; on the contrary, the conduction velocities did not recover easily to normal values and these measurements in the lower extremities were impossible, even after over 1 year from the onset.

(2) Study of 21 cases during rescreening in 1981

(a) Conventional electromyogram

Twenty-one cases with mild *n*-hexane polyneuropathy included 3 males and 19 females. Electromyographic study was done in the same 4 muscles in the distal parts of the limbs as mentioned above; the findings are summarized in Table VII. Denervation activity (fibrillation potentials and positive sharp waves) at rest was not

TABLE VII

NUMBER OF MUSCLES WITH ABNORMAL FINDINGS IN ELECTROMYOGRAPHY (1981)

Muscles	Upper extremity, flexor poll. brev., abductor digit. V	Lower extremity, tibialis anter., gastrocnemius	Total
Numbers of muscles examined	42	42	84
Fibrillation potentials	0	0	0
Positive sharp waves	0	0	0
Fasciculation potentials	0	0	0
Reduced interference pattern	23 (54.8)	32 (76.2)	55 (65.5)
Low amplitude potentials	0	0	0
High amplitude potentials	21 (50.0)	15 (35.7)	36 (42.9)
Polyphasic potentials	6 (14.3)	7 (16.7)	13 (15.5)

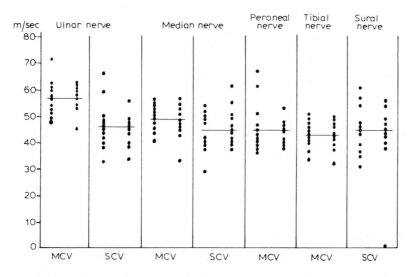

Fig. 2. Conduction velocities of *n*-hexane polyneuropathy in 1981. MCV, motor nerve conduction velocity; SCV, sensory nerve conduction velocity.

detected in this group, without any occurrence of fasciculation potentials. During voluntary effort reduced interference patterns were observed of slight degree, in 54.8% and 76.2% of the examined muscles of the upper and lower limbs; large amplitude potentials were seen in 50.0% and 35.7% and polyphasic potentials in 14.3% and 16.7%, without any volleys of low voltage potentials. This means that there may be different courses of regeneration of the nerve and muscle in the upper and lower extremities. This may suggest that the sandal workers did not complain of severe neurological symptoms because of working with a well equipped ventilation system; nevertheless, they had suffered from latent or mild intoxication by *n*-hexane, which acts strongly in a closed room in winter and does not in an open room in other seasons. Furthermore, they were sure that they had felt more severe numbness of the extremities in winter than at other times.

(b) Measurement of conduction velocities

Conduction velocities of the ulnar, median, peroneal, tibial and sural nerves in the present series are plotted in Fig. 2, in each of whose columns a small bar shows the average value which is seemingly within the normal range in all columns. The average value of the conduction velocity in each group in Table VIII shows a fairly good correlation with the severity of the disorders, although there was only 1 case in group II: more remarkable reduction and the difference between the severity of the disorder of MCV of the lower extremity and of SCV of both extremities. Pathological reduction below 45 m/sec of MCV in the ulnar and median nerves (elbow to wrist) was observed in 1 case (4.8%) and 4 cases (19.0%), respectively, and reduction below 40 m/sec of MCV in the tibial and peroneal nerves (knee to ankle) was present in 6 cases (28.5%). On SCV measurement of the ulnar and median

TABLE VIII

AVERAGE CONDUCTION VELOCITY IN EACH GROUP (m/sec) (1981)

	Number of cases	MCV				SCV		
		U	M	P	T	U	M	S
Group I	20	56.8	48.1	44.8	42.5	45.6	45.0	45.6
Group II	1	52.4	51.3	38.8	40.7	38.5	40.9	30.9
Group III	0	–	–	–	–	–	–	–

MCV, motor nerve conduction velocity; SCV, sensory nerve conduction velocity; U, ulnar nerve; M, median nerve; P, peroneal nerve; T, tibial nerve; S, sural nerve.

nerves (finger to wrist) pathological reduction below 40 m/sec was present in 9 (42.9%) and 10 cases (47.6%), respectively, and in the sural nerve (pedal dorsum to ankle) it was below 30 m/sec in 1 case (4.8%), which was the most remarkable finding in the study of sensory conduction velocities as compared with MCV measurements.

(c) Follow-up study of clinical course

From 1968 to 1980 after the large outbreak of *n*-hexane polyneuropathy only 2 cases visited the Nagoya University Hospital. One of these was included in the 21 cases found during the rescreening procedure. This case belonged to group II and was observed for one and a half years: during this period muscular weakness and sensory impairment of the lower extremities gradually improved and simultaneously the MCV and SCV of the distal portions recovered to the lower limit of the normal range, predominantly earlier in the upper extremity. This process and pattern during improvement were entirely the same as for the patients observed in 1968.

DISCUSSION

Hexacarbon (mainly *n*-hexane and methyl *n*-butyl ketone) neuropathy was first discovered through industrial exposure and sometimes encountered in individuals with inhalation. Each compound is metabolized to 2,5-hexanedione, responsible for the neurological effect.

Transient dizziness, headache and unconsciousness on exposure to *n*-hexane have been described as symptoms in an acute intoxication by this solvent (Spencer et al. 1980). As for chronic *n*-hexane intoxication, glove and stocking type polyneuropathy has been reported by several investigators in Japan (Oishi et al. 1964; Wada et al. 1965). A large outbreak of polyneuropathy due to *n*-hexane intoxication reported by Sobue et al. (1968) provided the most important literature in the field, including neurophysiological studies and follow-up of the patients with polyneuropathy. This is considered because *n*-hexane is widely used as an inexpensive solvent and is a minor component of gasoline and its combustion products. In widespread environmental contamination human neurological disease has been associated only with repetitive and prolonged exposure to levels in excess of 60–240 ppm. The United States threshold limit (air) value (TLV) for *n*-hexane in workroom air is 100 ppm (Spencer et al. 1981). In Japan recognition of the occurrence of *n*-hexane polyneuropathy around 1966 caused the maximal allowable concentration (TLV) to be changed from 500 ppm to 100 ppm.

Environmental, clinical and neurophysiological information on the 93 cases of *n*-hexane polyneuropathy during the large outbreak in 1968 greatly benefitted the understanding, treatment and counter-plan of the *n*-hexane intoxication. The first neurophysiological study was performed on this occasion in 1968 (Iida et al. 1969). The EMG findings among household workers in poorly ventilated small rooms with 500–2500 ppm of *n*-hexane revealed denervation activity (fibrillation potentials and positive sharp waves), reduced interference patterns, large amplitude potentials and polyphasic potentials as regenerating phenomenon in a high percentage of the cases, whose data corresponded well with the neurological disability of *n*-hexane polyneuropathy, especially with the more prominent features in the distal extremities. This study suggests that electromyography of the distal extremities is a simple and good screening technique to detect a latent or mild case of hexacarbon neuropathy, and carry out follow-up study of the neuropathic patient (Seppäläinen et al. 1980). Also, the rescreening in 1981 of 21 cases of mild *n*-hexane polyneuropathy showed no denervation activity but reduced interference pattern and large amplitude potentials in a fairly high percentage of the cases, suggesting a repetition of *n*-hexane intoxication.

As one of the neurophysiological studies, nerve conduction velocities (MCV, EP and SCV) were measured in the distal segments of the extremities. In each measurement for 44 cases during the large outbreak in 1968 a considerable reduction was apparent (Fig. 1). The frequency of reduction of the conduction velocities was, firstly SCV, secondly EP (compound nerve conduction velocity) and thirdly MCV, with the same type of electromyogram predominantly in the lower extremities. This type of study during the rescreening in 1981 had mostly the same features even from the cases with seemingly latent or mild *n*-hexane intoxication. Thus, measurement of conduction velocities as well as electromyography may be suggested as an excellent technique for screening the intoxication of nerves and for the follow-up study of these cases.

Biopsies of the sural nerves in 4 cases during the large outbreak in 1968 showed demyelination, axonal destruction and proliferation of Schwann cells with lymphocytic infiltration in 1 case and an outstanding decrease of the nerve fibres, especially with large diameters (Yamamura 1969; Sobue et al. 1978). In these cases, teased myelinated nerve fibre preparations clearly illustrated paranodal giant axonal swelling accompanied by myelin retraction, from which electron microscopy revealed the axonal swellings to consist of accumulations of 10 nm neurofilaments (Rizzuto et al. 1977). Giant axonal swellings were also found in the fasciculus gracilis of 1 case at autopsy. Histograms of the sural nerves in severely affected glue sniffing cases showed selective loss of the large myelinated fibres (Matsumura et al. 1972). These pathological features recently reported are identical to the abnormalities observed in experimental hexacarbon neuropathy (Spencer et al. 1977; Takeuchi et al. 1980b).

Ninety-three cases of *n*-hexane polyneuropathy were found during the large outbreak in 1968 and were taken care of for a few years. For about 10 years after that there were only 2 patients who visited the Nagoya University Hospital and were treated by vitamin B group. During the rescreening in 1981 21 cases with mild degrees of *n*-hexane polyneuropathy were found and clarified clinically and neurophysiologically the subclinical and mild pathological condition, although they had worked in conditions of less than 50 ppm of *n*-hexane concentration in the air. Accordingly, 100 ppm of maximal allowable concentration (air) of *n*-hexane (the present regulation) has to be reconsidered from the standpoint of the widespread environmental contamination potential of *n*-hexane, especially to man rather than the animal (Takeuchi et al. 1980a).

SUMMARY

Among 93 cases of *n*-hexane polyneuropathy during a large outbreak in 1968 44 cases were studied by conventional electromyogram and measurement of peripheral nerve conduction velocities, both of which showed remarkable changes, especially in the lower rather than the upper extremities. Over a few years since 1968 most of the cases completely recovered, except for a few with mild sensory impairment, after providing for 100 ppm as the maximal allowable concentration of *n*-hexane and well equipped ventilation systems in individual houses.

During the rescreening in 1981, before which there occurred only 2 patients, 21 cases with mild *n*-hexane polyneuropathy were clinically and neurophysiologically observed, revealing mostly the same features as in the previous outbreak in 1968. From these data it may be suggested that, in spite of less than 50 ppm of *n*-hexane concentration in a room, the sandal workers have suffered from neurotoxicity from this organic solvent and the appropriateness of the present regulation on *n*-hexane has to be reconsidered.

REFERENCES

Iida, M., Yamamura, Y. and Sobue, I. Electromyographic findings and conduction velocity on *n*-hexane polyneuropathy. Electromyography, 1969, 9: 247.

Matsumura, M., Inoue, N., Ohnishi, A., Santa, T. and Goto, I. Toxic polyneuropathy due to glue sniffing — 2 cases involving identical twins. Clin. Neurol., 1972, 12: 290.

Oishi, H., Mineno, K., Chiba, K. and Shibata, K. Polyneuropathy caused by an organic solvent (*n*-hexane). Saigai-Igaku, 1964, 7: 218.

Rizzuto, W., Terzian, H. and Galiazzo-Rizzuto, S. Toxic polyneuropathies in Italy due to leather cement poisoning in shoe industries. A light and electron-microscopic study. J. neurol. Sci., 1977, 31: 343.

Seppäläinen, A.M., Lindström, K. and Martelin, T. Neurophysiological and psychological picture of solvent poisoning. Amer. J. industr. Med., 1980, 1: 31.

Sobue, I., Yamamura, Y., Ando, K., Iida, M. and Takayanagi, T. n-Hexane polyneuropathy-outbreak among vinyl sandal manufacturers. Clin. Neurol., 1968, 8: 393.

Sobue, I., Iida, M., Yamamura, Y. and Takayanagi, T. n-Hexane polyneuropathy. Int. J. Neurol., 1978, 11: 1.

Spencer, P.S., Schaumberg, H.H., Sabri, M.I. and Veronesi, B. The enlarging view of hexacarbon neurotoxicity. In: L. Golberg (Ed.), Critical Review in Toxicology, Vol. 7. CRC Press, Boca Raton, Fla., 1980: 278.

Spencer, P.S., Couri, D. and Schaumburg, H.H. n-Hexane and methyl n-butyl ketone. In: P.T. Spencer and H.H. Schaumburg (Eds.), Experimental and Clinical Neurotoxicology. Williams and Wilkins, Baltimore, Md., 1980: 456.

Takeuchi, Y., Hisanaga, N., Ono, Y. and Inoue, T. Toxicity and dose-response (effect) relationship of n-hexane. Jap. J. industr. Hlth, 1980a, 22: 470.

Takeuchi, Y., Ono, Y., Hisanaga, N., Kitoh, J. and Sugiura, Y. A comparative study on the neurotoxicity of n-pentane, n-hexane, and n-heptane in the rat. Brit. J. industr. Med., 1980b, 37: 241.

Wada, Y., Okamoto, S. and Takagi, S. Intoxication polyneuropathy following exposure to n-hexane. Clin. Neurol., 1965, 5: 591.

Yamamura, Y. n-Hexane polyneuropathy, Folia psychiat. neurol. jap., 1969, 23: 45.

Kyoto Symposia (EEG Suppl. No. 36)
Editors: P.A. Buser, W.A. Cobb and T. Okuma
© 1982, Elsevier Biomedical Press, Amsterdam

Neurophysiological Effects of Methyl Mercury on the Nervous System

Y. MURAI, S. SHIRAISHI, Y. YAMASHITA, A. OHNISHI[1] AND K. ARIMURA

*Department of Neurology, University of Occupational and Environmental Health, Kitakyushu,
and [1]Department of Neuropathology, Neurological Institute, Faculty of Medicine, Kyushu University,
Fukuoka (Japan)*

Although sensory disturbances are one of the most frequent symptoms of organic mercury poisoning in man, the causative lesion of the symptom is still in controversy. Since Hunter et al. (1940) observed degeneration in the peripheral nerves of poisoned rats, the sensory symptoms have been attributed to a lesion of the primary sensory neurone. However, some of the recent studies performed in primates do not indicate the presence of sensory neuropathy (LeQuesne et al. 1974; Von Burg and Rustam 1974; Berlin et al. 1975; Snyder and Seelinger 1976). The purposes of this study are (1) to confirm the peripheral sensory nerve lesion in experimental rats and (2) to perform electrophysiological and morphological studies on poisoned monkeys, and find the causative lesion for the sensory symptoms of organic mercury poisoning in primates.

MATERIAL AND METHODS

Rats

Adult male Wistar rats, ranging in body weight from 200 to 217 g were used. The test group consisted of 9 rats and the control of 5 rats. To the test group, 5 mg/kg of methylmercuric chloride (CH_3HgCl) was given orally through a stomach tube every 2 days. The 9 rats in the test group were divided into 2 groups. Four rats of group A were studied electrophysiologically on the 32nd day, when the total dose of methylmercuric chloride was 80 mg/kg. After the electrophysiological study the rats were submitted to morphological study. Five rats of group B were studied on the 54th day, when the total dose of methylmercuric chloride was 135 mg/kg.

The method of the sural nerve conduction study was modified from that of DeJesus et al. (1978). Sodium pentobarbital was given intraperitoneally, and the sciatic and the sural nerves were surgically exposed. The sural nerve was stimulated at the ankle and the evoked nerve action potential was recorded from the sciatic nerve. Sensory conduction velocity of the sural nerve was calculated and the peak to peak amplitude of the sensory potential was measured.

For histological studies the sural nerve was fixed with 2% glutaraldehyde and divided into two portions, one for teased fibre preparations and one for epoxy sections, which were used for measurement of the density (the number per square millimeter of fascicular area) of total, large and small myelinated fibres and their size distribution.

Monkeys

Two monkeys (*Macaca fuscata*) were used. Five mg/kg of methylmercuric chloride was administered orally through a stomach tube once a week.

Motor conduction was studied in the median and the posterior tibial nerves, and sensory conduction was studied orthodromically in the median nerve and antidromically in the sural nerve. Somatosensory evoked potentials, visual evoked potentials and brain stem auditory evoked potentials were also measured. Methods used in these electrophysiological studies were essentially the same as those for humans. The measurements were performed under mild anaesthesia induced by ketamine hydrochloride.

Histological study was performed on their nervous systems including cerebrum, brain stem, cerebellum, spinal cord, cranial nerves, anterior and posterior spinal roots, posterior root ganglia and sural nerve.

RESULTS

Rats

Increase in body weight was less in the test group than in controls. Around the 20th day, rats in the test group showed less resistance when they were captured for the administration of the toxin. Increase of body weight ceased around the 30th day in the test group. Four rats of group A were studied on the 32nd day. On the 40th day there was an apparent clumsiness in their walking, and they became unable to walk on the 54th day. All of the 5 rats of group B were studied on the 54th day. Controls were also studied on the same day.

The amplitude of the sensory potential in 5 sural nerves of the control group averaged 346 μV (standard error 14), and that in 4 sural nerves of group A averaged 193 μV (standard error 28) ($P < 0.05$). No sensory potential was recorded from any sural nerve of group B. Conduction velocity in 5 sural nerves of the control group averaged 38.8 m/sec (standard error 1.4) and that in 4 sural nerves of group A averaged 36.0 m/sec (standard error 2.9) (not significant). Conduction velocity could not be measured in group B because of absence of the sensory potential. These electrophysiological data are suggestive of axonal degeneration.

Teased fibre analysis showed no condition E in control rats. However, condition E was observed in 21.5% (standard error 5.1) in group A and in 80.0% (standard error 5.0) in group B. There was no evidence of segmental demyelination in any of these 3 groups.

Monkeys

Ataxia developed acutely in both monkeys when the total dose was 30 and 35

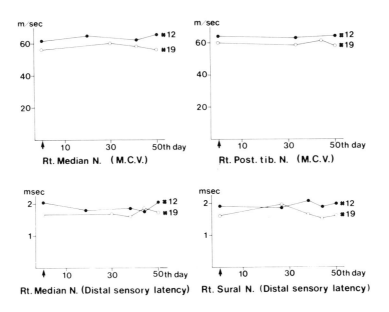

Fig. 1. Serial changes in motor conduction velocities in the median and posterior tibial nerves and sensory latencies of the median and sural nerves before (arrow) and after the administration of methyl mercury in 2 monkeys (Nos. 12, 19).

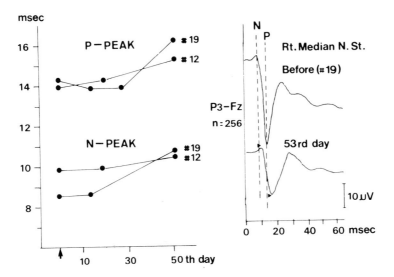

Fig. 2. Serial changes in the peak latencies of initial negative and positive cortical components of somatosensory evoked potentials to median nerve stimulation.

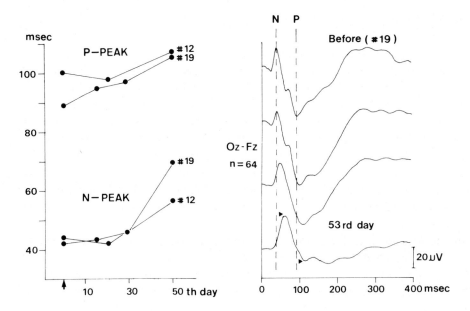

Fig. 3. Serial changes in the peak latencies of major negative and positive components of visual flash-evoked potentials.

mg/kg respectively. After the onset of the disease, monkeys could not walk or eat food by themselves.

Motor conduction velocity and distal motor latency in the median and posterior tibial nerves did not significantly change in the entire course of the study; the sensory latencies of the median and sural nerves were also unchanged (Fig. 1). The amplitude of the sensory potential was unchanged in the median nerve, but that in the sural nerve could not be used because it differed at each measurement, even on the same day. Therefore it was impossible to detect axonal degeneration of the sural nerve electrophysiologically. Somatosensory evoked potentials showed progressive slowing of major negative and positive peaks which correspond to the human N1 and Pl (Fig. 2). Visual evoked potentials also showed progressive slowing of the major negative and positive peaks, indicating dysfunction in the visual system (Fig. 3). The brain stem auditory evoked potential did not show any significant change in waves 1, 2 and 4.

Histological examination was performed 7 days after the onset of ataxia in 1 monkey. No pathological change was noticed in the cerebellum, brain stem, spinal cord and peripheral nerves on microscopic examination. However, examination of the cerebral cortex disclosed distinct change in the calcarine cortex. There were many vacuolations of the neurophils and neurones. In the other monkey there was a marked increase of proliferative astrocytes as well as vacuolation. Frontal, parietal and temporal cortices were within normal limits in both monkeys.

DISCUSSION

Nerve conduction and histological studies on the sural nerves of poisoned rats indicated axonal degeneration as previous investigators have already reported (Cavanagh and Chen 1971; Herman et al. 1973). In monkeys sensory latencies were normal and there was no histological evidence of sensory neuropathy. However, somatosensory and visual evoked potentials showed progressive slowing of their major components. The slowing of the somatosensory evoked potential could be attributed to dysfunction in some parts of the somatosensory system other than the peripheral sensory nerve, which showed normal latency. Histological abnormality was confined to the calcarine cortex. These data suggest that the visual cortex, and perhaps somewhere in the central portion of the somatosensory system as well, are much more vulnerable than the peripheral sensory nerve.

On reviewing the literature, most of the electrophysiological studies have failed to demonstrate peripheral sensory neuropathy in patients with organic mercury poisoning (LeQuesne et al. 1974; Von Burg and Rustam 1974; Snyder and Seelinger 1976; Nagaki 1981). Tokuomi (1981) also could not find anything abnormal in the sural nerve conduction and in the short latency components of the somatosensory evoked potential (N9, N11, N13 and N14), whereas N20 were abnormal in all cases, which suggests a central origin of the sensory symptoms of organic mercury poisoning in man. However, Cinca et al. (1979) reported 2 cases which showed definite abnormal sensory conduction and normal motor conduction velocities in the acute stage of the intoxication and recovered normal sensory conduction velocity 6 months later. These cases suggest that sensory neuropathy is detectable electrophysiologically in the early stage of severe intoxication by organic mercury.

Although some pathological studies failed to show definite lesions in sensory nerve, posterior root or posterior root ganglion in patients and experimental monkeys with organic mercury poisoning (Hunter and Russell 1954; Berlin et al. 1975), studies performed in Japan have demonstrated degeneration in both axon and myelin sheath of sensory nerve, posterior root or posterior root ganglion in patients with Minamata disease (Takeuchi et al. 1962; Etoh 1971; Ikuta et al. 1974; Myakawa et al. 1976). Sato (1979) demonstrated swelling and destruction of the myelin sheath and some change of the axon in the sural nerves of monkeys with long-term administration of small doses of methylmercuric chloride, in contrast to our acute study. A too large weekly dose of methylmercuric chloride was thought to be the reason why we could not demonstrate sensory neuropathy in poisoned monkeys.

From the review of the literature, we concluded that only in the early stage of patients with severe intoxication by organic mercury, the sensory nerve lesion could be detectable electrophysiologically. Pathologists also could observe old lesion even later in the course of the disease.

SUMMARY

There was electrophysiological and histological evidence of axonal degeneration in sural nerves of rats with methyl mercury intoxication. In monkeys, there was no sensory nerve involvement, whereas somatosensory and visual evoked potentials showed progressive slowing of their major peaks in the course of the intoxication. Pathological changes were confined to the calcarine cortex. The possibility of sensory nerve involvement in patients with organic mercury poisoning was discussed.

REFERENCES

Berlin, M., Grant, C.A., Hellberg, J., Hellström, J. and Schütz, A. Neurotoxicity of methylmercury in squirrel monkeys. Arch. environm. Hlth, 1975, 30: 340–348.

Cavanagh, J.B. and Chen, C.K. The effects of methyl-mercury-dicyandiamide on the peripheral nerves and spinal cord of rats. Acta neuropath. (Berl.), 1971, 19: 208–215.

Cinca, I., Dumitrescu, I., Onaca, P., Serbanescu, A. and Nestorescu, B. Accidental ethyl mercury poisoning with nervous system, skeletal muscle, and myocardium injury. J. Neurol. Neurosurg. Psychiat., 1979, 43: 143–149.

DeJesus, C.P.V., Towfighi, J. and Snyder, D.R. Sural nerve conduction study in the rat: A new technique for studying experimental neuropathies. Muscle Nerve, 1978: 1: 162–167.

Etoh, K. Pathological changes of peripheral nerve in human Minamata disease: An electron-microscopic observation. Adv. neurol. Sci. (Jap.), 1971, 15: 606–618 (in Japanese).

Herman, S.P., Klein, R., Talley, F.A. and Kriegman, M.R. An ultrastructural study of methylmercury-induced primary sensory neuropathy in the rat. Lab. Invest., 1973, 28: 104–118.

Hunter, D. and Russell, D.S. Focal cerebral and cerebellar atrophy in a human subject due to organic mercury compounds. J. Neurol. Neurosurg. Psychiat., 1954, 17: 235–241.

Hunter, D., Bomford, R.R. and Russell, D.S. Poisoning by methyl mercury compounds. Quart. J. Med., 1940, 9: 193–213.

Ikuta, F., Makifuchi, T., Ohama, E., Koga, M. et al. Morphological alterations in the autopsy cases of chronic organic mercury intoxication with minimal dose. Adv. neurol. Sci. (Jap.), 1974, 18: 861–881 (in Japanese).

LeQuesne, P.M., Damluji, S.F. and Rustam, H. Electrophysiological studies of peripheral nerves in patients with organic mercury poisoning. J. Neurol. Neurosurg. Psychiat., 1974, 37: 333–339.

Miyakawa, T., Murayama, E., Sumiyoshi, S., Deshimaru, M., Fujimoto, T., Hattori, E. and Shikai, I. Late changes in human sural nerves in Minamata disease and in nerves of rates with experimental organic mercury poisoning. Acta neuropath. (Berl.), 1976, 35: 131–138.

Nagaki, J. Sensory symptom and sensory action potential in Minamata disease. Jap. J. EEG EMG, 1981, X: 79 (in Japanese).

Sato, T. and Ikuta, F. Neuropathology of methylmercury intoxication in Niigata and chronic effect in monkeys. In: L. Roizin, H. Shiraki and N. Grčevič (Eds.), Neurotoxicology, Vol. 1. Raven Press, New York, 1977: 261–269.

Snyder, R.D. and Seelinger, D.F. Methylmercury poisoning. Clinical follow-up and sensory nerve conduction studies. J. Neurol. Neurosurg. Psychiat., 1976, 39: 701–704.

Takeuchi, T., Morikawa, N., Matsumoto, H. and Shiraishi, Y. A pathological study of Minamata disease in Japan. Acta neuropath. (Berl.), 1962, 2: 40–57.

Tokuomi, H. Pathophysiology of chronic neurotoxic disease (Minamata disease). Paper presented at 22nd Congr. Jap. Soc. Neurol. (Kumamoto), May 21, 1981.

Von Burg, R. and Rustam, H. Electrophysiological investigations of methylmercury intoxication in humans. Evaluation of peripheral nerve by conduction velocity and electromyography. Electroenceph. clin. Neurophysiol., 1974, 37: 381–392.

Kyoto Symposia (EEG Suppl. No. 36)
Editors: P.A. Buser, W.A. Cobb and T. Okuma
688

Quantified Electromyography as a Clinical Parameter of a Multifactorial Study of Workers Exposed to Different Toxic Agents

A. ARRIGO

Centro di Neurofisiologia Clinica, Università di Pavia, Pavia (Italy)

The research on workers exposed to the risk of poisoning by toxic agents is nowadays changing its goal. A few years ago, in fact, neurologists and electrophysiologists were requested to supply evidence of peripheral nervous system involvement, frequently for medico-legal controversies (Bergamini and Sibour 1960). As the industrial environment and the methods of working with toxic agents have improved, our task is more devoted to the aim of finding out earliest and minimal signs of neuropathies, defined by Thage et al. (1978) as "subclinical or minimal toxic neuropathies."

This kind of research needs, indeed, more accuracy in carrying out both clinical and electromyographic examinations and, in some ways, a better program than before. Referring to a paper by Le Quesne we deem it useful to underline some points: "Knowledge of the clinical features, previous electrophysiological studies, and pathological changes occurring in a particular neuropathy is important in choosing the most suitable approach." (Le Quesne 1978).

METHOD

Our plan of work is the following. Levels of the toxic substance in the environment should be noticed.

Personal anamnesis. Particular care should be devoted to family diseases, mainly diabetes, nephropathy and any other disease of neurological interest. It is important to know about arthropathies and limb trauma. The habits of the subjects should be investigated in order to find out drug or alcohol addiction, the amount of tobacco smoked and its quality.

Work anamnesis: period of exposure to the toxic substance expressed in hours per day, month and year. It is extremely important to know about the personal task of the worker in order to form an opinion of the subject's relationship to the toxic agent.

Subjective symptoms and complaints should be considered, bearing in mind both the characteristic symptoms of the peripheral nervous system involvement and the symptoms that are characteristic of poisoning by particular agents, such as gum inflammation by lead and mercury. Clinical examination should be accurately performed by a neurologist.

Blood and urine determinations of the levels of toxic substance are normally carried out (Arrigo et al. 1978; Kokodoko Dossé 1980; Pinelli 1980).

NEEDLE ELECTROMYOGRAPHY

Muscle at rest: presence or not of spontaneous pathological activity (fibrillation, fasciculation).

Low level of voluntary muscular contraction. MUAP parameters: duration, amplitude, number of phases (if possible number of peaks). A new method of automatic analysis (Arrigo et al. 1981, data not published) has been applied to some groups of subjects.

Maximum level of voluntary muscular contraction: interference pattern, reduced interference activity, discrete activity.

The presence of spontaneous activity in more than one muscle, in parallel with alterations of MUAP parameters, an increased number of polyphasic potentials and a reduced activity during strong effort are evaluated as signs of peripheral nervous involvement.

STIMULUS DETECTION ELECTROMYOGRAPHY

Maximum motor conduction velocity of nerves both in lower and in upper limbs (better in symmetrical nerves) (sometimes minimum motor conduction velocity of the same nerves).

Distal latency of M_{max} responses (Pinelli 1964).

M_{max} response amplitude.

Sensory conduction velocity with SAP amplitude.

H index.

Blink reflexes (when facial nerves might be involved).

A pathological value is given to those which are 2 S.D. outside the normal range.

CASES

All the subjects considered in this study underwent every examination voluntarily after previous agreement with the trade unions and the managing staffs of the firms. The cases were divided into 6 groups, as shown in Table I, according to toxic agents, age and period of exposure.

Lead. There were complaints from practically all the workers (one-third had symptoms related to the toxic activity of lead). Clinical examination showed reduced strength, slightly atrophic muscles, tendon reflexes not evoked in 40 cases. EMG

TABLE I

Toxic agent	Length of exposure			Total	Age range (years)
	A (long)	B (medium)	C (short)		
Lead	62	47	21	130	21–70
CS$_2$	20	29	99	148	16–57
Phthalate	14	13	15	42	24–57
Hg	77	51	45	173	20–29
DMF	3	2	5	10	21–53
Total	176	142	185	503	16–70

findings were within the normal range in 65 subjects. Needle EMG patterns were altered in 69 cases (51%). Maximum motor conduction velocity was reduced (20% normal values) in 35 (26%) cases, both in radial nerves and/or in peroneal nerves, bilaterally. No correlation was found between altered EMG patterns and the specific biohumoral indexes. On the contrary, pathological EMGs were found mainly in subjects exposed to the action of lead for a longer time.

CS$_2$. Subjective symptoms in practically all the subjects – without any clinical evidence.

Bilateral slowing of the maximum motor conduction velocity of the peroneal nerves was significant in 7 cases (4.3%); unilateral in 12. M_{max} wave amplitude was reduced in 2 cases (1.2%).

Needle EMG examinations showed alterations in 53 subjects (32%). No correlation was demonstrated with the level of CS$_2$ in the working environment; on the contrary, a relationship seemed to be possible between the reduction of maximum motor conduction velocity and the duration of exposure, even for the lower levels of the toxic agent.

Phthalate. Many subjects complained of muscle cramp, fatigue and paraesthesiae in their calves. Clinical examinations were normal. Needle EMG demonstrated 2 out of 3 alterations in 9 subjects (21%). Two subjects (4.6%) presented slight reduction of maximum motor conduction velocity and 2 (4.6%) had reduced amplitude of M_{max} wave.

Hg. Almost 50% of the subjects described different kinds of disturbance, not particularly related to signs of peripheral nervous system involvement. Twelve subjects had some gum inflammation or haemorrhage. The clinical examination can be summarized as normal.

Needle EMG showed alteration in 10 (5.7%) subjects. Two cases (1.2%) had slightly reduced maximum motor conduction velocity; no changes in M_{max} amplitude.

Eight cases (4.7%) presented a significantly (>2 S.D.) increased distal latency in the popliteal nerves, bilaterally.

All the parameters considered were within the normal range, with a high factor (>0.9) correlated with the age.

DMF. There were neither subjective complaints nor clinical evidence of peripheral nervous system involvement. Two out of 5 subjects had altered parameters on needle EMG examination. Maximum motor conduction velocity was within the normal range. M_{max} wave amplitude was slightly reduced in 3 out of 5 cases.

DISCUSSION

It is quite evident that, within the group of substances considered in our research, lead and CS_2 are the agents with high toxic activity (Seppäläinen and Tolonen 1974; Seppäläinen and Hernberg 1979; Moglia et al. 1980). In fact, even if most of our cases did not present any clinical evidence of peripheral nervous system involvement (except 40 cases exposed to lead), significant reductions of maximum MCV values were noticed in the subjects exposed to lead and CS_2.

Relatively few and scarce EMG signs of PNS involvement were evident in the group working with Hg. But it has not been clearly demonstrated that this kind of examination is the most sensitive to find signs of intoxication (Le Quesne et al., 1974).

As far as the automatic analysis of MUAP parameters is concerned, our opinion confirms that expressed in previous papers. The numbers of polyphasic MUAPs, carefully evaluated and expressed as percentages ($>15\%$), should be considered abnormal when it is found to be increased bilaterally in symmetric muscles, mainly if the number of peaks is also increased. These data must correlate with at least another of the following signs of peripheral nerve involvement (fibrillation, increased duration and amplitude of MUAPs, and reduced patterns of activity on maximal voluntary effort).

According to our experience needle EMG abnormal findings are the earliest signs allowing us to suspect a subclinical or minimal neuropathy.

REFERENCES

Arrigo, A., Moglia, A., Sandrini, G., Bernocchi, F. and Pernice, A. Methods of EMG quantitative analysis in the diagnosis of subclinical polyneuropathies. In: N. Canal and G. Plozza (Eds.), Peripheral Neuropathies. Elsevier/North-Holland Biomedical Press, Amsterdam, 1978: 63–68.

Bergamini, V. e Sibour, F. La diagnosi precoce di sofferenza nervosa periferica da intossicazione esogena (ricerche neurofisiologiche). Riv. Pat. nerv. ment., 1960, 81: 415–439.

Kokodoko Dossé, A. Studio clinico ed elettromiografico in 42 soggetti esposti in impianto di produzione a 2-etil-esil-ftalato, butil ed eso-butil-ftolato. Tesi di Specializzazione 1980. Università di Pavia, Italy.

Le Quesne, P.M. Neurophysiological investigation of subclinical and minimal toxic neuropathies. Muscle Nerves, 1978, 1: 392–395.

Le Quesne, P.M., Damluji, S.F. and Rustam, H. Electrophysiological studies of peripheral nerves in patients with organic mercury poisoning. J. Neurol. Neurosurg. Psychiat., 1974, 37: 333–339.

Moglia, A., Biscaldi, G.P., Sandrini, G., Pollini, G., Manni, R. and Arrigo, A. Clinical biohumoral electromyographic study in 100 workers exposed to lead poisoning risk. G. ital. Med. Lav., 1980, 2: 239–241.

Pinelli, P. Physical, anatomical and physiological factors in the latency measurement of the M response. Electroenceph. clin. Neurophysiol., 1962, 17: 86.

Pinelli, P. Errori concettuali e insufficienze metodologiche nella definizione di polineuropatia subclinica. G. ital. Med. Lav., 1980, 2: 1–4.

Seppäläinen, A.M. and Hernberg, S. Subclinical lead poisoning. Electrophysiological aspects at different blood lead levels. Abstracts, Int. Congress of Neurotoxicology, Varese, Italy, Sept. 1979: 29–32.

Seppäläinen, A.M. and Tolonen, M. Neurotoxicity of the long term exposure to carbon disulfide in the viscose rayon industry. A neurophysiological study. W.K. environm. Hlth, 1974, 2: 145–149.

Thage, O., Trojaborg, W. and Buchthal, F. Electromyographic findings in polineuropathy. Neurology (Minneap.), 1978, 13: 273–278.

Kyoto Symposia (EEG Suppl. No. 36)
Editors: P.A. Buser, W.A. Cobb and T. Okuma
© 1982, Elsevier Biomedical Press, Amsterdam

The Use of Clinical Neurophysiologial Methods in Studies of Workers Exposed to Solvents

ANNA MARIA SEPPÄLÄINEN

Institute of Occupational Health, Helsinki, Finland

Various solvents and their mixtures are widely used in industry. These solvents are usually hydrocarbons, and among them especially those with 6 carbon atoms – hexacarbons – have been shown to be neurotoxic, and many others have been suggested to have neurotoxic properties. Organic solvents are found, e.g., in paints, glues, cleaning and degreasing mixtures. They are used by small workshops and by large industrial plants, even at home, where people may glue sandals or other small leather items for commercial purposes.

Acute intoxications may occur, but they are exceptional in modern industrialized countries. At high concentrations many solvents are narcotic, many among them have been tested as anaesthetics. As such they depress the activity of the central nervous system (CNS) and some EEG changes could remain after accidental exposure to very high concentrations of solvent fumes in the air. Neurophysiological sequelae, e.g. EEG findings, after such episodes have not been thoroughly studied.

Chronic effects of occupational exposure to solvents are of greater practical and research interest. Patients with solvent poisoning and also workers with long-term exposure to solvents complain of various symptoms like headache, vegetative disorders, memory impairment, sleep disorders, paraesthetic sensations, muscle pain and diminished strength, suggestive of CNS or peripheral nervous system (PNS) involvement.

Axonopathy is thought to be the basic neurotoxic effect of solvents. The distal portions of the longest and largest axons are the most vulnerable, and thus the process has been referred to as distal axonopathy. The axons in the central tracts are, however, also affected (Schaumburg and Spencer 1978; Cavanagh and Bennetts 1981), and thus these neurotoxic phenomena have also been termed central-peripheral distal axonopathy. The prominent feature in these cases is accumulation of 10 nm neurofilaments within axons. Widespread microscopic changes of this type can be detected even at early stages of poisoning, without major functional disturbances being observed in the affected animals (Cavanagh and Bennetts 1981).

Nerve conduction velocities are only slightly affected in axonopathies. Individual patients may, however, show abnormally slow nerve conduction and epidemiological studies reveal differences in conduction velocities between exposed workers and appropriate age-matched reference groups.

Several Italian studies have reported neuropathic findings among workers exposed to mixtures of solvents in small workshops. It was considered that the polyneuropathy frequently found among shoe-workers was caused by paraffinic hydrocarbons of a low boiling point (pentane, isopentane, 2-methyl-pentane, 3-methyl-pentane, n-hexane, heptane, isoheptane) (Cianchetti et al. 1976) among which n-hexane alone or potentiated by methyl-ethyl-ketone has been shown to be neurotoxic (Yamamura 1969; Herskowitz et al. 1971; Altenkirch et al. 1977). Methyl n-butyl ketone which has a common metabolite – 2,5-hexanedione – with n-hexane (Spencer and Schaumburg 1975) is neurotoxic as well and caused an industrial outbreak of neuropathy in an American industrial plant producing plastic-coated and colour-printed fabrics (Allen et al. 1975). Electro-neuromyography has been shown to be a sensitive and useful method of identifying and diagnosing patients with mild toxic polyneuropathy (Allen et al. 1975; Cianchetti et al. 1976).

The prominent feature in neuropathy caused by various solvents has been distally accentuated slowing of both motor and sensory conduction velocities. Slowing of the motor conduction velocity (MCV) was noted especially in the peroneal nerve, although it was usually mild or moderate in degree; 50% slowing was exceptional (Allen et al. 1975; Cianchetti et al. 1976). The motor distal latency of the peroneal nerve was often clearly prolonged, and in more severe cases it was not possible to elicit a motor response from the extensor digitorum brevis muscle by stimulating the peroneal nerve at the ankle, although a stimulus at the knee level resulted in a response (Cianchetti et al. 1976). In many cases the slowing of the MCV in the peroneal nerve deteriorated further during the first months after stopping the occupational exposure, even to the point where no response was evocable with stimulation at the knee level. In 12–18 months after cessation of exposure, a clear improvement was usually noted in the MCVs, although symptoms like weakness, paraesthesiae and cramp-like muscular pain could remain unchanged for months or even years (Cianchetti et al. 1976). Slowing of conduction velocity has also been found in the ulnar, tibial and sural nerves (Allen et al. 1975) as well as in the femoral nerve (Cianchetti et al. 1976). Sensory conduction velocity (SCV) has been found to be slow in the distal portions especially (Allen et al. 1975).

The duration of the evoked motor action potential (MAP) from peroneal nerve stimulation was abnormally long in many patients and it further lengthened during the follow-up period (Cianchetti et al. 1976). In voluntary contraction the number of motor unit potentials was clearly diminished in the affected patients and often the amplitude and duration of motor unit potentials were increased as well (Allen et al. 1975). All these findings are typical of distally accentuated motor and sensory neuropathy of predominantly axonal degeneration.

Even more severe, progressive, ascending and mainly motor polyneuropathy, leading to pronounced muscle atrophy and characteristic vegetative alterations, in the most severe cases to tetraplegia, was observed in 18 juvenile patients who had sniffed a glue thinner (Altenkirch et al. 1977). Improvement was slow. Motor and sensory conduction velocities were reduced in proportion to the degree of paresis, especially distal latencies were prolonged. Nerves of the lower extremities were affected more severely, in part to the point where no response could be elicited. In

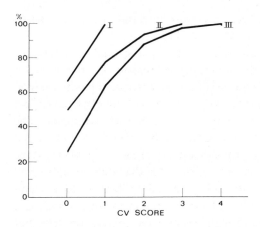

Fig. 1. Cumulative percentage distribution of CV scores (indicating the number of abnormally slow nerve conduction velocities) of 77 patients with solvent poisoning at exposure levels I = low, II = intermediate, and III = high. (From Seppäläinen et al. 1980a.)

the EMG denervation activity, fibrillations and positive sharp waves were found as well as signs of reinnervation in the form of small, polyphasic motor unit potentials of long duration. All the patients had abused thinner for long periods but the composition of the thinner had been changed a few months before the symptoms appeared and the new thinner contained methyl-ethyl-ketone and *n*-hexane. Sniffing thinner containing a higher concentration of *n*-hexane but no methyl-ethyl-ketone had not caused neuropathy, so the combination of methyl-ethyl-ketone and *n*-hexane was incriminated. Neuropathies occurred in patients who had abused only the new combination for 3–4 months. Equally striking reports of polyneuropathy caused by solvents have been published on American sniffers (Prockop et al. 1974; Korobkin et al. 1975) or after accidental exposure to a narcotic concentration of trichlorethylene (Sagawa et al. 1973) and rarely after occupational exposure to *n*-hexane in very poor working conditions (Takeuchi et al. 1975).

In milder cases of solvent poisoning, when symptoms mainly consisted of memory and sleep disorders, headache, vertigo, occasional numbness and weakness, abnormally slow MCVs and SCVs were found, and the frequency of abnormally slow conduction velocities tended to increase if the exposure level was higher (Fig. 1) (Seppäläinen et al. 1980a). Among 117 solvent-exposed workers who had come for periodic health examination or because of suspected solvent poisoning to the Institute of Occupational Health, Helsinki and who presented with some mild symptoms like paraesthetic feelings or muscular pain, 61 or 52% had at least one abnormally slow nerve conduction velocity, often in combination with some neurogenic EMG abnormality like a diminished number of motor units or denervation activity (Seppäläinen 1973). Swedish epidemiological studies have revealed that mean conduction velocities of several nerves were significantly slower in a group of 80 industrial and car painters in comparison with a reference group of 80 workers matched for age, education and job qualification (Elofsson et al. 1979).

In the same study the amplitude of the sensory action potential of the sural nerve was significantly smaller among solvent-exposed workers.

As nerve conduction velocities usually slow only slightly in axonal neuropathies, it would seem advantageous to measure amplitudes of sensory or motor action potentials elicited by nerve stimulation. The amplitude of motor action potentials is, however, easily affected by technical placement of the recording electrodes, skin resistance etc., and minor changes in it cannot be regarded as significant. The amplitude of sensory action potentials could be more reliable, especially if measured from needle records. Needle electrodes, on the other hand, are less suitable for large epidemiological studies, although they are appropriate for the study of individual patients. In a study of workers occupationally exposed to styrene Rosen and coworkers (1978) found statistically significant differences in the amplitudes and durations of sensory action potentials, although actual nerve conduction velocities did not differ from those in the control group. Styrene, which is a solvent widely used in the plastic and rubber industries, has been claimed to show toxic effects in the peripheral nervous system (Lilis et al. 1978), although it may be more toxic to the CNS (Seppäläinen and Härkönen 1976).

Carbon disulphide, which is at present used in the viscose rayon industry for the production of artificial fibres, causes a similar type of axonal degeneration to hexacarbons. Polyneuropathic symptoms are prominent features of chronic carbon disulphide poisoning and nerve conduction studies as well as EMG have been successfully applied for diagnostic purposes and in epidemiological studies (for reference see Seppäläinen and Haltia 1980).

Neurotoxic effects of solvents are not limited to PNS; as previously mentioned, CNS type symptoms are frequent complaints of workers exposed to solvents or suffering from solvent poisoning. EEG abnormalities are frequent among patients with relatively mild solvent poisoning (Seppäläinen et al. 1980a). The abnormalities are usually slow waves, one third of these being local and about two-thirds being diffuse or generalized in character. About 5% of patients with solvent poisoning have shown paroxysmal abnormalities as well, either generalized spike and wave discharges or focal sharp waves. A certain dose-response relationship was noted concerning abnormal EEGs in a group of 233 workers exposed to various solvents and their mixtures (Seppäläinen 1973) and having various symptoms of possible CNS affections. The subjects were divided into 3 exposure categories based on information collected from their work places, exposure levels being I (low), II (intermediate), and III (high). Exposure level III was close to the threshold limit according to the Finnish regulations, seldom exceeding it. Exposure level I referred to a working situation in which the exposure was generally low or occasional, and repeated high-peak exposures improbable. Subjects at exposure level III had abnormal EEGs in over 70% and this was statistically highly significantly different from the frequency of abnormal EEGs among subjects at exposure levels I or II ($P < 0.001$) (Fig. 2).

In an Italian series of 125 shoe factory workers (Giuliano et al. 1974) abnormal EEGs were found in 27% and borderline findings in 32%. Among 96 male workers

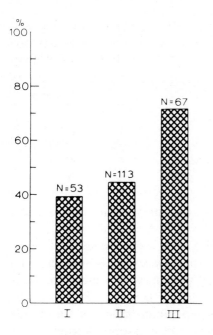

Fig. 2. Percentage of abnormal EEGs among 233 solvent exposed workers with symptoms divided into 3 exposure categories: I = mild, II = intermediate, and III = high. N notes the number of subjects in each category. The difference is statistically significant between exposure levels I and III (χ^2 = 11.14, $P<0.001$) and between levels II and III (χ^2 = 11.65, $P<0.001$).

exposed to styrene in the plastic industry the frequency of abnormal EEGs was significantly higher (around 30%) among those subjects whose individual exposure to styrene (measured by mandelic acid concentration in the urine) exceeded a certain threshold level than among those with lower styrene exposures, who had abnormal EEGs in about 10% (Seppäläinen and Härkönen 1976).

No actual increase in the frequency of abnormal EEGs has been found among industrial or car painters (Elofsson et al. 1979; Seppäläinen et al. 1978) in comparison to reference groups comprising manual workers without solvent exposure. However, a certain dose-response relationship emerges between groups of workers arranged according to the average exposure level within the worker group (Table I). Painters in the construction industry have the lowest solvent exposure and also the lowest frequency of abnormal EEGs, while car painters have a somewhat higher frequency and patients or subjects with symptoms of solvent exposure the highest.

When actual EEG abnormalities have been lacking, some other differences have been noted in the EEGs of solvent-exposed workers in comparison with a reference group. For example workers exposed to jet fuel (a mixture of solvents) had EEGs with poorer organization of the alpha activity than the referents (Knave et al. 1978). An increased amount of fast activity in the central and fronto-central areas was seen in 27% of styrene-exposed workers in comparison with one among 6 normal

TABLE I

PERCENTAGE OF ABNORMAL EEGs AMONG SOLVENT EXPOSED WORKERS IN VARIOUS
STUDIES CONDUCTED AT THE INSTITUTE OF OCCUPATIONAL HEALTH, HELSINKI,
FINLAND

	Percentage
72 painters in building industry (Seppäläinen and Lindström 1982)	17
102 car painters (Seppäläinen et al. 1978)	31
233 solvent-exposed workers with symptoms (Seppäläinen 1973)	40–72
107 patients with solvent poisoning (Seppäläinen et al. 1980a)	65

controls (Rosen et al. 1978). The relationship of the latter findings to the health situation of the subjects remains open.

Involvement of central axons can be studied with evoked potentials. These techniques have rarely been applied to solvent-exposed workers. A Swedish group studied 80 industrial and car painters and used pattern-evoked visual potentials (VEP). The main components tended to have longer latencies among solvent-exposed subjects, the difference from a reference group being not statistically significant (Elofsson et al. 1979). On the other hand, the peak-to-peak amplitude of N80 to P100 was significantly greater among solvent-exposed workers; this finding can hardly signify axonal degeneration.

Our group (Seppäläinen et al. 1979) has studied 15 industrial workers with 10 years (on the average) exposure to technical grade n-hexane, either in a vegetable oil extraction plant or in factories manufacturing adhesive tapes. Although overall exposure was low, certain peak exposure periods lasting minutes to perhaps 1 h had occurred in plants probably weekly; during peak exposures the air concentration may have reached 2500–3250 ppm, while the threshold limit value for n-hexane is 500 ppm in Finland. n-Hexane-exposed workers had flash-evoked visual potentials (VEPs) of small amplitude and the latencies of P45 and N65 were statistically significantly longer among n-hexane-exposed workers. Also the peak-to-peak amplitudes of electroretinograms (ERG) were significantly smaller among exposed workers. The findings were interpreted to represent either partial axonal degeneration or conduction block in the intracerebral axons. The same workers often had abnormally slow nerve conduction velocities as well as abnormal EEGs (Seppäläinen et al. 1980b); Fig. 3 represents the combinations of various neurophysiological findings. Electroneuromyographic findings compatible with neuropathy were more often found with small amplitude VEPs than abnormal EEGs, which further supports the idea of axonal involvement in both CNS and PNS.

Clinical neurophysiological methods are non-invasive and can furnish information on the functions of both PNS and CNS. It would be advisable to apply various techniques to the same patients or solvent-exposed workers, as has been done in a few studies (Elofsson et al. 1979; Seppäläinen et al. 1980b) and thus map lesions in various parts of the nervous system. Cavanagh and Bennetts (1981) have

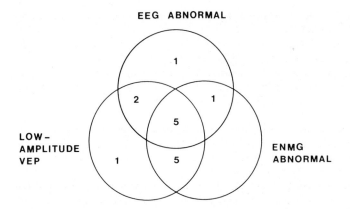

Fig. 3. Abnormal EEG and ENMG findings and low amplitude flash VEPs among 15 workers with long occupational exposure to *n*-hexane. (Seppäläinen et al. 1980b.)

emphasized the neuropathological study of various parts of the nervous system in experimental animal studies on the effects of solvents. Different solvents may have different distributions of toxic effects in the human being; some sites may escape, while others suffer from deleterious effects. Neurophysiological methods yield objective and quantitative data and exposed and reference groups can easily be compared. These methods are applicable to epidemiological studies and individual diagnosis. In individual patients mildly abnormal findings should be interpreted with caution, since multiple aetiological factors may cause, e.g., slight neuropathy and thus result in similar findings. The distal parts of nerves and intrinsic hand muscles are predilection sites for peripheral axonopathy and similarly also the sural nerve and foot muscles. However, extensor digitorum brevis muscle very often shows neurogenic abnormalities based on perhaps peripheral compression neuropathy (heavy shoes etc.) or discopathy, hence abnormal findings limited to that muscle should not be regarded as evidence of polyneuropathy. Entrapment neuropathies in other regions should also be ruled out. Other possible aetiologies for neuropathy should be kept in mind as well as various reasons for encephalopathy in cases with mainly CNS symptoms.

Signs of multiple lesion within CNS and PNS are suggestive of neurotoxic effects also in individual cases. Good epidemiological and clinical studies in combination with experimental studies increase our knowledge about aetiological factors too. In all these fields clinical neurophysiological methods offer sensitive and applicable measures.

REFERENCES

Allen, N., Mendell, J.R., Billmaier, D.J., Fontaine, R.E. and O'Neill, J. Toxic polyneuropathy due to methyl *n*-butyl ketone. Arch. Neurol. (Chic.), 1975, 32: 209–218.

Altenkirch, H., Mager, J., Stoltenburg, G. and Helmbrecht, J. Toxic polyneuropathies after sniffing a glue thinner. J. Neurol., 1977, 214: 137–152.

Cavanagh, J.B. and Bennetts, R.J. On the pattern of changes in the rat nervous system produced by 2,5-hexanediol. Brain, 1981, 104: 297–318.

Cianchetti, C., Abbritti, G., Perticoni, G., Siracusa, A. and Curradi, F. Toxic polyneuropathy of shoe-industry workers. A study of 122 cases. J. Neurol. Neurosurg. Psychiat., 1976, 39: 1151–1161.

Elofsson, S.-A., Gamberale, F., Hindmarsch, T., Iregren, A., Johansson, I., Knave, B., Lydahl, E., Mindus, P., Persson, H., Philipson, B., Steby, M.T., Struwe, G., Söderman, E., Wennbeg, A. och Widen, L. En epidemiologisk undersökning av yrkesmässigt exponerade bil- och industrilackerare. Läkartidningen, 1979, 46: 4127–4148.

Giuliano, G., Iannaccone, A. e Zappoli, R. Ricerche electroencefalografiche di operai di calzaturifici esposti al rischio di intossicazione da solventi. Lav. umano, 1974, 26: 33–42.

Herskowitz, A., Ishii, N. and Schaumburg, H. n-Hexane neuropathy. A syndrome occurring as a result of industrial exposure. New Engl. J. Med., 1971, 285: 82–85.

Knave, B., Anshelm-Olson, B., Elofsson, S., Gamberale, F., Isaksson, A., Mindus, P., Persson, H.E., Struwe, G., Wennberg, A. and Westerholm, P. Long term exposure to jet fuel. II. A cross-sectional epidemiologic investigation on occupationally exposed industrial workers with special reference to the nervous system. Scand. J. Work environm. Hlth, 1978, 4: 19–45.

Korobkin, R., Asbury, A.K., Sumner, A.J. and Nielsen, S.L. Glue-sniffing neuropathy. Arch. Neurol. (Chic.), 1975, 32: 158–162.

Lilis, R., Lorimer, W.V., Diamond, S. and Selikoff, I.J. Neurotoxicity of styrene in production and polymerization workers. Environm. Res., 1978, 15: 133–138.

Prockop, L.D., Alt, M. and Tison, J. "Huffers's" neuropathy. J. Amer. med. Ass., 1974, 229: 1083–1084.

Rosen, I., Haeger-Aronsen, B., Rehnström, S. and Welinder, H. Neurophysiological functions of workers occupationally exposed to styrene. Scand. J. Work environm. Hlth, 1978, 4, Suppl. 2: 184–194.

Sagawa, K., Nishitani, H., Kawai, H., Kuge, Y. and Ikeda, M. Transverse lesion of spinal cord after accidental exposure to trichloroethylene. Int. Arch. Arbeitsmed., 1973, 31: 257–564.

Schaumburg, H.H. and Spencer, P.S. Environmental hydrocarbons produce degeneration in cat hypothalamus and optic tract. Science, 1978, 199: 199–200.

Seppäläinen, A.M. Neurotoxic effects of industrial solvents. Electroenceph. clin. Neurophysiol., 1973, 34: 702–703.

Seppäläinen, A.M. and Haltia, M. Carbon disulfide. In: P.S. Spencer and H.H. Schaumburg (Eds.), Experimental and Clinical Neurotoxicology. Williams and Wilkins, Baltimore, Md., 1980: 356–373.

Seppäläinen, A.M. and Härkönen, H. Neurophysiological findings among workers occupationally exposed to styrene. Scand. J. Work environm. Hlth, 1976, 2: 140–146.

Seppäläinen, A.M. and Lindström, K. Neurophysiological findings among house painters exposed to solvents. Scand. J. Work environm. Hlth, 1982, 8 (Suppl. 1): 131–135.

Seppäläinen, A.M., Husman, K. and Mårtenson, C. Neurophysiological effects of long-term exposure to a mixture of organic solvents. Scand. J. Work environm. Hlth, 1978, 4: 304–314.

Seppäläinen, A.M., Raitta, Ch. and Huuskonen, M.S. n-Hexane-induced changes in visual evoked potentials and electroretinograms of industrial workers. Electroenceph. clin. Neurophysiol., 1979, 47: 492–498.

Seppäläinen, A.M., Lindström, K. and Martelin, T. Neurophysiological and psychological picture of solvent poisoning. Amer. J. industr. Med., 1980a, 1: 31–42.

Seppäläinen, A.M., Raitta, Ch. and Huuskonen, M.S. Nervous and visual effects of occupational n-hexane exposure. In: H. Lechner and A. Aranibar (Eds.), ICS 526, Excerpta Medica, Amsterdam, 1980b: 656–661.

Spencer, P.S. and Schaumburg, H.H. Experimental neuropathy produced by 2,5-hexanedione − a major metabolite of the neurotoxic industrial solvent methyl n-butyl ketone. J. Neurol. Neurosurg. Psychiat,., 1975, 38: 771–775.

Takeuchi, Y., Mabuchi, C. and Takagi, S. Polyneuropathy caused by petroleum benzine. Int. Arch. Arbeitsmed., 1975, 34: 185–197.

Yamamura, Y. n-Hexane polyneuropathy. Folia psychiat. neurol. jap., 1969, 23: 45–57.

Kyoto Symposia (EEG Suppl. No. 36)
Editors: P.A. Buser, W.A. Cobb and T. Okuma
© 1982, Elsevier Biomedical Press, Amsterdam

Peripheral Nerve Conduction and Toxic Effects on the Motor Unit

RICHARD F. MAYER

University of Maryland Hospital and School of Medicine, Baltimore, Md. (U.S.A.)

PERIPHERAL NERVE CONDUCTION

It is well known now that a number of industrial toxins and drugs affect the peripheral nervous system in man (Spencer and Schaumburg 1980). These neurotoxins affect specific parts of the peripheral nerves, i.e., neuronal cell body, axon (proximal or distal), Schwann cell-myelin sheath, nerve terminals or postsynaptic membrane (Table I). Most of the toxins which have been studied in man and experimental animals involve the neuron-axon primarily (dying back or distal axonal neuropathy, axonopathy) and few involve myelin or Schwann cells selectively (demyelinative neuropathy, myelinopathy). The effects of these toxins on nerve conduction and impulse generation depend primarily on whether they produce axonal degeneration or demyelination. However, some neurotoxins (e.g., *n*-hexane, glue sniffing and other hexacarbons (Spencer and Schaumburg 1977); B,B′-iminodipropionitrile (Clark et al. 1980)) as well as some metabolic disorders (e.g., uraemia (Dyck et al. 1976)), which cause axonal degeneration, also produce paranodal retraction of myelin or segmental demyelination (secondary demyelination). The effects of these toxins on conduction are more complex, reflecting changes in both the axon and myelin sheath.

The major effect of an axonal degenerative process on peripheral nerve conduction is to block conduction in the distal degenerated segment. Nerve fibres not involved in the process will conduct at normal velocities provided the metabolic environment is not altered. Toxins which selectively affect large, fast conducting axons, leaving intact smaller, slower conducting fibres (e.g., acrylamide), will produce slow nerve conduction velocities (NCV). Those toxins which have a greater effect on small or unmyelinated nerve fibres, however, may not alter the conduction velocity of the whole nerve. Associated with the loss of nerve fibres in axonopathies there is a decrease in amplitude of the whole nerve action potential (NAP). Thus, toxic neuropathies with axonal degeneration may have small NAPs and reduced NCVs.

With continued toxic exposure the distal segments of peripheral nerves degenerate in a centripetal direction toward the cell body (Cavanagh 1964). However, it is likely that the initial axonal changes occur over many distal nodal segments rather than at the distal tip of the axon (Spencer and Schaumburg 1976). Electrophysiological changes manifested by increased electrical threshold to excitation and reduced

TABLE I

REGIONAL PATHOPHYSIOLOGY OF THE LOWER MOTOR OR SENSORY NEURONE

Site	Agent	Mechanism
Nerve cell body	Polio virus, mercury	Neurone degeneration, conduction block, motor unit atrophy
Proximal axon	B,B′-Iminodipropionitrile	Proximal neurofilamentous swelling, conduction slowed
Axon	Trauma-section	Wallerian degeneration, conduction block
Distal axon	Acrylamide, hexacarbons carbon disulphide, TOCP	Distal conduction block, regeneration-reinnervation
Nodes of Ranvier	Tetrodotoxin	Na^+ channels blocked, conduction block
Schwann cell-myelin sheath	Diphtheria toxin, Buckthorn toxin	Demyelination-remyelination, nerve conduction slowed, block
Presynaptic nerve terminal	Botulinum toxin, neomycin	{ ACh release blocked, NMT defect, incremental response
	Black widow spider venom	Massive release of ACh, muscle cramps
Postsynaptic membrane	α-Bungarotoxin, curare, cobra toxin	ACh receptors blocked, NMT defect, decremental response

TOCP, tri-ortho-cresyl phosphate; ACh, acetylcholine; NMT, neuromuscular transmission.

conduction velocity occur in the distal segment of the degenerating nerves fibres, possibly secondary to paranodal demyelination. These changes in nerve conduction which occur in toxic distal axonopathies have been studied in some detail in the experimental animal by Sumner (1980).

Following removal of the neurotoxin, peripheral nerve fibres regenerate. Recovery of function may be complete if few fibres have degenerated but it is often incomplete when there is extensive nerve degeneration. With regeneration, the diameters of nerve fibres increase and, although they may return to normal, the internodal distances remain short (Sanders and Whitteridge 1946). Conduction velocities increase slowly with regeneration and enlargement of the axon but remain slower than normal, possibly as a result of the increased number and short internodes. Some nerve fibres may remain hypoplastic, especially if exposed to the toxin during regeneration, and this may be an additional factor to account for the persistent slow NCVs in chronic toxic neuropathies (Morgan-Hughes et al. 1974).

An example of a toxic polyneuropathy secondary to glue sniffing, with incomplete recovery and nerve regeneration is presented as follows: a 23-year-old male, who indulged in heavy glue sniffing, presented with a severe motor polyneuropathy involving lower more than upper extremities. He improved slowly over many months but weakness persisted in small foot and leg muscles 4 years after onset. Nerve conduction velocities, motor more than sensory, were reduced markedly when first examined. Four years later, the posterior tibial nerves remained inexcitable and the NCVs, although improved, remained slightly reduced (Table II).

In the more common toxic-metabolic distal axonopathies in man, the pathological

TABLE II

CONDUCTION VELOCITIES IN A GLUE SNIFFER WITH POLYNEUROPATHY

Date	Nerve	Segment	Type	Velocity (m/sec)	Latency (m/sec)	Controls
7/1974	Median	Elbow-wrist	Motor	34.6		59 ± 3.0
		Wrist-muscle	Motor		5.8	3.2 ± 0.3
		Digit-wrist	Sensory	52.0		65 ± 5.0
7/1974	Ulnar	Elbow-wrist	Motor	27.5		59 ± 2.5
		Wrist-muscle	Motor		4.8	2.7 ± 0.3
		Digit-wrist	Sensory	50.0		65 ± 5.0
		Wrist-muscle	F response		45.2	26-32
7/1974	Tibial	Knee-ankle	Motor	No response		45.5 ± 3.8
		Ankle-muscle	Motor		11.3	5.9 ± 3.0
8/1978	Median	Elbow-wrist	Motor	51.8		59 ± 3.0
		Wrist-muscle	Motor		3.7	3.2 ± 0.3
		Digit-wrist	Sensory	58.0		65 ± 5.0
8/1978	Ulnar	Elbow-wrist	Motor	49.1		59 ± 2.5
		Wrist-muscle	Motor		2.8	2.7 ± 0.3
		Digit-wrist	Sensory	66.7		65 ± 5.0
		Wrist-muscle	F response		29.0	26-32
8/1978	Tibial	Knee-ankle	Motor	No response		45.5 ± 3.8
		Ankle-muscle	Motor	No response		5.9 ± 1.3
		Ankle-knee	Sensory	55.6		55.0 ± 5.0

process evolves slowly, affecting conduction in distal segments apparently before that in more proximal segments. This in part reflects size (diameter) as well as length of fibres and is especially prominent in those neuropathies which affect large fibres before small ones. With the slowly evolving neuropathies, the effects of axonal degeneration are altered by the regenerative capacity of nerve fibres. It is also likely that in most of the toxic-metabolic neuropathies in man (e.g., uraemic, diabetic and alcoholic-nutritional) there is some degree of secondary demyelination and remyelination, possibly as a consequence of axonal atrophy (Dyck et al. 1981). Thus changes in nerve conduction and NAP amplitude reflect the overall results of nerve degeneration and regeneration and some demyelination and remyelination.

The effects of demyelination on peripheral nerve conduction are multiple and varied. The association of slow nerve conduction velocities with segmental demyelination of peripheral nerve has long been recognized in man and experimental animals (Bannister and Sears 1962; McDonald 1963; Mayer 1963; Mayer and Denny-Brown 1964). Demyelination of all nerve fibres results in a complete conduction block, which may be focal or diffuse. Less severe demyelination produces slow conduction velocities and temporally dispersed nerve action potentials. In a number of elegant studies Rasminsky and Sears (1972) have shown that conduction remains saltatory in demyelinated peripheral nerve fibres. However, in small diameter nerve fibres (<6 μm) Bostock and Sears (1976) have shown that conduction may be continuous over short lengths of demyelination.

Demyelinated nerve fibres have also been shown to have the following: prolonged refractory periods, impaired ability to transmit trains of impulses, post-tetanic depression of the action potential, increased sensitivity to rises in temperature and local generation of nerve impulses (Rasminsky 1978).

With remyelation of nerve fibres, conduction velocity returns toward normal and the nerve action potential is enlarged and less dispersed. Conduction velocities may remain reduced for long periods of time following recovery of function and remyelination (Mayer and Denny-Brown 1964). However, conduction velocities have been reported to return to normal following recovery from diphtheritic polyneuritis (McDonald and Kocen 1975). The conduction velocities remain reduced in most human polyneuropathies in which there is prominent demyelination and remyelination (e.g., chronic inflammatory polyradiculoneuropathy and hereditary hypertrophic polyneuropathy).

MOTOR UNIT CONTRACTILE PROPERTIES

Less is known about the effects of toxins on the contractile properties of muscle units, which consist of all the muscle fibres innervated by one axon and motoneurone (a motor unit). Muscle units (MUs) in man, like those in cat, can be classified physiologically by using the isometric twitch contraction time (Tc) and the resistance to fatigue (i.e., the effect of 2 min of repetitive electrical stimulation at 30–40 Hz on the isometric tension (Burke et al. 1973; Garnett et al. 1978; Mayer and Young 1979)). Three types of muscle unit have been identified in human muscle utilizing intramuscular microstimulation and classified as follows: (1) type FF units with fast Tc and high fatigability, (2) type FR units with fast Tc and resistance to fatigue, and (3) type S units with slow Tc and resistance to fatigue. It is also presumed in man, as in the cat, that type FF MUs consist of muscle fibres high in alkaline myofibrillar ATPase activity and low in oxidative activity (type IIB, classification of Brooke and Kaiser 1970); type FR MUs consist of muscle fibres high in alkaline myofibrillar ATPase activity and high to intermediate in oxidative activity (type IIA) and type S units consist of fibres low in alkaline myofibrillar ATPase activity and high in oxidative activity (type I). It is likely, therefore, in man as in other mammals, that there is a strong functional-biochemical correlation between a muscle unit's contractile properties and its histochemical profile (Garnett et al. 1978).

Recent studies in our laboratory of the contractile properties of the first dorsal interosseous muscle (FDI) in man have demonstrated considerable variability in normal MU properties and their plasticity in altered motor function (Young and Mayer 1981, 1982). Although motor units can be separated by their Tc and fatigue index (FI, the ratio of the isometric twitch tension, Pt, averaged 32 times following 2 min of repetitive electrical stimulation at 30 Hz for a third of a second in each second, to the initial Pt), there is overlap in their unpotentiated Pt (Table IIIA). There is a trend, however, for type FF units to have larger Pt, shorter distal

TABLE IIIA

CONTRACTILE PROPERTIES OF SINGLE MOTOR UNITS IN THE FIRST DORSAL INTEROSSEOUS MUSCLE

Control adults, aged 23–78 years.

Unit type	Distal motor latency (msec)	Twitch contraction time (msec)	Half relaxation time (msec)	Twitch tension (g)
F*	3.24 ± 0.98 (84)	57.1 ± 8.3 (93)	56.3 ± 14.9 (91)	3.83 ± 5.2 (93)
S**	3.10 ± 0.85 (27)	87.3 ± 18.0 (33)	71.9 ± 21.8 (31)	2.53 ± 3.2 (33)
FF	3.04 ± 0.4 (8)	57.6 ± 7.6 (9)	59.4 ± 14.2 (7)	8.89 ± 13.5 (9)
FR	3.44 ± 1.04 (28)	54.8 ± 10.3 (29)	51.1 ± 17.0 (24)	2.39 ± 2.3 (29)
S	3.66 ± 0.56 (8)	83.0 ± 11.8 (13)	75.2 ± 25.9 (13)	2.91 ± 3.6 (13)

All values are mean ± 1 S.D., unpotentiated twitches.
( ), number of units recorded
* F units include all units with twitch contraction times less than 70 msec.
**S units include all units with twitch contraction times 70 msec or greater.

latencies, faster axonal conduction velocities and higher thresholds to recruitment than type S units (Milner-Brown et al. 1973; Freund et al. 1975; Stephens and Usherwood 1977).

The number and percentage of each unit type in human muscle is difficult to estimate because of technical and sampling problems. In the FDI approximately 43% of muscle fibres are type II (Johnson et al. 1973) but approximately 70% of the MUs sampled have fast Tc. Of this sample, relatively few are type FF MUs (approximately 18%, 9 of 51 units). Whether this reflects the sampling problem of the microstimulation technique or other factors such as overlap of Tc of FR and S MUs or small innervation ratios in fast twitch units remains to be determined. The percentages of type IIB and IIA fibres in the FDI are not available, however, for comparison with the percentages of type FF and FR units.

In evaluating the effects of toxins or drugs on the contractile properties of motor units it is essential to separate those effects that are directed primarily at the muscle and its contractile elements from those that are directed primarily at the nerve. However, it is likely that many toxins and drugs affect both muscle and peripheral nerve because of similarities in structure and biochemical reaction. In this presentation, I shall discuss only those effects on muscle units secondary to axonal or demyelinative neuropathies (indirect effects). Since the indirect effects on the contractile properties of motor units may be similar in toxic (e.g., glue sniffing (1 patient), alcohol (1 patient)) and other types (e.g., traumatic (2 patients), hereditary hypertrophic (4 patients), acute or recurrent polyradiculoneuropathy (4 patients)) of polyneuropathies, these will be discussed together depending on whether they are predominantly axonal or demyelinative.

TABLE IIIB

CONTRACTILE PROPERTIES OF SINGLE MOTOR UNITS IN THE FIRST DORSAL
INTEROSSEOUS MUSCLE

Patients with demyelinative neuropathy, aged 19–67 years.

Unit type	Distal motor latency (msec)	Twitch contraction time (msec)	Half relaxation time (msec)	Twitch tension (g)
F*	5.35 ± 2.81***	56.34 ± 9.2	63.67 ± 16.3	5.13 ± 6.6
	(36)	(35)	(33)	(35)
S**	4.61 ± 2.22***	81.37 ± 10.3	79.89 ± 22.9	4.98 ± 4.8
	(30)	(31)	(31)	(31)
FF	8.25 ± 6.66***	53.7 ± 9.7	64.55 ± 23.1	8.68 ± 10.75
	(4)	(4)	(4)	(4)
FR	4.72 ± 1.81	57.27 ± 9.3	63.26 ± 17.6	4.48 ± 6.1
	(22)	(22)	(21)	(22)
S	4.25 ± 1.47	81.43 ± 11.5	72.18 ± 20.0	5.22 ± 2.1
	(18)	(18)	(18)	(18)
SF	6.36 ± 3.95***	78.24 ± 4.4	109.56 ± 17.9***	4.29 ± 2.1
	(5)	(5)	(5)	(5)

All values are mean ± 1 S.D., unpotentiated twitches.
( ), number of units recorded.
*   F units include all units with twitch contraction times less than 70 msec.
** S units include all units with twitch contraction times 70 msec or greater.
***Significant at the $P < 0.01$ compared with controls.

In distal axonal neuropathies single motor units may be difficult to activate in the FDI due to the degeneration and loss of nerve fibres. There is a wide variability of twitch tensions in single MUs (ranging from 0.77 to 15.26 g, mean 3.36 g in 3 patients compared with controls of 3.49 ± 4.8 g). Many of the MUs generate small amounts of tension and few generate large tensions (giant motor units). The Tcs tend to be slightly prolonged but within the range of control values (range 55–80 msec, mean 67.7 msec). In 1 patient with a chronic, predominantly motor, distal axonal neuropathy of undetermined aetiology both Tc (mean 72.8 msec) and half relaxation times (mean 110.5 msec; mean control, 60.3 ± 18.1 msec) were prolonged and twitch tensions were all moderately large (mean 4.2. g, range 2.7–5.45 g). Similar observations have been reported in patients with ulnar entrapment neuropathies or amyotrophic lateral sclerosis (Milner-Brown et al. 1974).

In patients with demyelinative neuropathies, records of single MUs in the FDI reveal the same 3 types of MU recorded in controls. However, a few units characterized by slow twitch contraction times (range 74.0–84.7 msec) and high fatigability (FI less than 1, range 0.06–0.89) were recorded (Table IIIB). This type of unit (type SF, slow twitch fatigable unit) has not been observed in the control sample, but has been recorded in patients with chronic spastic hemiplegia (Young and Mayer 1982). Distal motor latencies are prolonged (64% of fast twitch and 52% slow twitch units recorded) in those patients with decreased distal motor conduction velocities, evidence of demyelination of distal nerve fibres. This increase in distal latency is highly significant ($P < 0.001$) for the fast twitch and SF MUs. No significant change in either mean Tc or mean Pt was observed in single MUs in the FDI in the patients studied with demyelinative neuropathies. Half relaxation times tended to be prolonged but this was significant in only the SF units (Table IIIB).

Studies to date of motor units in the human FDI muscle suggest that the basic properties of MUs in man, as in the cat (Mayer et al. 1981), are maintained following a variety of manipulations (e.g. immobilization and muscle atrophy). The potential effects of an axonal or demyelinative neuropathy on motor units are complex and must be interpreted in regard to the specific muscle's location and function as well as motor unit type and size. These may vary in different species and results obtained in one species may not apply to all. The effects of denervation followed by reinnervation on MU properties depend greatly on the type of motoneurone innervating the unit. A number of other factors which affect the contractile properties of skeletal muscle must also be considered. These include the following: (1) the frequency, pattern and amount of muscle activity; (2) muscle length and tension; (3) muscle temperature and environment; (4) muscle size − atrophy or hypertrophy and subsequent changes in the sarcolemmal membrane, contractile proteins and sarcoplasmic reticulum; (5) the active state mechanism (Ca^{2+} uptake and release); and (6) trophic factors (nerve-muscle interactions). Most of these have yet to be studied in any detail in patients with neuropathy.

REFERENCES

Bannister, R.G. and Sears, T.A. The changes in nerve conduction in acute idiopathic polyneuritis. J. Neurol. Neurosurg. Psychiat., 1962, 25: 321–328.

Bostock, H. and Sears, T.A. Continuous conduction in demyelinated mammalian nerve fibers. Nature (Lond.), 1976, 263: 786–787.

Brooke, M.H. and Kaiser, K.K. Muscle fiber types: How many and what kind? Arch. Neurol. (Chic.), 1970, 23: 369–379.

Burke, R.E., Levine, D.N., Tsairis, P. and Zajac, F.E. Physiological types and histochemical profiles in motor units of the cat gastrocnemius. J. Physiol. (Lond.), 1973, 234: 723–748.

Cavanagh, J.B. The significance of the "dying-back" process in experimental and human neurological disease. Int. Rev. exp. Pathol., 1964, 3: 219–267.

Clark, A., Griffin, J.W. and Price, D.L. The axonal pathology in chronic B,B'-iminodipropionitrile intoxication. J. Neuropath. exp. Neurol., 1980, 39: 42–55.

Dyck, P.J., Johnson, W.J., Lambert, E.H. and O'Brien, P.C. Segmental demyelination secondary to axonal degeneration in uremic neuropathy. Mayo Clin. Proc., 1976, 46: 400–431.

Dyck, P.J., Lais, A.C., Karnes, J.L., Sparks, M., Hunder, H., Low, P.A. and Windebank, A.J. Permanent axotomy, a model of axonal atrophy and secondary segmental demyelination and remyelination. Ann. Neurol., 1981, 9: 575–583.

Freund, H.J., Budingen, H.J. and Dietz, V. Activity of single motor units from human forearm muscles during voluntary isometric contractions. J. Neurophysiol., 1975, 38: 933–946.

Garnett, R.A.F., O'Donovan, M.J., Stephens, J.A. and Taylor, A. Motor unit organization of human medial gastrocnemius. J. Physiol. (Lond.), 1978, 287: 33–43.

Johnson, M.A., Polgar, J., Weightman, D. and Appleton, D. Data on the distribution of fiber types in thirty-six human muscles. An autopsy study. J. neurol. Sci., 1973, 18: 111–129.

Mayer, R.F. Nerve conduction studies in man. Neurology (Minneap.), 13: 1021–1030.

Mayer, R.F. and Denny-Brown, D. Conduction velocity in peripheral nerve during experimental demyelination in the cat. Neurology (Minneap.), 1964, 14: 714–726.

Mayer, R.F. and Young, J.L. Physiological properties of muscle units in humans. Trans. Amer. neurol. Ass., 1979, 104: 193–196.

Mayer, R.F., Burke, R.E., Toop, J., Hodgsen, J.A., Kanda, K. and Walmsley, B. The effect of long-term immobilization on the motor unit population of the cat medial gastrocnemius muscle. Neuroscience, 1981, 6: 725–739.

McDonald, W.I. The effects of experimental demyelination on conduction in peripheral nerve. A histological and electrophysiological study. Brain, 1963, 86: 481–524.

McDonald, W.I. and Kocen, R.S. Diphtheritic neuropathy. In: P.J. Dyck, P.K. Thomas and E.H. Lambert (Eds.), Peripheral Neuropathy, Vol. 2. Saunders, Philadelphia, Pa., 1975: 1281–1300.

Milner-Brown, H.S., Stein, R.B. and Yemm, R. The orderly recruitment of human motor units during voluntary isometric contractions. J. Physiol. (Lond.), 1973, 230: 359–370.

Milner-Brown, H.S., Stein, R.B. and Lee, R.G. Contractile and electrical properties of human motor units in neuropathies and motor neurone disease. J. Neurol. Neurosurg. Psychiat., 1974, 37: 670–676.

Morgan-Hughes, J.A., Sinclair, Sally and Durston, J.H.J. The pattern of peripheral nerve regeneration induced by crush in rats with severe acrylamide neuropathy. Brain, 1974, 97: 235–250.

Rasminsky, M. Physiology of conduction in demyelinated axons. In: S.G. Waxman (Ed.), Physiology and Pathobiology of Axons. Raven Press, New York, 1978: 361–376.

Rasminsky, M. and Sears, T.A. Internodal conduction in undissected demyelinated nerve fibers. J. Physiol. (Lond.), 1972, 277: 323–350.

Sanders, F.K. and Whitteridge, D. Conduction velocity and myelin thickness in regenerating nerve fibers. J. Physiol. (Lond.), 1946, 105: 152–174.

Spencer, P.S. and Schaumburg, H.H. Central and peripheral distal axonopathy – The pathology of dying-back polyneuropathies. In: H.M. Zimmerman (Ed.), Progress in Neuropathology, Vol. III. Grune and Stratton, New York, 1976: 235–295.

Spencer, P.S. and Schaumburg, H.H. Ultrastructural studies of the dying-back process; III. The evolution of experimental peripheral giant axonal degeneration. J. Neuropath. exp. Neurol., 1977, 36: 276–299.

Spencer, P.S. and Schaumburg, H.H. Experimental and Clinical Neurotoxicology. Williams and Wilkins, Baltimore, Md., 1980.

Stephens, J.A. and Usherwood, T.P. The mechanical properties of human motor units with special reference to their fatigability and recruitment threshold. Brain Res., 1977, 125: 91–97.

Sumner, A.J. Axonal polyneuropathies. In: A.J. Sumner (Ed.), The Physiology of Peripheral Nerve Disease. Saunders, Philadelphia, Pa., 1980: 340–357.

Young, J.L. and Mayer, R.F. Physiological properties and classification of single motor units activated by intramuscular microstimulation in the first dorsal interosseous muscle in man. In: J.E. Desmedt (Ed.), Progress in Clinical Neurophysiology, Vol. 9. Karger, Basel, 1981: 17–25.

Young, J.L. and Mayer, R.F. Physiological alterations of motor units in hemiplegia. J. neurol. Sci., 1982, 54: 401–412.

Kyoto Symposia (EEG Suppl. No. 36)
Editors: P.A. Buser, W.A. Cobb and T. Okuma

Circadian Rhythm Disturbances and Sleep Disorders in Shift Workers

CHRISTIAN GUILLEMINAULT, CHARLES CZEISLER, RICHARD COLEMAN
and LAUGHTON MILES

*Stanford University Disorders Center, Stanford University School of Medicine, Stanford, Calif. 94305
(U.S.A.)*

Several reports have been published indicating that shift work results in changes in total sleep disorder time and the distribution of sleep states and stages. Not much is known, however, of the impact of these changes on a shift worker's well being, mental state and daytime performance.

We shall report on the role of shift work in the onset of two specific sleep disorders.

SHIFT WORK AND DELAYED SLEEP PHASE INSOMNIA (DSP INSOMNIA)

In 1979 Weitzman et al. reported a new sleep disorder characterized by difficulty in initiating sleep when desired ("sleep onset insomnia") but with no difficulty in maintaining sleep once initiated. This latter point distinguishes this disorder from other forms of insomnia. Normal life styles require that an individual be awake at certain hours if he is to pursue gainful employment and satisfying social activities. If a person is required to awaken at a specific time, but has difficulty falling asleep, total sleep time may be curtailed greatly. Individuals with this complaint tend to rely heavily on external means of awakening (such as alarm clocks, automatic radios), and experience not only tiredness, fatigue and sleepiness but also feelings of depression during their "daytime."

We had the opportunity to study 12 subjects who were employed on shift work and who suffered from this form of sleep disturbance intermittently.

MATERIALS AND METHODS

The 12 subjects were referred to our Stanford Sleep Disorders Clinic for intermittent greatly curtailed total sleep time associated with intermittent severe insomnia. Many of the subjects had taken hypnotic medications and found that

Address for correspondence: Christian Guilleminault, M.D., Stanford Sleep Disorders Center, TD114, Stanford University Medical Center, Stanford, Calif. 94305, U.S.A.

their condition was not adequately controlled. Their sleep disorder had had a very detrimental effect on their daytime functioning; half of the total population either had lost or had nearly lost their jobs because of their sleep disorder.

There were 8 men and 4 women whose ages ranged from 16 to 58 years. Their professions were as follows: medical resident (1), nurse (4), casino employee (2), baker (1), flight attendant (2), bartender (1), and switchboard operator (1). All subjects were submitted to changes in schedule fairly regularly. The nurses, casino employees, and switchboard operator (7) switched shifts every 3–4 weeks; the baker (1) switched every 3 months; the others (4) had more variable shift changes. The flight attendants, of course, had the additional complication of time zone changes. All subjects had been doing shift work for no longer than 4 years 8 months and not less than 1 year. Some rotated through the standard daytime (7:00–15:00)/afternoon (15:00–23:00)/night (23:00–7:00) shifts, while others had less clear-cut schedule changes (for example, the bartender worked shifts such as 10:00–18:00, 12:00–20:00, or 18:00–2:00). All patients had progressively developed problems in falling asleep, and all had been using sleeping pills (prescription or over the counter medications) on a more or less regular basis. In all cases, there was a general trend toward progressively heavier use of sleeping medications. All reported the greatest difficulty in sleeping when on "day shift." Typically, subjects reported functioning best at work when on a late shift schedule (i.e., working afternoons or nights). When they switched to a day shift and attempted to fall asleep between 22:00 and midnight, they usually were unable to sleep until 4:00, 5:00, or even 7:00, and thus had to get up after only 2–4 h of sleep. Subjects used sleeping medication most when working day shift and experienced continual problems in waking up at appropriate times. They reported sleeping through alarm clock wake-ups, being late for work often, and feeling "drugged" during the day.

Each patient was asked to keep a sleep/waking diary while working a day shift and while abstaining from sleeping medication for 2–3 weeks. Pre-printed forms were supplied for them to record clock times for the following each day: bedtime, estimated sleep onset, nocturnal awakenings (time and length), waking time and time of arising from bed. Times of meals (and snacks), alcoholic drinks, and exercise (if any) were also requested.

During one of the weeks the subjects wore an ambulatory monitor (Vitalog Co.) consisting of an activity/non-activity sensor the size of a watch which was worn on the non-dominant arm, and a smooth, flexible temperature probe which was placed in the rectum. Both monitors were linked by small cables taped on the subject's skin to a cassette-type microcomputer which was worn on the side and held in place by a belt. The microcomputer was programmed before being given to the patient. This battery operated microcomputer had sufficient memory to store and analyse data collected every 2 min over a period of 5 days (Miles et al. 1978; Miles and Rules 1982). The device allows intelligent processing of the sensors' information in real time. Only the most pertinent information is stored. The probes can be detached by subjects for showering, using the bathroom, etc., but time tracking is maintained automatically by the microcomputer.

Each subject underwent a nocturnal polysomnogram, scheduled during the sleep period in which the subject experienced the most difficulty in sleeping (i.e., the nocturnal period). The following variables were monitored: electroencephalogram (EEG), C_3-A_2 and C_4-A_1 of the 10-20 system; electro-oculogram (EOG); chin electromyogram (EMG); electrocardiogram (ECG) lead II; respiratory effort monitored by thoracic and abdominal strain gauges and airflow measured by nasal and buccal thermistors.

ANALYSIS OF DATA

Sleep diaries were reviewed with each subject and were compared to the ambulatory monitoring records. The ambulatory records were analysed with a program written for an Apple II computer, and the results of the 5 days' monitoring of the subject's activity/non-activity and core temperature during each 24 h period were obtained and were plotted automatically. These results were available within minutes of the return of the ambulatory monitor. The all night polygraphic records were scored for sleep and sleep stages and for cardio-respiratory changes using the standard criteria of Rechtschaffen and Kales (1968).

RESULTS

During polygraphic monitoring, all subjects demonstrated long sleep latency (several hours); i.e., the time from lights out until sleep onset was unusually long.

Four patients were allowed to sleep under monitoring until they awakened spontaneously. In these cases, subjects presented a total sleep time of over 6.5 h. In the other 8 cases, the monitoring ended and the subjects were awakened at 7:30 (as is done for our normal all night polygraphic recording); in these cases, a total sleep time between 1 and 3 h was noted.

The sleep diaries and ambulatory monitoring records demonstrated that, when subjects were working day shift, there was a dissociation between temperature curve and activity/non-activity plot, with a switch to the right of the peaks and troughs of the temperature values. That is, the highest and lowest monitored temperatures were recorded at later times than would be expected in an individual appropriately synchronized with a day/night schedule (see Fig. 1).

FOLLOW UP

Once diagnosed, patients were advised to seek employment where abrupt schedule changes would not be required, or to ask their current employers for permission to work on no more than 2 consecutive shifts (such as day and evening or evening and

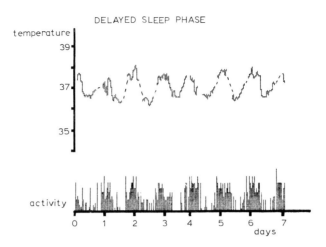

Fig. 1. Activity/non-activity and temperature monitoring records obtained using a portable microcomputer (Vitalog Co.). Note the dissociation between peak temperature and greatest activity level, and between lowest temperature and rest. There is a delay in the core temperature cycle as compared to the activity cycle.

night). Letters from our clinic were sent to employers to aid subjects in getting approval for these changes.

All subjects were advised to select a fixed bedtime, to be kept regardless of their work schedule or their days off. After these recommendations had been instituted, we recommended that our subjects undergo chronotherapy (Czeisler et al. 1981). Five patients agreed to chronotherapy at the Stanford Sleep Disorders Clinic.

The techniques used for chronotherapy changed slightly as we gained insight into what was most feasible. Originally, 3 patients were given therapy to "reset" their biological clocks, using daily scheduled changes of 1 h in their bedtimes (i.e., they went to bed 1 h later each night until they reached a bedtime which was acceptable). The last 2 patients, following the recommendations of Czeisler et al. (1981), underwent the same therapy with a scheduled change of 3 h per day in their bedtimes. This latter approach, which proved to be just as successful as the first, allows a complete "resetting" of a subject to any selected bedtime within 5 or 6 days of treatment. As described by Czeisler et al. (1981), each subject went to bed 3 h later each day, slept for a mean of 7.5 h, and then stayed awake until the next (3 h later) bedtime. When the subject's bedtime approached the selected goal, he was placed under a strict schedule for bedtime, morning awakening and meals so that daytime cues would be reinforced. All patients achieved well adapted, normal sleep with this method. However, after 2 years of good sleeping patterns, the youngest subject neglected to follow our recommendations, began to follow an irregular bedtime schedule, and eventually shifted his bedtime from midnight to the early morning hours. He again developed delayed sleep phase insomnia and recently has again undergone chronotherapy and has been rescheduled to an appropriate, earlier, bedtime.

SHIFT WORK AND THE ONSET OF NARCOLEPTIC SYNDROME

The Association of Sleep Disorders Center's "Diagnostic Classification of Sleep and Arousal Disorders" (1979) gives criteria for "narcolepsy" (demonstration of sleep onset rapid eye movement periods on objective polygraphic recording) and "idiopathic central nervous system hypersomnia" (polygraphically monitored short sleep latency (less than 5 min) using the multiple sleep latency test (MSLT)); at the present time, over 500 of our patients have received one or the other diagnosis. In 50 of these patients, we have found that onset of the syndrome was directly associated with rapid changes in their work shift assignments. Ten of them presented onset of clinical symptoms while working on board a ship, where they were subjected to rotating 6 h shifts. Five other individuals experienced onset of symptoms while serving in the Air Force when assigned to radar watch or other types of shift work duties. In the remaining 35 civilians, onset of clinical symptoms occurred while they were employed in occupations requiring frequent changes in work shift assignments, often associated with periods of sleep deprivation.

In 23 cases a positive family history of a disorder of excessive daytime sleepiness was elicited. "Family" for this study was defined as including not only parents and siblings but also first degree cousins and aunts and uncles in both the maternal and paternal lines.

COMMENTS

When individuals are submitted to rapidly changing shift work, substantial disruption of the sleep-waking cycle occurs. Studies of circadian rhythms have demonstrated that, in the absence of periodic environmental cues, the circadian cycle length or "free running period length" (τ) of periodic physiological functions is no longer "entrained," or synchronized, to a 24 h period. It is conceivable that some individuals, when submitted to abrupt and frequent shift changes, may not respond appropriately to known synchronizers of human circadian rhythms, such as the light-dark cycle, which is an effective synchronizer (Czeisler 1978). Patients with DSP insomnia have developed a sleep scheduling disorder characterized by inappropriate temporal relationships between the periodic environment and their circadian sleep-waking cycle.

Our DSP insomnia patient population presented the most severe complaints during one type of schedule only (i.e., day shift work). When these patients are on the day work-night off schedule, their sleep is in an inappropriate phase. These patients are better able to adapt to the other 2 shift schedules (i.e., evening and night shifts), as their bedtimes can remain the same for either shift.

The relationship between various sleep disorders and disruptions of the circadian "timing" system is not yet clear; however, these interactions deserve further study. Rotating shift work may increase the risk of developing certain sleep disorders, or may lead to these sleep disorders occurring earlier in life than would have been the case had the individual maintained a normal sleep-waking schedule. Industrial and military physicians responsible for examining candidates for shift work should inquire whether there is a family history of narcolepsy or CNS hypersomnia. They should also understand that there is a possibility that abrupt and frequent changes in sleep phase may be responsible for specific sleep complaints. Sleep disorders with this aetiology should not be controlled by medication.

SUMMARY

Employment which requires frequent shift rotation may lead to the development of specific sleep disorders. Delayed sleep phase (DSP) insomnia, a syndrome identified recently, can greatly impair an individual's circadian rhythm-dependent functions; it can occur when shift work disrupts normal sleep-waking schedules. Disorders of excessive daytime sleepiness, such as narcolepsy, occur in some subjects after they have been subjected to frequently rotating shifts. Understanding the problems associated with circadian rhythm disturbances and their interaction with sleep disorders is particularly important in industrial medicine; any clinician whose patients are subjected to frequent shift rotations should consider the effects of disrupted sleep-waking schedules.

REFERENCES

Association of Sleep Disorders Centers. Diagnostic classification of sleep and arousal disorders. 1st Ed., prepared by the Sleep Disorders Classification Committee, H.P. Roffwarg, Chairman. Sleep, 1979, 2: 1–137.

Czeisler, C.A. Human Circadian Physiology: Internal Organization of Temperature, Sleep-Wake and Neuroendocrine Rhythms Monitored in an Environment Free of Time Cues. Ph.D. Dissertation, Stanford University, 1978.

Czeisler, C.A., Richardson, G.S., Coleman, R.M., Zimmerman, J.C., Moore-Ede, M.C., Dement, W.C. and Weitzman, E.D. Chronotherapy: resetting the circadian clocks of patients with delayed sleep phase insomnia. Sleep, 1981, 4: 1–21.

Miles, L. and Rule, B.R. Long term monitoring of multiple physiologic parameters using a programmable portable micro-computer. In: E.D. Stott, E.B. Raftery and E. Goulding (Eds.), ISAM 1981 4th International Symposium on Ambulatory Monitoring. Academic Press, New York, 1982, in press.

Miles, L., Cutler, R., Drake, K., Rule, B.R. and Dement, W. Use of a temperature/activity monitor to investigate chronobiological dysfunction in patients presenting to a sleep disorders clinic. Sleep Res., 1978, 7: 293 (abstr.).

Rechtschaffen, A. and Kales, A. A Manual of Standardized Terminology, Techniques and Scoring System for Sleep Stages of Human Subjects. Brain Information Service/Brain Research Institute, University of California, Los Angeles, Calif., 1968.

Weitzman, E.D., Czeisler, C.A., Coleman, R.M., Dement, W.C., Richardson, G.S. and Pollack, C.P. Delayed sleep phase syndrome: a biological rhythm sleep disorder. Sleep Res., 1979, 8: 221 (abstr.).

Kyoto Symposia (EEG Suppl. No. 36)
Editors: P.A. Buser, W.A. Cobb and T. Okuma
© 1982, Elsevier Biomedical Press, Amsterdam

Neurophysiological Effects of Electromagnetic Fields. A Critical Review

KJELL HANSSON MILD[1] and P. ÅKE ÖBERG[2]

[1] *National Board of Occupational Safety and Health, Department of Occupational Health, Umeå, and*
[2] *Department of Biomedical Engineering, University of Linköping, Linköping (Sweden)*

Human exposure to non-ionizing electromagnetic (EM) fields occurs in various industrial processes as well as in everyday life. It is known that such exposure can affect the health conditions of human beings. The effects reported in the literature range from high level microwave overexposure with lethal outcome to low level long-term radiation characterized by the neurasthenic syndrome (Barański and Czerski 1976).

For high intensity fields the resulting biological-thermal effect can be predicted by applying classical biophysical theory, but the question of whether low intensity EM field can interact with biological material on a non-thermal basis is still not settled.

The number of papers on biological effects of EM fields is rapidly increasing and the latest index of publications lists 3627 articles in the world literature (Kinn and Postow 1981). Many of the earlier reports are insufficient in details of the exposure conditions to make it possible to rule out that the effect seen was due to a thermal interaction. Several reviews and monographs on general biological effects of EM fields have been published (Barnothy 1964, 1969; Presman 1970; Cleary 1977; Sheppard and Eisenbud 1977; Stuchly 1978; Gandhi 1980; Adey 1981). In this review neurophysiological effects resulting from exposure to EM fields at levels considered to be non-thermal and with exposure conditions well controlled will be discussed. The effects are seen at various levels of organization of the living organism: subcellular, cellular, organic, systemic or organismic. Among the numerous reports of neurophysiological effects of EM fields only the most pertinent will be discussed. A schematic presentation of some of the better established effects is given in Table I.

Effects of EM fields have been reported for the whole frequency range from 0 Hz up to several GHz. The terms and concepts used to describe the fields are different for the various frequency ranges and therefore this review starts with a section where the characteristics of the fields are briefly given. In this section ranges of field intensities typically encountered in occupational exposure are also given.

Address all correspondence to: Dr. Kjell Hansson Mild, National Board of Occupational Safety and Health, Department of Occupational Health, Box 6104, S-900 06 Umeå, Sweden.

TABLE I

NEUROPHYSIOLOGICAL EFFECTS OF EM FIELDS OF VARIOUS FREQUENCIES AND
INTENSITIES AS SEEN AT VARIOUS BIOLOGICAL LEVELS OF ORGANIZATION

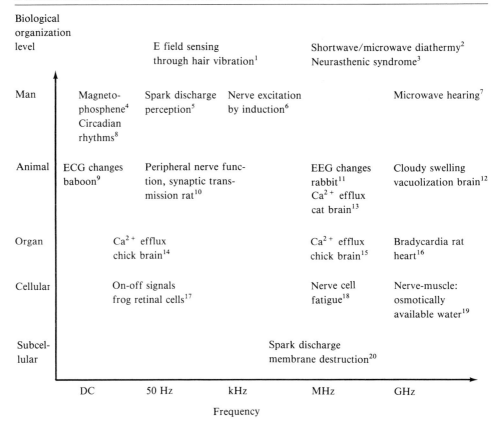

References to Table I: [1] Deno (1978); [2] Stillwell (1965); [3] Silverman (1973); [4] Lövsund et al. (1980); [5] Deno (1978); [6] Lövsund and Hansson Mild (1978); [7] Lin (1980); [8] Wever (1974); [9] Beischer and Knepton (1964); [10] Jaffe et al. (1980): [11] Takashima et al. (1979); [12] Tolgskaya and Gordon (1973); [13] Adey (1980, preliminary results); [14] Adey (1980); [15] Adey (1980); [16] Olsen et al. (1977); [17] Lövsund et al. (1980); [18] McRee and Wachtel (1980): [19] Portela et al. (1975); [20] Zimmerman et al. (1978).

EM FIELD AND OCCUPATIONAL EXPOSURE

The non-ionizing part of the electromagnetic spectrum can be divided into different regions in order of increasing frequencies: static, quasistatic, microwave, quasioptical, and optical. In this text only the three first regions will be discussed, i.e., the frequency range 0 Hz up to 300 GHz.

An electromagnetic field is characterized by both an electric and a magnetic field. The electric field (E) is expressed in volts per meter (V/m) and the magnetic field (H) is given in amperes per meter (A/m). In some situations the magnetic field is described by the flux density, B, measured in Tesla (T) or Gauss.

The E and H fields are not independent of each other but related through Maxwell's equations. When an electromagnetic wave propagates in free space the E and H fields are perpendicular to each other and to the direction of propagation of the wave. The magnitudes of the fields are related through $E = Z \cdot H$, where Z is the impedance; for free space its numerical value is 377 Ω. The energy transferred per unit time and unit area by an EM wave is given by the power flux density $S = EH$, measured in W/m^2, or, more commonly in the western literature, mW/cm^2 (1 mW/cm^2 = 10 W/m^2).

When an EM wave impinges upon a biological object, in general a large part of the wave is reflected at the surface and the rest is transmitted into the object with a change in both propagation direction and wave length. The ratio between reflected and transmitted waves is highly dependent on the geometrical shape of the object and its dielectric properties. The energy transmitted into the object is progressively absorbed so that the wave decreases in magnitude as it penetrates the material. The depth at which the power level is decreased by 86.5% ($1/e^2$) is called the skin depth (D). The magnitude of D depends on the dielectric properties of the material. Tissues with high water content — muscle — have a high dielectric constant and tissues with low water content — fat — have a low value for the constant. Since these constants are frequency dependent, D will also show such a dependence. For muscle tissue radiated at 27 MHz D is 14 cm, which is reduced to 1.7 cm at 2450 MHz. The corresponding figures for fat are 160 cm and 11 cm at 27 and 2450 MHz, respectively (Johnson and Guy 1972). The power absorbed by the body as the microwaves attenuate produces a local heating at a rate called specific absorbtion rate (SAR) and it can be shown that the SAR is proportional to the square of the internal E field at the point in question. SAR is given in watts/kg (W/kg). The SAR distribution in humans and animals resulting from microwave radiation will generally be highly non-uniform due to the complex dependence on geometrical shape and dielectrical properties of the body. However, considerable information on SAR distribution from plane wave exposure has been gained in the last decade (Durney et al. 1980).

Occupational exposure to microwaves can occur, for instance, around radar equipment, broadcasting transmitters and antennae for UHF-TV, and microwave diathermy apparatus. The term radiation can usually be applied in these situations since the distance from the radiation source is usually of the order of several wave lengths. To assess the health hazard involved measurements of the power density are sufficient. For radar equipment also the pulse modulation of the signal has to be taken into account.

The intensities of microwave exposure which can be encountered near these sources range from a few μW/cm^2 around generators in cabinets with good shielding up to several hundreds of mW/cm^2 in front of the antenna systems of radar or diathermy apparatus. Usually the occupational exposure levels for extended periods of time are below 1 mW/cm^2. The exposure standards for microwaves differ by 3 orders of magnitude between the U.S.A. and the Soviet Union. In the U.S.A. 10 mW/cm^2 is allowed for a working day whereas in the U.S.S.R. the corresponding value is only 10 μW/cm^2. This large difference can be taken as an indication of our incomplete knowledge of the possible health effects of the microwaves, but it also reflects, to some extent, the different philosophies behind the standard settings in the two countries.

For frequencies below about 300 MHz, i.e. wave lengths longer than 1 m, the situation becomes more complex. Practically all occupational exposure then takes place near the radiation source, usually within one wave length, a situation termed near-field radiation. The waves then have not been fully developed and the field configuration is characterized by components which decrease rapidly with increasing distance from the source. Usually no fixed relation can be established for E and H, in either magnitude or direction. The dosimetry for near-fields is still very much in its initial stage and only a few papers have been published on near-field SAR distributions. It is however quite clear today that to assess the health hazard in a near-field exposure both E and H fields have to be taken into account.

In this frequency range the main sources of radiation are plastic welding machines, glue dryers, short wave diathermy apparatus, and broadcasting equipment for FM radio and VHF-TV. The field strengths in the vicinity of these sources range from over 1000 V/m and 2 A/m very close to the electrodes or antennae down to some 10 V/m and 0.1 A/m at 1–2 m from the sources (Hansson Mild 1980).

At still lower frequencies – from the kHz range down to about 100 Hz – the occupational exposure in industry to EM fields is dominated by magnetic fields from various sources. Lövsund (1980) found field flux densities in the range 0–10 mT in welding and in the steel industry, where electric currents are used for a variety of heating purposes. The H field at these frequencies induces eddy currents in the exposed tissue. To get some idea of the possible biological effects of such an exposure, the induced current density (j) is usually estimated. For j < 1 mA/cm^2 no acute effect – such as nerve excitation – is expected (Bernhart 1979).

At AC power distribution frequencies both electric and magnetic field exposure can occur. Near the high voltage lines the E field exposure dominates over H field exposure. However, due to the electrical properties of the body at this frequency the E field is shielded or reflected. The ratio of internal E field to incident external field is only about 10^{-8}. The distribution of this capacitively coupled current has recently been estimated by Kaune and Phillips (1980) and, as an example, it can be mentioned that for a man standing in a vertical E field of strength 10 kV/m the current density in the neck region will be about 0.5 μA/cm^2.

NEUROPHYSIOLOGICAL EFFECTS

Effects at the cellular level

Only a very limited number of papers has so far been published describing the effects of magnetic fields at the cellular level of the nervous system. Schwartz (1980, 1981) has studied the effects of strong constant magnetic fields on conduction velocity, membrane potentials and transmembrane currents in the nerve trunk and the giant axon of the lobster. In a well controlled experiment he compared conduction velocity before and after field exposure for 5–10 min using a flux density of 1.2 Tesla. The nerve trunk was exposed, with the field perpendicular as well as parallel to the nerve fibres. Schwartz did not discover any significant changes in the studied variables related to the field.

Ueno et al. (1981, 1982) recently studied the influence of alternating magnetic fields (10–50 Hz) on the lobster giant axon. The authors used an intracellular recording technique and were primarily interested in membrane phenomena such as changes in excitability, permeability or action potential changes. In this study the axon was perpendicular to the direction of magnetic flux, which was maximally 1.2 T. No significant magnetic field effects were found.

These model experiments showed, however, that eddy currents induced in tissue surrounding the nerve fibre could generate activity in the fibre under certain conditions. The preliminary results from the studies quoted indicate that the peripheral nerve axon itself is insensitive to strong magnetic fields. However, effects at the cellular level can be induced via the surrounding tissue.

A number of reports describe stimulatory responses from a time-varying magnetic field using nerve preparations of different kinds. Kolin et al. (1959) reported that a nerve-muscle preparation from the bullfrog could be stimulated by a magnetic field. Stimulation of the nerve resulted in intense tetanic contractions of the muscle. These authors used 2 frequencies, 60 and 1000 Hz, and flux densities of 200–800 mT. Muscular contractions occurred when the nerve was formed into a one-turn loop functioning as a "secondary winding" to the electromagnet used. It was also possible to stimulate the muscle directly by submerging it in Ringer's solution and placing it in the air gap of the electromagnet. The mechanism behind the stimulation effect is probably eddy currents induced in the nerve and muscle tissue. However, the flux densities used in these experiments by far exceed those usually found in industry today. Even from other viewpoints this result is not directly applicable to human beings and in vivo situations.

Using a nerve-muscle preparation from the frog Öberg (1973) showed that it was possible to induce contractions in the muscle by the rapid switching of a magnetic field across the nerve perpendicular to the long axis. The nerve was positioned in an air gap in a ferrite core and isolated from the core. A coil wound on the core was energized with currents at 1–20 kHz. At moderate to low flux densities it was possible to elicit muscle contractions. The probable mechanism in this case is the same as in the experiment reported by Kolin, i.e. the induction of eddy currents in the nerve bundle and the surrounding tissue.

Gengerelli and Holter (1941) stimulated the sciatic nerve of the frog by placing the nerve in an electrical field of 60 Hz and 55 kV/m. The authors showed that the stimulatory effect occurred directly on the nerve and not on the muscle. In Ringer's solution it was no longer possible to stimulate the nerve. The electrostatic shielding effect of the solution may explain the lack of stimulation in this experiment.

Lövsund et al. (1980) used the frog retina for studies of ganglion cell activity and its dependence on a magnetic field to which the preparation was exposed. The ganglion cell activity was recorded extracellularly by glass microelectrodes. A group of active ganglion cells was identified by means of a light stimulus. The retina was then exposed to a time-varying magnetic field with a frequency of 20–30 Hz and a flux density around 20 mT for 20 sec. When the magnetic field was switched off it was possible to record an increased ganglion cell activity for some seconds. The intensity of the cellular discharge depended on the frequency and the intensity of the magnetic field. The frequency of the field giving the maximal post-stimulus discharge (20 Hz) agreed with that giving maximal sensitivity for magnetophosphenes in human volunteers (see below).

The effects of microwaves on isolated nerves and muscles have been investigated rather extensively both in acute irradiation and in long-term experiments. Chou and Guy (1978) used isolated frog sciatic nerves, cat saphenous nerves, rabbit vagus nerves and superior cervical ganglia, as well as rat diaphragm muscle in their study. In a specially designed wave guide apparatus, which allowed control of the temperature of the bathing solution, the nerves and muscles were exposed to 2450 MHz continuous waves (CW) with SARs from 0.3 to 1500 W/kg and pulsed with peak SARs from 0.3 to 220 kW/kg. The compound action potential (CAP) of the nerves and the contractile tension of the muscles were recorded before, during and after the exposure. No effect was seen on the CAP as long as the temperature was held constant. At high power levels a slight increase in conduction velocity was seen, but this could be reproduced by raising the temperature of the bathing solution. No direct stimulation of nerve cells by either CW (1500 W/kg) or pulsed (peak 220 kW/kg) microwaves could be observed. The exposure of the isolated muscle preparations did not result in any significant changes in the measured parameter.

In order to study in more detail the effects of microwaves on excitable cells, Seaman and Wachtel (1978) exposed the abdominal ganglion of *Aplysia californica* and measured the firing rate of individual beating pacemakers. Exposure for 2–3 min at an SAR of only a few mW/g was capable of changing the firing rate of some pacemaker cells. Two types of response were seen; one developed slowly – of the order of minutes – in all neurones. These changes were mostly a decrease in firing rate, but also increased rates were seen. The other response occurred a few seconds after onset of the irradiation as an increase in firing rate. Pulsed radiation induced rapid changes in firing rate more readily than did CW at the same mean SAR. The slow response is believed to result largely from a thermal interaction; on the other hand the rapid change cannot readily be explained as a thermal effect.

McRee and Wachtel (1980) studied the effects of microwave radiation, 2.45 GHz CW, on isolated frog sciatic nerves using SARs ranging from 0 to 100 mW/g. The effect on the viability of the nerves was measured in terms of the ability of the nerve trunks to sustain a high firing rate over prolonged periods without suffering appreciable changes in excitability. The nerves were stimulated with twin pulses separated by a 5 msec interval at a rate of 50 pps. The exposed nerves underwent a prolongation of the refractory period as evidenced by a decrease in size of the second CAP. This effect was usually observable after 20–30 min of exposure for SARs greater than 10 mW/g. The investigators did not find any indication of an immediate microwave effect, such as a sudden jump in the CAP size at the start of the exposure. The gradual loss of viability led McRee and Wachtel to suggest that the observed effect is based on interference with long-term regulatory mechanisms, such as the maintenance of the ionic concentration gradients across the membranes.

Portela et al. (1975) reported on the effect of pulsed microwaves on a nerve-muscle preparation from frog skeletal muscle. The muscle fibres were exposed in vitro for 2 h at 10 mW/cm^2 in a chamber containing Ringer solution. Transient changes of 10–30% were detected in a number of passive and dynamic electrical parameters of the cell membrane, the propagation velocity of the action potential, and the water permeability. Also the osmotically available cell volume was transiently increased. No details of the dosimetry of the system were provided.

Effects at the organ level

Adey and collaborators have, in an extensive series of papers, described changes in the efflux of calcium in brain tissue following the application of an electromagnetic field. Electrical gradients of the order of 50 mV/cm pulses increased the calcium efflux in the cat brain. Similar experiments were carried out with extremely low frequency fields with field strengths between 5 and 100 V/m and frequencies between 6 and 32 Hz. The results were decreased efflux of calcium for 6 and 16 Hz and nearly unchanged conditions for the rest of the frequencies. Frequency as well as amplitude "windows" were observed.

Experiments have also been carried out with low intensity amplitude-modulated RF fields, in which an enhanced release of calcium ions was seen (Bawin et al. 1975). Neonatal chick forebrain was irradiated with an amplitude-modulated 147 MHz carrier wave at intensities of 1–2 mW/cm^2. Radioactive $^{45}Ca^{2+}$ fluxes from the irradiated brain were compared with those of the controls. At modulation frequencies around 16 Hz a significant increase in efflux (20%) was seen. These findings have been confirmed in independent work by Blackman et al. (1979). Using a carrier wave frequency of 450 MHz Bawin et al. (1978) showed the existence of a frequency window as well as a power window. The effects disappeared gradually for intensities above 2 mW/cm^2 and were not significant at 5 mW/cm^2. For recent reviews of this work, see Adey (1979, 1980, 1981).

Recently Blackman et al. (1980) found that 50 MHz modulated 16 Hz, at certain power levels produced changes in the Ca^{2+} efflux from chick brains exposed in vitro. The enhanced efflux occurred within at least two distinctly separated ranges of power density. The first effective range spanned from 1.44 to 1.67 mW/cm^2 and the other included 3.64 mW/cm^2, which were bracketed by no-effect results at 0.72, 2.17 and 4.32 mW/cm^2. The dosimetry used in these experiments has recently been worked out by Joines and Blackman (1980). The results show that the average electrical field intensity within the sample remained the same at different carrier frequencies if the incident power density for which an effect was seen was adjusted by an amount that compensated for the frequency dependence of the electrical properties of the tissue. All experimental results so far obtained at the different carrier frequencies are in complete agreement with this interpretation.

Some suggestions have been made to explain the fairly complicated result of interaction between the EM fields and brain tissue, but it still awaits full explanation.

It has been shown that microwave irradiation can influence the heart rate of isolated perfused hearts. Olsen et al. (1977) found that in rat hearts bradycardia results after radiation with SARs of 1.3 and 2.1 mW/g, values which are too low to give a measurable temperature increase during the experiment. The interaction mechanism causing the effect is not known, but the authors hypothesized that the microwave energy interacts with the remaining portion of the autonomic nervous system within the heart to produce the chronotropic effect.

Effects at the organismic level

The literature on electromagnetic field effects on animals are sizeable but only a few reports give reliable evidence on the extent and nature of the interactions. The existing knowledge can be described as a variety of observations with great differences in flux density, frequency and exposure duration. The results give a rather confused picture which is difficult to use, at least so far, for drawing any definite conclusions.

However, some examples of results should be given. Beischer and Knepton (1966) discovered large effects on EEG amplitudes and power spectra when squirrel monkeys were exposed to very high fields 2–9 T. In a series of studies DeLorge (1972, 1973a, b) exposed rhesus monkeys to combined electric and magnetic fields to study possible behavioural effects. The fields used had a relatively small amplitude. The behaviour of the animals was examined by 3 tests in which the animals responded to different signals. No positive effects were found. The summary ends: "the present study, in addition to previous work provides cumulative evidence that Elf (extremely low frequency) non-ionizing radiation as produced in our laboratory does not influence animal behaviour in either a beneficial or detrimental manner."

Beischer and Knepton (1964) have studied the influence of a strong static (DC) magnetic field on the ECG of squirrel monkeys. The animals were placed in 2–7 T fields. The ECG was recorded before and after the exposure. The most interesting result was an increased T wave amplitude during the field exposure. This change disappeared when the field was switched off. The effect could probably be explained by the induction law, the blood acting as a moving conductor in the field and generating a potential which was added to the ECG.

Chronic exposure of rats to a 60 Hz electrical field have been shown by Jaffe et al. (1980) to affect synaptic transmission. The rats were housed and exposed individually in polycarbonate cages. The undisturbed field strength was measured to be 100 kV/m, but due, among other things, to interaction by animals in adjacent cages, the "effective" field strength was estimated to be about 65 kV/m. The animals were exposed 20 h/day for 30 days. No clinically observable effects of the exposure were seen. Several measures and tests were performed of synaptic transmission and peripheral nerve function. The result showed that only synaptic transmission was significantly affected by the exposure. A conditioning-test (C-T) response was used to measure excitability and refractory period of the synapses of the superior cervical sympathetic ganglia. The postganglionic action potentials were measured as a function of the time interval between 2 stimuli applied to the preganglionic nerve. The curves thus obtained were consistently higher at every point for the exposed animals. In 7 of the 11 tested C-T intervals the spike height ratio was significantly higher in exposed than in sham-exposed animals. The mechanism through which the effect was produced is not known, and furthermore the biological significance of the effect in terms of health and well-being of the organism is not clear.

The effect of amplitude-modulated radio frequency fields on mammalian EEGs has been investigated by Takashima et al. (1979). Rabbits were chronically irradiated for 2 h a day for 6 weeks at 1–10 MHz, 15 Hz modulation. The exposure took place between two large aluminium plates separated by a distance of 20 cm. The RF field strengths ranged from 0.5 to 1 kV/m. For EEG recording silver electrodes were placed on the skull; they were removed after the initial recordings and reinserted before the intermediate and final EEG recordings. After about 2 or 3 weeks of exposure an abnormal EEG pattern developed. A low frequency component around 4 Hz was enhanced and the high frequency components decreased. These experiments were later corroborated by Takashima and Schwan (1979). In particular, after long irradiation at 100–200 V/m the EEG was characterized by the presence of spindle-like signals with a frequency of 14–16 Hz. These spindles had large amplitudes and appeared with a mean interval of 20–30 sec.

No effect was noticed by Takashima et al. (1979) from acute irradiations of the rabbits at levels 0.5–1 kV/m, 1–30 MHz, 60 Hz modulation. If the recording electrodes were left in place during exposure an abnormal EEG pattern could be seen with both 60 Hz modulation and CW acute RF exposure. Repeating these experiments with the metal electrodes removed during the exposure caused no abnormality and the investigators thus concluded that the effect on the EEG was due to the local fields created by the presence of metal electrodes in the cranial cavity.

Histological studies of brain tissues after microwave exposure have shown pathological changes. Tolgskaya and Gordon (1973) reported on morphological changes in irradiated rabbits, rats and mice. The type of change seen was dependent on intensity, frequency and duration of irradiation. One common feature in almost all cases was swelling of the cytoplasm of the nerve cells with vacuolation, marked in the hypothalamic region. Corresponding pathological changes were observed by Albert and DeSantis (1975) in a study of Chinese hamsters radiated 14 h/day for 22 days at 25 mW/cm^2, 2.45 GHz. The hypothalamus and subthalamus were consistently altered, showing vacuoles and chromatolysis. It is known that the first response of a cellular system to a disturbance is a cloudy swelling of the cytoplasm and if the disturbance is prolonged or increased in intensity vacuolation follows (Hill and LaVia 1980). However, since the dosimetry of these investigations is not clear it cannot be excluded that the effects have a thermal cause.

Effects on humans

Magnetophosphenes

A well established biomagnetic effect is the so called magnetophosphene (for review see Lövsund et al. 1980). Phosphenes can be described as faint flickering visual sensations generated by stimuli other than photons. Examples of such stimuli are pressure upon the eye, mechanical shocks, sudden fright and also electric currents and magnetic fields applied to the eye. This phenomenon is very reproducible and has been studied by many groups during the years. The magnetophosphene is a "model phenomenon" which may give interesting results concerning the interaction between an electromagnetic field and nervous tissue (Lövsund et al. 1980). Recent studies (Lövsund et al. 1979) have confirmed that the phosphenes are generated in the retina and not in the optic nerve or visual cortex as suggested by earlier authors.

Especially the threshold of phosphenes and its variation with the frequency of the field is of particular interest. A sharp sensitivity maximum at 20–30 Hz has been found by Lövsund et al. (1980). The minimum flux density is as low as 10 mT. The same sensitivity maximum can be studied if electric currents at the same frequencies are passed through the retina.

The same authors also studied the difference in threshold curves between deutan (colour defective) volunteers and volunteers with normal colour vision. The difference is reproducible and an interesting finding that could give new information about how the field interacts with the nervous structures in the retina.

Induction heating

We know of 2 near-accidents with induction furnaces which may be of some interest to report in this context (Lövsund and Hansson Mild 1978). Both cases occurred during repair of furnaces when the current in the induction coil was accidently turned on while a maintenance man was still down in the furnace. In the first case it was a 2 ton furnace with a power of 1100 kW, working at 890 Hz. The flux density was estimated at 40 mT. The person afterwards said that he had a feeling of panic and felt weightless. He also lost his bearings. The discomfort did not remain after the exposure. In the second case a man was exposed to 60 mT 50 Hz. He experienced this in the form of trembling all over. Calculations of the induced current density give values of the order of $0.1–0.3$ mA/cm^2.

Therapeutic use

Short-wave and microwave diathermy have been in therapeutic use for over half a century. The main effect of this type of therapy is to produce heat in deep tissues. The necessary SAR value is of the order of 50–100 W/kg leading to local tissue temperatures of 40–42°C. One of the most common indications for treatment is relief of pain (Stillwell 1965). However, this is not an effect specifically induced by the EM field, but merely a result of local heating.

Microwave hearing

It is now well established that when humans are exposed to pulse-modulated microwaves above certain intensity levels, an audible sound occurs which appears to originate from within or near the head. The threshold for various pulse widths and frequencies have recently been given by Lin (1980). The estimated peak SAR in the head at threshold was of the order of 0.5–1 W/g. The time-averaged incident power density was about 0.1 mW/cm^2. The interaction mechanism behind the phenomenon is thought to be purely thermal. The pulsed microwave energy initiates a thermoelastic wave of pressure in brain tissue and that activates the inner ear receptors via bone conduction. It is not likely that the sound results from a direct interaction between the microwaves and the cochlear nerve or neurones along the auditory pathway (Lin 1980). At the moment the health hazard of this effect is under discussion.

Epidemiological studies

Several investigators have performed epidemiological studies on workers exposed to radio frequency and microwave radiation. The complex exposure situations in various occupational environments make it very difficult to determine the level of exposure. In most cases only a rough estimate is possible because of the wide variation in the field intensity over the dimension of the body. It is furthermore difficult to specify exposure time since most processes have intermittent duty cycles. Many of the epidemiological studies have been criticized on the ground that other environmental factors, which might influence the outcome, have been neglected. Specifically, such factors as noise, vibration, ventilation, lighting and shift work should be paid more attention. Information on the control groups with regard to age distribution and occupation are also inadequately given in most studies (Silverman 1973). However, in spite of this criticism it is remarkable how often the clinical findings are in accordance to a certain extent. The symptoms and signs commonly found more frequently in the exposed groups than in the controls include headache, irritability, dizziness, loss of appetite, sleeplessness, sweating, difficulties in concentration or memory, depression, emotional instability, dermographism, thyroid gland enlargement and tremor of extended fingers. These disturbances are called the neurasthenic syndrome (cf. Silverman 1973).

In recent years some new epidemiological studies have been published. Djordjević et al. (1979) studied 322 radar workers with a history of occupational exposure from 5 to 10 years. No remarkable changes in the health status of the observed workers were found, yet subjective complaints such as headache, fatigue and irritability were more frequent in the exposed group than in controls. The authors conclude that these findings may very well be attributed to other environmental factors and not solely to the microwaves. Bielski et al. (1980) showed changes in the EEG in 2 groups of workers, one of which was exposed to microwave 3–7 GHz and the other to RF fields 7–30 MHz. The authors state in their conclusion that larger groups and analysis according to age, time of exposure and social standards are needed before this type of EEG change can be related to RF exposure.

DISCUSSION

A general consensus among scientists today is that the majority of biological effects of RF and microwave fields can be explained by thermal energy conversion. However, this does not mean that it is possible to give a predictive model of the interaction, since the energy absorbtion in humans and animals is highly non-uniform and at present the energy distribution is unpredictable. The energy absorbtion may give rise to temperature gradients in the body and cause alterations whose extent and implications have not yet been fully recognized. As an indication of the importance of the thermal effects it can be mentioned that the proposed new American national standard ANSI C-95.4 is based on an average SAR for the whole body or parts thereof of not more than 0.4 W/kg.

For frequencies in the kHz range the possibility exists of direct nerve excitation by induced eddy currents. However, the H field strengths needed are so high that they might be encountered accidently in few occupations. The effects are as far as we know reversible, but since the current density needed for excitation is of the order of 1 mA/cm^2 the thermal risk should also be taken into account in long-term exposure.

From the literature surveyed for this review article it seems as if modulated fields have a greater capacity for interfering with biological material than do CW. In the case of pulse-modulated fields it can be speculated that thermal mechanisms are involved as in microwave hearing (Lin 1980).

Both amplitude-modulated UHF fields and ELF fields with frequencies in the range 6–30 Hz have been shown to affect brain tissue and the bioelectrical activity. The intensites of these fields in situ have been calculated to be of the same order of magnitude as those occurring naturally from the EEG activity.

Schmitt et al. (1976) point out the important role played by neuronal local circuits and dendro-dendritic contacts in higher brain functions, and that the language of much of the central nervous system may be graded electrotonic potentials rather than regenerative spikes. For the retina and the olfactory bulb local circuits and the role of dendritic interaction are well illustrated. In view of this it is very interesting to note that Lövsund et al. (1980) found in the thresholds for magnetophosphenes and retinal ganglion cell activity the same general type of frequency sensitivity, with a maximum around 20 Hz, as did Adey and collaborators for the Ca^{2+} efflux from brain tissues and Takashima et al. for the EEG changes in rabbit. The induced current density in the retina at threshold for the magnetophosphenes is low;

estimates by Lövsund (1980) gave values of the order of 1 mA/m^2, which corresponds to an electrical gradient of 5 mV/m.

Our level of knowledge of the mechanisms behind electromagnetic field effects on biological systems is still unsatisfactorily low. The branch of physics studying the bioeffects of fields has collected and described observations from a wide variety of experimental conditions without, so far, being able to summarize and explain the effects in a conclusive way. Table I is one way of presenting some of these "islands of knowledge;" we still lack the "bridges of knowledge" between these findings, necessary to formulate more general conclusions.

The way to a better understanding probably goes via the study of reproducible effects in as easily understandable an experimental model as possible. So far the influence of low frequency magnetic fields on living tissue has been studied mainly on very complex biological systems concerning experimental animals or human volunteers. Very often the method of investigation has had an epidemiological approach. It seems that this way of exploring field effects could make it difficult to detect the specific effect of the field, since these effects are of the same order of magnitude as other systemic responses with different genesis. The magneto-biological responses may be buried in "the physiological noise."

REFERENCES

Adey, W.R. Long-range electromagnetic field interactions at brain cell surfaces. In: T.S. Tenforde (Ed.), Magnetic Field Effect on Biological Systems. Plenum Press, New York, 1979: 57–77.

Adey, W.R. Frequency and power windowing in tissue interaction with weak electromagnetic fields. Proc. IEEE, 1980, 68: 119–125.

Adey, W.R. Tissue interactions with nonionizing electromagnetic fields. Physiol. Rev., 1981, 61: 435–514.

Albert, E.N. and DeSantis, M. Do microwaves alter nervous system structure? Ann. N.Y. Acad. Sci., 1975, 247: 87–106.

Barański, S. and Czerski, P. Biological Effects on Microwaves. Dowden, Hutchinson and Ross, Stroudsburg, Pa., 1976.

Barnothy, M.F. (Ed.) Biological Effects of Magnetic Fields, Vol. 1. Plenum Press, New York, 1964.

Barnothy, M.F. (Ed.) Biological Effects of Magnetic Fields, Vol. 2. Plenum Press, New York, 1969.

Bawin, S.M., Kaczmarek, L.K. and Adey, W.R. Effects of modulated VHF fields on the central nervous system. Ann. N.Y. Acad. Sci., 1975, 247: 74–81.

Bawin, S.M., Sheppard, A.R. and Adey, W.R. Possible mechanisms of weak electromagnetic field coupling in brain tissue. Bioelectrochem. Bioenerg., 1978, 5: 67–76.

Beischer, D.E. and Knepton, Jr., J.C. Influence of strong magnetic fields on the electrocardiogram of squirrel monkeys (Saimiri sciureus). Aerospace Med., 1964, 35: 939–944.

Beischer, D.E. and Knepton, Jr., J.C. The electroencephalogram of the squirrel monkey (Saimiri sciureus) in a very high magnetic field. Naval Aerospace Medical Institute, Pensacola, Fla., 1966: Rep. NAMI-972.

Bernhart, J. The direct influence of electromagnetic fields on nerve and muscle cells of man within the frequency range of 1 Hz to 30 MHz. Radiat. environm. Biophys., 1979, 16: 309–323.

Bielski, J., Sawinska, A. and Pianowska, J. Bioelectrical activity in employees exposed to various frequencies of electromagnetic fields. In: A.-J. Berteaud and B. Servantie (Eds.), Symposium URSI "Ondes Electromagnétiques et Biologie", Jouy-en-Josas. 1980: 193–195.

Blackman, C.F., Elder, J.A., Weil, C.M., Benane, S.G., Eichinger, D.C. and House, D.E. Induction of calcium-ion efflux from brain tissue by radio-frequency radiation: Effects of modulation frequency and field strength. Radio Sci. 1979, 14: 93–98.

Blackman, C.F., Benane, S.G., Joines, W.T., Hollis, M.A. and House, D.E. Calcium-ion efflux from brain tissue: power density versus internal field-intensity dependencies at 50-MHz RF radiation. Bioelectromagnetics, 1980, 1: 277–283.

Chou, C.-K. and Guy, A.W. Effects of electromagnetic fields on isolated nerve and muscle preparations. IEEE Trans. Microwave Theory Tech., 1978, MTT-26: 141–147.

Cleary, S.F. Biological effects of microwaves and radiofrequency radiation. CRC crit. Rev. environm. Control, 1977, 7: 121–165.

DeLorge, J. Operant behaviour of rhesus monkeys in the presence of extreme low frequency-low intensity magnetic and electric fields: Experiment 1. Naval Aerospace Medical Research Laboratory, Pensacola, Fla., 1972: Rep. NAMRL-1179.

DeLorge, J. Operant behaviour of rhesus monkeys in the presence of extreme low frequency-low intensity magnetic and electric fields: Experiment II. Naval Aerospace Medical Research Laboratory, Pensacola, Fla., 1973a: Rep. NAMRL-1179.

DeLorge, J. Operant behaviour of rhesus monkeys in the presence of extreme low frequency-low intensity magnetic and electric fields: Experiment III. Naval Aerospace Medical Research Laboratory, Pensacola, Fla., 1973b: Rep. NAMRL-1196.

Deno, D.W. Electrostatic and electromagnetic effects of ultrahigh-voltage transmission lines. EL-802, Research Project 566-1, Electric Power Research Institute, Palo Alto, Calif., 1978.

Djordjević, Z., Kolak, A., Stojković, M., Ranković, N. and Ristić, P. A study of the health status of radar workers. Aviat. Space environm. Med., 1979, 50: 396–398.

Durney, C.H., Iskander, M.F., Maasoudi, H., Allen, S.J. and Mitchell, J.C. Radiofrequency Radiation Dosimetry Handbook, 3rd Ed. USAF School of Aerospace Medicine, Brooks Air Force Base, Texas, 1980: Rep. SAM-TR-80-32.

Gandhi, O.P. (Ed.) Special issue on "Biological effects and medical applications of electromagnetic energy". Proc. IEEE, 1980, 68: 1–169.

Gengerelli, J.A. and Holter, N.J. Experiments on stimulation of nerves by alternating electrical fields. Proc. Soc. exp. Biol. Med. (N.Y.), 1941, 46: 532.

Hansson Mild, K. Occupational exposure to radio-frequency electromagnetic fields. Proc. IEEE, 1980, 68: 12–17.

Hill, R.B. and LaVia, M.F. (Eds.) Principles of Pathobiology, 3rd Ed. Oxford University Press, Oxford, 1980.

Jaffe, R.A., Laszewski, B.L., Carr, D.B. and Phillips, R.D. Chronic exposure to a 60-Hz electric field: Effects on synaptic transmission and peripheral nerve function in the rat. Bioelectromagnetics, 1980, 1: 131–147.

Johnson, C.C. and Guy, A.W. Nonionizing electromagnetic wave effects in biological materials and systems. Proc. IEEE, 1972, 60: 692–718.

Joines, W.T. and Blackman, C.F. Power density, field intensity, and carrier frequency determinants of RF-energy-induced calcium-ion efflux from brain tissue. Bioelectromagnetics, 1980, 1: 271–275.

Kaune, W.T. and Phillips, R.D. Comparison of the coupling of grounded humans, swine and rats to vertical, 60-Hz electric fields. Bioelectromagnetics, 1980, 1: 117–129.

Kinn, J.B. and Postow, E. Index of Publications on Biological Effects of Electromagnetic Radiation (0–100 GHz). United States Environmental Protection Agency, EPA-600/9-81-011, 1981: 567 pp.

Kolin, A., Brill, N.Q. and Broberg, P.J. Stimulation of irritable tissues by means of an alternating magnetic field. Proc. Soc. exp. Biol. Med. (N.Y.), 1959, 102: 251–252.

Lin, J.C. The microwave auditory phenomena. Proc. IEEE, 1980, 68: 67–73.

Lövsund, P. Biological Effects of Alternating Magnetic Fields with Special Reference to the Visual System. Ph.D. Thesis, Linköping Studies in Science and Technology. Dissertations No. 47, Linköping University, Sweden, 1980.

Lövsund, P. and Hansson Mild, K. Low frequency electromagnetic fields near some induction heaters. Nat. Board Occup. Safety and Health, Sweden, 1978, Invest. Rep. 1978: 38.

Lövsund, P., Öberg, P.Å. and Nilsson, S.E.G. Quantitative determination of thresholds of magnetophosphenes. Radio Sci., 1979, 14, no. 6S: 199–200.

Lövsund, P., Nilsson, S.E.G., Reuther, T. and Öberg, P.Å. Magnetophosphenes. A quantitative analysis of thresholds. Med. biol. Engng Comput., 1980, 18: 326–334.

McRee, D.I. and Wachtel, H. The effects of microwave radiation on the vitality of isolated frog sciatic nerves. Radiat. Res., 1980, 82: 536–546.

Öberg, P.Å. Magnetic stimulation of nerve tissue. Med. biol. Engng, 1973, 11: 55–64.

Olsen, R.G., Lords, J.L. and Durney, C.H. Microwave-induced chronotropic effects in the isolated rat heart. Ann. Biomed. Engng, 1977, 5: 395–409.

Portela, A., Llobera, O., Michaelson, S.M., Stewart, P.A., Perez, J.C., Guerrero, A.H., Rodriguez, C.A. and Perez, R.J. Transient effects of low-level microwave irradiation on bioelectric muscle cell properties and on water permeability and its distribution. In: S.M. Michaelson et al. (Eds.), Fundamental and Applied Aspects of Nonionizing Radiation. Plenum Press, New York, 1975: 93–127.

Presman, A.S. Electromagnetic Fields and Life. Plenum Press, New York, 1970.

Schmitt, F.O., Dev, P. and Smith, B.H. Electrotonic processing of information by brain cells. Science, 1976, 193: 114–120.

Schwartz, J.-L. Influence of a constant magnetic field on nervous tissues: I. Nerve conduction velocity studies. IEEE Trans. biomed. Engng, 1980, BME-25: 467–473.

Schwartz, J.-L. Influence of a constant magnetic field on nervous tissues: II. Voltage Clamp Studies. IEEE Trans. biomed. Engng, 1981, BME-26: 238–243.

Seaman, R.L. and Wachtel, H. Slow and rapid response to CW and pulsed microwave radiation by individual *Aplysia* pacemakers. J. Microwave Power, 1978, 13: 77–86.

Silverman, C. Nervous and behavioral effects of microwave radiation in humans. Amer. J. Epidemiol., 1973, 97: 219–224.

Sheppard, A.R. and Eisenbud, M. Biological Effects of Electric and Magnetic Fields of Extremely Low Frequency. New York University Press, New York, 1977.

Stillwell, G.K. General principles of thermotherapy. In: S. Licht (Ed.), Theurapeutic Heat and Cold, 2nd Ed. Waverly Press, Baltimore, Md., 1965: 232–239.

Stuchly, M.A. Health aspects of radio frequency and microwave exposure, Part. 2. Environmental Health Directorate, Canada, 1978: Rep. 78-EHD-22.

Takashima, S. and Schwan, H.P. Effects of radio frequency fields on the EEG of rabbit brains. In: Program and Abstracts from the 1979 Spring Meeting, International Union of Radio Science, Seattle, Wash., 1979.

Takashima, S., Onaral, B. and Schwan, H.P. Effects of modulated RF energy on the EEG of mammalian brains. Effects of acute and chronic irradiations. Radiat. environm. Biophys., 1979, 16: 15–27.

Tolgskaya, M.S. and Gordon, Z.V. Pathological effects of radio waves. Consultants Bureau, New York, 1973.

Ueno, S., Lövsund, P. and Öberg, P.Å. On the effect of alternating magnetic fields on action potentials in lobster giant axon. Proc. Vth Nordic Meeting on Medical and Biological Engineering, 1981, 12: 7, 262.

Ueno, S., Lövsund, P. and Öberg, P.Å. On the effect of alternating magnetic fields on action potentials in lobster giant axon. Bioelectromagnetics, 1982, in press.

Wever, R. ELF-effects on human circadian rhythms. In: M.A. Persinger (Ed.), ELF and ULF Electromagnetic Field Effects. Plenum Press, New York, 1974: 101–144.

Zimmerman, U., Pilwat, G., Holzaptel, C. and Rosenheck, K. Electrical hemolysis of human and bovine red blood cells. J. Membrane Biol., 1978, 30: 135–152.

Kyoto Symposia (EEG Suppl. No. 36)
Editors: P.A. Buser, W.A. Cobb and T. Okuma
© 1982, Elsevier Biomedical Press, Amsterdam

730

Effects of Solid Vibrations on Balance and Spinal Reflexes in Man

MAURICE HUGON, GABRIEL M. GAUTHIER, BERNARD MARTIN and JEAN PIERRE ROLL

Laboratoire de Psychophysiologie, Université d'Aix-Marseille I, Centre St-Jérôme, Rue H. Poincaré, ERA 272, CNRS, 13397-Marseilles Cedex 13 (France)

Vehicles such as helicopters or trucks can generate vibration (V) which is transmitted to passengers and pilots through solid contacts (seat, floor, pedals, handles, etc.). Vibration signals enter the nervous system through various sensory receptors from skin, muscles and joints and induce reflex and perceptive effects (De Gail et al. 1966; Eklund 1972). The aim of this study was to detect per- and possibly post-vibration on the balance of standing subjects (Martin et al. 1980), and to identify their underlying mechanisms (Roll et al. 1980).

METHOD

Vibration was applied to the seated subject (whole body vibration: WBV) by means of a powerful vertical hydraulic jack acting on a rigid platform on which a heavily cushioned seat was bolted. At platform level, where the feet were resting, the vibration frequency and amplitude were respectively 18 Hz and $0.5 \times g$. Due to the filtering effect through body elements, the acceleration was generally lower at the knee, thorax and forehead levels. Vibration was also specifically applied to the feet and legs (LV), or to the head (HV) or trunk and head (THV). In a first series of experiments, postural equilibrium in standing subjects was studied before and after 30 min periods of V, using a stabilometer which displayed antero-posterior and lateral components of the postural forces.

RESULTS

The main observations may be summarized as follows. (1) During V, the subjects reported some discomfort and itching; after V, they experienced a feeling of comfort and perfect stability which lasted about 1 min. (2) The postural forces recorded in standing subjects with eyes closed were significantly larger in amplitude for at least 15 min after vibration. Similar perceptive and motor effects were obtained from LV but not from THV or HV. No deviation from reference (pre-V) was noticed in non-vibrated control subjects submitted to the noise of the running equipment. From such experiments we conclude that (1) the transitory perceptive alterations are not responsible for post-vibration motor defects; (2) some change in leg sensorimotor apparatus causes the post-vibration postural instability since stimulation of trunk-head (including labyrinthine apparatus) has no such effects.

The second set of experiments (Roll et al. 1980) was aimed at defining per- and post-vibration modifications of the monosynaptic reflexes (Hoffmann (H) and tendon (T) reflexes) elicited in the soleus muscle of a seated subject. Reflexes were elicited through a standard procedure with ankle and knee joint angles positioned respectively at 90° and 120°. The tonic vibration response (17–100 Hz) was induced in some experiments by Achilles tendon stimulation. Such a tonic response was investigated under WBV. The results were as follows: (1) WBV induced a dramatic reduction of H and T reflexes without any changes of the M response. This reduction lasted a few minutes after suppression of the vibration; (2) THV and HV resulted only in reduced depressive effects on the monosynaptic reflexes; (3) the TVR was also reduced by solid V (pre- and post-effects).

CONCLUSIONS

The close similarity between the effects of WBV and LV on H, T and TV responses suggests that similar mechanisms are responsible for the observed effects of vibration. Muscle spindles (primary and secondary afferent fibres) are especially sensitive to vibration (Burke et al. 1976). Such inputs are known to cause presynaptic inhibition of reflexes either by direct segmental action or by supraspinal control (i.e., spino-bulbo-spinal presynaptic inhibition of the H reflex after skin stimulation (Thoden et al. 1971)). Also, vibration-induced afferent may be interpreted by the central nervous system as an unpleasant noise which could result in protective motor and perceptive responses such as reduction of extensor reflexes, or loss of fine discrimination of postural sensations. Finally defects in balance during and after vibration may be induced by alteration of both central (perception) and peripheral (segmental reflexes) mechanisms.

Further studies (Gauthier et al. 1981) have described the effects of vibration on sensorimotor performance such as foot and hand tracking of a visual target and force control. The observed alterations may be interpreted in a manner similar to that developed earlier regarding postural and reflex alterations.

REFERENCES

Burke, D., Hagbarth, K.E., Lofsted, L. and Wallin, B.G. The response of human muscle spindle endings to vibration of non contracting muscles. J. Physiol. (Lond.), 1976, 261: 673–693.

De Gail, P.J., Lance, W.J. and Neilson, P.D. Differential effects on tonic and phasic reflex mechanisms produced by vibration of muscles in man. J. Neurol. Neurosurg. Psychiat., 1966, 29: 1–11.

Eklund, G. Position sense and state of contraction: The effects of vibrations. J. Neurol. Neurosurg. Psychiat., 1972, 35: 606–611.

Gauthier, G.M., Roll, J.P., Martin, B. and Harlay, F. Effects of whole-body vibrations on sensory motor performance in man. Aviat. Space environm. Med., 1981, 52: 473–479.

Hagbarth, K.E. and Eklund, G. Motor effects of vibratory stimuli in man. In: R. Granit (Ed.), Muscular Afferents and Motor Control, Nobel Symposium I. Almqvist and Wiksell, Stockholm, 1966: 177–186.

Hugon, M. Methodology of the H reflex in man. In: J.E. Desmedt (Ed.), New Developments in Electromyography and Clinical Neurophysiology, Vol. III. Karger, Basel, 1973: 277–293.

Martin, B., Gauthier, G.M., Roll, J.P., Hugon, M. and Harlay, F. Effects of whole-body vibrations on standing posture in man. Aviat. Space environm. Med., 1980, 51: 778–787.

Roll, J.P., Martin, B., Gauthier, G.M. and Mussa Ivaldi, F. Effects of whole-body vibration on spinal reflexes in man. Aviat. Space environm. Med., 1980, 51: 1227–1233.

Thoden, U., Magherini, D.C. and Pompeiano, O. Proprioceptive influence on supraspinal descending inhibitory mechanisms. Arch. ital. Biol., 1971, 109: 130–152.

Kyoto Symposia (EEG Suppl. No. 36)
Editors: P.A. Buser, W.A. Cobb and T. Okuma
© 1982, Elsevier Biomedical Press, Amsterdam

EMG Analysis of Muscle Function in Repetitive Tasks in Laboratories and in Industry

ILKKA KUORINKA

Institute of Occupational Health, Helsinki (Finland)

Many occupations both in modern industry and in services are characterised by repeated work movements and constrained working postures. Automation and mechanisation eliminate those tasks which involve the most elevated work paces and stereotyped movements, but new branches of industry appear with the health problems typical of semimechanised industry. One of the physical problems commonly encountered in repetitive tasks is disease which results from overstrain, such as tenosynovitis, epicondylitis, tension neck, etc.

The frequency of overstrain disease varies from one branch to another. The lack of a common basis for classification does not allow valid comparisons to be made. Some figures indicate that overstrain diseases are a significant problem. Maeda (1977) from Japan cited figures from the Ministry of Labour for 1970–1971. According to these data, there were about 10,000 cases of occupational cervico-brachial syndromes among 6.1 million workers, and the frequency was sharply increasing. In Finland, a survey of a female population working at repetitive tasks found that the prevalence of tension neck syndrome (which approximates to the cervico-brachial syndrome) was 37.5% and the prevalence of tenosynovitis was 55.9%. The corresponding prevalences among shop assistants were 27.8% and 13.5% (Luopajärvi et al. 1979). Komoike and his colleagues (1974) estimated that the prevalence of the cervico-brachial syndrome ranges from 4% to 21%, depending on the occupational group.

AETIOLOGY OF THE DISEASES OF OVERSTRAIN

The symptoms of overstrain in workers who perform repetitive tasks are commonly related to the repetitivity of the working movements. Although this may generally be true, other factors should also be considered. Individual predisposition is one causative factor which is often proposed, but little is known about the nature of individual predisposition. Hettinger (1958) proposed that neurovascular lability as revealed by a vibration test would be an important factor of predisposition. However, the method used in testing is open to criticism (Kuorinka et al. 1982). Direct trauma and microtrauma can explain some of the cases (Thompson 1951). Infectious agents, rheumatic factors and erroneous metabolism of the connective tissue have been proposed as aetiological factors.

Although the primary pathology of overstrain diseases in the upper limbs is often located in the connective tissue, muscle metabolism and especially static muscle load have been thought to play a role. Intramuscular processes may be important *per se* in affections of the neck and shoulder region. The mechanism through which static muscle load could be mediated to tendon injury is obscure. Static loading of the muscle-tendon unit may also affect the metabolism of the tendon itself. However, in cases of tendon injuries in overstrain diseases, the mechanical injury remains the most probable.

The above considerations have led to 2 questions. Do repetitive tasks contain a component of static muscle effort which would be measurable by myoelectric techniques? What type of muscle effort patterns are typical of repetitive tasks?

MUSCLE EFFORT AND STATIC WORK IN REPETITIVE TASKS IN INDUSTRY

Muscle effort and static work were investigated in a plant where female workers packed bread. The task comprised the manipulation and the packing of loaves of bread. The weight of the packs seldom exceeded 1 kg. The population of packers included numerous cases of tenosynovitis, which motivated the study. However, the subjects were healthy at the time of the investigation.

Continuous or periodic myoelectric records were made for 14 subjects covering one work shift for each subject. Myoelectric signals were registered from the biceps muscle (10 subjects), from the hand flexors (14 subjects) and from the adductor pollicis muscle (4 subjects). The signals were registered from the preferred hand, using surface electrodes, and recorded and analysed by conventional methods. A spectral analysis of the recorded signals was carried out by a method described elsewhere (Kuorinka 1976).

Spectral analysis of the signals did not reveal an increase in low frequency components as an indication of muscle fatigue. This was true for all of the muscles measured. Technical breaks in production might have interfered with the results, however.

While these direct measurements failed to reveal fatigue, hand grip tests were carried out on 6 of the subjects. The maximal grip force and an endurance test (50% of the maximum) were made at the beginning and at the end of the work shift. If cumulative fatigue developed during the work shift, it should have been reflected in the loss of maximal grip force and in a shorter endurance, and a concomitant change should have taken place in the frequency spectrum. No change was found in the grip endurance, nor was there a change in the myoelectric spectrum.

The maximal grip force showed a nearly significant decrease at the end of the shift. This finding is parallel to the findings of Moikin (1981). In his study of 1600 workers in manual occupations, Moikin found that muscle force at the end of the workday had decreased by 8.5–21.5%.

LABORATORY EXPERIMENTS WITH REPETITIVE TASKS

Studies carried out in factories are plagued by various disturbing factors, breaks in the production, variation in the work load, etc. Although a simulated task in the laboratory is less authentic, it offers better opportunities to control the experimental situation. In order that the experiment could be controlled better, we constructed a simulated repetitive task at a conveyor belt. The task consisted of assembling the components of water tubes. Additional static effort was introduced to the task by springs, as more force was then required to connect the parts.

After an instruction session the subjects had 5 sessions on 5 consecutive days. Each session comprised the assembly of 150 work pieces at a pace chosen by the subject. The subjects were young women who had no previous experience of industrial assembly work.

Among other variables, myoelectric signals were recorded from 4 muscles of the right hand: the hand flexor and extensor groups, the biceps muscle and the upper part of the trapezius.

A conventional EMG registration system was used, with polygraphic recording and magnetic tape storage. Spectral analysis of the stored signals was done using the system mentioned earlier (Kuorinka 1976). Since the biceps muscle did not show any variation of interest, it was omitted from further experiments.

In contrast to the phasic extensor and flexor muscles, the myoelectric activity of the trapezius muscle was continuous throughout the experiment; there was only a slight work-cycle-related variation, as judged visually.

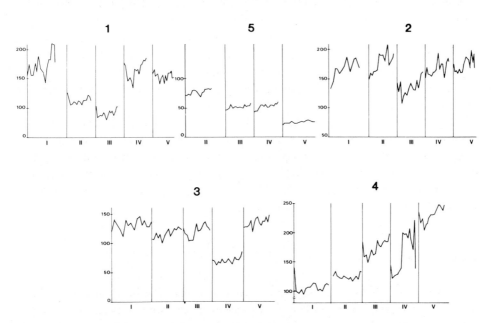

Fig. 1. Integrated EMG in arbitrary units as a function of time. Roman numerals indicate successive trials. X axis = time, y axis = IEMG, arbitrary units/time unit.

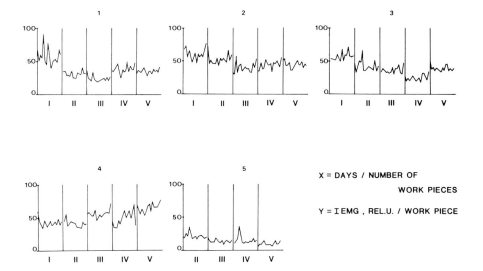

Fig. 2. Integrated EMG as a function of the number of completed work pieces. Roman numerals indicate successive trials. X axis = number of work pieces, Y axis = IEMG, arbitrary units/one work piece.

The integrated myoelectric signal from trapezius muscle was analysed in 2 cases: IEMG activity per unit time (1 min), and IEMG per time used to assymble one work piece (= IEMG per work piece). The previous set, IEMG per time unit, reflects the general work load and IEMG per work piece time reflects the muscle effort needed to complete one work piece. With a few exceptions, the IEMG for time unit curves from the trapezius muscle showed an ascending in-trial trend (Fig. 1).

There were great intra- and interindividual variations, but they had no relation to the other variables recorded. The ascending trend of the curves can be partly explained by the shortening cycle times (the subjects worked faster when trained, thus more work cycles were included in 1 time unit). The results partly reflect the increasing general muscle load.

In the IEMG per work piece, there was no clear cut trend in the trial (Fig. 2).

Spectral analysis was done from the myoelectric signals recorded from the hand flexors and extensors. There was considerable inter- and intraindividual variation in the spectra. The non-stationary nature of the signal from these phasic muscles partly explains the variation. There was no tendency in the spectra towards lower frequencies which would indicate muscle fatigue.

DISCUSSION

The analysis of myoelectric signals as a tool to reveal some background factors of overstrain diseases has proved to be valuable. In the studies cited above, much concern has been directed to the problem of the possible occurrence of static muscle work in repetitive tasks. The spectral analysis of myoelectric signals has proved to be − if not ideal − one of the methods available in the investigation of the muscle fatigue caused by static muscle load. Its special advantage is that it can be employed in the working situation. One of its drawbacks is the relative insensitivity caused by the characteristics of myoelectric signals.

The results from both the factory and the laboratory tasks seem to indicate that muscle fatigue, as revealed by the EMG spectrum in the hand flexors and extensors, is negligible. Thus, the evidence does not support the hypothesis that static work is the major aetiological factor for tenosynovitis and related affections in the wrist and the hand.

This result does not mean that muscle load itself would be minor. Moikin (1981) showed that work load in the upper limb muscles, both in the main and in the auxiliary muscles, can be high in repetitive tasks. The hypothesis that mechanical trauma is the main causal factor in tendon overstrain is compatible with the finding of elevated muscle load.

The strain on various structures in the shoulder and neck region can be high in repetitive tasks and relates to the work load as can be illustrated by the results of our laboratory experiment. The postural load on the neck and shoulder muscles seems to be intimately related not only to the physical work load but also to the psychological load, as found by Teiger et al. (1973) in their EMG studies of the neck. Research on the occupational musculo-skeletal diseases of overstrain will thus widely profit from kinesiological and biomechanical studies which use electrophysiological techniques.

REFERENCES

Hettinger, Th. Eine Modifikation des Hauttemperaturtests zur Erkennung der Disposition zu Sehnenscheidenentzundungen. Int. Z. angew. Physiol., 1958, 17: 271–275.

Komoike, Y., Miyoshi, K. and Nakamura, A. A report of health examinations on key punchers, typists and others. X. Reinstatement of patients with cervicobrachial syndrome. Sumimoto Bull. Hlth, 1974, 10: 159–171.

Kuorinka, I. Assessment of Muscular Fatigue with the Spectral Analysis of Myoelectric Potentials. Doctoral dissertation, Helsinki, 1976: 77 pp.

Kuorinka, I., Videman, T. and Lepistö, M. Reliability of a vibration test in screening for predisposition to tenosynovitis. Europ. J. appl. Physiol., 1981, 47: 365–376.

Luopajärvi, T., Kuorinka, I., Virolainen, M. and Holmberg, M. Prevalence of tenosynovitis and other injuries of the upper extremities in repetitive work. Scand. J. Work environm. Hlth, 1979, 5 (Suppl. 3): 48–55.

Maeda, K. Occupational cervicobrachial disorder and its causative factors. J. hum. Ergol., 1977, 6: 193–202.

Moikin, Yu. Conditions of the development of muscle overstrain in the process of local physical work. In: Proceedings, Finnish-Soviet Symposium on Occupational Hygiene and Work Physiology, Suzdahl, Moscow, 1981.

Teiger, C., Laville, A. et Duraffourg, J. Tâches Répétitives sous Contrainte de Temps et Charge de Travail. CNAM, Laboratoire de Physiologie de Travail et Ergonomie, Paris, 1973: Rapport No. 39.

Thompson, A.R., Plewes, L.W. and Shaw, E.G. Peritendinitis crepitans and simple tenosynovitis: a clinical study of 544 cases in industry. Brit. J. industr. Med., 1951, 8: 150–160.

Kyoto Symposia (EEG Suppl. No. 36)
Editors: P.A. Buser, W.A. Cobb and T. Okuma
© 1982, Elsevier Biomedical Press, Amsterdam

738

Finding Appropriate Work-Rest Rhythm for Occupational Strain on the Basis of Electromyographic and Behavioural Changes

KAZUTAKA KOGI

Division of Work Physiology and Psychology, Institute for Science of Labour, 1544 Sugao, Miyamae-ku, Kawasaki 213 (Japan)

In industrial work today, muscle fatigue usually results from intermittent static contractions or from repetitive dynamic work. Fatigue usually becomes excessive when the intervening periods of rest are too short to ensure its recovery. This condition of rest is dependent upon both the intensity of muscular load and its duration in either intermittent static contractions (Rohmert 1960; Kogi and Hakamada 1962; Bjorkstén and Jonsson 1977) or dynamic work (Numajiri 1968).

Fatigue of muscles in industrial conditions may lead to 2 kinds of negative consequences. First, it brings about stressful periods of work, in which the worker is compelled to continue to work with increasing fatigue or pain and with reduced capacity, the safety of work being sometimes endangered. Second, it may have long-term effects which often result in occupational impairments, such as low back pain and occupational neck-shoulder-arm disorder (Ohara et al. 1976; Onishi et al. 1976).

To prevent these negative consequences, it is very important to find appropriate work-rest rhythms which enable active muscles to work without falling into excessive fatigue. To find such rhythms, it is essential to identify stages of fatigue at which work should be discontinued for the active muscles. So this paper will discuss what kinds of fatigue indications are relevant to the need to take a rest and how we can use these indications for re-designing existing industrial work-rest cycles.

STAGES OF FATIGUE IN STATIC MUSCLE CONTRACTION

Fig. 1 shows cumulative frequency curves for various fatigue indications in sustained elbow flexion, time being expressed proportionally to the maximum endured time (Tanii et al. 1973). In the figure, degree 1 corresponds to initiation of local fatigue, 2 to onset of pain, 3 to distinct pain and 4 to intolerable pain. Other changes also seemed to appear in a consistent sequence. Significant increase of the integrated surface electromyogram, as evidenced by a trend test as well as increase in foot pressure was seen before the onset of local pain. Increase of synergistic activities of the brachio-radialis and other effort-depending changes came when distinct pain was already present. It is noteworthy that early indications of fatigue appeared at around two-tenths of the maximum endured time.

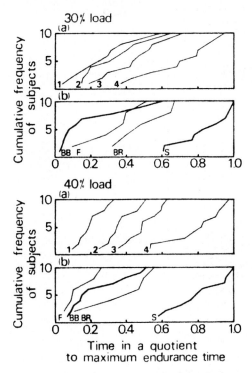

Fig. 1. Cumulative frequency curves of 10 subjects for various fatigue indications when the elbow flexion
was sustained until exhaustion at 30% or 40% of the maximum force. 1, onset of local fatigue; 2, onset
of muscle pain; 3, distinct muscle pain; 4, intolerable pain; F, significant change in foot pressure; BB,
significant increase of integrated EMG of brachial biceps; BR, of brachioradialis; S, onset of breath-
holding.

This confirms our earlier finding, shown in Fig. 2, that not only the maximum
endured time but also the time of onset of local pain from static contraction were in
a bilogarithmically linear relationship with sustained force expressed in percentage
of the maximum voluntary force (Kogi and Hakamada 1962). The onset of pain was
clearly linked with significant increase of low frequency components below 60 c/sec
of the surface electromyogram. Thus, even for the range of 10–20% force, pain
could be felt within several minutes.

SPONTANEOUS ALTERNATION OF WORKING MUSCLES

Fig. 3 shows how the working arm was alternated between right and left when
each of 7 subjects performed a tracking task using a lever with the arm raised
overhead and being freely exchanged (Tanii et al. 1972). The results were strikingly
similar between the two conditions of with or without display of tracking errors. The
mean interval of arm exchange was 185 sec without display of errors and 217 sec
with it. The interval until changing the arm was nearly equal for the 2 arms and did

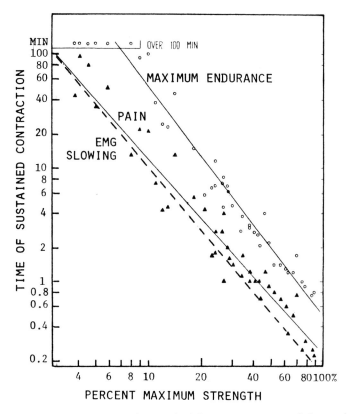

Fig. 2. Relation between the sustained force as percentage of the maximum force and the time of endurance (o) and time to onset of muscle pain (▲) when the elbow flexion was sustained until exhaustion. Regression lines for endurance time, onset time of pain and time to 25% increase of slow component below 60 c/sec of EMG of the brachial biceps are indicated.

not change significantly from the first to the latter half of the 30 min period. What interests us is at what stage of muscle fatigue did these changes of active muscle occur.

So we compared this result with the time course of various variables in forced operation, using only 1 arm continuously (Fig. 4). Using only 1 arm, all the subjects could endure the overhead work for more than 15 min. The mean time of arm alternation in free conditions corresponded to the stage of forced conditions at which the slow wave components below 40 c/sec of the surface EMG of the deltoid muscle were about 33% of all the components from 8 to 1000 c/sec. At this early stage, heart rate and respiration were still keeping steady states. Further, the mean interval of alternating the arms in free conditions was positively correlated with the individual time of onset of local fatigue sensation.

Similarly, alternation of the working arm in dynamic 1-arm cranking could also be seen to occur at an early stage of muscle fatigue (Tanii and Kogi 1976). This kind of spontaneous exchange of active muscles also seems to play a vital role in avoiding the impairing effect of advanced fatigue in industrial work.

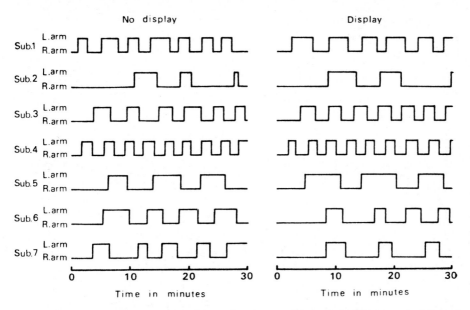

Fig. 3. Alternation of the working arm while performing a tracking task for 30 min manipulating a lever with the arm raised overhead. Results for 2 conditions, without and with display of tracking errors are shown for each subject. Exchange of arms was free. L. arm, raising the left arm; R. arm, raising the right arm.

Fig. 5 gives the gradual changes of the EMG stretch reflex pattern during a sustained contraction of 504 sec of the flexor pollicis longus, bending the interphalangeal joint of the thumb (Sadoyama and Kogi 1976). The load was 18% of the maximum voluntary force. Each line in the upper diagram of the figure shows the integrated surface EMG before stretch and each line in the lower diagram shows the integrated EMG during stretch. Each line represents 300 msec. The stretch was given at intervals of 4–12 sec. Augmentation of the stretch reflex started at the 4th min, when the integrated electrical activity before stretch also began to increase. This means that the gain of the stretch reflex loop, and thus the effort of sustaining the static contraction, gradually increased from an early phase of muscle fatigue. Spontaneous alternation of the active muscles, which we have seen, seems to be associated with such early changes. If active muscles are allowed to rest at this stage, fatigue will not develop. Therefore, it seems useful to use EMG findings corresponding to early fatigue as criteria pointing to the need to rest.

MUSCLE LOAD AND FATIGUE IN INDUSTRIAL REPETITIVE WORK

Fig. 6 summarizes results of EMG studies of arm and shoulder muscles in 8 different jobs (Onishi 1976). A, B, C and D were office machine jobs, A being typewriting in Japanese, B typewriting in English, C telephone operating and D telex operating; E, F, G and H were assembly line jobs in an electric appliance factory.

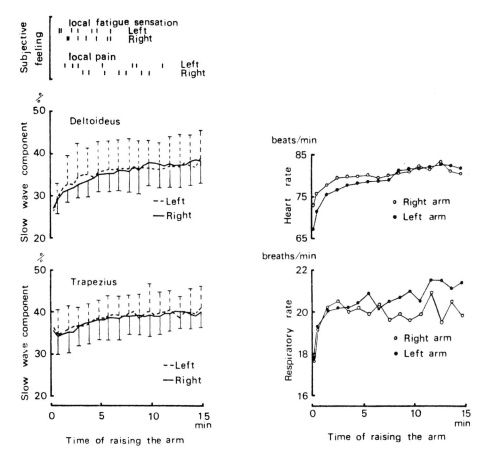

Fig. 4. Time of onset of subjective feelings and changes in the slow wave components below 40 c/sec of the deltoid and trapezius and in heart and respiratory rates while performing a tracking task manipulating a lever placed overhead, being forced to use only 1 arm continuously for 15 min.

In these office machine or assembly jobs, contractions reaching 10–30% or more of the maximum force were quite common. And many of them, shown by black dots, were of static nature usually lasting tens of seconds or more. These static contractions took the form of intermittent static contractions. While these types of work were mostly continuous for one to a few hours and reached several hours of such work a day, field investigations have revealed that the operators complained of arm and shoulder fatigue after work (Onishi et al. 1977).

An example of the EMG changes in this kind of repetitive work is shown in Fig. 7. It gives changes in the integrated EMG of subjects operating 3 different kinds of cash register machines. The mean counterpressure of the numerical keys was about 185 g for A and about 400 g for B and C. The forearm extensors and shoulder muscles were seen to make intermittent static contractions, especially when operations continued in sequence. Here, the operators worked continuously, dealing with goods of mostly 50–300 g with the left arm, but without counting the paid

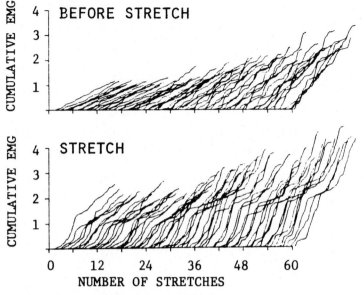

Fig. 5. Integrated EMG of the flexor pollicis longus for a 300 msec period before and immediately after a stretch was given while the muscle maintained a static contraction for 504 sec.

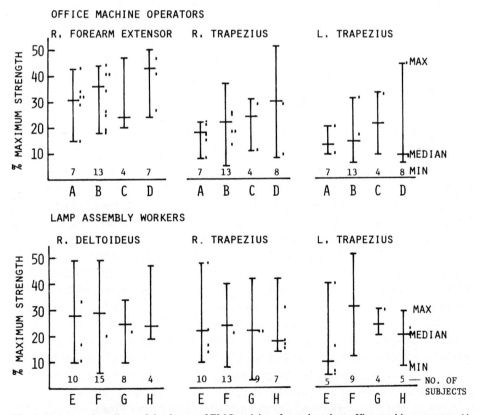

Fig. 6. Ranges and medians of the degree of EMG activity of muscles when office machine operators (A, B, C and D) and lamp assembly workers (E, F, G and H) continued their repetitive work. Number of subjects is given for each job group. Black dots show muscle activity of static nature.

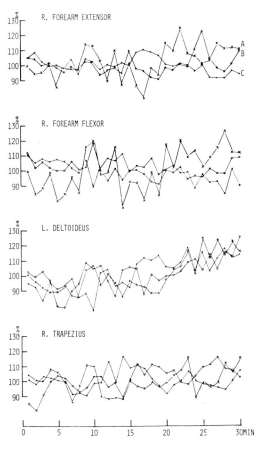

Fig. 7. Changes in average integrated EMG of the forearm extensor and flexor, deltoid, and trapezius when the subjects continued to operate 3 kinds of cash register.

money. In this experimental condition, the integrated EMG increased in the second half of the 30 min period in the case of the forearm extensors, deltoid and trapezius. It may be said that in densely repeated operations, muscles involved in operating keys could be easily fatigued as early as 15–30 min.

Fig. 8 gives changes in subsidiary behaviour due to the operation of a visual display unit (Sakai 1980). Among subsidiary behaviours such as looking aside, yawning, arm motions, shoulder motions and foot and leg movements, shoulder motions notably increased in the afternoon. In this and other studies of subsidiary behaviour during repetitive work, muscle fatigue, as observed in the form of increased compensatory motions of the neck, shoulders and arms, seemed to develop gradually towards the end of the afternoon work, a lunch break plus 1 or 2 short breaks being insufficient to prevent. These results are consistent with the finding that spontaneous rests of short duration interrupted repetitive factory work, especially in the later periods of a shift (Rutenfranz and Stoll 1966).

An interesting result was observed, as seen in Fig. 9, during a field study of female

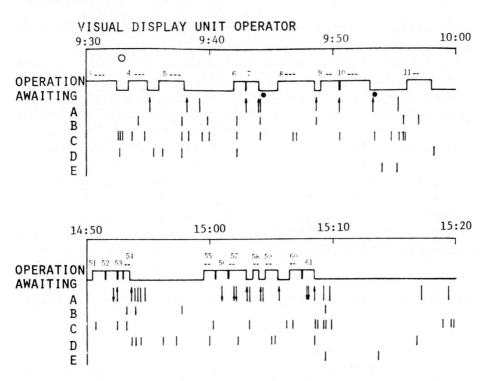

Fig. 8. Occurrence of various kinds of subsidiary behaviour of a visual display unit operator in the morning and in the afternoon. A, looking aside; B, changing working posture; C, motion of the upper extremities; D, neck and shoulder motion; E, yawning.

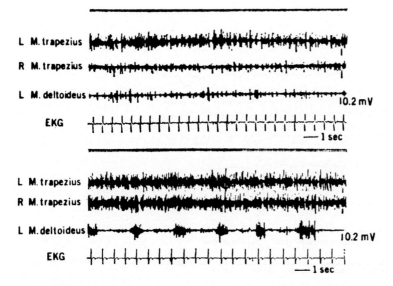

Fig. 9. EMGs and ECGs of 2 workers rolling films along a conveyor line using rolling and capping machines in a dark room.

factory workers, who were rolling films along a conveyor line, using rolling and capping machines in a dark room (Onishi et al. 1977). These 2 records were taken from 2 different job groups. But characteristically, the trapezius in both cases showed similar continuous contractions in sustaining the arm. The activity level reached 10–38% of the maximum voluntary force as expressed by the amount of integrated electrical activity. As Fig. 10 shows, the heart rate of these workers maintained a level of 15–25 beats/min above the resting level while processing 10–16 times a minute. But the activity of the trapezius in every 10 sec period was seen to fluctuate, gradually increasing for about 5–15 min, followed by a sudden decrease. This decrease after a period of gradual increase may imply an attempt to avoid increasing fatigue. In other words, the presence of fatigue in the shoulders necessitated changes of working positions. In fact, the local fatigue in the shoulders was significant at the end of the day's work. So we recommended insertion of short breaks and ergonomic improvements.

RECOMMENDATIONS ON WORK-REST CYCLES OF REPETITIVE WORK

As these results suggest, it is important to adjust the work-rest rhythms of working muscles at 2 different levels. First, regarding repeating contractions, the cycle period of each contraction must be suitable, so as to secure brief intra-work pauses in which the muscles involved can be free from static load. Secondly, there must be a break after a certain period of continuous work. Common work-rest systems consisting of a lunch break and 1 or 2 short breaks during a whole working day do not seem appropriate for such repetitive tasks.

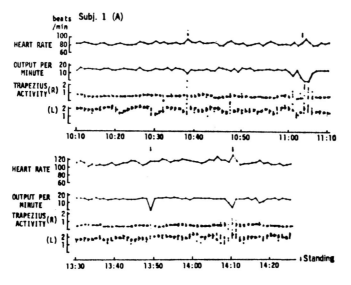

Fig. 10. Changes in heart rate, output and integrated EMG of the right and left trapezius while continuing film rolling work.

TABLE I

RECOMMENDATIONS FOR APPROPRIATE WORK-REST REGIMENS OF REPETITIVE WORK BASED ON FIELD STUDIES

Author	Year	Job	Criteria	Work-rest regime (min)	
				Work	Rest
Kano	1960	Typewriting, key punching	Flicker fusion, fatigue	60	20
Ishihara	1965	Key punching	Work rate, errors	45–60	–
Murokawa	1966	Key punching	Autonomic reactions	60	6–10
Saito	1973	Repetitive work	Fatigue, complaints	90	10
Suzuki	1973	Key operators	Cervico-brachial disorder	–	Voluntary rests
Maeda	1974	Assembly work	Motion study	60	10–15
Ohara et al.	1976	Cash register	Cervico-brachial disorder	60	15
Itani	1977	Film rolling	Cervico-brachial disorder	55	7 rests per day
Onishi et al.	1977	Office machine	EMG, muscle pain threshold	15–30	–

As for this second aspect, there are a number of recommendations on the basis of field studies on office machine and factory work, using hands and fingers intensively. These recommendations are listed in Table I (Kano 1960; Ishihara 1965; Murokawa 1966; Saito 1973; Suzuki 1973; Maeda 1974; Ohara et al. 1976; Itani 1977; Onishi et al. 1977). They commonly recommend a limit of continuous work of about 45–60 min. They all argue that this should be followed by a break of 10–20 min. These recommendations are based on evidence showing subacute fatigue in terms of fatigue complaints, autonomic reactions, work performance and errors, as well as EMG changes. Our results also support the limit of less than 60 min for continuous repetitive work. If the work were concentrated, however, an even shorter duration, going down to about 30 min, would be necessary.

In Japan, many workplaces of keyboard operations and similar work now comply with the 60 min work and 10–15 min rest cycles which have been recommended by the Ministry of Labour notifications of 1964 and 1973 (Saito et al. 1980). When the work-rest schedules of keyboard operators processing input data for computers were compared between 1962 and 1979, they were very different between the 2 periods. In 1962, keyboard operators had usually 1 or 2 short breaks in addition to a lunch break. In 1979, almost all the undertakings studied had 3 or more breaks of mostly 10–20 min in addition to a lunch break, clearly tending to limit the length of a work spell to around 60 min. About one-third of the undertakings had 5 or more short breaks. Most common were 2 breaks in the morning and 1–3 breaks in the afternoon. This insertion of frequent breaks for keyboard operators has come to be adopted as a preventive measure, being supported by the above mentioned Ministry of Labour notifications. Thus, if each break should last for at least 10–15 min, insertion of multiple breaks in this rather unusual form seems effective in reducing the occupational hazard of keyboard operating work.

As complaints of the neck-shoulder-arm region and general fatigue are still seen under such schedules, measures to change the fragmentary nature of the work and to ensure spontaneous pauses being more frequently taken would be essential to prevent excessive muscle fatigue. In our experience, EMG and behavioural data are certainly useful for finding more appropriate rhythms of work and rest at both of the above mentioned levels: that of repeated contractions and that of each continuously worked period.

REFERENCES

Bjorkstén, A. and Jonsson, B. Endurance limit of force in long-term intermittent static contractions. Scand. J. Work environm. Hlth, 1977, 3: 23–27.

Ishihara, Y. Kii-panchā no sagyō jōken (working conditions of key punchers). In: H. Kano (Ed.), Sangyō Shinrigaku kara Mita Rōdō to Ningen. Seishin Shobo, Tokyo, 1965: 265–286.

Itani, T. Keikenwan-shōgai no kenko kanri (health control against occupational cervico-brachial disorder). Rodo no kagaku, 1977, 32 (7): 45–56.

Kano, H. Flicker fusion frequency in a working spell. J. Sci. Labour, 1960, 36: 604–609.

Kogi, K. and Hakamada, T. Slowing of surface electromyogram and muscle strength in muscle fatigue. Rep. Inst. Sci. Labour, 1962, 60: 27–41.

Maeda, K. Konbea nagare-sagyō ni okeru keikenwan-shōgai (occupational cervico-brachial disorder in conveyor-belt work). Rodo no kagaku, 1974, 29 (10): 26–33.

Murokawa, M. Seishin-sagyō no teijō-jōtai seiritsuji ni okeru sagyōsha no shinpakusū: kokyū rizumu kansatsu ni yoru seiriteki futan no hyōka. Teishin Igaku, 1966, 18: 995–1006.

Numajiri, K. A study on the fatigue allowance for muscular work. J. Sci. Labour, 1968, 44: 567–576.

Ohara, H., Aoyama, H. and Itani, T. Health hazard among cash register operations and the effects of improved working conditions. J. hum. Ergol., 1976, 5: 31–40.

Onishi, N. Gendaiteki shugi sagyo no kinhirō (muscle fatigue in modern manipulative work). Rodo no kagaku, 1976, 32 (12): 31–40.

Onishi, N., Sakai, K., Itani, T. and Shindo, H. Muscle load and fatigue of film rolling workers. J. hum. Ergol., 1977, 6: 179–186.

Rohmert, W. Ermittlung von Erholungspausen für statische Arbeit des Menschen. Int. Z. angew. Physiol., 1960, 18: 123–169.

Rutenfranz, J. und Stoll, F. Untersuchungen über die Verteilung von Pausen bei freier Arbeit. Arbeitswissenschaft, 1966, 5: 132–135.

Sadoyama, T. and Kogi, K. Changes of electromyographic discharges by stretch reflex in the course of muscle fatigue. J. physiol. Soc. jap., 1976, 38: 382–385.

Saito, H. Studies on monotonous work: comparison of various types of monotonous work developed by the technical innovation and some considerations about the effects of several kinds of countermeasures. J. Sci. Labour, 1973, 49: 47–88.

Saito, H., Kogi, K., Sakai, K. and Ueno, Y. Work-rest schedules and related problems of key operators dealing with computer input data: results of a survey on 310 establishments. J. Sci. Labour, 1980, 56 (3), Part II: 1–16.

Sakai, K. Kōsoku-jōken ni okeru fukuji dōsa. Rōdō no Kagaku, 1980, 35 (4): 16–23.

Suzuki, H. Work loads and occupational health impairment in business machine operators. Jap. J. industr. Hlth, 1973, 15: 637–647.

Tanii, K. and Kogi, K. Spontaneous alternation of the working arm in one-arm cranking. J. hum. Ergol., 1976, 5: 41–50.

Tanii, K., Kogi, K. and Sadoyama, T. Spontaneous alternation of the working arm in static overhead work. J. hum. Ergol., 1972, 1: 143–155.

Tanii, K., Sadoyama, T., Sanjo, Y. and Kogi, K. Appearance of effort-depending changes in static local fatigue. J. hum. Ergol., 1973, 3: 31–45.

Kyoto Symposia (EEG Suppl. No. 36)
Editors: P.A. Buser, W.A. Cobb and T. Okuma
© 1982, Elsevier Biomedical Press, Amsterdam

750

Electromyographic Studies of Muscle Strain in Industrial Work

ROLAND KADEFORS* AND INGEMAR PETERSÉN**

* *Projekt Lindholmen Center, Göteborg, and* ** *Laboratory of Clinical Neurophysiology, Sahlgren Hospital, Göteborg (Sweden)*

In 1970, the Swedish Trade Union Confederation (LO) issued to all of its members a questionnaire on work environment problems, in which the workers could mark which problems they were confronted with in their work, to a large extent, to some extent, or not at all. Included were physical and chemical factors, and some symptoms as well. The results of the questionnaire were used to set priorities by the labour unions to press for elimination of work environment problems in Swedish industry.

Ten years later, in 1980, a similar survey was carried out again, and the results are now being published (Bolinder 1981, personal communication). It is of interest to compare the 2 investigations in terms of, for instance, the most common complaints. Table I shows a 1970 top-twelve list, together with the corresponding 1980 figures.

The 10 year time span represents a period of continuous modernization of Swedish industry, when great emphasis was given to improvements of working conditions. Of particular interest in the present context is that physical workload complaints are still the most common. There seems to be a general conception that with the advent of automation and mechanization, arduous work is gradually becoming eliminated in industry. On the contrary, it is evident that physical workload must still be termed a top priority occupational health concern. Methods for evaluation of workload and assessment of working situations from the point of view of the musculo-skeletal system are as important as ever.

Effects of physical workload on muscles and associated structures include *acute effects* on the organism and *long-term effects* as well. Since both aspects can, at least to some extent, be elucidated using similar electromyographic methods, and since these aspects are of importance from an ergonomic and occupational health point of view, they will both be touched upon below. Examples concern current projects related to welding work, but the conclusions apply to studies of any work where acceleration forces can be neglected, to a first approximation.

COMPARATIVE STUDIES: WORKPLACE DESIGN

The reason why the electromyogram is of such interest in ergonomics and occupational health applications is the well known relation to muscle mechanical

TABLE I

PERCENTAGE OF WORK ENVIRONMENT COMPLAINTS IN SURVEYS IN 1970 AND 1980 DIRECTED TO MEMBERS OF THE SWEDISH TRADE UNION CONFEDERATION

Factor	1970 survey	1980 survey	Index 1980/1970
Physical workload	51	71	1.39
Noise	41	54	1.32
Draft	40	45	1.13
Temperature	29	42	1.45
Skin irritations	26	43	1.65
Dust	14	26	1.86
Vibrations	14	24	1.71
Gases	12	21	1.75
Lighting	11	21	1.91
Welding fumes	10	14	1.40
Metal fumes	10	15	1.50
Humidity	9	17	1.89
Solvents	8	21	2.63

output: the root mean square (or the full-wave rectified and smoothed) value of the EMG signal reflects muscle force. We shall not be concerned here with details of the relation between EMG ($E_{r.m.s.}$) and force (F), and make only a couple of observations. The form of the relation is

$$E = KF^r,$$

K and r being constants, $0.5 < r < 2$ (Bigland and Lippold 1954; Moore 1967; Grieve and Pheasant 1976). The common assumption $r = 1$ holds reasonably well in many practical measurement situations, but in quantitative studies this should be checked by a calibration procedure (Jonsson 1976), in which readings are taken at various output forces relative to the maximal voluntary contraction. Such a calibration is not valid under fatiguing conditions, since K will then increase markedly (Kadefors 1978).

With these reservations, electromyographic methods may contribute substantially in ergonomic studies related to assessment of working situations. One of the most straightforward applications is to monitor the change in the level of activity, given a certain subject and a certain electrode position, as a result of a modification in, say, the workplace layout, the working posture or the design of a hand tool. Here, it is necessary to be aware of the fact that relative movements between muscle tissue and the electrode site introduce signal level shifts (Lindström and Kadefors 1974). Whenever possible such studies should therefore be carried out using fine wire electrodes. Fig. 1 presents the results of an investigation on the effect on back muscle activity of introducing a new prototype welding chair for use in overhead welding tasks (Lundgren 1981). It is seen in the figure that the new chair entails a marked decrease in muscle activity. Based on these measurements, and on subjective assessment by the welders, it was decided to introduce the chair in the workshops of the company concerned.

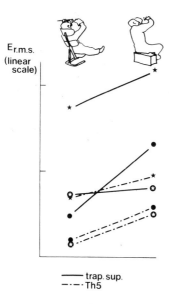

Fig. 1. Change in myoelectric activity level at 2 electrode sites as a result of workplace design modification. 3 subjects, left side.

A similar use of the EMG in ergonomics is the study of the effect of working techniques on muscle strain. As an example, Fig. 2 shows the results of an investigation of the effect on muscle strain in welding by the conformation attained in the arm, i.e., the positioning of the elbow, given a position and attitude in the hand. The figure depicts $E_{r.m.s.}$ from the anterior deltoid muscle in 5 subjects, in 8 different welding positions: 2 in waist level welding (1:1, 1:2), 3 in shoulder level welding (2:1, 2:2, 2:3), and 3 in overhead welding (3:1, 3:2, 3:3). No normalization was carried out. It is seen that the levels are reasonably coherent in the different subjects, suggesting that there is a consistent pattern in how the muscles are recruited and employed in certain welding postures. Waist level welding seems to be an exception to this (1:1). It is often noticed that there are vast differences between activity levels in different subjects in less taxing work. The conclusion to be drawn is that elbow position very definitely influences the strain on the deltoid muscle and its associated structures. The same is true also in other muscles of the shoulder complex (Kadefors et al. 1976a; Herberts et al. 1980; Herberts et al. 1982). In a clinical perspective, this is of interest since it has been shown that shoulder pain is a common syndrome in welders (Herberts and Kadefors 1976; Herberts et al. 1982).

EVALUATION OF LOAD DISTRIBUTION

Since the EMG reflects muscle force, registration of myoelectric activity during periods of work provides information on the distribution of load on a certain

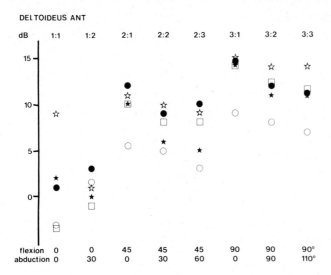

Fig. 2. Myoelectric activity level ($E_{r.m.s.}$) of the deltoid anterior muscle in 5 subjects, holding a welding holder (weight: 2 kg). 1:1 and 1:2 depict waist level welding with 0 and 30° humeral abduction; 2:1 to 2:3 shoulder level welding, and 3:1 to 3:3 overhead welding.

muscle. From an ergonomic point of view, the occurrence of high peak loads, as well as the extent of static load at lower effort, are of interest. Here, the well known strength-duration curve provides a basis for judgement and, based on a calibration procedure as indicated above, it is possible to check if there are periods of static load exceeding the 20% of maximum voluntary contraction threshold implied in the curve.

Because of the large mass of data collected, and the need for quality check, evaluation of lengthy records proves very time consuming. In a current project, methods have been developed which facilitate the analysis (Almström et al. 1980; Arvidsson et al. 1981). The analysis package, which was developed on a PDP 11 minicomputer, includes a real-time operating quality control program, as well as a number of statistical evaluation programs. The quality control check is based on spectral analysis; the parameters for acceptance can be set according to, for example, the type of electrode employed. There is automatic rejection of records with disturbing hum, artefacts or noise. A useful asset in the analysis package is the r.m.s. amplitude histogram; this makes possible a summary evaluation of load variation during a work period. Fig. 3 shows a print-out from the plotter, resulting from a measurement carried out during a welding task (and during welding simulation) on the trapezius muscle. The different traces depict $E_{r.m.s.}$ after quality control (A), amplitude distribution summarizing 5 overhead welds (B), and fatigue assessment (see below). Mean values and standard deviations are given separately. It is seen in the example that overhead welding presents continuous load on the muscle concerned, with little time for relaxation, but with considerable amplitude variation range due to the slow change in arm elevation as welding proceeds.

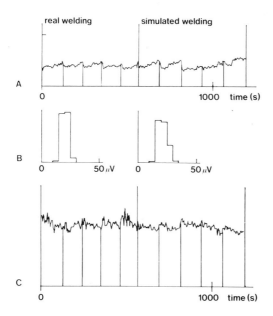

Fig. 3. Recording of myoelectric activity from (left) actual welding work overhead; (right) simulated welding work in a similar position. (A) $E_{r.m.s.}$ as a function of time, (B) amplitude densitograms, (C) mean frequency. Linear amplitude scales. M. trapezius. Electrode changing periods are neglected for clarity.

MODELS: AN APPROACH TOWARDS GENERALIZATION

One of the basic problems encountered when using electromyographic methods as a tool for ergonomic assessment is the need for highly qualified persons to carry out the practical investigations. Pitfalls tend to hamper the applicability markedly. During the last few years, some interesting attempts have been made to overcome this problem by using the information achieved by electromyography and other means to construct mathematical models for parts of the musculo-skeletal system. The goal is to arrive at a description of the system which allows calculation in quantitative terms of the forces acting on various structures, knowing the body posture, the masses and geometrical properties of the body segments, and the resulting forces (for instance, the tool mass or the pushing force against a workpiece).

Arriving at a reliably useful mathematical model is not a trivial task in any part of the musculo-skeletal system. A model with practical applicability was developed recently incorporating the lumbar spine (Schultz and Andersson 1981). The model, which is based on thorough knowledge of the functional anatomy, is arrived at in several steps: computation of the net reaction forces and moments; computation of the internal forces providing the net reaction; and validation of internal force estimates.

The critical stage in the formulation of the model is the computation of internal forces. In general, the system considered is statistically indeterminate, which means that additional assumptions must be made to account for the optimization criteria to be used in the model. Here, monitoring the relative myoelectric signal activity in different muscles and different postures can provide relevant information.

The model, once established, should be able to predict the internal loads on different structures over a great range of loads and in a number of positions. The predicted values must be checked in a validation stage before the model is put to use. Such validation may involve intrusive mechanical measurements on body tissues, which present a multitude of problems. In the case of the lumbar spine model, intradiscal pressure, intra-abdominal pressure and EMG were used in the validation stage. A problem using EMG in this context is the incomplete knowledge of the constants K and r, and much would be gained if reliable measurements could be made to establish such relations.

In current projects, independent measurements of mechanical parameters include measurement of the acoustic transmission properties of tendinous tissue and measurement of intramuscular pressure. Preliminary investigations in vivo on these methods have revealed that the phase shift of transverse acoustic waves varies significantly in the low audio frequency range as the muscle force is changing. In an experiment on the Achilles tendon, excitation with a 500 Hz acoustic wave entailed a phase shift change of $+10-12°/kp$ plantar force. Likewise, intramuscular pressure is dependably related to muscle force (Mubarak et al. 1976). Current work is focussed on establishing the relations between measurable parameters, classification of mechanisms involved, and analysis of the information content of the different signals to arrive at quantitative information in absolute terms to be included in future mathematical models.

FATIGUE ASSESSMENT USING ELECTROMYOGRAPHY

It is well known that the electromyogram modifies under fatiguing conditions, and that spectral measurements are effective in quantification of these changes. From an occupational health point of view, the presence of electromyographically evidenced fatigue gives an indication of the muscle's acute response to strain during work. There are several reasons why this information is of profound interest. In addition to the pain and discomfort associated with muscle fatigue, the motor skill is affected, tremor increases, clumsiness leads to a high risk of accidents, and there are adverse effects on the physiological system at large. Since the electromyographic changes are caused by partial or total ischaemia in the muscle tissue (Mortimer et al. 1970), there is direct information on muscle physiology available in the EMG. The mean frequency f_m of the EMG power spectrum is, according to the model presented by Lindström and Magnusson (1977), proportional to the muscle fibre conduction velocity.

An example of the practical evaluation of a working task (overhead welding) using f_m calculation is given in Fig. 3C. Here, a special mean frequency analyser (Broman and Kadefors 1979) was employed. The graph gives current f_m measures; it is seen that there is a consistent pattern in the f_m development during welding: the mean frequency tends to decrease. In order to avoid fatigue, better working positions (Herbert et al. 1980) and improved working techniques should be sought (Petersén and Kadefors 1977).

It is probably true that, since the electromyographically evidenced fatigue correlates with perceived exertion (Lindström and Petersén 1981), fatigue investigations could be carried out by interview techniques. However, in many cases it remains necessary to have the possibility to localize the perceived exertion to a specific muscle, and to measure the effect of changes in the working situation directly on this muscle.

OCCUPATIONAL TRAINING: AN INTEGRATED APPROACH

It was observed in an investigation on shipyard welders (Kadefors et al. 1976a) that the degree of skill played an important role in the extent of muscle fatigue in standardized tasks. It was concluded that the technique of working is, in part, determining the amount of strain on vulnerable structures in the musculo-skeletal system. In a current project, the acquisition of skill in welding is being studied. The basic concept is that, through ergonomically planned training, the welder-to-be may be able to attain a high degree of skill combined with a comparably low strain on individual muscles. In order to test to what extent this is possible, measurements on experienced welders and trainees are being carried out. A test set-up has been designed, where the operator performs a welding task on a modified welding simulator according to Tredre and Collins (1980). The simulator contains a moving target, and a welding pistol with a moving rod miming actual welding equipment, with the electrode gradually melting away. The precision with which the electrode tip points at the target is measured. EMGs from relevant muscles of the arm and shoulder are monitored, recorded and analysed, using a PDP 11/40 minicomputer.

Fig. 3 shows (to the left) the processed EMG in welding overhead, and (to the right) the similarly processed EMG recorded during a corresponding simulated task. The analysis package provides $E_{r.m.s.}$ and fatigue measures. It is seen that there are similar signs of fatigue in real and in simulated welding; in other words, the simulator seems to copy real work reasonably well from this particular point of view. In the project, the fatigued muscles are monitored, and information on the activity level is fed back to the operator in order to facilitate acquisition of a relaxed way of performing welding in the position concerned.

CONCLUSION

The above projects illustrate how EMG methods can be put to use, particularly to serve in preventive medicine applications. It is felt that electromyography may not, within the foreseeable future, become an easily applicable method to be used by relatively uninformed investigators; rather, EMG may continue to prove valuable mainly as a research tool. The approach to be taken is to employ EMG particularly to arrive at results of enough principal interest to be referred to and applied in practical ergonomic work in the field. It is vital that the information is presented and made available in such a form that it will help make ergonomic evaluation of working situations less arbitrary and more reliable than it is today.

REFERENCES

Almström, C., Arvidsson, A., Kadefors, R., Petersen, I., de Walden-Galuszko, K. and Droszcz, J. Evaluation of working positions in industrial work by means of electromyography, Part 1. Methods. Bull. Inst. trop. Med. Hyg. (Gdansk), 1980, 12: 177–184.

Arvidsson, A., Lindström, L. and Örtengren, R. Automatic detection of signal disturbances. Application to myoelectric signals from a work-place environment. Proc. 5th Nordic Meeting Med. Biol. Engng, 1981, 2: 34–36.

Bigland, B. and Lippold, O.C.J. The relation between force, velocity and integrated electrical activity in human muscles. J. Physiol. (Lond.), 1954, 123: 214–224.

Bolinder, E. The Swedish Trade Union Confederation. Personal communication. 1981.

Broman, H. and Kadefors, R. A spectral moment analyzer for quantification of electromyograms. Proc. 4th Congr. ISEK, Boston, 1979.

Grieve, D.W. and Pheasant, S.T. Myoelectric activity, posture and isometric torque in man. Electroenceph. clin. Neurophysiol., 1976, 16: 3–21.

Herberts, P. and Kadefors, R. A study of painful shoulder in welders. Acta orthop. scand., 1976, 47: 381–387.

Herberts, P., Kadefors, R. and Broman, H. Arm positioning in manual tasks. An electromyographic study of localized muscle fatigue. Ergonomics, 1980, 23: 655–665.

Herberts, P., Kadefors, R., Andersson, G. and Petersén, I. Shoulder pain in industry: an epidemiological study on welders. Acta orthop. scand., 1981, 52: 299–306.

Herberts, P., Almström, C., Högfors, C., Kadefors, P., Palmerud, G. and Sigholm, G. Shoulder muscle load in different working postures. Proc. World Congr. med. Phys. biomed. Engng, Hamburg, 1982: 6.12.

Jonsson, B. Methodological aspects on contraction level estimation from myoelectric signals. In: A. Arrigo (Ed.), Abstr. Comm. 3rd int. Congress of ISEK. G. Polli, Pavia, 1976, 73–75.

Kadefors, R. Application of electromyography in ergonomics: new vistas. Scand. J. rehab. Med., 1978, 10: 127–133.

Kadefors, R., Petersén, I. and Herberts, P. Muscular reaction to welding work: an electromyographic investigation. Ergonomics, 1976a, 19: 543–558.

Kadefors, R., Herberts, P. and Lindström, L. On the use of fine wires in applied electromyography. Digest 11th ICMBE, 1976b: 224–225.

Lindström, L. and Kadefors, R. A model describing the power spectrum of myoelectric signals. Part IV. Total power. Res. Lab. Med. Electr., Chalmers Univ. of Technology, Göteborg, 1974.

Lindström, L. and Magnusson, R. Interpretation of myoelectric power spectra: a model and its applications. Proc. IEEE, 1977, 65: 653–662.

Lindström, L. and Petersén, I. Power spectra of myoelectric signals: motor unit activity and muscle fatigue. In: E. Stålberg and R. Young (Eds.), Clinical Neurophysiology, Neurology I. Butterworths, London, 1981: 66–87.

Lundgren, C.G. Svetsstolar. Thesis, Work Physiology Division, National Board of Occupational Safety and Health, Umeå, Sweden, 1981.

Moore, A.D. Synthetic EMG waves. In: J.V. Basmajian (Ed.), Muscles Alive. Williams and Wilkins, Baltimore, 1967: 53–70.

Mortimer, J.T., Magnusson, R. and Petersén, I. Conduction velocity in ischemic muscle: effect on EMG frequency spectrum. Amer. J. Physiol., 1970, 219: 1324–1329.

Mubarak, S., Hargens, A., Owen, C., Garetto, L. and Akeson, W. The wick catheter technique for measurement of intramuscular pressure. J. Bone Jt Surg., 1976, 58A: 1011–1019.

Petersén, I. and Kadefors, R. Electromyographic study of training technique in welding. Electroenceph. clin. Neurophysiol., 1977, 43: 594.

Schultz, A. and Andersson, G. Analysis of loads on the lumbar spine. Spine, 1981, 6: 76–82.

Tredre, B. and Collins, J.C. A tracking task used for the simulation of manual metal arc welding. Ergonomics, 1980, 23: 401–404.